THE GENETICS OF NEURODEVELOPMENTAL DISORDERS

THE GENETICS OF NEURODEVELOPMENTAL DISORDERS

Edited by

KEVIN J. MITCHELL

WILEY Blackwell

Published by John Wiley & Sons, Inc., Hoboken, New Jersey

Published simultaneously in Canada

For general information on our other products and services or for technical support, please contact our Customer Care Department within the United States at (800) 762-2974, outside the United States at (317) 572-3993 or fax (317) 572-4002.

Wiley also publishes its books in a variety of electronic formats. Some content that appears in print may not be available in electronic formats. For more information about Wiley products, visit our web site at www.wiley.com.

Library of Congress Cataloging-in-Publication Data:

The genetics of neurodevelopmental disorders / edited by Kevin J. Mitchell.
    p. ; cm.
Includes bibliographical references and index.
ISBN 978-1-118-52488-6 (cloth)
I. Mitchell, Kevin J. (Professor of genetics), editor. [DNLM: 1. Intellectual Disability–genetics. 2. Developmental Disabilities–genetics. WM 300]
    RJ496.N49
    618.92′80475–dc23

2015006778

Printed in Singapore by C.O.S. Printers Pte Ltd

10 9 8 7 6 5 4 3 2 1

1   2015

CONTENTS

List of Contributors   vii

Foreword   *Kevin J. Mitchell*   ix

1   **The Genetic Architecture of Neurodevelopmental Disorders**   1
Kevin J. Mitchell

2   **Overlapping Etiology of Neurodevelopmental Disorders**   29
Eric Kelleher and Aiden Corvin

3   **The Mutational Spectrum of Neurodevelopmental Disorders**   49
Nancy D. Merner, Patrick A. Dion, and Guy A. Rouleau

4   **The Role of Genetic Interactions in Neurodevelopmental Disorders**   69
Jason H. Moore and Kevin J. Mitchell

5   **Developmental Instability, Mutation Load, and Neurodevelopmental Disorders**   81
Ronald A. Yeo and Steven W. Gangestad

6   **Environmental Factors and Gene–Environment Interactions**   111
John McGrath

7   **The Genetics of Brain Malformations**   129
M. Chiara Manzini and Christopher A. Walsh

8   **Disorders of Axon Guidance**   155
Heike Blockus and Alain Chédotal

9   Synaptic Disorders   195
     Catalina Betancur and Kevin J. Mitchell

10   Human Stem Cell Models of Neurodevelopmental Disorders   239
     Peter Kirwan and Frederick J. Livesey

11   Animal Models for Neurodevelopmental Disorders   261
     Hala Harony-Nicolas and Joseph D. Buxbaum

12   Cascading Genetic and Environmental Effects on Development: Implications for
     Intervention   275
     Esha Massand and Annette Karmiloff-Smith

13   Human Genetics and Clinical Aspects of Neurodevelopmental Disorders   289
     Gholson J. Lyon and Jason O'Rawe

14   Progress Toward Therapies and Interventions for Neurodevelopmental Disorders   319
     Ayokunmi Ajetunmobi and Daniela Tropea

Subject Index   345
Gene Index   353

LIST OF CONTRIBUTORS

Ayokunmi Ajentunmobi, *Nanomedicine and Molecular Imaging Group, Department of Clinical Medicine, School of Medicine, Trinity College Dublin, Dublin, Ireland*

Catalina Betancur, *INSERM U1130, Paris, France; CNRS UMR 8246, Paris, France; Sorbonne Universités, UPMC Univ Paris 6, Neuroscience Paris Seine, Paris, France*

Heike Blockus, *Sorbonne Universités, UPMC Univ Paris, UMRS968 and CNRS, UMR 7210, Institut de la Vision, Paris, France; INSERM, Institut de la Vision, UMRS_968, Paris, France; CNRS, UMR_7210, Paris, France*

Joseph D. Buxbaum, *Seaver Autism Center for Research and Treatment, Departments of Psychiatry, Neuroscience, and Genetics and Genomic Sciences, The Friedman Brain Institute and the Mindich Child Health and Development Institute, Icahn School of Medicine at Mount Sinai, New York, NY, USA*

Alain Chédotal, *Sorbonne Universités, UPMC Univ Paris, UMRS968 and CNRS, UMR 7210, Institut de la Vision, Paris, France; INSERM, Institut de la Vision, UMRS_968, Paris, France; CNRS, UMR_7210, Paris, France*

Aiden Corvin *Department of Psychiatry and Neuropsychiatric Genetics Research Group, Institute of Molecular Medicine, Trinity College Dublin, Dublin 2, Ireland*

Patrick A. Dion, *Department of Pathology and Cellular Biology, Université de Montréal, Montréal, QC, Canada; Montreal Neurological Institute, McGill University, Montréal, QC, Canada*

Steven W. Gangestad, *Department of Psychology, University of New Mexico, Albuquerque, NM, USA*

Hala Harony-Nicolas, *Seaver Autism Center for Research and Treatment, Departments of Psychiatry, Neuroscience, and Genetics and Genomic Sciences, The Friedman Brain Institute and the Mindich Child Health and Development Institute, Icahn School of Medicine at Mount Sinai, New York, NY, USA*

Annette Karmiloff-Smith, *Centre for Brain and Cognitive Development of Psychological Sciences, School of Sciences, Birkbeck, Birkbeck University of London, London, UK*

Eric Kelleher *Department of Psychiatry and Neuropsychiatric Genetics Research Group, Institute of Molecular Medicine, Trinity College Dublin, Dublin 2, Ireland*

Peter Kirwan, *Gurdon Institute, Department of Biochemistry and Cambridge Stem Cell Institute, University of Cambridge, Cambridge, UK*

Frederick J. Livesey, *Gurdon Institute, Department of Biochemistry and Cambridge Stem Cell Institute, University of Cambridge, Cambridge, UK*

Gholson J. Lyon, *Stanley Institute for Cognitive Genomics, Cold Spring Harbor Laboratory, Cold Spring Harbor, NY, USA; Institute for Genomic Medicine, Utah Foundation for Biomedical Research, E 3300˜S, Salt Lake City, UT, USA; Department of Psychiatry, Stony Brook University, Stony Brook, NY, USA*

M. Chiara Manzini, *Department of Pharmacology and Physiology, and Integrative Systems Biology, The George Washington University, Washington, DC, USA*

Esha Massand, *Centre for Brain and Cognitive Development, Department of Psychological Sciences, School of Sciences, Birkbeck, University of London, London, UK*

John McGrath, *Queensland Brain Institute, The University of Queensland, St. Lucia, QLD, Australia; Queensland Centre for Medical Health Research, The Park Centre for Mental Health, Richlands, QLD, Australia*

Nancy D. Merner, *CHUM Research Center, Université de Montréal, Montréal, QC, Canada; Department of Drug Discovery and Development, Harrison School of Pharmacy, Auburn University, Auburn, AL, USA*

Kevin J. Mitchell, *Smurfit Institute of Genetics and Institute of Neuroscience, Trinity College Dublin, Dublin, Ireland*

Jason H. Moore, *Institute for Quantitative Biomedical Sciences, Departments of Genetics and Community and Family Medicine, Geisel School of Medicine, Dartmouth College, Hanover, NH, USA*

Jason O'Rawe, *Stanley Institute for Cognitive Genomics, Cold Spring Harbor Laboratory, Cold Spring Harbor, NY, USA; Graduate Program in Genetics, Stony Brook University, Stony Brook, NY, USA*

Guy A. Rouleau, *Montreal Neurological Institute, McGill University, Montréal, QC, Canada*

Daniela Tropea, *Department of Psychiatry, Trinity Centre for Health Sciences, St. James Hospital, Dublin, Ireland*

Christopher A. Walsh, *Division of Genetics, The Manton Center for Orphan Disease Research and Howard Hughes Medical Institute, Boston Children's Hospital, Boston, MA, USA*

Ronald A. Yeo, *Department of Psychology, University of New Mexico, Albuquerque, NM, USA*

FOREWORD

Kevin J. Mitchell

The term "neurodevelopmental disorders" is clinically defined in psychiatry as *"a group of conditions with onset in the developmental period... characterized by developmental deficits that produce impairments of personal, social, academic, or occupational functioning"*.[1] This term encompasses the clinical categories of intellectual disability (ID), developmental delay (DD), autism spectrum disorders (ASD), attention-deficit hyperactivity disorder (ADHD), speech and language disorders, specific learning disorders, tic disorders, and others.

However, the term can be defined differently, not based on age of onset or clinical presentation, but by an etiological criterion, to mean disorders arising from aberrant neural development. This definition includes many forms of epilepsy (considered either as a distinct disorder or as a comorbid symptom) as well as disorders such as schizophrenia (SZ), which have later onset but which can still be traced back to neurodevelopmental origins. Though the symptoms of SZ itself typically arise only in late teens or early twenties, convergent evidence of epidemiological risk factors during fetal development and very early deficits apparent in longitudinal studies strongly indicate that SZ is a disorder of neural development, though its clinical consequences may remain latent for many years.

Collectively, severe neurodevelopmental disorders affect ~5% of the population (though exact numbers are almost impossible to obtain, due to changing diagnostic criteria and substantial comorbidity between clinical categories). These disorders impact on the most fundamental aspects of human experience: cognition, language, social interaction, perception, mood, motor control, and sense of self. They impair function, often severely, and restrict opportunities for sufferers, as well as placing a heavy burden on families and caregivers. As lifelong illnesses, they also give rise to a substantial economic burden, both in direct health-care costs and indirect costs due to lost opportunity.

The treatments currently available for neurodevelopmental disorders are very limited and problematic. Intensive educational interventions may help ameliorate some cognitive or behavioral difficulties, such as those associated with ID or ASD, but to a limited extent and without addressing the underlying pathology. With respect to psychiatric symptoms, the mainstays of pharmacotherapy (antipsychotic medication, mood stabilizers, antidepressants, and anxiolytics) all emerged between the 1940s and 1960s

[1] Diagnostic and Statistical Manual of Mental Disorders, 5th Edition

with almost no new drugs being developed since. Most of these treatments were discovered serendipitously, and their mechanisms of action remain poorly understood. In most cases, the existing treatments are only partially effective and can induce serious side effects. This is also true for the range of anticonvulsants, and, for all these drugs, it is typically impossible to predict from symptom profiles alone whether individual patients will benefit from a particular drug or possibly be harmed by it. These difficulties and the attendant poor outcomes for many patients arise from not knowing the causes of disease in particular patients and not understanding the underlying pathogenic mechanisms. Genetic research promises to address both these issues.

Neurodevelopmental disorders are predominantly genetic in origin and have often been thought of as falling into two groups. The first includes a very large number of individually rare syndromes with known genetic causes. Examples include Fragile X syndrome, Down syndrome, Rett syndrome, and Angelman syndrome but there are literally hundreds of others. Each of these is clearly caused by a single genetic lesion, sometimes involving an entire chromosome or a section of chromosome, sometimes affecting a single gene. Most are characterized by ID, but many also show high rates of epilepsy, ASD or other neuropsychiatric symptoms.

The second group comprises idiopathic cases of ID, ASD, SZ, or epilepsy – those with no currently known cause. Despite the lack of an identified genetic lesion, there is still very strong evidence of a genetic etiology across these categories. All of these conditions are highly heritable, showing high levels of twin concordance, much higher in monozygotic than in dizygotic twins, substantially increased risk to relatives and typically zero effect of a shared family environment, indicating strong genetic causation.

What has not been clear is whether these so-called "common disorders" are simply collections of rare genetic syndromes that we cannot yet discriminate, or whether they have a very different genetic architecture. The dominant paradigm in the field has held that the idiopathic, non-syndromic cases of common disorders such as ASD or SZ reflect the extreme end of a continuum of risk across the population. This is based on a model involving the segregation of a very large number of genetic variants, each of small effect alone, which can, above a collective threshold of burden in individuals, result in frank disease.

Recent genetic discoveries are prompting a re-evaluation of this model, as well as casting doubt on the biological validity of clinical diagnostic categories. After decades of frustration, the genetic secrets of these conditions are finally yielding to new genomic microarray and sequencing technologies. These are revealing a growing list of rare, single mutations that confer high risk of ASD, ID, SZ, or epilepsy, particularly epileptic encephalopathies.

These findings strongly reinforce a model of genetic heterogeneity, whereby common clinical categories do not represent singular biological entities, but rather are umbrella terms for a large number of distinct genetic conditions. These conditions are individually rare but collectively common. Strikingly, almost all of the identified mutations are associated with variable clinical manifestations, conferring risk across traditional diagnostic boundaries. These findings fit with large-scale epidemiological studies that also show shared risk across these disorders. Thus, while current diagnostic categories may reflect more or less distinct clinical states or outcomes, they do not reflect distinct etiologies.

The "genetics of autism" is thus neither singular nor separable from the "genetics of intellectual disability," the "genetics of schizophrenia," or the "genetics of epilepsy." The more general term of *developmental brain dysfunction*" has been proposed to encompass disorders arising from altered neural development, which can manifest clinically in diverse ways. This book is about the genetics of developmental brain dysfunction.

A lot can go wrong in the development of a human brain. The right numbers of hundreds of distinct types of nerve cells have to be generated in the right places, they have to migrate to form highly organized structures, and they must extend nerve fibers, which navigate their way through the brain to ultimately find and connect with their appropriate partners, avoiding wrong turns and illicit interactions. Once they find their partners they must form synapses, the incredibly complex and diverse cellular structures that mediate communication between nerve cells. These synapses are also highly dynamic, responding to patterns of activity by strengthening or weakening the connection.

The instructions to carry out these processes are encoded in the genome of the developing embryo. Each of these aspects of neural development requires the concerted action of the protein products of thousands of distinct genes. Mutations in any one of them (or sometimes in several at the same time) can lead to developmental brain dysfunction.

The identification of numerous causal mutations has focused attention on the roles of the genes affected, with a number of prominent classes of neurodevelopmental genes emerging. These include genes involved in early brain patterning and proliferation, those mediating later events of cell migration and axon guidance, and a major class involved in synapse formation and subsequent activity-dependent synaptic refinement, pruning, and plasticity. Also highlighted are a number of biochemical pathways and networks that appear especially sensitive to perturbation.

Genetic discoveries thus allow an alternate means to classify disorders, based on the underlying neurodevelopmental processes affected. This provides more etiologically valid and arguably more biologically coherent categories than those based on clinical outcome. For individual patients, the application of microarray and sequencing technologies is already changing clinical practice in diagnosis and management of neurodevelopmental disorders. This will only increase as more and more pathogenic mutations are identified.

Such discoveries also provide entry points to enable the elucidation of pathogenic mechanisms, where exciting progress is being made using cellular and animal models. For any given mutation, this involves defining the defects at a cellular level (in the right cells), and working out how such defects propagate to the levels of neural circuits and systems, ultimately producing pathophysiological states that underlie neuropsychiatric symptoms. Definition of these pathways will hopefully lead to a detailed enough understanding of the molecular or circuit-level defects to rationally devise new therapeutics.

The elucidation of the heterogeneous genetic and neurobiological bases of neurodevelopmental disorders should thus enable a much more personalized approach to diagnosis and treatment for individual patients, and a shift in clinical care for these disorders from an approach based on superficial symptoms and generic medicines, to one based on detailed knowledge of specific causes and mechanisms.

The book is organized into several sections:

Chapters 1–6 cover broad conceptual issues relevant to neurodevelopmental disorders in general. These are informed by recent advances in genomic technologies, which have transformed our view of the genetic architecture of both rare and so-called "common" neurodevelopmental disorders. These chapters will consider the genetic heterogeneity of clinical categories such as ASD or SZ, the relative importance of different types of mutations (common vs rare; single-gene vs large deletions or duplications; inherited vs *de novo*), etiological overlap between clinical categories and complex interactions between two or more mutations or between genetic and environmental factors.

Chapters 7–11 present our current understanding of several different types of disorder, grouped by the neurodevelopmental process impacted. Consideration of disorders from this angle provides a more rational and biologically valid approach than consideration from the point of view of clinical symptoms, which can be arrived at through various routes.

Chapters 12–14 deal with the elucidation of pathogenic mechanisms, following genetic discoveries. They include chapters on cellular models (using induced pluripotent stem cells derived from patients) and animal models (recapitulating pathogenic mutations in mice), which are revealing the routes of pathogenesis, from defects in diverse cellular neurodevelopmental processes to resultant alterations in neural circuits and brain systems, which ultimately impinge on behavior. The manifestation of these defects in humans also depends on processes of learning and experience-dependent development that proceed for many years after birth. Taking this aspect of development seriously is essential as it is a critical period where symptoms can be exacerbated if neglected or potentially improved by intensive interventions.

Chapters 15–16 consider the clinical implications of recent discoveries and of the general principles described in earlier chapters. Foremost among these is the recognition of extreme genetic heterogeneity, meaning that understanding what is going on in any particular patient requires knowledge of the specific underlying genetic cause. The dramatic reductions in cost for whole-genome sequencing mean such diagnoses will become far easier to make, with important implications for clinical genetic practice (including preimplantation or prenatal screening or diagnosis). Finally, the study of cellular and animal models of specific disorders is already suggesting potential therapeutic avenues for some conditions. These advances illustrate a general principle – to treat these conditions we need to identify and understand the underlying biology and design therapies to treat the specific cause in each patient and not just the generic symptoms.

1

THE GENETIC ARCHITECTURE OF NEURODEVELOPMENTAL DISORDERS

KEVIN J. MITCHELL

Smurfit Institute of Genetics and Institute of Neuroscience, Trinity College Dublin, Dublin, Ireland

1.1 INTRODUCTION

There are several hundred known genetic syndromes that affect neural development and result in intellectual disability (ID), epilepsy, or other neurological or psychiatric symptoms. These include recognized syndromes that often manifest with symptoms of autism spectrum disorders (ASD) or schizophrenia (SZ), such as Fragile X syndrome, Rett syndrome, tuberous sclerosis, velocardio-facial syndrome, and many others. For ASD, it has been known for many years that these syndromes account for a significant but still small fraction (5–10%) of all cases (Miles, 2011). What has not been clear is whether such cases, associated with single mutations, represent a typical mode by which such conditions arise or are, alternatively, exceptional and quite distinct from the general etiology of idiopathic ASD, epilepsy, SZ, or ID (Wray and Visscher, 2010). Other common disorders including dyslexia, specific language impairment, obessive-compulsive disorder, and so on, will not be considered here in detail, though the general principles probably apply.

In general, the genetic architecture of common NDDs has been considered to be "complex" or multifactorial (Plomin et al., 2009; Sullivan et al., 2003). This is usually taken to mean that many causal factors, both genetic and nongenetic, are involved in each affected individual. Under this view, the large group of currently idiopathic cases have a very different genetic architecture from the small number of known monogenic cases. An alternative view is that the vast majority of cases of these conditions are caused by independent mutations in any one of a very large number of genes. According to this model, these diagnostic categories of idiopathic cases represent artificial groupings reflecting our current ignorance, rather than natural kinds.

Here, I consider the theoretical underpinnings and empirical evidence relating to the genetic architecture of NDDs. These have been greatly influenced by technological advancements which have allowed various types of

The Genetics of Neurodevelopmental Disorders, First Edition. Edited by Kevin J. Mitchell.
© 2015 John Wiley & Sons, Inc. Published 2015 by John Wiley & Sons, Inc.

genetic variation to be assayed. Studies over the past several years have revealed an extreme level of genetic heterogeneity and complexity for common NDDs, with the discovery of high-risk mutations in a large number of single loci and additional complexities in the causal architecture in individuals.

1.2 THEORETICAL CONSIDERATIONS

Linkage studies have clearly shown that common NDDs are not caused by mutations in one particular gene, leading to the unchallenged conclusion that variants at many loci must be involved *across the population* (e.g., (O'Rourke et al., 1982; Szatmari, 1999)). However, models of the genetic architecture of these conditions differ in two additional, independent parameters: (i) the number of variants thought to contribute to disease *in any individual* (from one or a few to many, possibly thousands), and (ii) the presumed frequency of risk alleles (from very rare to very common). The differences between models have profound implications for finding causal variants, predicting disease risk, discovering underlying biology, and developing treatments for particular patients. More fundamentally, they represent very different ways of conceptualizing these conditions.

1.2.1 Number of Causal Alleles Per Individual

At one extreme, a model of Mendelian inheritance with genetic heterogeneity proposes that each case is caused by a single mutation, but that these can occur in any one of a large number of different loci (McClellan and King, 2010; Mitchell, 2011; Wright and Hastie, 2001). The types of mutations could include chromosomal aberrations that change the copy number of multiple genes, or mutations affecting a single gene. This model also encompasses diverse modes of inheritance, from *de novo* mutations to dominant or recessive inheritance. Fundamentally, this model conceives of common clinical categories such as SZ, ASD, epilepsy, ID, and so on, as

umbrella terms for large numbers of distinct conditions that happen to manifest with similar symptoms (Betancur, 2011; McClellan et al., 2007; Mitchell, 2012; Mitchell and Porteous, 2011; Ropers, 2008).

There are many precedents for this kind of genetic heterogeneity, including the genetics of congenital deafness (Lenz and Avraham, 2011), various forms of blindness, such as retinitis pigmentosa (Wright et al., 2010) and the many known Mendelian forms of intellectual disability (Ellison et al., 2013) and epilepsy (Poduri and Lowenstein, 2011). What differs with these conditions is that they typically display clear-cut Mendelian modes of inheritance, which is rarely the case for NDDs.

Moreover, linkage studies have been highly successful in identifying causal loci involved in specific Mendelian sub-types of these disorders, whereas they have produced highly inconsistent findings for common diagnostic categories, such as ASD and SZ (see below). Partly due to the failure of linkage studies to zero in on specific causal loci, an alternative model of polygenic inheritance became the dominant paradigm in the field (Risch, 1990).

The polygenic model proposes that common disorders arise from the combined action of a large number of risk alleles in each affected individual (Falconer, 1965; Plomin et al., 2009). Regrettably, the term polygenic has been used more loosely in recent literature to refer simply to the involvement of many loci across the population, where the number of contributing loci per individual remains unknown and could be as low as one (Purcell et al., 2014; Sullivan et al., 2012). I use polygenic here in the original sense to refer to conditions caused by the combined effects of multiple variants per individual.

Under the polygenic model, many risk variants are floating through the population and their independent segregation generates a continuous distribution of risk variant burden. Individuals at the extreme end of this distribution are thought of as passing a threshold and consequently developing disease (Falconer, 1965) (Fig. 1.1). This model views common disorders effectively as unitary conditions, reflecting a common

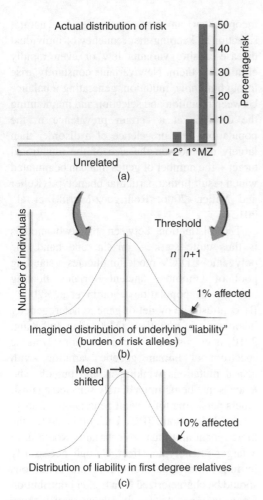

Fig. 1.1 *The liability-threshold model.* A discontinuous distribution of observed risk across the population (a) is represented as reflecting an underlying latent variable, the "liability", which is assumed to be normally distributed (b). A threshold of burden is invoked to regenerate the observed discontinuity. The mean liability of siblings of affected individuals is presumed to be shifted toward the threshold (c), explaining the greater disease incidence in this group compared to the population average. This yields a scenario analogous to response to selection for a quantitative trait, enabling heritability to be estimated (Falconer, 1965). (Reproduced, with permission, from (Mitchell, 2012).) *(See insert for color representation of this figure.)*

etiology – people with disease are simply at the tail end of a single distribution that extends continuously across the whole population. The distribution in this case is of the imagined latent variable, "liability," which is presumed to exist and to be normally distributed, but which cannot be measured directly. It can be translated, statistically, into the highly discontinuous distribution of observed risk in relatives of affected individuals, for example, by invoking an essentially arbitrary threshold, above which disease results. This liability-threshold model is statistically convenient but highly abstract (Mitchell, 2012).

An extension of this model considers the disorder as arising from the extremes of a number of actual quantitative traits, or endophenotypes (Gottesman and Gould, 2003; Meyer-Lindenberg and Weinberger, 2006). Common neuropsychiatric conditions affect multiple cognitive or social functions or faculties, such as working memory, executive function, sociability, and so on. All of these traits also show a distribution across the unaffected population and all show moderate heritability. This led to the suggestion that individuals diagnosed with conditions such as ASD or SZ may simply be at the extreme end of the normal distributions for several of these traits at the same time (Gottesman and Gould, 2003; Meyer-Lindenberg and Weinberger, 2006).

The corollary of that idea is that the genetic variants contributing to variation in such traits across the normal population will be the risk variants for such disorders. The hope was that such traits might have simpler genetic architectures than clinical diagnoses or at least that any genetic associations would be more obvious, as these traits reflect functions supposedly closer to the action of the genes.

1.2.2 Frequency of Risk Alleles – Evolutionary Considerations

In addition to the number of loci involved, the frequency of each causal allele in the population is an independent parameter of models of genetic architecture. Polygenic models could involve rare or common alleles, or a mixture of both. The common disease/common variants (CD/CV) model proposes that common diseases arise from the cumulative burden of a number of common risk variants that float through the population, or at least that some of the causal variants would be common (Reich and Lander, 2001).

When applied to NDDs, a major problem arises for the CD/CV hypothesis. Such disorders significantly reduce fitness, with early onset, higher than average mortality and much lower than average fecundity (Keller and Miller, 2006). The CD/CV hypothesis must therefore address how genetic variants that predispose to the disorder could become common in the population in the face of negative selection (Keller and Miller, 2006). Various explanations have been invoked, including different forms of balancing selection, where the disease-causing variants are beneficial in another context. They could, for instance, increase fitness in a subset of individuals with a different genomic context, that is, those who do not develop disease but carry some of the risk variants. Or it could be that such risk variants were beneficial in a different environment, such as our species' recent past. There is, however, no evidence to support either of these contentions (Keller and Miller, 2006), and examples of balancing selection remain exceptional (Mayo, 2007; Olson, 2012).

An alternative explanation is that in situations where the effects on risk of each common variant are very small, and only expressed in a minority of carriers for any one variant, they are effectively invisible to selection. This may well apply under a model involving a huge number of loci with infinitesimal effect sizes. It could also arise if common alleles act as modifiers of rare mutations, but have no effect in most carriers. On the other hand, given a large effective population size, even a small average decrease in fitness across all carriers of a genetic variant means that natural selection can quite effectively keep its frequency low (Agarwala et al., 2013; Eyre-Walker, 2010; Gazave et al., 2013).

By contrast, a model involving multiple rare variants/mutations is completely congruent with evolutionary genetics as it explicitly

incorporates an important role for natural selection in keeping the frequency of individual disease-causing variants low or even rapidly eliminating them. New variants constantly arise through *de novo* mutation, generating a balance between mutation and selection and maintaining the disorder at a certain prevalence in the population. The prevalence of a disorder then largely depends on the size of the mutational target – the number of genes that can be mutated which result in that particular phenotype (Keller and Miller, 2006; Rodriguez-Murillo et al., 2012).

The distinction between the two models is thus quite stark – on the one hand, the polygenic, CD/CV model implicates a standing pool of common, ancient variants floating through the population (Plomin et al., 2009). By contrast, the model of genetic heterogeneity involving rare mutations (McClellan and King, 2010) is consistent with a much more dynamic spectrum of human genetic variation, with causal mutations winking in and out of existence, some being immediately selected against, others persisting for several generations (Lupski et al., 2011; Olson, 2012). Under this model, the more recent and thus rarer variants would have a larger phenotypic effect, though necessarily in fewer individuals. More severe conditions should be characterized by a higher contribution from *de novo* or recent alleles, while those where the effects of fitness are lower could involve a greater contribution from less rare (possibly even common) alleles, which could persist in the population for longer (Agarwala et al., 2013; Eyre-Walker, 2010; Simons et al., 2014).

This model fits with recent data showing the extent of rare variation in human populations and the frequency distribution of deleterious alleles (Abecasis et al., 2012; Gravel et al., 2011; Keinan and Clark, 2012; MacArthur et al., 2012). Rare alleles collectively make up 90% of the variation across the population. There is, moreover, a strong skew toward rarer, more recent alleles among those predicted to deleteriously affect a protein (including nonsense mutations, frameshifts, and those affecting splicing particularly) (Keinan and Clark, 2012; Kryukov et al., 2007). This implies that such alleles tend to be under strong negative selection and, conversely, that alleles with large biological effects tend to be rare. Because *de novo* mutations have not yet been subject to negative selection, they are likely to include the most highly penetrant alleles.

The aforementioned descriptions represent the extreme versions of these two models. As we will see subsequently, the empirical evidence actually favors an integrative model for the genetic architecture of NDDs. This encompasses a heterogeneity of causal architectures across individual cases, with some being more genetically complex than others. It also combines effects of multiple variants in individuals to explain observed complexities in relating genotypes to phenotypes. This model applies not just to common clinical categories but also to rare, identified syndromes, where phenotypic variability and genetic modifier effects are becoming more apparent.

1.3 EMPIRICAL EVIDENCE

1.3.1 Familiality

Several characteristics of the observed familiality of common disorders have been taken as evidence against a model of simple Mendelian inheritance with genetic heterogeneity and in favor of a polygenic burden model of inheritance.

1. With rare exceptions, most families do not show an obviously Mendelian pattern of inheritance – these disorders are characterized by familial *aggregation*, rather than consistent patterns of *segregation*.
2. There is a high rate of sporadic cases – most affected children have normal parents and no affected first-degree relatives.
3. Recurrence risk increases with the number of affected children in a family.

4. Recurrence risk to siblings typically increases with severity of the defect in the proband.
5. Risk is greater when both parents are affected.
6. Risk to relatives falls off sharply with increasing degree of relationship to an affected proband.

All of these observations are consistent with the idea of an increased burden of risk alleles in some families, which would be indicated by both increased number of affected individuals and increased clinical severity and which would manifest as increased risk to subsequent children.

However, these observations are also consistent with a scenario where (i) many cases are caused by *de novo* mutations, explaining the high incidence of sporadic cases and rapid fall off in risk with increasing genetic distance, and, (ii) many causal mutations are incompletely penetrant for any particular clinical category. More highly penetrant mutations segregating in a family would lead to greater severity and a greater proportion of individuals reaching the criteria for a clinical diagnosis. The observed patterns of familiality thus do not distinguish between models of genetic heterogeneity and polygenic burden (Mitchell and Porteous, 2011).

In fact, the association of increased risk to siblings with increasing severity in the proband likely does not hold for all NDDs. The relative risk to siblings of patients with intellectual disability is paradoxically much lower (no higher than population average in fact) if their relative has severe intellectual disability than if they are only mildly affected (Roberts, 1952). This is consistent with a scenario where mutations causing intellectual disability with high penetrance are effectively immediately selected against and thus must arise *de novo*, while those causing only mild impairment are far more likely to be inherited.

1.3.2 Linkage Studies

Linkage studies for specific rare syndromes have been highly successful in identifying causal loci. Examples include Rett syndrome, tuberous sclerosis, Hirschsprung's disease, and many others (e.g., (Amir et al., 1999; Escayg et al., 2000; Luo et al., 1993; Wan et al., 1999)). In these cases, the fact that they were discrete conditions was recognized *a priori* on the basis of typical symptom clusters, thus permitting the grouping of patients from different families.

By contrast, linkage studies based on common, broader clinical diagnostic categories were not so successful. Given the scarcity of large pedigrees with multiple affecteds, it was necessary to pool samples from large numbers of smaller families in the hopes of identifying common loci. Though many linkage peaks were reported, these were often not replicated in subsequent studies and generally did not lead to the identification of specific genes.

These results, along with segregation analyses, clearly rule out mutations in one or a small number of specific loci as causing the majority of cases of any common NDD. The inconsistency of linkage results for common NDDs such as SZ has been given as evidence in favor of a polygenic model of inheritance (Risch, 1990). However, negative linkage results are also fully expected under a model of extreme genetic heterogeneity (Agarwala et al., 2013; Mitchell and Porteous, 2011) and thus do not distinguish between models.

1.3.3 Endophenotypes

The endophenotype model for the genetic architecture of NDDs predicts that the mean phenotypic value of unaffected relatives of patients should be shifted toward the extreme end of the distribution of the endophenotype trait in question. This does appear to be the case for some endophenotypes, though not for all. For example, relatives of patients with SZ show mean values for some psychological measures that are lower than the population average, falling between the means of patients and controls (Allen et al., 2009; Braff et al., 2008). This trend extends to certain motor abilities and sensory processing measures and even various brain imaging measures.

What is not clear from those studies is whether this represents a consistent shift across all relatives or an effect seen in only a subset. The latter scenario appears to hold for ASD, where only a subset of relatives display what has been termed the Broad Autism Phenotype, scoring above a threshold on measures of autistic-like traits. For example, the BAP was apparent in 14–23% of parents of autistic children, compared to 5–9% of parents from a community sample (Sasson et al., 2013), with the remainder scoring in the normal range.

This more bimodal distribution of effects in relatives is consistent with a model of causation by rare mutations, with incomplete penetrance. Many relatives would not carry the causal mutation and would thus not differ from controls. Others would carry the mutation without developing the full clinical condition, but could show more subtle effects. This has been observed in clinically "unaffected" carriers of many pathogenic CNVs, for example (Stefansson et al., 2014). Alternatively, in cases caused by two or more mutations, relatives might carry only one of those and thus show a lesser effect (Berg and Geschwind, 2012; Girirajan et al., 2012) (Fig. 1.2). The fact that the values of some endophenotypes are altered in some relatives thus does not distinguish between models of genetic architecture.

In a related vein, studies of the heritability of autistic-like traits across the general population have been taken by some as arguing that the genetics of these traits generally overlaps with the genetics of ASD. These studies have found that the heritability is about the same at the extremes of the normal distribution of these traits, where patients with ASD diagnoses tend to score, as in the middle (Lundstrom et al., 2012; Robinson et al., 2011).

By itself, this does not prove, or even really argue for, a model whereby patients with ASD are those who fall at the extreme end of a unitary population distribution. The phenotypic values of ASD patients on those traits may fall at that position of the distribution for a different reason. If we consider an analogy with height, for example, it is clear that the genetics of dwarfism

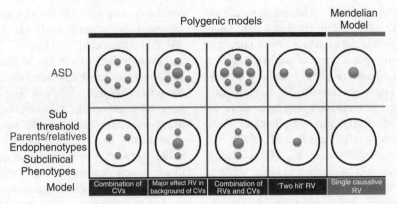

Fig. 1.2 *Expectations of risk allele burden and endophenotypes in relatives under a range of models of genetic architecture.* Large red circles represent high-risk mutations, small blue circles represent common variants. The top row shows possible causal architectures for patients with ASD. The bottom row shows the expected distributions of causal variants in clinically unaffected relatives for each of these scenarios. (Reproduced, with permission, from (Berg and Geschwind, 2012).) *(See insert for color representation of this figure.)*

or gigantism are quite distinct from the genetics of the normal distribution. A similar situation holds for the genetics of severe intellectual disability, which is clearly distinct from the genetics of IQ generally.

In addition, many single mutations are highly pleiotropic, affecting multiple endophenotypes at once, even though the genetics of such traits across the general population are largely nonoverlapping. Overall, there is thus little support for the model that clinical patients with diverse symptoms happen to lie at the extreme end of the normal distributions of multiple independent traits.

1.3.4 Common Variants – Genome-Wide Association Studies

Direct tests of the hypothesis that common variants contribute to risk of disease were made possible by the development of the human Haplotype Map (Consortium, 2003), which enabled genome-wide association studies (GWAS) (Hardy and Singleton, 2009). These studies assay the frequencies of different alleles at hundreds of thousands of single-nucleotide polymorphisms (SNPs), distributed across the genome. These are positions where two alternative DNA bases are both at high frequency in the population. They reflect an ancient mutation that

has spread to some extent throughout the population, typically due to genetic drift. There are tens of millions of such sites across the genome, but, due to uneven patterns of recombination across the genome, many such SNPs fall into haplotype blocks that tend to be co-inherited. As a result, sampling hundreds of thousands of SNPs, defined by the HapMap Project (Consortium, 2003), allows one to assay common variants across a much larger proportion of the genome.

The idea behind GWAS is very simple: if a common variant increases risk of disease, then the frequency of that variant should be higher in cases with the disease than in healthy controls (Hardy and Singleton, 2009; Risch and Merikangas, 1996). So, if an SNP shows that pattern, then either that SNP, or a variant that tends to be co-inherited with it, can be said to be associated with greater statistical risk of the disease. The problem is that if that statistical increase in risk is very small, then it requires a massive sample to detect it. This problem is greatly exacerbated by the statistical burden of correcting for all the multiple tests performed when assaying hundreds of thousands of SNPs at once.

Initial GWAS for NDDs, such as SZ, epilepsy and ASD, revealed no genome-wide significant hits (Anney et al., 2010; Kasperaviciute et al.,

2010; Need et al., 2009). The sample sizes of these studies were relatively small but large enough to exclude the existence of any common variants with even a modest statistical effect on risk (increased risk of 2-fold or more). Somewhat larger studies for SZ have identified statistical associations with a number of common SNPs, with quite small effect sizes (odds ratios of <1.2) (Purcell et al., 2009; Shi et al., 2009; Stefansson et al., 2009). Along with additional loci implicated in larger studies, these collectively account for ~3% of the total genetic variance affecting disease risk (Purcell et al., 2009; Ripke et al., 2013). At the time of writing, results from even larger GWAS for SZ have been reported, though not yet published. These mention over 100 associated SNPs, with even smaller individual effect sizes, though the overall genetic variance explained has not increased from earlier studies (Wright, 2014).

Recognizing the etiological overlap between diagnostic categories, a recent study conducted a cross-disorder GWAS, encompassing cases with ASD, SZ, ADHD, bipolar disorder, and major depression. Four loci gave genome-wide significant hits and seven others approached this level. Some signals were associated with single disorders, but most gave signal across disorders (Consortium, 2013). Moreover, the effect sizes were very small and the overall variance explained was less than 3%.

GWAS have also been conducted for a number of clinical or psychlogical endophenotypes. A small number of statistically significant hits have been found (Alliey-Rodriguez et al., 2011; Connolly et al., 2013; Goodbourn et al., 2014; Knowles et al., 2014). These should be interpreted with caution; however, as they derive from small samples, have not been replicated and test for association with multiple traits at once. GWAS with larger samples, looking at individual dimensions of clinical symptoms, have not detected any hits at genome-wide significance (Bramon et al., 2014; Fanous et al., 2012). In addition, a large number of candidate gene associations with diverse endophenotypes have been reported in the literature. These have typically not held up well in subsequent replication attempts and the vast majority likely represent false positives (Flint and Munafo, 2013; Ioannidis et al., 2011).

Given the lack of variance in disease liability explained by currently identified SNPs and the possibility that studies to date have simply been underpowered, it is interesting to ask more generally, how much variance could theoretically be explained by common alleles collectively? A new quantitative genetics technique, which does not rely on individual SNPs reaching genome-wide significance, has been applied to GWAS results to attempt to estimate this quantity (Yang et al., 2010; Yang et al., 2011). This method of genome-wide complex trait analysis (GCTA) looks for a signature of increased (but still distant) relatedness among cases, compared to that among controls, and uses such a signature to estimate heritability. Estimates from this method for the overall percentage of genetic variance that is tagged by common SNPs are quite high for SZ and ASD (23% and 40–60%, respectively) (Klei et al., 2012; Lee et al., 2012). However, confidence in these figures is undermined by questions about the methodology and underlying assumptions of this technique and the interpretation of the results (Browning and Browning, 2011; Lee et al., 2012). In particular, the idea that a hypothetical, minuscule increase in risk could be detected in people cryptically related at only the fourth or fifth cousin level, when the increase in risk for the first cousins is only about twofold for SZ and ASD (Lichtenstein et al., 2006; Sandin et al., 2014), appears to warrant some skepticism. Moreover, despite claims that this method indicates a large collective role for many common variants, it actually cannot distinguish either the number of loci involved or the frequency of causal alleles (discussed in more detail in Box 1).

Returning to those SNPs that do show genome-wide significant hits, what do these statistical associations mean? First, they do not imply that the SNP that is assayed is necessarily the causal variant itself. Each SNP tags an extended haplotype with many other common variants, so that the GWAS signal only implicates a general locus in the genome as containing some variant (or variants) affecting risk. Moreover, from that signal alone, it is impossible to infer how common the causal variant is. Modeling suggests that some GWAS signals may tag rare variants at a locus, which may by chance be more associated with one haplotype over another (Chang and Keinan, 2012; Dickson et al., 2010; Wang et al., 2010). Others have countered that rare variants cannot explain GWAS signals (Wray et al., 2011), but simulations incorporating the important parameter of negative selection suggest that GWAS signals across a locus can indeed be quite consistent with the presence of multiple, rare causal variants at that locus in the population (Thornton et al., 2013).

Empirical studies, involving resequencing of GWAS loci, have now found several instances where GWAS signals for various disorders or traits can be partially or largely attributed to effects of rare variants at the associated locus (Oosterveer et al., 2013; Sanna et al., 2011; Saunders et al., 2014; Thun et al., 2013). This effect has not been seen in all cases, however (Hunt et al., 2013). Furthermore, the general level of consistency of direction of allelic associations across distant populations, though by no means universal (Ntzani et al., 2012), is somewhat higher than expected under a model of synthetic associations as the sole drivers of GWAS signals (Carlson et al., 2013; Marigorta and Navarro, 2013). Overall, it thus appears likely that at least some of the reported GWAS signals for many disorders reflect a functional role for associated common variants.

This leads to the question of how to interpret the effect sizes of associated SNPs in GWAS. These are usually expressed as odds ratios, which summarize the statistical increase in relative frequency of one SNP allele in cases versus controls. For disorders that are not very common, this approximates the relative risk – the increased likelihood of being a case, given the presence of the risk allele. Most odds ratios from GWAS are in the range of 1.05 to 1.2-fold increased risk. How can this statistical effect across the population be related to biological effects in individuals?

The most straightforward possibility is that everyone who carries that risk allele is at very slightly higher risk of developing disease than those who carry the alternate allele. An alternative interpretation is that average signal reflects a much more potent effect, but in far fewer people. Such a situation could arise where: (i) rare variants of larger effect fall predominantly on that common haplotype, that is, the signal is driven by synthetic associations, as described earlier, or, (ii) a common allele acts as a strong genetic modifier of particular rare mutations, at the same or different loci, but has essentially no effect in most individuals, who do not carry such mutations. Examples of such modifiers will be discussed in the following sections.

1.3.5 Rare Mutations – Copy Number Variants

Many rare neurodevelopmental syndromes (such as Down, Williams, Angelman, Prader-Willi syndromes, and many others) are associated with specific chromosomal anomalies, including deletions or duplications of sections of chromosomes (also known as copy number variants, as they change the number of copies of genes within the deleted or duplicated segment). These conditions were initially distinguished by the consistent clustering of behavioral and nonpsychological symptoms, such as typical facial morphology, for example. The causal chromosomal anomalies were discovered by classical cytogenetics and subsequently defined molecularly.

The development of array technologies for detecting CNVs across the genome allowed these efforts to become far more systematic and powerful (Sebat et al., 2004). The application of these technologies and the realization that CNVs could also be detected using SNP arrays led to the discovery of numerous additional CNVs that are associated with increased incidence of various common NDDs (e.g., (Cooper et al., 2011; Kirov et al., 2009; Marshall et al., 2008; Mefford et al., 2010; Sebat et al., 2007; Walsh et al., 2008); reviewed in (Cook and Scherer, 2008; Grayton et al., 2012; Merikangas et al., 2009)). The risk associated with such CNVs is recognizable because they recur at a low but detectable frequency at particular sites in the genome, due to local properties of genomic organization (Liu et al., 2012). It is thus possible to find many people with effectively the same chromosomal deletion or duplication and assess rates of illness in this group.

Though individually rare, the CNVs so far identified can collectively account for a significant proportion of previously idiopathic cases of conditions such as ASD (>10%) and SZ (>5%). One of the most striking findings from this work has been the lack of respect for clinical diagnostic boundaries in the effects of such CNVs. The same CNVs have been detected in patients with ASD, SZ, epilepsy, ADHD, ID, and other clinical presentations (Cook and Scherer, 2008; Grayton et al., 2012; Merikangas et al., 2009). The genetic etiology of these conditions is thus clearly overlapping (Coe et al., 2012; Craddock and Owen, 2010; Moreno-De-Luca et al., 2013), a finding that is reinforced by large-scale epidemiological studies and by analyses of mutations in single genes (see Chapter 2).

1.3.6 Single-Gene Mutations

CNVs delete or duplicate chunks of chromosomes and typically affect more than one gene. But NDDs can also be caused by mutations in single genes, which are now also being discovered at an increasing rate, thanks to the development of next-generation sequencing technologies. In addition to those associated with syndromic forms of mental illness, such as Fragile X syndrome and Rett syndrome, early studies had identified a small number of single-gene mutations associated mainly with psychiatric manifestations in particular families. These include DISC1, where carriers in a large Scottish pedigree of a translocation that disrupts the gene manifest with a variety of psychiatric diagnoses (Millar et al., 2000), and genes encoding neuroligin-3 and neuroligin-4, mutations in which were found in families with

multiple individuals affected by ASD (Jamain et al., 2003).

As with the initially identified chromosomal syndromes, some argued that these might be isolated examples that are not relevant to the majority of idiopathic cases. This idea has turned out to be untenable, as more and more cases associated with single-gene mutations are discovered. Next-generation sequencing studies, using both family and case-control designs, have identified numerous point mutations, or single-nucleotide variants (SNVs), associated with high risk of NDDs (Allen et al., 2013; Chahrour et al., 2012; Cukier et al., 2014; Fromer et al., 2014; Iossifov et al., 2012; Lim et al., 2013; Neale et al., 2012; O'Roak et al., 2011; O'Roak et al., 2012; Piton et al., 2010; Purcell et al., 2014; Sanders et al., 2012; Xu et al., 2011; Yu et al., 2013). As with CNVs, most of these mutations are associated with diverse clinical manifestations. Mutations in any one gene are individually very rare, as expected, but an overall excess of damaging SNVs in patients with NDDs compared to controls suggests that a large portion of the burden of disease may be accounted for by such rare mutations collectively (Allen et al., 2013; Cukier et al., 2014; Fromer et al., 2014; Kenny et al., 2013; Purcell et al., 2014).

One of the most important findings from studies of CNVs and SNVs is that a significant proportion of the pathogenic mutations arise *de novo*, in the generation of sperm or eggs, rather than being inherited from a carrier parent (Ku et al., 2012) (Chapter 3). Typically, mutations that have higher penetrance for more severe phenotypes will be more likely to have arisen *de novo* than to have been inherited, as carriers are less likely to have children. Current estimates suggest that as many as 50% of cases of ASD may be attributable to *de novo* mutations (Ronemus et al., 2014). This is likely to be even higher for severe forms of ID (Vissers et al., 2010), but lower for later-onset disorders with smaller effects on fitness, such as SZ and bipolar disorder.

This finding has several general implications. First, it illustrates the general point that even common NDDs can be caused by single, dominant mutations. Second, it shows that such conditions can be genetic but not inherited, reconciling high heritability (based on MZ twin concordance) with the high level of sporadic cases. Finally, it further undermines the quantitative genetics framework, which is premised on the idea of a standing pool of variation that simply gets shuffled around from generation to generation.

As more and more high-risk mutations are identified, more and more cases will move from the idiopathic pool to the pool with known high-risk mutations (Fig. 1.3). However, while some such mutations will define new syndromes, it would be a mistake to think of causality generally in such simple terms. The incomplete penetrance and variable phenotypic expressivity of many single mutations, whether *de novo* or inherited, suggests additional layers of complexity in relating genotypes to phenotypes.

1.4 COMPLEX GENOTYPE–PHENOTYPE RELATIONSHIPS

1.4.1 Incomplete Penetrance and Variable Expressivity

While the list of high-risk mutations is growing all the time, it is also clear that simple models relating genotypes at single loci to clinical phenotypes generally do not hold. The phenotypic expression of most such mutations is quite variable and penetrance for any specific diagnosis is typically incomplete. Of course, penetrance can be defined in other ways, which do not rely on reified clinical categories. For example, while the penetrance for many CNVs for SZ is relatively low (Vassos et al., 2010), the penetrance for a broader category including ASD and developmental delay is much higher (Kirov et al., 2014). In addition, while such CNVs are also detected at reduced frequency in healthy controls, a recent study has found that many are associated with general decreases in

cognitive ability, even in clinically "unaffected" carriers (Stefansson et al., 2014).

Variability in phenotypic expression is also now becoming apparent even for mutations associated with specific syndromes, such as VCFS, Williams syndrome, Angelman syndrome, and others. Prospective screening of psychiatric patients without syndromic diagnoses has revealed that the CNVs causing these syndromes also are found in patients with idiopathic symptoms of autism, epilepsy, or other neurological or psychiatric manifestations (Grayton et al., 2012). The initial, narrow definition of specific syndromes thus likely reflects an ascertainment bias, in that discovery of these mutations was based on grouping together those patients with the most recognizably similar pattern of symptoms. A similar situation is observed for mutations causing inborn errors of metabolism. Though these are typically recognized due to their phenotypic effects in young infants, many such mutations are now also being implicated in adult-onset psychiatric patients with no previous diagnosis (Kayser, 2008; Sedel, 2012).

Another important factor in relating mutations in specific genes to specific clinical outcomes is allelic heterogeneity. Not all mutations at a particular gene will alter protein production or function in the same way. This is classically exemplified by mutations in different parts of the dystrophin gene, which cause the clinically distinct conditions of Duchenne or Becker muscular dystrophy. Many genes show a similar diversity of outcomes associated with mutations in different regions of the gene (Walsh and Engle, 2010). In addition, some mutations associated with severe cortical malformations or other developmental syndromes when homozygous, have now been found in heteroyzgous condition in less severely affected patients, manifesting mainly with psychiatric symptoms (Walsh and Engle, 2010).

1.4.2 Genetic Modifiers and Oligogenic Effects

The effects of primary mutations are commonly modified by genetic background. This is a truism

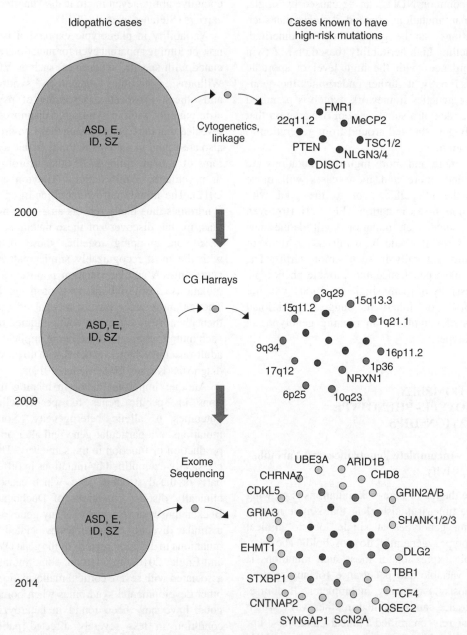

Fig. 1.3 *The cumulative identification of genetic causes of neurodevelopmental disorders.* The circle on the left represents the current pool of idiopathic cases, reflecting the level of ignorance at the time. The small circles on the right represent cases carrying rare, high-risk mutations. New technologies including comparative genome hybridization (CGH) arrays and next-generation sequencing of exomes or genomes have allowed a continuing stream of discoveries of new risk mutations (lighter circles), thus shrinking the pool of idiopathic cases. Note that only an arbitrary set of examples of such mutations are shown; the real list runs to many hundreds. *(See insert for color representation of this figure.)*

in experimental genetics with model organisms, where strain background effects are commonplace – almost ubiquitous, in fact (Mackay, 2009; Nadeau, 2001; Phillips, 2008; Spiezio et al., 2012). The phenotypic effects of many mutations vary – sometimes hugely – between strains of mice or flies, for example. This has several interesting implications: first, and most obviously, the phenotype in individuals is often determined by more than one genetic variant. Second, some of the variants involved have little or no phenotypic effect alone (in cases where the phenotype in question does not vary between two strains in the absence of a major mutation, for example). Third, the existence of such cryptic genetic variation is evidence that the developmental system is capable of buffering substantial genetic variation without altering the phenotype (Gibson and Dworkin, 2004; Wagner, 2007). The latent effects of such variation may be released, however, in the presence of a serious mutation.

This is also true in human genetics. Many mutations associated with distinct Mendelian conditions are strongly modified by additional genetic variants (Badano and Katsanis, 2002; Cooper et al., 2013; Dipple and McCabe, 2000). This is true even for conditions associated with mutations in a single gene, such as sickle cell anemia, cystic fibrosis, and Huntington's disease, where severity, age of onset, and progression can all be modified by specific variants in other genes. The manifestation of various NDDs also depends on background variants, as in Rett syndrome (Grillo et al., 2013; Renieri et al., 2003), Dravet syndrome (Singh et al., 2009), and Kallmann syndrome (Shaw et al., 2011), for example. Specific modifying variants have been identified for many genetic conditions (Cooper et al., 2013). Some of the modifying variants are themselves rare, but common variants can often make important contributions, significantly modifying the risk of specific mutations.

This scenario is exemplified by Hirschsprung's disease, a neurodevelopmental disorder affecting the enteric nervous system (Alves et al., 2013). Rare mutations in 18 genes have been associated with this condition, including the RET and NRG1 genes. Importantly, common variants in both those genes also increase risk and are much more frequent in affected carriers of the rare mutations than in unaffected carriers. However, in the absence of a rare mutation, these common variants have little or no phenotypic consequence. These effects thus exemplify epistatic, or nonadditive genetic interactions in determining individual phenotypes (Chapter 4).

To date, no specific modifying mutations have been definitively identified for more common NDDs, but this may reflect a lag in discovery, exacerbated by the higher level of primary genetic heterogeneity. It appears quite possible that some of the common variants identified by GWAS may be acting in this fashion – that is, the small statistical effects associated with some common SNPs, when averaged across the population, could be due to much larger effects in only a subset of individuals carrying rare mutations. Interestingly, GWAS signals for common NDDs have shown up in a number of loci in which rare mutations are associated with specific syndromes with neurological and psychiatric symptoms, such as Pitt-Hopkins syndrome (TCF4) (Forrest et al., 2014), Timothy syndrome (CACNA1C) (Bhat et al., 2012), and cerebellar ataxia (SYNE1) (Consortium, 2013; Noreau et al., 2013). These GWAS signals could be due to synthetic associations, but could alternatively reflect a situation such as that in observed in Hirschsprung's disease, where common variants have strong modifying effects. It will likely be necessary to first define carriers of specific primary mutations before these kinds of specific modifying effects can be recognized.

One common variant that has been demonstrated to have a large effect on the phenotypic outcome associated with neurodevelopmental mutations is the Y chromosome. This is most evident in ASD, where males are much more commonly affected than females (a 4:1 ratio) (Ronemus et al., 2014), but can also be observed in sex differences in the rates of many NDDs, including ADHD, dyslexia, SZ, and others

(Cahill, 2006). Analyses of the spectrum of mutations in autistic patients reveal that affected females tend to have more severe mutations than affected males. This is true for both CNVs (which affect many more genes on average in females) (Levy et al., 2011) and SNVs (which include more potentially deleterious mutations in females) (Jacquemont et al., 2014). Importantly, these effects extend to broader categories of NDDs and are also seen in the previous generation. When the mutation is inherited, it is significantly more likely to come from the mother than the father (Jacquemont et al., 2014; Ronemus et al., 2014). This suggests that men who carried such a mutation were more severely affected and thus less likely to become fathers in the first place.

These findings indicate that it takes a more severe mutation to push a female brain into an autistic state, or, conversely, that males are more susceptible to the effects of such mutations. This sex difference could be due to the Y chromosome itself, through its known influences on brain development and connectivity (Gilmore et al., 2007; Ingalhalikar et al., 2014; McCarthy et al., 2012; Wu and Shah, 2011). Alternatively, it may be not the presence of the Y, but the lack of one X chromosome that is important – this may make male development intrinsically less robust to the effects of mutations anywhere in the genome. However, the facts that not all developmental disorders show this male bias, and that the bias is uneven for different NDDs, appear more consistent with a Y chromosome effect.

In addition to modifying effects of common variants, a growing number of cases of NDDs are now turning up with more than one severe rare mutation. This has been observed for CNVs, where affected individuals who have inherited a CNV with relatively low penetrance more often have a second, potentially pathogenic CNV elsewhere in the genome (Bassuk et al., 2013; Girirajan et al., 2012; Girirajan et al., 2010). Similar events have been observed for known pathogenic single-gene mutations with incomplete penetrance alone (Chilian et al., 2013; Leblond et al., 2012; Schaaf et al., 2011).

In these cases, both CNVs or mutations are likely having an effect alone and these may combine, additively or nonadditively, to cause frank disease. By contrast, mutations with higher penetrance tend to arise *de novo* and are not associated with an excess of secondary events (Girirajan et al., 2012).

1.4.3 Nongenetic Sources of Variance

The fact that concordance for NDD diagnoses is not complete between MZ twins indicates the presence of additional sources of variance beyond overall genotype. These may include environmental risk factors but can also reflect an often neglected nongenetic source of variance, which is intrinsic developmental variation.

Environmental factors: Epidemiological studies have associated a number of environmental risk factors, such as maternal infection during gestation, preterm delivery, obstetric complications, and others with statistically significant increased risk for NDDs ((Hamlyn et al., 2013), Chapter 6). The odds ratios for each of these broad categories of risk factors are typically low (less than twofold). However, such risks may be unevenly distributed across the population. In particular, pathogenic mutations could make the developing brain more susceptible to the effects of such environmental insults, leading to a greater effect in genetically vulnerable individuals. While plausible, and arguably more likely than a uniform effect, this kind of gene-by-environment interaction remains to be directly demonstrated for NDDs (Chapter 6).

Intrinsic developmental variation. The outcome of development is inherently variable, as evidenced by physical differences between isogenic organisms, including monozygotic twins, or even between the two sides of nominally symmetrical organisms (Leamy and Klingenberg, 2005). Such differences are also observed at the neuroanatomical level, as in agenesis of the corpus callosum, for example, where this structure may be absent in one twin and present in the other (Mitchell, 2007; Ruge and Newland, 1996; Wahlsten, 1989). On a finer scale, the effects of many mutations are played out at a cellular level in a probabilistic fashion across the developing brain, so that the pattern of abnormalities may vary widely from one brain to the next (as with mutations causing cortical heterotopia, to take an obvious example). Thus, even in nonpathogenic circumstances, by the time they emerge from the womb, the brains of monozygotic twins are already quite unique (Clarke, 2012; Mitchell, 2007).

Such effects could presumably contribute to differences in emergent psychological traits and neuropsychiatric disorders between MZ twins.

For example, while the heritability of epilepsy is quite high, the heritability of the specific anatomical focus is much lower (Corey et al., 2011), likely reflecting such stochastic events in neurodevelopment. Intrinsic developmental variability may thus make a large contribution to the nongenetic variance observed for NDDs, which can be sizeable.

Behavioral genetics studies typically divide the sources of phenotypic variance into genetic variance, shared family environment effects and a third term, called the "nonshared environment" (Plomin and Daniels, 2011). This term mathematically accounts for the incomplete heritability of a trait or lack of full concordance between monozygotic twins, reflecting an additional nongenetic source of variance in the population generally (Turkheimer and Waldron, 2000). The phrase nonshared environment is somewhat regrettable, as it implies an origin outside the organism. This has often been interpreted as reflecting an important role for personal experiences, such as interactions with peers or teachers, which may help to differentiate MZ twins from each other (Harris, 1998; Plomin and Daniels, 2011). Given the strong and consistent evidence that family environment has little or no effect on phenotypic outcome for NDDs, there appears little reason to think that peer interactions or other, nontraumatic, personal experiences would make such an important contribution. Nor is there any reason to expect differential exposure to environmental toxins or other risk factors would be greater between MZ twins than between different families.

In fact, the nonshared environment term also encompasses: (i) measurement error or misclassification (an important source of variance for behavioral traits or psychiatric diagnoses especially), and, (ii) chance, or, in this case, intrinsic developmental variation. The developmental program is quite robust and, under normal circumstances, strongly canalizes development toward a species-typical outcome (Wagner, 2007). This idea is captured in the epigenetic landscape, a metaphor developed by Conrad Waddington, to conceptualize the probabilistic, but also canalized nature of development (Waddington, 1957). (This original usage of epigenetic derives from the Greek term "epigenesis," meaning the emergence of the organism, and does not relate to the molecular genetic usage of the term, referring to mitotically stable chromatin states).

The developmental program is robust to small changes (as evidenced by the presence of cryptic genetic variation (Gibson and Dworkin, 2004)) but this robustness is challenged by severe mutations. These tend to not only decrease the probability of a species-typical phenotype, but also increase the phenotypic variance, making the outcome more susceptible to noise and stochastic events (Wagner, 2007; Yeo et al., 2007). Interestingly, the ability of a developing organism to buffer the effects of specific mutations may itself be a genetic trait, reflecting what we might call "genomic reserve." The possibility that such a trait reflects the general mutational load in the genetic background is explored in Chapter 5.

1.4.4 Heterogeneity and Complexity of Causal Factors in Individuals

The preceding sections paint a picture of the etiology of NDDs that involves complexities on many levels. First, there is tremendous underlying locus and allelic heterogeneity. This reinforces the view that many broad clinical categories of common NDDs do not represent natural kinds, at least in terms of etiology. The distinction between cases whose symptoms are associated with known causes and the much larger group of idiopathic cases is simply an expression of current ignorance, not a reifying principle that justifies treating diagnoses of exclusion as natural kinds. This heterogeneity largely undermines the quantitative genetics framework (Mitchell, 2012), which lumps together patients with common diagnoses under the assumption of a shared and unitary etiology (Robinson et al., 2014).

Second, there is heterogeneity in modes of causality across individuals (Fig. 1.4). In some cases, a primary mutation will be readily recognizable. In others, multiple mutations or modifying variants may be at play. Conditions that are more severe are more likely to have a greater proportion of cases caused by individual, recent mutations (often *de novo*), while those with less severe manifestations are more likely to have one or more inherited mutations and modifying variants.

Third, the sharp dichotomy between rare and common disorders has become blurred. On the one hand, we can now recognize within the broad categories of common disorders a growing number of distinct, very rare conditions (Fig. 1.3). On the other, even the formerly

recognized rare conditions show a previously unappreciated level of genetic complexity, with important contributions from genetic modifiers. Digenic or oligogenic causality, with a few contributing variants, is thus likely in many cases.

Whether the range of modes of causality extends to a highly polygenic architecture, involving a very large number of variants in some individuals, remains an open question. The statistical association of some variants of small effect across the population does not mean that they must act in this collective fashion. Rather than supposing a division whereby some cases are caused by mutations of large effect and others by the combined action of a very large number of mutations of small effect, an integrative model incorporates variants of low statistical effect size across the population (common or rare) as epistatic modifiers of major mutations (Mitchell and Porteous, 2011), as demonstrated for disorders such as Hirschsprung's disease.

The extreme level of locus heterogeneity is reflected in the diversity of functions of the genes implicated, which encode proteins acting in many different cellular processes. While many of the implicated genes encode proteins

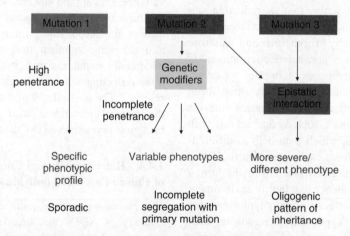

Fig. 1.4 *Heterogeneity of causal architectures across individuals.* High penetrance mutations will most often be immediately selected against and so will typically arise *de novo*, rather than being inherited. Lower penetrance mutations will be more likely to be inherited and will often be modified by additional common or rare variants in the genetic background. (Reproduced, with permission, from (Mitchell, 2011).) *(See insert for color representation of this figure.)*

involved in neural development or synaptic function (discussed in detail in Chapters 7–9), others include chromatin regulatory proteins, basal translation factors, metabolic enzymes and miscellaneous proteins whose functions are not obviously neurodevelopmental. This raises an interesting and important question: how could disruption of so many different genes, with such diverse functions, lead to such similar outcomes – the states we recognize as ASD or SZ or epilepsy? An answer may lie in considering the symptoms of these disorders as emergent phenotypes.

1.4.5 The Genetics of Emergent Phenotypes

We already know of hundreds of different genes in which mutations can cause intellectual disability. This is perhaps not surprising, given the complexity of the human brain – it appears reasonable to expect that mutations in many different genes could impair its function. Somewhat more surprising is the idea that a similarly diverse set of mutations could give rise to the apparently much more specific phenotypes associated with common NDDs, such as autistic behavior, psychosis, depression, hyperactivity, or seizures. The symptoms of these conditions appear to reflect not just a decrement in function but the emergence of qualitatively novel brain states.

Understanding how mutations in so many diverse genes can give rise to these states involves the recognition that the relationship between the normal functions of genes and their resultant mutant phenotypes can be extremely indirect. This is especially true for phenotypes that reflect very high-level, emergent functions of complex systems. The kinds of cognitive processes impaired in ASD and SZ represent the highest-level functions of the human mind. These processes rely on the functions of myriad distinct systems, each composed of multiple brain regions and fiber pathways, hundreds of cell types, and thousands of gene products. Like "performance" of a fighter jet, high-level cognitive operations rely on the complex and dynamic interactions between all these components.

The fact that these systems are susceptible to mutations in many different genes is thus not so shocking. The upgrades to our cognitive hardware which arose through evolution may carry with them a certain vulnerability – the price of increasing complexity may be more ways to break down. We may in addition, as a social species, be highly attuned to notice subtle differences in function of the brain, which might be far less evident for other organs.

However, the fact that our neural systems tend to fail in particular ways, generating qualitatively novel brain states, remains an interesting puzzle. It appears likely, though, that this reflects organizational properties of the brain, rather than the functions of the perturbed genes. In particular, maladaptive reactivity of the brain to early differences may channel development toward discrete pathological states (Ben-Ari, 2008; Hulme et al., 2013; Lisman et al., 2008; Lodge and Grace, 2011).

The functions of the disease-associated genes are thus too diverse and too far removed from the emergent effects of the pathogenic mutations to think of them as "genes for" ASD, SZ, or epilepsy. Nor is it accurate to conceive of them as genes for working memory or executive function or other high-level cognitive operations. The proximal effects of mutations in various genes, which arise at the molecular and cellular levels, will have cascading consequences over neural and cognitive development, with the phenotype of the organism sometimes being channeled by developmental systems and neural architectures to produce emergent states that we recognize as psychiatric or neurological conditions.

1.4.6 Implications for Research and Clinical Practice

The genetic architecture of NDDs is characterized by heterogeneity of causes across individuals and complexity of causes within individuals. This has a number of important implications for both research and for clinical practice:

1. Finding additional high-risk mutations by case-control comparisons will likely

require very large samples, in order to distinguish the cuplrits from the innocent bystanders (Zuk et al., 2014). It may be possible and necessary to bootstrap our way from mutations that were strongly implicated under more specific study designs and to use biological knowledge to generate priors for inference of pathogenicity.

2. The identification of high-risk mutations in enough people may enable the secondary discovery of genetic modifiers. With increasing knowledge of such interactions, this may allow more accurate prediction of individual risks based on genome-types, not just single-mutation-genotypes.

3. Inferring genetic causality will likely remain a matter of probabilities. Nevertheless, as genetic information becomes available for more and more patients, it should be possible to discern which pieces of information are relevant for treatment (Box 2) (Chapter 13).

4. The segregation of patients based on genetic knowledge should greatly enhance the ability to define clinical subsyndromes (Bruining et al., 2014) and also to investigate the neurobiological phenotypes associated with specific mutations (Consortium, 2012; Stessman et al., 2014). It should be much more informative to characterize patients with the same mutation than to analyse patients grouped solely by broad clinical diagnosis, with high underlying heterogeneity.

5. The identification of high-risk mutations offers a proven discovery route to the underlying biological processes. Cellular and animal models with direct etiological validity, combined with our growing general understanding of how the brain works, should reveal pathogenic mechanisms and cascading pathways through which various mutations presumably converge on a narrower set of pathophysiological states (Arguello and Gogos, 2012; Mitchell et al., 2011) (Chapters 10, 11).

6. Combined, all these approaches offer the hope of rationally designing new therapies and intervention strategies based on a detailed understanding of the pathogenic and pathophysiological mechanisms in individual patients (Chapters 12, 14).

1.4.7 Box 1 Estimating the Overall Contribution of Common Variants

Recently, a new type of analysis of GWAS data has been developed that purports to estimate how large a contribution common alleles could collectively make to quantitative traits, including the modeled liability to complex disorders (Lee et al., 2011; Yang et al., 2011). Genome-wide complex trait analysis, or GCTA, analyses SNP data from case-control datasets, but, rather than looking for signatures of association with individual SNPs, it uses these data merely to estimate genetic similarity between ostensibly unrelated pairs of individuals. This can then be correlated with phenotypic similarity, where continuous traits are concerned, to estimate how heritable the trait is. The logic for continuous traits is thus the same as with twin or family studies – the comparison is just carried out over much larger genetic distances, with correspondingly smaller phenotypic similarity.

For dichotomous traits, such as disease diagnosis, however, the logic is inverted from that of twin studies. Here, you start with people with a certain degree of phenotypic similarity (they all have the disease) and ask if they have higher genetic similarity (to each other than to a set of controls). A signature of increased mean genetic similarity across all pairs of cases is taken as evidence of heritability of risk for the disorder over large genetic distances. According to this method, a quantitative value for the percent of genetic variance tagged by common SNPs can be derived from the similarity matrix. The application of this method to SZ datasets has led to the assertion that 23% of the variance in liability to SZ is captured by SNPs and that a substantial proportion of this variation must be the result of common causal variants (Lee et al., 2012). A similar analysis for cases diagnosed with

ASD concludes that "common genetic polymorphisms exert substantial additive genetic effects on ASD liability" and estimate the magnitude of these effects as explaining between 40 and 60% of additive genetic variance (Klei et al., 2012).

These values are obviously very substantial, but how much confidence can we have in their estimation and interpretation? The values are extrapolated from a tiny signal of increased (but still very distant) genetic similarity among cases, compared to controls, raising a general concern that such a signal may reflect artefacts or noise. There are a number of methodological concerns with this approach, to do, for example, with the statistical corrections required to exclude effects of cryptic population stratification (Browning and Browning, 2011) and to correct for highly skewed ascertainment of cases and controls relative to the true population prevalence of the disorder (Lee et al., 2011).

More generally, recurrence risks for SZ and ASD decrease sharply with increasing genetic distance and are only on the order of 1.5 to 2-fold for first cousins (Lichtenstein et al., 2006; McGue et al., 1983; Sandin et al., 2014). It appears likely, therefore, that any increased risk to fourth or fifth cousins would be negligible. The idea that a statistical signature of such an effect, if it exists at all, could be detected, measured accurately and extrapolated to give a definitive value of variance tagged by common SNPs thus appears inherently questionable.

Even taking the data at face value, however, it is not possible to infer that these signals are driven by causal effects of common variants, as stated by the authors of one of these studies: "From the analyses we have performed, we cannot estimate a distribution of the allele frequency of causal variants" (Lee et al., 2012). Allele-sharing between distant relatives is often concentrated in one or two genomic segments derived from a common ancestor (Ralph and Coop, 2013), meaning that increased sharing of rare variants in such segments could explain the supposed tiny average increased risk of disease among distant relatives (or, conversely, increased distant relatedness among cases). Using common SNPs to estimate heritability across distant relatives thus simply does not inform on the number of causal variants in the population or in individuals or the frequency of causal alleles.

1.4.8 Box 2 Causality and Genetic Diagnoses

Given the incomplete penetrance and variable expressivity of the known mutations implicated in NDDs, how should we think about genetic causality? In considering this issue, a clear distinction should be drawn between explanation versus prediction of illness, as the probability relationships are entirely different in these two directions.

In terms of predicting illness based on the presence of a known disease-associated mutation, the only information we have to go on is the penetrance of the mutation for the disorder in question. For the well known 22q11.2 deletion, for example, the risk of psychosis is about 30% (though the risk of any clinical diagnosis is much higher). By contrast, the rate of SZ in carriers of the NRXN1 deletion is about 6%. These increased risks may be deemed actionable in terms of reproductive decisions but would provide less justification, for example, for drastic preemptive clinical intervention in currently unaffected carriers.

On the other hand, the presence of these mutations in individuals who are *already affected* allows stronger inferences to be drawn about their contribution to illness. Here, one can compare the odds of someone having the illness, given the presence of the mutation, with the odds of them having the illness for some other reason (i.e., the population prevalence). For 22q11 deletions, the odds in favor of that deletion being a primary contributor to schizophrenic symptoms in that individual are thus around 30:1. For NRXN1 deletions, where prediction is quite weak, the inference of causality, given the illness having occurred, is considerably stronger: about 6:1 odds of the patient having the disease due to the NRXN1 mutation, as opposed to some other reason. This approach defines causality in a counterfactual rather than a reductive sense – it does not imply that the mutation in question was a sufficient cause, but does estimate the likelihood that it was a necessary cause in that patient.

However, patients with low penetrance mutations are more likely to also have a secondary mutation or additional genetic variants contributing to pathogenesis. This has been observed empirically (Girirajan et al., 2012) and fits generally with the known high concordance levels of MZ twins for common NDDs such as ASD and SZ. Simply put, most individuals who develop these diseases were at high risk of having done so. Though ascertainment biases likely inflate these figures somewhat (only seeing pairs condordant for illness, not for health), this does imply that most patients with these conditions carry high-risk *genome-types*. If the primary mutation is not potent enough on its own, this suggests the presence of additional accomplices.

The definition of discrete genetic syndromes and the assignment of categorical genetic diagnoses may be somewhat justified for high penetrance mutations but is thus less appropriate for patients with lower penetrance mutations. A more pragmatic approach will be simply to consider the potential relevance of any piece of genetic information to clinical management based on empirical observation, such as whether patients with mutations in Gene X tend to show particular symptoms or respond better to particular treatments.

Genetic information can thus be incorporated into clinical management without falling into the conceptual trap of issuing overly categorical genetic diagnoses (Chapter 13). In the future, the identification of modifying mutations, as for Hirschsprung's disease, for example, should make it possible to make more accurate predictions of risk based on an individual's entire genome-type, and not just with a single mutation.

REFERENCES

Abecasis, G.R., Auton, A., Brooks, L.D., DePristo, M.A., Durbin, R.M., Handsaker, R.E., Kang, H.M., Marth, G.T., and McVean, G.A. (2012). An integrated map of genetic variation from 1,092 human genomes. Nature 491, 56–65.

Agarwala, V., Flannick, J., Sunyaev, S., and Altshuler, D. (2013). Evaluating empirical bounds on complex disease genetic architecture. Nat Genet 45, 1418–1427.

Allen, A.J., Griss, M.E., Folley, B.S., Hawkins, K.A., and Pearlson, G.D. (2009). Endophenotypes in schizophrenia: a selective review. Schizophr Res 109, 24–37.

Allen, A.S., Berkovic, S.F., Cossette, P., Delanty, N., Dlugos, D., Eichler, E.E., Epstein, M.P., Glauser, T., Goldstein, D.B., Han, Y., et al. (2013). De novo mutations in epileptic encephalopathies. Nature 501, 217–221.

Alliey-Rodriguez, N., Zhang, D., Badner, J.A., Lahey, B.B., Zhang, X., Dinwiddie, S., Romanos, B., Plenys, N., Liu, C., and Gershon, E.S. (2011). Genome-wide association study of personality traits in bipolar patients. Psychiatr Genet 21, 190–194.

Alves, M.M., Sribudiani, Y., Brouwer, R.W., Amiel, J., Antinolo, G., Borrego, S., Ceccherini, I., Chakravarti, A., Fernandez, R.M., Garcia-Barcelo, M.M., et al. (2013). Contribution of rare and common variants determine complex diseases-Hirschsprung disease as a model. Dev Biol 382, 320–329.

Amir, R.E., Van den Veyver, I.B., Wan, M., Tran, C.Q., Francke, U., and Zoghbi, H.Y. (1999). Rett syndrome is caused by mutations in X-linked MECP2, encoding methyl-CpG-binding protein 2. Nat Genet 23, 185–188.

Anney, R., Klei, L., Pinto, D., Regan, R., Conroy, J., Magalhaes, T.R., Correia, C., Abrahams, B.S., Sykes, N., Pagnamenta, A.T., et al. (2010). A genome-wide scan for common alleles affecting risk for autism. Hum Mol Genet 19, 4072–4082.

Arguello, P.A., and Gogos, J.A. (2012). Genetic and cognitive windows into circuit mechanisms of psychiatric disease. Trends Neurosci 35, 3–13.

Badano, J.L., and Katsanis, N. (2002). Beyond Mendel: an evolving view of human genetic disease transmission. Nat Rev Genet 3, 779–789.

Bassuk, A.G., Geraghty, E., Wu, S., Mullen, S.A., Berkovic, S.F., Scheffer, I.E., and Mefford, H.C. (2013). Deletions of 16p11.2 and 19p13.2 in a family with intellectual disability and generalized epilepsy. Am J Med Genet Part A 161A, 1722–1725.

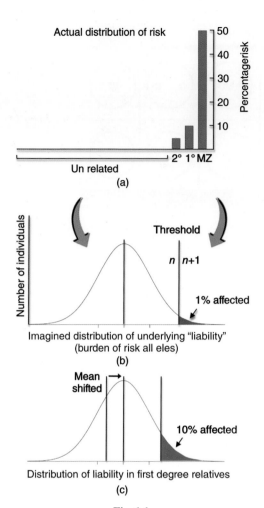

Actual distribution of risk

Percentage risk

50
40
30
20
10

2° 1° MZ

Un related

(a)

Number of individuals

Threshold

n | n+1

1% affected

Imagined distribution of underlying "liability"
(burden of risk all eles)

(b)

Mean shifted →

10% affected

Distribution of liability in first degree relatives

(c)

Fig. 1.1

The Genetics of Neurodevelopmental Disorders, First Edition. Edited by Kevin J. Mitchell.
© 2015 John Wiley & Sons, Inc. Published 2015 by John Wiley & Sons, Inc.

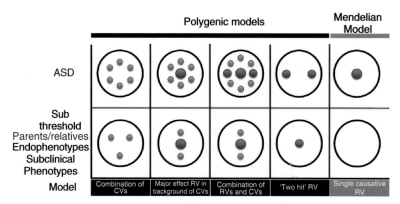

Fig. 1.2

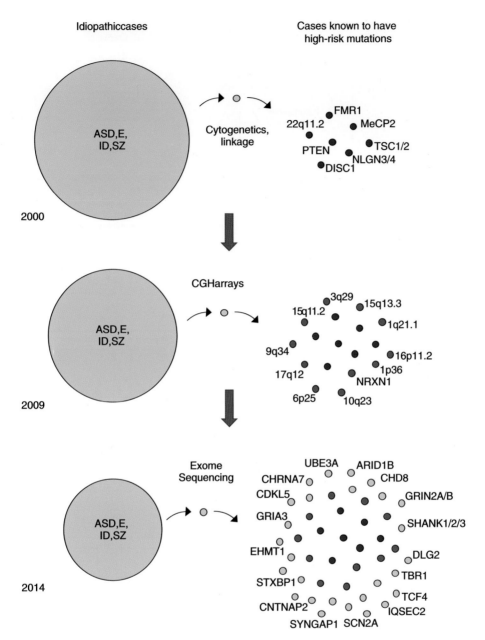

Fig. 1.3

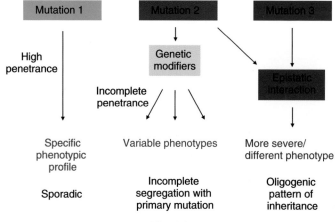

Fig. 1.4

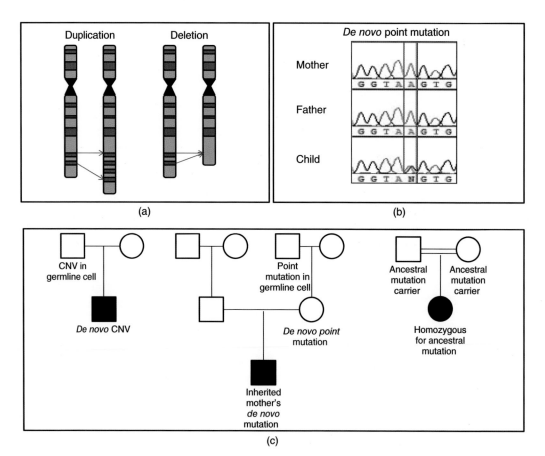

Fig. 3.1

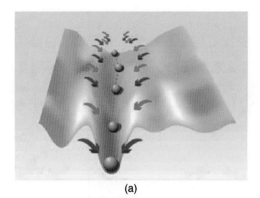

(a)

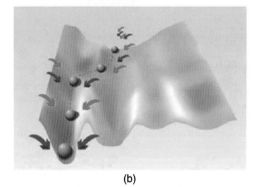

(b)

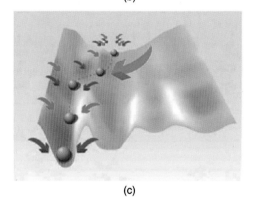

(c)

Fig. 5.1

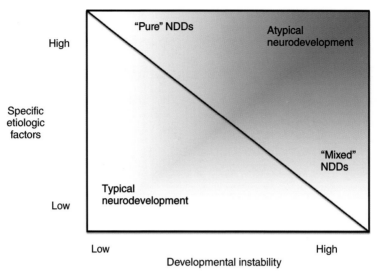

Fig. 5.3

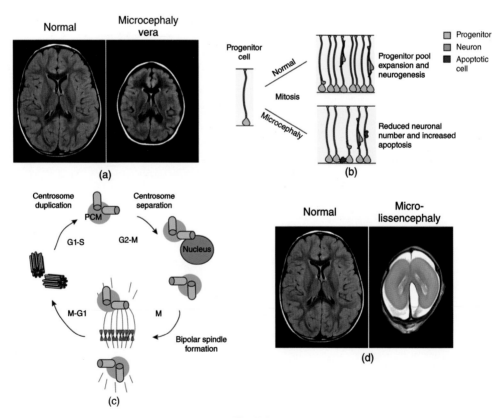

Fig. 7.1

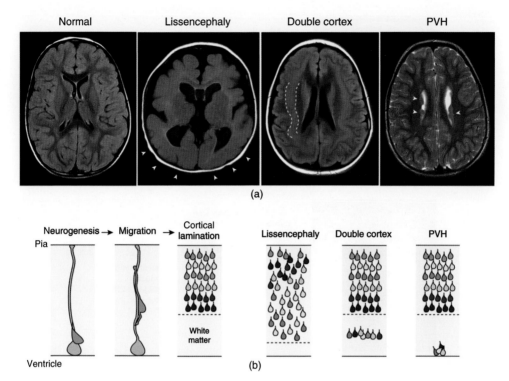

Fig. 7.2

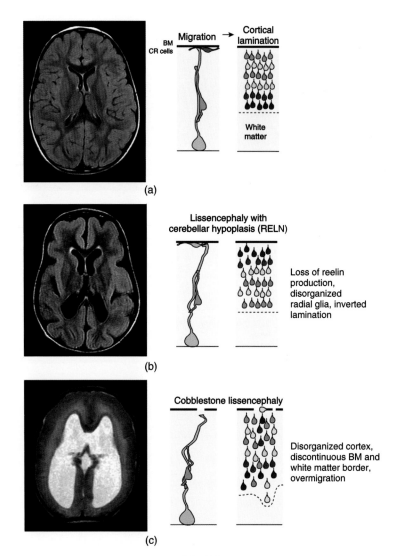

Fig. 7.3

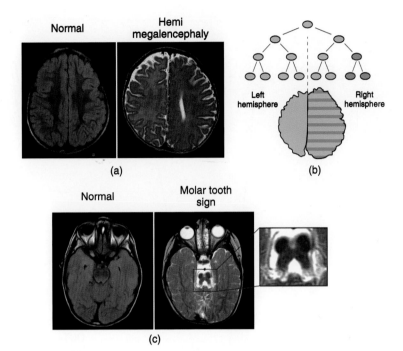

Fig. 7.4

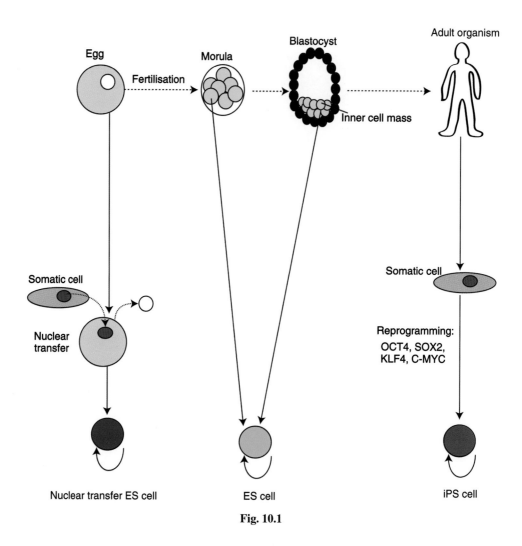

Fig. 10.1

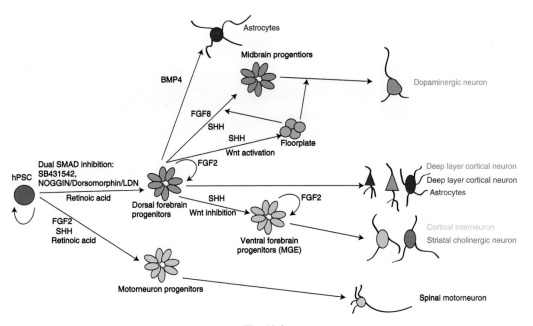

Fig. 10.2

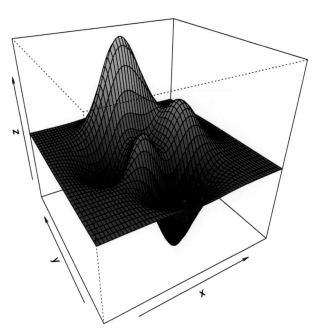

Fig. 13.1

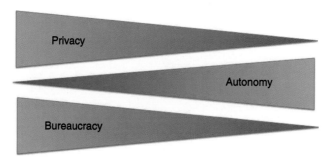

Fig. 13.2

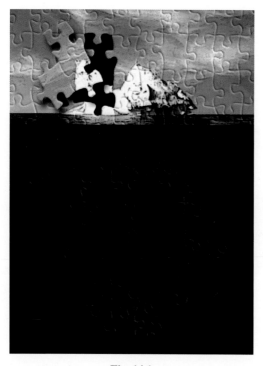

Fig. 14.1

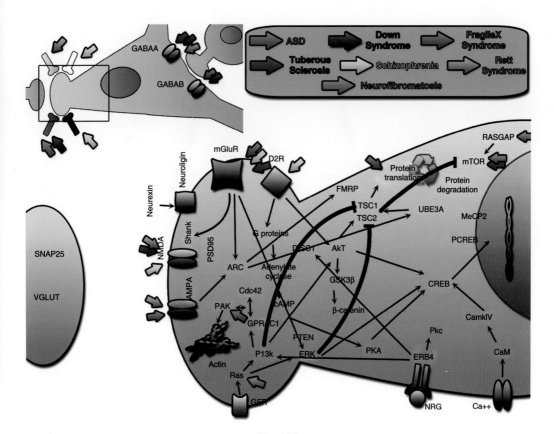

Fig. 14.2

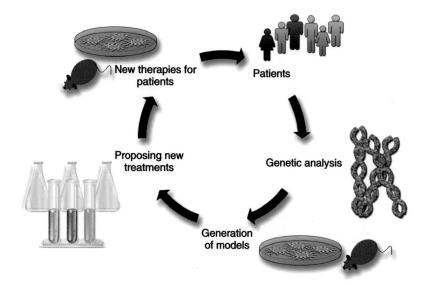

Fig. 14.3

Ben-Ari, Y. (2008). Neuro-archaeology: pre-symptomatic architecture and signature of neurological disorders. Trends Neurosci 31, 626–636.

Berg, J.M., and Geschwind, D.H. (2012). Autism genetics: searching for specificity and convergence. Genome Biol 13, 247.

Betancur, C. (2011). Etiological heterogeneity in autism spectrum disorders: more than 100 genetic and genomic disorders and still counting. Brain Res 1380, 42–77.

Bhat, S., Dao, D.T., Terrillion, C.E., Arad, M., Smith, R.J., Soldatov, N.M., and Gould, T.D. (2012). CACNA1C (Cav1.2) in the pathophysiology of psychiatric disease. Prog Neurobiol 99, 1–14.

Braff, D.L., Greenwood, T.A., Swerdlow, N.R., Light, G.A., and Schork, N.J. (2008). Advances in endophenotyping schizophrenia. World Psychiatry 7, 11–18.

Bramon, E., Pirinen, M., Strange, A., Lin, K., Freeman, C., Bellenguez, C., Su, Z., Band, G., Pearson, R., Vukcevic, D., et al. (2014). A genome-wide association analysis of a broad psychosis phenotype identifies three loci for further investigation. Biol Psychiatry 75, 386–397.

Browning, S.R., and Browning, B.L. (2011). Population structure can inflate SNP-based heritability estimates. Am J Hum Genet 89, 191-193; author reply 193–195.

Bruining, H., Eijkemans, M.J., Kas, M.J., Curran, S.R., Vorstman, J.A., and Bolton, P.F. (2014). Behavioral signatures related to genetic disorders in autism. Mol Autism 5, 11.

Cahill, L. (2006). Why sex matters for neuroscience. Nat Rev Neurosci 7, 477–484.

Carlson, C.S., Matise, T.C., North, K.E., Haiman, C.A., Fesinmeyer, M.D., Buyske, S., Schumacher, F.R., Peters, U., Franceschini, N., Ritchie, M.D., et al. (2013). Generalization and dilution of association results from European GWAS in populations of non-European ancestry: the PAGE study. PLoS biology 11, e1001661.

Chahrour, M.H., Yu, T.W., Lim, E.T., Ataman, B., Coulter, M.E., Hill, R.S., Stevens, C.R., Schubert, C.R., Greenberg, M.E., Gabriel, S.B., et al. (2012). Whole-exome sequencing and homozygosity analysis implicate depolarization-regulated neuronal genes in autism. PLoS Genet 8, e1002635.

Chang, D., and Keinan, A. (2012). Predicting signatures of "synthetic associations" and "natural associations" from empirical patterns of human genetic variation. PLoS Comput Biol 8, e1002600.

Chilian, B., Abdollahpour, H., Bierhals, T., Haltrich, I., Fekete, G., Nagel, I., Rosenberger, G., and Kutsche, K. (2013). Dysfunction of SHANK2 and CHRNA7 in a patient with intellectual disability and language impairment supports genetic epistasis of the two loci. Clin Genet 84, 560–565.

Clarke, P.G. (2012). The limits of brain determinacy. Proc Biol Sci/ R Soc 279, 1665–1674.

Coe, B.P., Girirajan, S., and Eichler, E.E. (2012). The genetic variability and commonality of neurodevelopmental disease. Am J Med Genet C Semin Med Genet 160C, 118–129.

Connolly, J.J., Glessner, J.T., and Hakonarson, H. (2013). A genome-wide association study of autism incorporating autism diagnostic interview-revised, autism diagnostic observation schedule, and social responsiveness scale. Child Dev 84, 17–33.

Consortium, C.-D.G.o.t.P.G. (2013). Identification of risk loci with shared effects on five major psychiatric disorders: a genome-wide analysis. Lancet 381, 1371–1379.

Consortium, I.H. (2003). The international HapMap project. Nature 426, 789–796.

Consortium, S.V. (2012). Simons Variation in Individuals Project (Simons VIP): a genetics-first approach to studying autism spectrum and related neurodevelopmental disorders. Neuron 73, 1063–1067.

Cook, E.H., Jr., and Scherer, S.W. (2008). Copy-number variations associated with neuropsychiatric conditions. Nature 455, 919–923.

Cooper, D.N., Krawczak, M., Polychronakos, C., Tyler-Smith, C., and Kehrer-Sawatzki, H. (2013). Where genotype is not predictive of phenotype: towards an understanding of the molecular basis of reduced penetrance in human inherited disease. Human Genet 132, 1077–1130.

Cooper, G.M., Coe, B.P., Girirajan, S., Rosenfeld, J.A., Vu, T.H., Baker, C., Williams, C., Stalker, H., Hamid, R., Hannig, V., et al. (2011). A copy number variation morbidity map of developmental delay. Nat Genet 43, 838–846.

Corey, L.A., Pellock, J.M., Kjeldsen, M.J., and Nakken, K.O. (2011). Importance of genetic factors in the occurrence of epilepsy syndrome type: a twin study. Epilepsy Res 97, 103–111.

Craddock, N., and Owen, M.J. (2010). The Krae-pelinian dichotomy - going, going … but still not gone. Br J Psychiatry 196, 92–95.

Cukier, H.N., Dueker, N.D., Slifer, S.H., Lee, J.M., Whitehead, P.L., Lalanne, E., Leyva, N., Konidari, I., Gentry, R.C., Hulme, W.F., et al. (2014). Exome sequencing of extended families with autism reveals genes shared across neurodevelopmental and neuropsychiatric disorders. Mol Autism 5, 1.

Dickson, S.P., Wang, K., Krantz, I., Hakonarson, H., and Goldstein, D.B. (2010). Rare variants create synthetic genome-wide associations. PLoS Biol 8, e1000294.

Dipple, K.M., and McCabe, E.R. (2000). Modifier genes convert "simple" Mendelian disorders to complex traits. Mol Genet Metab 71, 43–50.

Ellison, J.W., Rosenfeld, J.A., and Shaffer, L.G. (2013). Genetic basis of intellectual disability. Annu Rev Med 64, 441–450.

Escayg, A., MacDonald, B.T., Meisler, M.H., Baulac, S., Huberfeld, G., An-Gourfinkel, I., Brice, A., LeGuern, E., Moulard, B., Chaigne, D., et al. (2000). Mutations of SCN1A, encoding a neuronal sodium channel, in two families with GEFS+2. Nat Genet 24, 343–345.

Eyre-Walker, A. (2010). Evolution in health and medicine Sackler colloquium: Genetic architecture of a complex trait and its implications for fitness and genome-wide association studies. Proc Natl Acad Sci U S A 107 Suppl 1, 1752–1756.

Falconer, D.S. (1965). The inheritance of liability to certain diseases, estimated from the incidence among relatives. Ann Hum Genet Lond 29, 51–76.

Fanous, A.H., Zhou, B., Aggen, S.H., Bergen, S.E., Amdur, R.L., Duan, J., Sanders, A.R., Shi, J., Mowry, B.J., Olincy, A., et al. (2012). Genome-wide association study of clinical dimensions of schizophrenia: polygenic effect on disorganized symptoms. Am J Psychiatry 169, 1309–1317.

Flint, J., and Munafo, M.R. (2013). Candidate and non-candidate genes in behavior genetics. Curr Opin Neurobiol 23, 57–61.

Forrest, M.P., Hill, M.J., Quantock, A.J., Martin-Rendon, E., and Blake, D.J. (2014). The emerging roles of TCF4 in disease and development. Trends Mol Med.

Fromer, M., Pocklington, A.J., Kavanagh, D.H., Williams, H.J., Dwyer, S., Gormley, P., Georgieva, L., Rees, E., Palta, P., Ruderfer, D.M., et al.

(2014). De novo mutations in schizophrenia implicate synaptic networks. Nature 506, 179–184.

Gazave, E., Chang, D., Clark, A.G., and Keinan, A. (2013). Population growth inflates the per-individual number of deleterious mutations and reduces their mean effect. Genetics 195, 969–978.

Gibson, G., and Dworkin, I. (2004). Uncovering cryptic genetic variation. Nature reviews genetics 5, 681–690.

Gilmore, J.H., Lin, W., Prastawa, M.W., Looney, C.B., Vetsa, Y.S., Knickmeyer, R.C., Evans, D.D., Smith, J.K., Hamer, R.M., Lieberman, J.A., et al. (2007). Regional gray matter growth, sexual dimorphism, and cerebral asymmetry in the neonatal brain. J Neurosci: Off J Soc Neurosci 27, 1255–1260.

Girirajan, S., Rosenfeld, J.A., Coe, B.P., Parikh, S., Friedman, N., Goldstein, A., Filipink, R.A., McConnell, J.S., Angle, B., Meschino, W.S., et al. (2012). Phenotypic heterogeneity of genomic disorders and rare copy-number variants. N Engl J Med 367, 1321–1331.

Girirajan, S., Rosenfeld, J.A., Cooper, G.M., Antonacci, F., Siswara, P., Itsara, A., Vives, L., Walsh, T., McCarthy, S.E., Baker, C., et al. (2010). A recurrent 16p12.1 microdeletion supports a two-hit model for severe developmental delay. Nat Genet 42, 203–209.

Goodbourn, P.T., Bosten, J.M., Bargary, G., Hogg, R.E., Lawrance-Owen, A.J., and Mollon, J.D. (2014). Variants in the 1q21 risk region are associated with a visual endophenotype of autism and schizophrenia. Genes brain behav 13, 144–151.

Gottesman, I.I., and Gould, T.D. (2003). The endophenotype concept in psychiatry: etymology and strategic intentions. Am J Psychiatry 160, 636–645.

Gravel, S., Henn, B.M., Gutenkunst, R.N., Indap, A.R., Marth, G.T., Clark, A.G., Yu, F., Gibbs, R.A., and Bustamante, C.D. (2011). Demographic history and rare allele sharing among human populations. Proc Natl Acad Sci U S A 108, 11983–11988.

Grayton, H.M., Fernandes, C., Rujescu, D., and Collier, D.A. (2012). Copy number variations in neurodevelopmental disorders. Prog Neurobiol 99, 81–91.

Grillo, E., Lo Rizzo, C., Bianciardi, L., Bizzarri, V., Baldassarri, M., Spiga, O., Furini, S., De Felice, C.,

Signorini, C., Leoncini, S., et al. (2013). Revealing the complexity of a monogenic disease: rett syndrome exome sequencing. PLoS One 8, e56599.

Hamlyn, J., Duhig, M., McGrath, J., and Scott, J. (2013). Modifiable risk factors for schizophrenia and autism–shared risk factors impacting on brain development. Neurobiol Dis 53, 3–9.

Hardy, J., and Singleton, A. (2009). Genomewide association studies and human disease. N Engl J Med 360, 1759–1768.

Harris, J.R. (1998). The Nurture Assumption: Why Children Turn Out the Way They Do. New York: Free Press.

Hulme, S.R., Jones, O.D., and Abraham, W.C. (2013). Emerging roles of metaplasticity in behaviour and disease. Trends Neurosci 36, 353–362.

Hunt, K.A., Mistry, V., Bockett, N.A., Ahmad, T., Ban, M., Barker, J.N., Barrett, J.C., Blackburn, H., Brand, O., Burren, O., et al. (2013). Negligible impact of rare autoimmune-locus coding-region variants on missing heritability. Nature 498, 232–235.

Ingalhalikar, M., Smith, A., Parker, D., Satterthwaite, T.D., Elliott, M.A., Ruparel, K., Hakonarson, H., Gur, R.E., Gur, R.C., and Verma, R. (2014). Sex differences in the structural connectome of the human brain. Proc Natl Acad Sci U S A 111, 823–828.

Ioannidis, J.P., Tarone, R., and McLaughlin, J.K. (2011). The false-positive to false-negative ratio in epidemiologic studies. Epidemiology 22, 450–456.

Iossifov, I., Ronemus, M., Levy, D., Wang, Z., Hakker, I., Rosenbaum, J., Yamrom, B., Lee, Y.H., Narzisi, G., Leotta, A., et al. (2012). De novo gene disruptions in children on the autistic spectrum. Neuron 74, 285–299.

Jacquemont, S., Coe, B.P., Hersch, M., Duyzend, M.H., Krumm, N., Bergmann, S., Beckmann, J.S., Rosenfeld, J.A., and Eichler, E.E. (2014). A higher mutational burden in females supports a "female protective model" in neurodevelopmental disorders. Am J Hum Genet 94, 415–425.

Jamain, S., Quach, H., Betancur, C., Rastam, M., Colineaux, C., Gillberg, I.C., Soderstrom, H., Giros, B., Leboyer, M., Gillberg, C., et al. (2003). Mutations of the X-linked genes encoding neuroligins NLGN3 and NLGN4 are associated with autism. Nat Genet 34, 27–29.

Kasperaviciute, D., Catarino, C.B., Heinzen, E.L., Depondt, C., Cavalleri, G.L., Caboclo, L.O., Tate, S.K., Jamnadas-Khoda, J., Chinthapalli, K., Clayton, L.M., et al. (2010). Common genetic variation and susceptibility to partial epilepsies: a genome-wide association study. Brain.

Kayser, M.A. (2008). Inherited metabolic diseases in neurodevelopmental and neurobehavioral disorders. Semin Pediatr Neurol 15, 127–131.

Keinan, A., and Clark, A.G. (2012). Recent explosive human population growth has resulted in an excess of rare genetic variants. Science 336, 740–743.

Keller, M.C., and Miller, G. (2006). Resolving the paradox of common, harmful, heritable mental disorders: which evolutionary genetic models work best? Behav Brain Sci 29, 385–404; discussion 405–352.

Kenny, E.M., Cormican, P., Furlong, S., Heron, E., Kenny, G., Fahey, C., Kelleher, E., Ennis, S., Tropea, D., Anney, R., et al. (2013). Excess of rare novel loss-of-function variants in synaptic genes in schizophrenia and autism spectrum disorders. Mol Psychiatry.

Kirov, G., Grozeva, D., Norton, N., Ivanov, D., Mantripragada, K.K., Holmans, P., Craddock, N., Owen, M.J., and O'Donovan, M.C. (2009). Support for the involvement of large copy number variants in the pathogenesis of schizophrenia. Hum Mol Genet 18, 1497–1503.

Kirov, G., Rees, E., Walters, J.T., Escott-Price, V., Georgieva, L., Richards, A.L., Chambert, K.D., Davies, G., Legge, S.E., Moran, J.L., et al. (2014). The penetrance of copy number variations for schizophrenia and developmental delay. Biol Psychiatry 75, 378–385.

Klei, L., Sanders, S.J., Murtha, M.T., Hus, V., Lowe, J.K., Willsey, A.J., Moreno-De-Luca, D., Yu, T.W., Fombonne, E., Geschwind, D., et al. (2012). Common genetic variants, acting additively, are a major source of risk for autism. Mol Autism 3, 9.

Knowles, E.E., Carless, M.A., de Almeida, M.A., Curran, J.E., McKay, D.R., Sprooten, E., Dyer, T.D., Goring, H.H., Olvera, R., Fox, P., et al. (2014). Genome-wide significant localization for working and spatial memory: Identifying genes for psychosis using models of cognition. Am J Med Genet Part B, Neuropsychiatric Genet: Off Publ Int Soc Psychiatr Genet 165, 84–95.

Kryukov, G.V., Pennacchio, L.A., and Sunyaev, S.R. (2007). Most rare missense alleles are deleterious in humans: implications for complex disease and association studies. Am J Hum Genet 80, 727–739.

Ku, C.S., Polychronakos, C., Tan, E.K., Naidoo, N., Pawitan, Y., Roukos, D.H., Mort, M., and Cooper, D.N. (2012). A new paradigm emerges from the study of de novo mutations in the context of neurodevelopmental disease. Mol Psychiatry.

Leamy, L.J., and Klingenberg, C.P. (2005). The genetics and evolution of fluctuating asymmetry. Annu Rev Ecol Evol Syst 36, 1–21.

Leblond, C.S., Heinrich, J., Delorme, R., Proepper, C., Betancur, C., Huguet, G., Konyukh, M., Chaste, P., Ey, E., Rastam, M., et al. (2012). Genetic and functional analyses of SHANK2 mutations suggest a multiple hit model of autism spectrum disorders. PLoS Genet 8, e1002521.

Lee, S.H., DeCandia, T.R., Ripke, S., Yang, J., Sullivan, P.F., Goddard, M.E., Keller, M.C., Visscher, P.M., and Wray, N.R. (2012). Estimating the proportion of variation in susceptibility to schizophrenia captured by common SNPs. Nat Genet 44, 247–250.

Lee, S.H., Wray, N.R., Goddard, M.E., and Visscher, P.M. (2011). Estimating missing heritability for disease from genome-wide association studies. Am J Hum Genet 88, 294–305.

Lenz, D.R., and Avraham, K.B. (2011). Hereditary hearing loss: from human mutation to mechanism. Hear Res 281, 3–10.

Levy, D., Ronemus, M., Yamrom, B., Lee, Y.H., Leotta, A., Kendall, J., Marks, S., Lakshmi, B., Pai, D., Ye, K., et al. (2011). Rare de novo and transmitted copy-number variation in autistic spectrum disorders. Neuron 70, 886–897.

Lichtenstein, P., Bjork, C., Hultman, C.M., Scolnick, E., Sklar, P., and Sullivan, P.F. (2006). Recurrence risks for schizophrenia in a Swedish national cohort. Psychol Med 36, 1417–1425.

Lim, E.T., Raychaudhuri, S., Sanders, S.J., Stevens, C., Sabo, A., MacArthur, D.G., Neale, B.M., Kirby, A., Ruderfer, D.M., Fromer, M., et al. (2013). Rare complete knockouts in humans: population distribution and significant role in autism spectrum disorders. Neuron 77, 235–242.

Lisman, J.E., Coyle, J.T., Green, R.W., Javitt, D.C., Benes, F.M., Heckers, S., and Grace, A.A. (2008). Circuit-based framework for understanding neurotransmitter and risk gene interactions in schizophrenia. Trends Neurosci 31, 234–242.

Liu, P., Carvalho, C.M., Hastings, P.J., and Lupski, J.R. (2012). Mechanisms for recurrent and complex human genomic rearrangements. Curr Opin Genet Dev 22, 211–220.

Lodge, D.J., and Grace, A.A. (2011). Hippocampal dysregulation of dopamine system function and the pathophysiology of schizophrenia. Trends Pharmacol Sci 32, 507–513.

Lundstrom, S., Chang, Z., Rastam, M., Gillberg, C., Larsson, H., Anckarsater, H., and Lichtenstein, P. (2012). Autism spectrum disorders and autistic like traits: similar etiology in the extreme end and the normal variation. Arch Gen Psychiatry 69, 46–52.

Luo, Y., Ceccherini, I., Pasini, B., Matera, I., Bicocchi, M.P., Barone, V., Bocciardi, R., Kaariainen, H., Weber, D., Devoto, M., et al. (1993). Close linkage with the RET protooncogene and boundaries of deletion mutations in autosomal dominant Hirschsprung disease. Hum Mol Genet 2, 1803–1808.

Lupski, J.R., Belmont, J.W., Boerwinkle, E., and Gibbs, R.A. (2011). Clan genomics and the complex architecture of human disease. Cell 147, 32–43.

MacArthur, D.G., Balasubramanian, S., Frankish, A., Huang, N., Morris, J., Walter, K., Jostins, L., Habegger, L., Pickrell, J.K., Montgomery, S.B., et al. (2012). A systematic survey of loss-of-function variants in human protein-coding genes. Science 335, 823–828.

Mackay, T.F. (2009). The genetic architecture of complex behaviors: lessons from Drosophila. Genetica 136, 295–302.

Marigorta, U.M., and Navarro, A. (2013). High trans-ethnic replicability of GWAS results implies common causal variants. PLoS Genet 9, e1003566.

Marshall, C.R., Noor, A., Vincent, J.B., Lionel, A.C., Feuk, L., Skaug, J., Shago, M., Moessner, R., Pinto, D., Ren, Y., et al. (2008). Structural variation of chromosomes in autism spectrum disorder. Am J Hum Genet 82, 477–488.

Mayo, O. (2007). The rise and fall of the common disease-common variant (CD-CV) hypothesis: how the sickle cell disease paradigm led us all astray (or did it?). Twin Res Hum Genet : Off J Int Soc Twin Stud 10, 793–804.

McCarthy, M.M., Arnold, A.P., Ball, G.F., Blaustein, J.D., and De Vries, G.J. (2012). Sex differences in the brain: the not so inconvenient truth. J Neurosci: Off J Soc Neurosci 32, 2241–2247.

McClellan, J., and King, M.C. (2010). Genetic heterogeneity in human disease. Cell 141, 210–217.

McClellan, J.M., Susser, E., and King, M.C. (2007). Schizophrenia: a common disease caused by multiple rare alleles. Br J Psychiatry 190, 194–199.

McGue, M., Gottesman, II, and Rao, D.C. (1983). The transmission of schizophrenia under a multifactorial threshold model. Am J Hum Genet 35, 1161–1178.

Mefford, H.C., Muhle, H., Ostertag, P., von Spiczak, S., Buysse, K., Baker, C., Franke, A., Malafosse, A., Genton, P., Thomas, P., et al. (2010). Genome-wide copy number variation in epilepsy: novel susceptibility loci in idiopathic generalized and focal epilepsies. PLoS Genet 6, e1000962.

Merikangas, A.K., Corvin, A.P., and Gallagher, L. (2009). Copy-number variants in neurodevelopmental disorders: promises and challenges. Trends Genet: TIG 25, 536–544.

Meyer-Lindenberg, A., and Weinberger, D.R. (2006). Intermediate phenotypes and genetic mechanisms of psychiatric disorders. Nat Rev Neurosci 7, 818–827.

Miles, J.H. (2011). Autism spectrum disorders--a genetics review. Genet Med: Off J Am Coll Med Genet 13, 278–294.

Millar, J.K., Wilson-Annan, J.C., Anderson, S., Christie, S., Taylor, M.S., Semple, C.A., Devon, R.S., Clair, D.M., Muir, W.J., Blackwood, D.H., et al. (2000). Disruption of two novel genes by a translocation co-segregating with schizophrenia. Hum Mol Genet 9, 1415–1423.

Mitchell, K.J. (2007). The genetics of brain wiring: from molecule to mind. PLoS Biol 5, e113.

Mitchell, K.J. (2011). The genetics of neurodevelopmental disease. Curr Opin Neurobiol 21, 197–203.

Mitchell, K.J. (2012). What is complex about complex disorders? Genome Biol 13, 237.

Mitchell, K.J., Huang, Z.J., Moghaddam, B., and Sawa, A. (2011). Following the genes: a framework for animal modeling of psychiatric disorders. BMC Biol 9, 76.

Mitchell, K.J., and Porteous, D.J. (2011). Rethinking the genetic architecture of schizophrenia. Psychol Med 41, 19–32.

Moreno-De-Luca, A., Myers, S.M., Challman, T.D., Moreno-De-Luca, D., Evans, D.W., and Ledbetter, D.H. (2013). Developmental brain dysfunction: revival and expansion of old concepts based on new genetic evidence. Lancet Neurol 12, 406–414.

Nadeau, J.H. (2001). Modifier genes in mice and humans. Nat Rev Genet 2, 165–174.

Neale, B.M., Kou, Y., Liu, L., Ma'ayan, A., Samocha, K.E., Sabo, A., Lin, C.F., Stevens, C., Wang, L.S., Makarov, V., et al. (2012). Patterns and rates of exonic de novo mutations in autism spectrum disorders. Nature 485, 242–245.

Need, A.C., Ge, D., Weale, M.E., Maia, J., Feng, S., Heinzen, E.L., Shianna, K.V., Yoon, W., Kasperaviciute, D., Gennarelli, M., et al. (2009). A genome-wide investigation of SNPs and CNVs in schizophrenia. PLoS Genet 5, e1000373.

Noreau, A., Bourassa, C.V., Szuto, A., Levert, A., Dobrzeniecka, S., Gauthier, J., Forlani, S., Durr, A., Anheim, M., Stevanin, G., et al. (2013). SYNE1 mutations in autosomal recessive cerebellar ataxia. JAMA Neurol 70, 1296–1231.

Ntzani, E.E., Liberopoulos, G., Manolio, T.A., and Ioannidis, J.P. (2012). Consistency of genome-wide associations across major ancestral groups. Hum Genet 131, 1057–1071.

O'Roak, B.J., Deriziotis, P., Lee, C., Vives, L., Schwartz, J.J., Girirajan, S., Karakoc, E., Mackenzie, A.P., Ng, S.B., Baker, C., et al. (2011). Exome sequencing in sporadic autism spectrum disorders identifies severe de novo mutations. Nat Genet 43, 585–589.

O'Roak, B.J., Vives, L., Girirajan, S., Karakoc, E., Krumm, N., Coe, B.P., Levy, R., Ko, A., Lee, C., Smith, J.D., et al. (2012). Sporadic autism exomes reveal a highly interconnected protein network of de novo mutations. Nature 485, 246–250.

O'Rourke, D.H., Gottesman, II, Suarez, B.K., Rice, J., and Reich, T. (1982). Refutation of the general single-locus model for the etiology of schizophrenia. Am J Hum Genet 34, 630–649.

Olson, M.V. (2012). Human genetic individuality. Annu Rev Genomics Hum Genet 13, 1–27.

Oosterveer, D.M., Versmissen, J., Defesche, J.C., Sivapalaratnam, S., Yazdanpanah, M., Mulder, M., van der Zee, L., Uitterlinden, A.G., van Duijn, C.M., Hofman, A., et al. (2013). Low-density lipoprotein receptor mutations generate synthetic genome-wide associations. Eur J Hum Genet: EJHG 21, 563–566.

Phillips, P.C. (2008). Epistasis--the essential role of gene interactions in the structure and evolution of genetic systems. Nat Rev Genet 9, 855–867.

Piton, A., Gauthier, J., Hamdan, F.F., Lafreniere, R.G., Yang, Y., Henrion, E., Laurent, S., Noreau, A., Thibodeau, P., Karemera, L., et al. (2010). Systematic resequencing of X-chromosome synaptic genes in autism spectrum disorder and schizophrenia. Mol Psychiatry.

Plomin, R., and Daniels, D. (2011). Why are children in the same family so different from one another? Int J Epidemiol 40, 563–582.

Plomin, R., Haworth, C.M., and Davis, O.S. (2009). Common disorders are quantitative traits. Nat Rev Genet 10, 872–878.

Poduri, A., and Lowenstein, D. (2011). Epilepsy genetics--past, present, and future. Curr Opin Genet Dev 21, 325–332.

Purcell, S.M., Moran, J.L., Fromer, M., Ruderfer, D., Solovieff, N., Roussos, P., O'Dushlaine, C., Chambert, K., Bergen, S.E., Kahler, A., et al. (2014). A polygenic burden of rare disruptive mutations in schizophrenia. Nature 506, 185–190.

Purcell, S.M., Wray, N.R., Stone, J.L., Visscher, P.M., O'Donovan, M.C., Sullivan, P.F., and Sklar, P. (2009). Common polygenic variation contributes to risk of schizophrenia and bipolar disorder. Nature 460, 748–752.

Ralph, P., and Coop, G. (2013). The geography of recent genetic ancestry across Europe. PLoS biology 11, e1001555.

Reich, D.E., and Lander, E.S. (2001). On the allelic spectrum of human disease. Trends Genet 17, 502–510.

Renieri, A., Meloni, I., Longo, I., Ariani, F., Mari, F., Pescucci, C., and Cambi, F. (2003). Rett syndrome: the complex nature of a monogenic disease. J Mol Med (Berl) 81, 346–354.

Ripke, S., O'Dushlaine, C., Chambert, K., Moran, J.L., Kahler, A.K., Akterin, S., Bergen, S.E., Collins, A.L., Crowley, J.J., Fromer, M., et al. (2013). Genome-wide association analysis identifies 13 new risk loci for schizophrenia. Nat Genet 45, 1150–1159.

Risch, N. (1990). Genetic linkage and complex diseases, with special reference to psychiatric disorders. Genet Epidemiol 7, 3–16; discussion 17–45.

Risch, N., and Merikangas, K. (1996). The future of genetic studies of complex human diseases. Science 273, 1516–1517.

Roberts, J.A. (1952). The genetics of mental deficiency. Eugen Rev 44, 71–83.

Robinson, E.B., Koenen, K.C., McCormick, M.C., Munir, K., Hallett, V., Happe, F., Plomin, R., and Ronald, A. (2011). Evidence that autistic traits show the same etiology in the general population and at the quantitative extremes (5%, 2.5%, and 1%). Arch Gen Psychiatry 68, 1113–1121.

Robinson, M.R., Wray, N.R., and Visscher, P.M. (2014). Explaining additional genetic variation in complex traits. Trends Genet: TIG 30, 124–132.

Rodriguez-Murillo, L., Gogos, J.A., and Karayiorgou, M. (2012). The genetic architecture of schizophrenia: new mutations and emerging paradigms. Annu Rev Med 63, 63–80.

Ronemus, M., Iossifov, I., Levy, D., and Wigler, M. (2014). The role of de novo mutations in the genetics of autism spectrum disorders. Nat Rev Genet 15, 133–141.

Ropers, H.H. (2008). Genetics of intellectual disability. Curr Opin Genet Dev 18, 241–250.

Ruge, J.R., and Newland, T.S. (1996). Agenesis of the corpus callosum: female monozygotic triplets. Case Report. J Neurosurg 85, 152–156.

Sanders, S.J., Murtha, M.T., Gupta, A.R., Murdoch, J.D., Raubeson, M.J., Willsey, A.J., Ercan-Sencicek, A.G., DiLullo, N.M., Parikshak, N.N., Stein, J.L., et al. (2012). De novo mutations revealed by whole-exome sequencing are strongly associated with autism. Nature 485, 237–241.

Sandin, S., Lichtenstein, P., Kuja-Halkola, R., Larsson, H., Hultman, C.M., and Reichenberg, A. (2014). The familial risk of autism. JAMA 311, 1770–1777.

Sanna, S., Li, B., Mulas, A., Sidore, C., Kang, H.M., Jackson, A.U., Piras, M.G., Usala, G., Maninchedda, G., Sassu, A., et al. (2011). Fine mapping of five loci associated with low-density lipoprotein cholesterol detects variants that double the explained heritability. PLoS genetics 7, e1002198.

Sasson, N.J., Lam, K.S., Parlier, M., Daniels, J.L., and Piven, J. (2013). Autism and the broad autism phenotype: familial patterns and intergenerational transmission. J Neurodev Disord 5, 11.

Saunders, E.J., Dadaev, T., Leongamornlert, D.A., Jugurnauth-Little, S., Tymrakiewicz, M., Wiklund, F., Al Olama, A.A., Benlloch, S., Neal, D.E., Hamdy, F.C., et al. (2014). Fine-mapping the HOXB region detects common variants tagging a rare coding allele: evidence for synthetic association in prostate cancer. PLoS Genet 10, e1004129.

Schaaf, C.P., Sabo, A., Sakai, Y., Crosby, J., Muzny, D., Hawes, A., Lewis, L., Akbar, H., Varghese, R., Boerwinkle, E., et al. (2011). Oligogenic heterozygosity in individuals with high-functioning autism spectrum disorders. Hum Mol Genet 20, 3366–3375.

Sebat, J., Lakshmi, B., Malhotra, D., Troge, J., Lese-Martin, C., Walsh, T., Yamrom, B., Yoon, S., Krasnitz, A., Kendall, J., et al. (2007). Strong association of de novo copy number mutations with autism. Science 316, 445–449.

Sebat, J., Lakshmi, B., Troge, J., Alexander, J., Young, J., Lundin, P., Maner, S., Massa, H., Walker, M., Chi, M., et al. (2004). Large-scale copy number polymorphism in the human genome. Science 305, 525–528.

Sedel, F. (2012). Inborn errors of metabolism in adults: a diagnostic approach to neurological and psychiatric presentations. In: Fernandes J, Saudubray JM, van den Berghe G, Walter JH, eds. Inborn Metabolic Diseases: Diagnosis and Treatment, 5th edn. Berlin: Springer, pp. 56–74.

Shaw, N.D., Seminara, S.B., Welt, C.K., Au, M.G., Plummer, L., Hughes, V.A., Dwyer, A.A., Martin, K.A., Quinton, R., Mericq, V., et al. (2011). Expanding the phenotype and genotype of female GnRH deficiency. J Clin Endocrinol Metab 96, E566–E576.

Shi, J., Levinson, D.F., Duan, J., Sanders, A.R., Zheng, Y., Pe'er, I., Dudbridge, F., Holmans, P.A., Whittemore, A.S., Mowry, B.J., et al. (2009). Common variants on chromosome 6p22.1 are associated with schizophrenia. Nature 460, 753–757.

Simons, Y.B., Turchin, M.C., Pritchard, J.K., and Sella, G. (2014). The deleterious mutation load is insensitive to recent population history. Nat Genet 46, 220–224.

Singh, N.A., Pappas, C., Dahle, E.J., Claes, L.R., Pruess, T.H., De Jonghe, P., Thompson, J., Dixon, M., Gurnett, C., Peiffer, A., et al. (2009). A role of SCN9A in human epilepsies, as a cause of febrile seizures and as a potential modifier of Dravet syndrome. PLoS Genet 5, e1000649.

Spiezio, S.H., Takada, T., Shiroishi, T., and Nadeau, J.H. (2012). Genetic divergence and the genetic architecture of complex traits in chromosome substitution strains of mice. BMC Genet 13, 38.

Stefansson, H., Meyer-Lindenberg, A., Steinberg, S., Magnusdottir, B., Morgen, K., Arnarsdottir, S., Bjornsdottir, G., Walters, G.B., Jonsdottir, G.A., Doyle, O.M., et al. (2014). CNVs conferring risk of autism or schizophrenia affect cognition in controls. Nature 505, 361–366.

Stefansson, H., Ophoff, R.A., Steinberg, S., Andreassen, O.A., Cichon, S., Rujescu, D., Werge, T., Pietilainen, O.P., Mors, O., Mortensen, P.B., et al. (2009). Common variants conferring risk of schizophrenia. Nature 460, 744–747.

Stessman, H.A., Bernier, R., and Eichler, E.E. (2014). A genotype-first approach to defining the subtypes of a complex disease. Cell 156, 872–877.

Sullivan, P.F., Daly, M.J., and O'Donovan, M. (2012). Genetic architectures of psychiatric disorders: the emerging picture and its implications. Nat Rev Genet 13, 537–551.

Sullivan, P.F., Kendler, K.S., and Neale, M.C. (2003). Schizophrenia as a complex trait: evidence from a meta-analysis of twin studies. Arch Gen Psychiatry 60, 1187–1192.

Szatmari, P. (1999). Heterogeneity and the genetics of autism. J Psychiatry Neurosci: JPN 24, 159–165.

Thornton, K.R., Foran, A.J., and Long, A.D. (2013). Properties and modeling of GWAS when complex disease risk is due to non-complementing, deleterious mutations in genes of large effect. PLoS Genet 9, e1003258.

Thun, G.A., Imboden, M., Ferrarotti, I., Kumar, A., Obeidat, M., Zorzetto, M., Haun, M., Curjuric, I., Couto Alves, A., Jackson, V.E., et al. (2013). Causal and synthetic associations of variants in the SERPINA gene cluster with alpha1-antitrypsin serum levels. PLoS Genet 9, e1003585.

Turkheimer, E., and Waldron, M. (2000). Nonshared environment: a theoretical, methodological, and quantitative review. Psychol Bull 126, 78–108.

Vassos, E., Collier, D.A., Holden, S., Patch, C., Rujescu, D., St Clair, D., and Lewis, C.M. (2010). Penetrance for copy number variants associated with schizophrenia. Hum Mol Genet 19, 3477–3481.

Vissers, L.E., de Ligt, J., Gilissen, C., Janssen, I., Steehouwer, M., de Vries, P., van Lier, B., Arts, P., Wieskamp, N., del Rosario, M., et al. (2010). A de novo paradigm for mental retardation. Nat Genet 42, 1109–1112.

Waddington, C.H. (1957). The Strategy of the Genes. George Allen & Unwin Ltd.

Wagner, A. (2007). Robustness and Evolvability in Living Systems. Princeton University Press.

Wahlsten, D. (1989). Deficiency of the corpus callosum: incomplete penetrance and substrain differentiation in BALB/c mice. J Neurogenet 5, 61–76.

Walsh, C.A., and Engle, E.C. (2010). Allelic diversity in human developmental neurogenetics: insights into biology and disease. Neuron 68, 245–253.

Walsh, T., McClellan, J.M., McCarthy, S.E., Addington, A.M., Pierce, S.B., Cooper, G.M., Nord, A.S., Kusenda, M., Malhotra, D., Bhandari, A., et al. (2008). Rare structural variants disrupt multiple genes in neurodevelopmental pathways in schizophrenia. Science 320, 539–543.

Wan, M., Lee, S.S., Zhang, X., Houwink-Manville, I., Song, H.R., Amir, R.E., Budden, S., Naidu, S., Pereira, J.L., Lo, I.F., et al. (1999). Rett syndrome and beyond: recurrent spontaneous and familial MECP2 mutations at CpG hotspots. Am J Hum Genet 65, 1520–1529.

Wang, K., Dickson, S.P., Stolle, C.A., Krantz, I.D., Goldstein, D.B., and Hakonarson, H. (2010). Interpretation of association signals and identification of causal variants from genome-wide association studies. Am J Hum Genet 86, 730–742.

Wray, N.R., Purcell, S.M., and Visscher, P.M. (2011). Synthetic associations created by rare variants do not explain most GWAS results. PLoS Biol 9, e1000579.

Wray, N.R., and Visscher, P.M. (2010). Narrowing the boundaries of the genetic architecture of schizophrenia. Schizophr Bull 36, 14–23.

Wright, A.F., Chakarova, C.F., Abd El-Aziz, M.M., and Bhattacharya, S.S. (2010). Photoreceptor degeneration: genetic and mechanistic dissection of a complex trait. Nat Rev Genet 11, 273–284.

Wright, A.F., and Hastie, N.D. (2001). Complex genetic diseases: controversy over the Croesus code. Genome Biol 2, COMMENT2007.

Wright, J. (2014). Genetics: unravelling complexity. Nature 508, S6–S7.

Wu, M.V., and Shah, N.M. (2011). Control of masculinization of the brain and behavior. Curr Opin Neurobiol 21, 116–123.

Xu, B., Roos, J.L., Dexheimer, P., Boone, B., Plummer, B., Levy, S., Gogos, J.A., and Karayiorgou, M. (2011). Exome sequencing supports a de novo mutational paradigm for schizophrenia. Nat Genet 43, 864–868.

Yang, J., Benyamin, B., McEvoy, B.P., Gordon, S., Henders, A.K., Nyholt, D.R., Madden, P.A., Heath, A.C., Martin, N.G., Montgomery, G.W., et al. (2010). Common SNPs explain a large proportion of the heritability for human height. Nat Genet 42, 565–569.

Yang, J., Manolio, T.A., Pasquale, L.R., Boerwinkle, E., Caporaso, N., Cunningham, J.M., de Andrade, M., Feenstra, B., Feingold, E., Hayes, M.G., et al. (2011). Genome partitioning of genetic variation for complex traits using common SNPs. Nat Genet 43, 519–525.

Yeo, R.A., Gangestad, S., and Thoma, R. (2007). Developmental instability and individual variation in brain development - implications for the origin of neurodevelopmental disorders. Curr Dir Psychol Sci 16, 245–249.

Yu, T.W., Chahrour, M.H., Coulter, M.E., Jiralerspong, S., Okamura-Ikeda, K., Ataman, B., Schmitz-Abe, K., Harmin, D.A., Adli, M., Malik, A.N., et al. (2013). Using whole-exome sequencing to identify inherited causes of autism. Neuron 77, 259–273.

Zuk, O., Schaffner, S.F., Samocha, K., Do, R., Hechter, E., Kathiresan, S., Daly, M.J., Neale, B.M., Sunyaev, S.R., and Lander, E.S. (2014). Searching for missing heritability: designing rare variant association studies. Proc Natl Acad Sci U S A 111, E455–464.

2

OVERLAPPING ETIOLOGY OF NEURODEVELOPMENTAL DISORDERS

ERIC KELLEHER AND AIDEN CORVIN

Neuropsychiatric Genetics Research Group, Department of Psychiatry, Trinity Centre for Health Sciences, St James' Hospital, Dublin, Ireland

2.1 INTRODUCTION

Neurodevelopmental disorders (NDDs) are relatively common but represent a wide range of different etiologies. Temporally, NDDs include events from early neural tube defects in the first trimester, to subtle anomalies of executive cognitive processing emerging in early adulthood as synaptic maturation is completed. The phenotypic effects vary from the profound (e.g., severe intellectual disability, severe physical disability) to the relatively subtle (e.g., dyslexia, dyspraxia) impacting a broad range of functions including motor function, learning, memory and perception; but also emotional regulation, social interaction, and communication. Investigation of NDD etiology has benefited enormously from what can be learned from studying model systems (from yeasts to mice), but also brings into stark relief the challenge of understanding what makes us uniquely human.

For some individuals, environmental causes are readily identifiable such as toxins (e.g., fetal alcohol syndrome); maternal nutritional deficiency (e.g., neural tube defects with folic acid deficiency); infection *in utero* or in early childhood (e.g., toxoplasmosis); brain trauma (e.g., cerebral palsy); metabolic disorders (e.g., maternal diabetes); and sensory or emotional deprivation (e.g., disorders of attachment). In other cases, a clear genetic etiology can be elucidated, examples being the many rare Mendelian disorders associated with intellectual disability (de Ligt et al., 2012), for example, Fragile X syndrome (Kremer et al., 1991), Rett syndrome (Amir et al., 1999), or ataxia (Lim et al., 2006).

Most of the burden associated with NDDs involves disorders defined as having a complex etiology involving environmental risk and a substantial genetic contribution. Understanding the architecture of this genetic risk has been challenging, but with substantial collaborative initiatives and technological progress, significant discoveries are being made in intellectual disability (ID); specific disorders of learning

The Genetics of Neurodevelopmental Disorders, First Edition. Edited by Kevin J. Mitchell.
© 2015 John Wiley & Sons, Inc. Published 2015 by John Wiley & Sons, Inc.

(e.g., dyslexia) or communication; autism spectrum disorder (ASD); attention-deficit hyperactivity disorder (ADHD); epilepsy; and other psychiatric disorders (e.g., schizophrenia and bipolar disorder). From this work, novel and often unexpected overlaps across NDDs are being identified (as we discuss below) (Corvin, 2011; Moore et al., 2011). In fact, such is the extent of overlap that shared molecular mechanisms may operate across disorder boundaries and in the future these may be defined as pathological deviation of specific developmental processes or be seen to represent stages on a continuum of neurodevelopmental causality (Owen, 2012).

In one sense, this is expected as the same symptoms co-occur across diagnoses, and there is also substantial diagnostic overlap between disorders (Reiss, 2009). Individual disorders can also be clinically heterogeneous and patients' symptom profiles may differ substantially. As currently defined the common NDDs (e.g., autism or schizophrenia) are syndromes rather than specific disease entities, defined by symptoms and course of illness, rather than on the basis of known etiology and pathophysiology. Identifying pathophysiological mechanisms, to identify specific neurodevelopmental disease entities, is a critical aim for translational neuroscience research. Data emerging from genetics and work from other fields (e.g., neuroimaging) will challenge how these disorders are defined in the future. For example, it may be the case that the current syndromal diagnoses capture many different etiologies, as is being suggested by genetic studies of ASD. But to begin, we review the history of what we term NDDs to appreciate how they came to be regarded as distinct conditions.

2.2 A BRIEF HISTORY OF NEURODEVELOPMENTAL DISORDERS

The recognition of neurodevelopmental disorders is likely to be as old as humanity itself. For instance, the earliest recorded reference to intellectual disability dates to the Papyrus of Thebes in 1552 BC. But through to the early Middle Ages, these disorders were bound up with beliefs about witchcraft, evil spirits, or Galen's theories of the four humors (black bile, yellow bile, blood, and phlegm). "Malleus Malefactorium" (1494), a manual pertaining to allow the identification of witches contained early descriptions of "possession" states which retrospectively may be taken as descriptions of people with persecutory delusions and seizures (Institoris et al., 1978). By the eighteenth century, work by Pinel (1801) and Cullen (1769), consolidated the idea of "Neuroses" as nervous diseases of altered "sensitivity" in the function of the nervous system. Morel (1857) and Neumann (1859) postulated hereditary concepts of epilepsy and insanity and of progressive intellectual degeneration associated with epilepsy. This inherited tendency, manifest in various members of the same family became known as "neurological taint" and was early evidence for a heritable contribution to brain disorders (Johnson and Shorvon, 2011).

The earliest description of what came to be described as Schizophrenia (Bleuler, 1911) was made by Emil Kraepelin who termed the disorder "Dementia Praecox", which translates as premature dementia (1893). Kraepelin viewed Dementia Praecox as being a lifelong, predominantly degenerative condition, but estimated that intellectual disability was the basis for approximately 3.5% of cases. Others, prominently Thomas Clouston (1891), argued that at least some "insanities" were developmental in origin and today few would doubt a developmental contribution to schizophrenia etiology (Church et al., 2002). The modern conceptualization of epilepsy emerged through the work of neurologists including Hughlings Jackson (1870), who both defined seizures and recognized that they could alter consciousness and behavior. Confirmation of this theory came with the development of EEG studies, the first recording on humans was being administered by Berger and described in 1929.

Childhood psychiatric disorders have a much more recent history. The concept of "Autism" emerged from descriptions by Bleuler (1911) of behavior observed in some of his schizophrenia patients, whom he described as having an "absolute predominance of the inner life, we term Autism". The term re-surfaced in the work of Kanner (1943) and subsequently by Asperger (1944), in their description of groups of children with impaired social functioning and particularly a lack of empathy. Both Kanner and Asperger believed that the syndrome of Autism was distinct from schizophrenia; this has been formalized in diagnostic classification systems since the 1970s. Children with excessive hyperactivity, inattentive, and impulsivity have been reported in the literature since the nineteenth century. Initially described by Weikard (1775) and Crichton (1798) who characterized the features of sustained inattention, it was later believed to be due to a "defect of moral control" as noted by Still (1902) who recognized the further symptoms of hyperactivity and who displayed normal intellect. In the twentieth century descriptions of hyperkinetic reaction of childhood (American Psychiatric Association, 1968) and the subsequent combination of hyperkinetic symptoms with attention-deficit disorder led to the current conceptualization of the disorder in (American Psychiatric Association, 1987).

In the 1960s and 1970s, Zigler and colleagues (1967) found that some children with an intellectual disability could not be definitely traced to organic causes. Instead development followed sequences that were qualitatively similar to typically developing individuals, differing only in the rate of development achieved. This model recognized the importance of genetic background, particularly cognitive abilities of the parents and the effect of genetic abnormalities on patterns of cognition and behavior.

The development of these historical, clinical distinctions has shaped modern health services organized into medical and psychiatric specialties on the basis of primary symptoms, course of the disorders, and age of the patient. Therefore, learning disability services are separate from child psychiatric services, based on the presence of pervasive impairment in cognitive function. Whereas disorders such as schizophrenia and epilepsy are treated by general adult psychiatry and neurology services respectively. This reflects how clinical diagnoses are made in the standard diagnostic manuals for example, Diagnostic And Statistical Manual of Mental Disorders 5 (American Psychiatric Association, 2013). Such a system is helpful to both manage and target treatments for these disorders and to develop expertise in each field. However, it also supports the conceptualization of these disorders as discrete categories when in fact, as this chapter outlines, there is significant overlap between entities. This includes symptom overlap, but also evidence of comorbidity between NDDs, which we consider in the next section.

2.3 EVIDENCE OF COMORBIDITY IN INDIVIDUAL PATIENTS

Essentially all neurodevelopmental disorders exist with other neurodevelopmental disorders much more commonly than would be expected by chance alone (Yeargin-Allsopp, 2008). While the prevalence of psychiatric illness in the general population has been estimated as 14% (Alonso et al., 2004), in ID populations psychiatric comorbidity is estimated as being between 44 and 46% (Whitaker and Read, 2006). ID co-occurs with approximately two thirds of individuals with ASD (Dykens and Lense, 2011), and the presence/absence of ID is considered to be the most critical factor affecting outcomes in this population (Howlin et al., 2004). Numerous studies have found evidence of overlap between ADHD and ASD: with up to 20–50% and children with ADHD meeting the criteria for ASD (Rommelse et al., 2009). Within the ADHD population, up to 90% of children are also diagnosed with a co-morbid disorder (Willcutt et al., 1999). Additionally, epilepsy is more common in children with ASD but estimates of the rate vary from 5 to 46% (Spence and Schneider, 2009).

As early as 1919, Kraepelin noted an overlap between ID and schizophrenia, estimating that ID formed the basis for at least 3.5% of cases of schizophrenia (Kraepelin, 1919). This observation is supported by more recent work, which indicates a 3–5 fold increased risk of ID in schizophrenia populations (Penrose, 1938; Hemmings et al., 2006; Morgan et al., 2008). Individuals with epilepsy also have a 5.5-fold increase in the risk of having a broadly defined psychotic disorder, an almost 8.5-fold increase in the risk of having schizophrenia, and a 6.3-fold increase in the risk of having bipolar disorder (Qin et al., 2005; Clarke et al., 2012).

If shared symptoms, or comorbidity between NDDs are common, this begs the question as to whether overlap represents different processes converging on the same neural mechanisms or a common etiology. An example of the former may be the comorbidity between psychosis and temporal lobe epilepsy. This is consistent with the medial temporal lobe structural alterations reported in both disorders, but does not necessarily the same etiology (Shenton et al., 2010). By contrast, some of the genomic syndromes discussed in the following sections (e.g., velocardiofacial syndrome) are associated with many different NDD outcomes, despite having a very similar genetic lesion. More generally, one might expect that disorders with overlapping etiology are likely to share genetic or environmental risk factors.

2.4   FAMILIAL CO-OCCURRENCE OF NDDs

Since Kraepelin, if not before, there has been a strong research interest in the identification of familial co-occurrence of NDDs. Since the 1960s a large number of genetic epidemiological studies have investigated specific disorders. Schizophrenia, Autism, ADHD and epilepsy has shown heritability through family studies (Kendler et al 1993a, Kendler et al, 1993c), twin studies (Cardno and Gottesman, 2000; Bailey et al, 1995; Lichtenstein et al, 2010; Faraone et al, 2005; Berkovic et al, 1995) and adoption studies (Ingraham and Kety, 2000; Sprich et al, 2000). Furthermore, for individual disorders (e.g., schizophrenia or ASD), less severe phenotypic forms also cluster within affected families. Taking schizophrenia as an example, within affected families there are increased rates

of a spectrum of clinical syndromes including schizoaffective disorder (Kendler et al., 1993a), nonaffective psychoses (Kendler et al., 1993b) and schizotypal personality disorder (Kendler et al., 1993c). Similarly, a spectrum of milder manifestations is recognized within families of ASD probands (Piven et al., 1997).

Extending beyond the concept of a "spectrum" of phenotypic expression for a given disorder, there is increasing awareness of how NDDs cluster together within the same families. With high-throughput genomics research, substantial progress has been made in addressing the molecular genetics of more common NDD phenotypes including ASD, ID, and schizophrenia. This is discussed subsequently, but as a consequence, there has been a reappraisal of the genetic epidemiology of what had previously been conceptualized as distinct disorders. Analysis from larger studies, with national case register data has shown that the presence of schizophrenia in parents is associated with a threefold increased risk of ASD in offspring (Sullivan et al., 2012b). A similar pattern, but of smaller effect, has also been shown for bipolar disorder, which shares genetic etiology with schizophrenia (Sullivan et al., 2012b; Lichtenstein et al., 2009). The reverse is also true, as elevated rates of schizophrenia have been reported in both the mothers (OR = 1.9) and fathers (OR = 2.1) of individuals with autism (Daniels et al., 2008).

But the shared genetic risk is also likely to extend more broadly as increased rates of ID, epilepsy, and ASD have also been identified in children of mothers with schizophrenia, bipolar disorder, and depression, respectively (Morgan et al., 2012; Clarke et al., 2012). The overlap extends to include epilepsy, as suggested by evidence of clustering of epilepsy and psychosis within the same families. Having a parental history of epilepsy doubles lifetime risk of developing psychosis. Reciprocally, those with a parental history of psychosis have a 2.7-fold increased risk of generalized epilepsy (Clarke et al., 2012). Overlapping genetic influences contributing to ADHD and autism have also been reported from twin research (Ronald et al.,

2008), as have increased rates of epilepsy in ADHD (adjusted HR 3.94) and of ADHD in epilepsy (Chou et al., 2013). Additionally, there is a broader phenotype including speech and learning disorders as well as intellectual deficits in ADHD families (Lauritsen and Ewald, 2001).

2.5 ENVIRONMENTAL RISK FACTORS IN NEURODEVELOPMENTAL DISORDERS

Neurodevelopmental disorders vary in their prevalence, gender, geography, and ethnicity. Even a cursory examination of the literature for individual disorders rapidly identifies key thematic areas: poor maternal health; prenatal exposure to toxins (including alcohol and tobacco), infection or other insult (e.g., obstetric complications); neonatal or early life exposure to toxins; poor nutrition and infection also feature prominently. Additionally, more complex psychological risk factors in early life (e.g., chronic family conflict, exposure to parental psychopathology, and abuse (Biederman et al., 1995a; Biederman et al., 1995b) contribute to the risk of developing many NDDs from developmental delay to psychiatric disorders. Early insults to the developing brain can compound genetic factors leading to the manifestation of psychopathology. Notably these risk factors are not specific for any one particular diagnostic category. Here are a few examples, but other environmental risk factors including the effects of drug exposure or urban environment are considered more comprehensively in another chapter of this volume.

2.5.1 Season of Birth

Season of birth has long been associated with the risk of developing mental illness. Systematic reviews of individuals born in winter and spring show that they tend to have a slightly increased risk of developing schizophrenia (McGrath and Welham, 1999; Davies et al., 2003). There is some (inconsistent) evidence to suggest that the risk of autism fluctuates across season of birth, and that the nature of this relationship is related to latitude (Grant and Soles, 2009).

It has been suggested that this effect relates to *in utero* exposure to seasonal infections.

2.5.2 Prenatal Infection

Maternal infection during pregnancy with Toxoplasmosis gondii, rubella, cytomegalovirus, herpes simplex, and other microbes is associated with a range of outcomes including ID, cerebral hypoplasia, schizophrenia, and ASD (Remington et al., 2006; Brown et al., 2004; Brown et al., 2001; Mortensen et al., 2007). Exposure to infection necessitating maternal hospitalization in the first or second trimester of pregnancy has also been associated with an increased risk of ASD in offspring (Atladottir et al., 2010) as has evidence for maternal immune activation in pregnancy (Canetta and Brown, 2012).

2.5.3 Obstetric Complications

Based on prospective population-based studies obstetric complications can be broadly grouped into three categories namely (1) complications of pregnancy such as bleeding, preeclampsia, and diabetes; (2) abnormal fetal growth and development such as low birth weight, congenital malformations; (3) complications of delivery such as asphyxia and uterine atony (Cannon et al., 2002). Evidence from meta-analyses and systematic reviews indicates an association between obstetric complications (OR < 2.0) and the subsequent risk of developing schizophrenia (Clarke et al., 2006; Geddes, 1999). A similar relationship has been reported for ASDs, in particular with maternal bleeding in pregnancy (Gardener et al., 2009) and with neonatal seizures, in particular for late (>42 weeks) delivery (Glass et al., 2009).

2.5.4 Migrant Status

There is a well documented association between migrant status and the risk of developing schizophrenia. Large scale meta-analysis (Cantor-Graae and Selten, 2005) and systematic review (McGrath et al., 2004) reported that the relative risk of developing schizophrenia among first generation migrants was 2.7, which almost doubled for second-generation migrants, who reported a relative risk of 4.5. The risk was the highest for Afro-Caribbean migrants. This has been less extensively investigated for ASD, but offspring of dark-skinned migrants to cold countries seem to be at higher risk (Eyles, 2010; Humble et al., 2010).

2.5.5 Nutrition

As highlighted in Chapter 6, the links between periconceptual folate supplementation and the risk of spina bifida has galvanized the field to consider nutritional candidates and a wider spectrum of neurodevelopmental disorders. Individuals who were in utero during the Dutch famine (Susser and Lin, 1992) and famine in China during the Cultural Revolution (St Clair et al., 2005) showed an increased risk of schizophrenia and schizophrenia spectrum personality disorders. With respect to autism, prenatal nutrition has been proposed as a candidate risk factor with a growing body of evidence linking the use of prenatal folate use and a reduced risk of autism and autism-related outcomes (Roth et al., 2011; Suren et al., 2013).

2.6 GENOMICS STUDIES OF NDDs

2.6.1 Genome-Wide Association Studies (GWAS)

Identifying risk genes and molecular pathways that contribute to specific NDDs or explain overlap between disorders is a critical step in understanding disease etiology. ID is genetically heterogeneous and captures at least hundreds of discrete syndromes. Before the publication of the first paper of the GWAS-era in 2005, progress had been made in identifying risk genes for many rare Mendelian NDD disorders, particularly presenting with ID. A working assumption for ASD, ADHD, schizophrenia, bipolar disorder, or epilepsy was that these represented independent core syndromes in each case involving a more homogeneous, less complex genetic architecture. This was considered likely to encompass a wide spectrum of risk variation, from highly penetrant rare

mutations to common risk variants contributing much smaller effects to disease risk. Only in the last decade has it become possible to systematically test this hypothesis, starting with common risk variants.

From the publication of the Human Genome sequence, and subsequent HapMap project, emerged high-throughput assays of single nucleotide polymorphisms (SNPs) capturing information on a relatively high proportion of common risk variation in the human genome (Barrett and Cardon, 2006). To test for association with human disease, the standard approach taken is the familiar cross-sectional case control study (Corvin et al., 2010). GWAS studies now routinely test for association at millions of individual SNPs, but because of the requirement to adjust for such a large number of tests to reduce Type I error when looking for relatively small effects ($p < 5 \times 10^{-8}$ is the standard cutoff taken), sample sizes are by necessity large. This has resulted in unprecedented levels of collaboration among researchers, for example, through the EPICURE Epilepsy Consortium (2012) and Psychiatric Genomics Consortium (PGC) (Cross-Disorder Group of the Psychiatric Genomics Consortium et al., 2013).

In one of the first reported GWAS efforts in schizophrenia, O'Donovan et al. (2008) performed a relatively small initial scan of 479 cases and 2937 controls identifying modest evidence of association at 12 loci. Examining these loci in up to 16,726 subjects, they identified suggestive evidence of association around the gene *ZNF804A* and this effect reached genome-wide significance when the affected phenotype included bipolar disorder, a finding supported by a large replication study (Steinberg et al., 2011a). In bipolar disorder, a GWAS meta-analysis including 4387 cases identified support for two loci containing the genes *ankyrin G (ANK3)* and the *alpha 1C subunit of the L-type voltage-gated calcium channel gene (CACNA1C)*. This was not the first evidence for involvement of *CACNA1C* in NDD as mutations in the gene are implicated in Timothy syndrome, a condition characterized by cognitive impairments, ASD symptoms, syndactyly, and cardiac defects. Through the PGC, large meta-analyses of schizophrenia and bipolar disorder GWAS data identified seven significant schizophrenia loci (including 1p21.3 containing the primary transcript for *MIR137* and 18q21.2 (*TCF4*)), and a novel risk locus for bipolar disorder (*ODZ4*) (Schizophrenia Psychiatric Genome-Wide Association Study (GWAS) Consortium, 2011; Psychiatric GWAS Consortium Bipolar Disorder Working Group, 2011). Null and missense mutations of the *TCF4* gene have been implicated in Pitt-Hopkins syndrome a severe form of epileptic encephalopathy with ID and intermittent hyperventilation (Blake et al., 2010). In a joint analysis, three loci were significant across both disorders (*ANK3*, *CACNA1C*, and *ITIH3-ITIH4*).

By comparison, sample sizes for GWAS of other disorders (e.g., in ASD and ADHD) have been insufficient to allow definitive comment on the presence or absence of the type of small common effects that contribute to complex disorders (Stergiakouli et al., 2012; Anney et al., 2012). The Cross Disorder Group of the PGC recently performed a combined GWAS including more than 33,000 cases with five major psychiatric disorders (schizophrenia, bipolar disorder, major depressive disorder (MDD), ADHD, and ASD) (Cross Disorder Group of the PGC et al., 2013). Four independent regions contained genome-wide significant loci, including *CACNA1C* and another calcium channel subunit gene, *CACNB2*. There was also some evidence of association at *MIR137*, *TCF4*, the Major Histocompatibility Complex (*MHC*) region and *SYNE1*. Again this gene was not new to the NDD literature, as mutations of the *SYNE1* gene cause autosomal recessive cerebellar ataxia type 1 (ARCA1) a disorder presenting with ataxia and dysarthria. But two recent sequencing studies have found mutations of this gene in ASD patients (O'Roak et al., 2011; Yu et al., 2013) and association with a common risk variant at the locus has been reported in bipolar disorder (Green et al., 2013).

Despite a relatively modest sample size, four susceptibility loci have emerged for genetic generalized epilepsies (Epicure Consortium et al., 2012). Of these, the association at chromosome 2p16.1 is of particular interest, as it includes the gene *vaccine-related serine/threonine kinase 2 (VRK2)*: significant association has also been reported near *VRK2* in schizophrenia, with an SNP correlated with the most strongly associated variants in epilepsy (Steinberg et al., 2011b). Haploinsufficiency of this gene may impair cortical development and this locus is also implicated in the 2p15-p16.1 microdeletion syndrome characterized by ID, microcephaly, and seizures (Chabchoub et al., 2008).

These data suggest at least some degree of overlap in common risk loci among NDDs and several of the common risk loci identify genes previously implicated in rare Mendelian NDDs (e.g., *TCF4*, *VRK2*, *SYNE1*). It is important to note that even in schizophrenia where the largest number of risk variants is reported, the GWAS findings explain a relatively modest proportion of total heritability for the disorder (<3%). This has prompted alternative approaches to explore the extent of Type II error within the "noisy" signal that emerges from GWAS analysis. By examining large numbers of genetic markers to generate risk scores, the "polygene score method" was developed to test for the presence of hundreds, or even thousands of small effects within the large number of weakly associated loci that are identified by GWAS analysis. Applying this approach, the International Schizophrenia Consortium reported replication of risk scores from their discovery dataset in other schizophrenia and bipolar samples, but not in other nonpsychiatric diseases, suggesting that the risk score included many real associations (International Schizophrenia Consortium, 2009). This finding has been widely replicated and the proportion of schizophrenia risk explained by, possibly thousands, of small effects is estimated as being at least 25% (Lee et al., 2012).

This begs a wider question as to the extent of overlap across disorders. A recent analysis by the Cross-Disorder Group of the PGC has confirmed that common SNPs also make an important contribution to the overall variance in susceptibility to bipolar disorder, MDD,

ASD, and ADHD (Cross Disorder Group of the PGC et al., 2013). Across disorders, the total variance in liability explained by SNPs (SNP heritability h^2_{SNP}) ranged from 0.17 (ASD) to 0.28 (ADHD). The study also provided evidence of substantial sharing of genetic risk variants tagged by SNPs between schizophrenia and bipolar disorder, bipolar disorder and MDD, schizophrenia and MDD, ADHD and MDD, and, to a lesser extent, schizophrenia and ASD. Yet to be reported is an analysis between these psychiatric disorders and epilepsy, but this is underway.

2.6.2   Rare Genetic Variants and NDDs

Common risk variants, by their nature are likely to have subtle effects on illness. By contrast, low frequency variants are enriched for the potentially functional mutations most likely to help study the molecular basis of disease (1000 Genomes Project Consortium et al., 2012; Karayiorgou et al., 2012). Rapid progress in methods to assess this type of variation has been developed in the last decade, transitioning from cytogenetics and array-based studies of structural variation (copy number variation (CNV) to exome and whole-genome sequencing.

Significant, albeit indirect evidence for the involvement of rare mutations in NDDs came from the observation that advanced paternal age is associated with a wide range of neurodevelopmental and neurocognitive defects (e.g., neural tube defects, epilepsy, autism, and schizophrenia). Men transmit a much higher number of mutations to their children and the age of the father plays a critical role in determining the number of *de novo* mutations in the child. Whole-genome sequencing has made it possible to accurately measure mutation rates and confirm that the variance in mutation rates is predominantly explained by the age of the father at conception (Kong et al., 2012). Supporting the paternal age data, increased rates of *de novo* point and structural mutations have now been identified in ASD and schizophrenia (Pinto et al., 2010; Sanders et al., 2012; O'Roak et al., 2012; Neale et al., 2012; Girard et al., 2012; Xu et al., 2012).

The rates of mutation may be higher, but do the impacted genes overlap between disorders? Studies of chromosomal duplications, deletions and translocations make a strong case. Velocardiofacial syndrome (VCFS) is the most common known microdeletion syndrome and is caused by a 1.503 Mb hemizygous deletion of chromosome 22q11.2. Despite the relative uniformity of this event, the syndrome is associated with a highly variable phenotype including developmental delay, ID, cardiac anomalies, dysmorphology, and psychiatric features including a 20-fold increased risk of psychosis (Murphy et al., 1999), increased rates of ASD and ADHD (Gothelf et al., 2004). A similar, classical example from the psychiatric literature is the balanced translocation at 1:11 (q42; q14.3) initially reported in a Scottish individual with conduct disorder. This event, which disrupts the gene *DISC1*, was later found to cosegregate with major psychiatric disorders including schizophrenia, bipolar disorder and depression in the extended family of that proband (St Clair et al., 1990; Blackwood et al., 2001). With the development of array-base technologies, a number of smaller recurrent CNV loci have been identified including 1q21.1, 15q11.2, 15q13.3, 16p11.2, 16p13.1, and 17q12. In each case, the identified locus has been found to increase susceptibility to a range of NDD phenotypes including developmental delay, ID, ASD, schizophrenia, and seizure disorder (see Table 2.1, from an et al., 2012a). As these technologies are applied to clinical genetics referrals (mostly for ID and developmental delay), a more complete picture of the genes (or loci) affected by CNVs in developmental morbidity is emerging (Cooper et al., 2011) and it will be interesting to see the range of NDD phenotypes associated with these events.

Three large CNV studies in ASD have identified ~20 genes disrupted by rare de novo CNVs in ASD (Berg and Geschwind, 2012). The list includes presynaptic neurexin (*NRXN1*) and post neuroligin (*NLGN3*) genes, to which they bind in modulating excitatory and inhibitory synaptic functions, but also other related synaptic proteins (e.g., *CNTNAP2*, *SHANK3*).

TABLE 2.1 Structural variation associated with psychiatric disorders

Structural variant	Location, Mb	Genes	Type	Disorder	Frequency in cases	Frequency in controls	Odds ratio	P value	Other associations
1q21.1	chr1:145.0–148.0	34	Deletion	SCZ	0.0018	0.0002	9.5	8×10^{-6}	Developmental delay, intellectual disability, micro-and macrocephaly, dysmorphia, epilepsy, cataracts, cardiac defects, possibly ASD thrombocytopenia-absent radius syndrome
2p16.3	chr2:50.1–51.2	NRXN1 exons	Duplication Deletion	SCZ ASD	0.0013	0.0004	4.5	0.02 0.004	Developmental delay, intellectual disability, epilepsy, Pitt–Hopkins-like syndrome
3q29	chr3:195.7–197.3	19	Deletion Deletion	SCZ SCZ	0.0018 0.0010	0.0002 0.0	7.5 3.8	1×10^{-6} 4×10^{-4}	Developmental delay, intellectual disability, possibly ASD
7q11.23	chr7:72.7–74.1	25	Duplication	ASD	0.0011			0.003	Developmental delay, intellectual disability. Deletion: Williams–Beuren syndrome
7q36.3 15q11.2	chr7:158.8–158.9 chr15:23.6–28.4	VIPR2 70	Duplication Duplication	SCZ ASD	0.0024 0.0018	0.0001	16.4	4×10^{-5} 4×10^{-9}	Developmental delay, intellectual disability, Prader–Willi and Angelman syndromes

(*continued*)

TABLE 2.1 (*Continued*)

Structural variant	Location, Mb	Genes	Type	Disorder	Frequency in cases	Frequency in controls	Odds ratio	P value	Other associations
15q13.3	chr15:30.9–33.5	12	Duplication	ADHD	0.0125	0.0061	2.1	2×10^{-4}	Developmental delay, intellectual disability, epilepsy
16p13.11	chr16:15.4–16.3	8	Duplication	ASD	0.0013			2×10^{-5}	Deletion: developmental delay, epilepsy
			Deletion	SCZ	0.0019	0.0002	12.1	7×10^{-7}	
			Duplication	ADHD	0.0164	0.0009	13.9	8×10^{-4}	
16p11.2	chr16:29.5–30.2	29	Deletion	ASD	0.0037			5×10^{-29}	Developmental delay, intellectual disability, epilepsy, macrocephaly, obesity
			Duplication	ASD	0.0013			2×10^{-5}	Developmental delay, intellectual disability, epilepsy, microcephaly, low body mass index
17q12	chr17:34.8–36.2	18	Duplication	SCZ	0.0031	0.0003	9.5	3×10^{-8}	
			Deletion	ASD	0.0017	0.0	6.12	9×10^{-4}	
			Deletion	SCZ	0.0006	0.0	4.49	3×10^{-4}	
22q11.21	chr22:18.7–21.8	53	Deletion or duplication	ASD	0.0013			0.002	Developmental delay, intellectual disability, velocardiofacial-DiGeorge syndrome
			Deletion	SCZ	0.0031	0.0	20.3	7×10^{-13}	

Source: from Sullivan et al., 2012a

38

Nonrecurrent CNVs disrupting *NRXN1* are also reported in schizophrenia and deletions of the gene are associated with developmental delay and Pitt-Hopkins-like syndrome 2. Rare exonic deletions in a key postsynaptic membrane scaffolding protein gene (*GPHN*), linked to the neuroligins, are also implicated in ASD, schizophrenia, and seizures (Lionel et al., 2013).

The development of high-throughput sequencing methods has allowed more detailed assessment of rare variation at the much more fine-grained level of point mutations. Initially, this was applied to identify mutations in target genes (e.g., *NLGN3*, *NLGN4* in ASD (Jamain et al., 2003) and as a next step to target multiple regions. A good example is the identification of 50 novel candidate genes for recessive forms of ID based on sequencing of linkage intervals in consanguineous families (Najmabadi et al., 2011). But sequencing methodology has now moved on to exome or whole-genome sequencing. A relatively small number of ASD and schizophrenia studies have been performed. These come with the challenge of establishing causality for what are rare events, likely to be impacting many genes, set across the "noise" generated by the background mutation rate in the human genome. Despite, these caveats three recent ASD papers provide supportive evidence for three genes (*SCN2A*, *KATNAL2*, and *CHD8*) (Sanders et al., 2012; Neale et al., 2012; O'Roak et al., 2012). In keeping with the theme of overlap, mutations of the *SCN2A* gene, coding for a subunit of the voltage-gated sodium channel, have also been implicated in epilepsy.

2.6.3 The Path Ahead: Future Directions

The last five years has seen remarkable progress. The hypothesis that for ASD, ADHD, schizophrenia, bipolar disorder, or epilepsy there are core, independent syndromes involving independent genetic architectures and disease processes has been severely tested. Although there are likely to be common variants contributing liability to these disorders, the boundaries between them are not distinct. These broad NDD categories are also likely to capture many rare genomic disorders involving high penetrance mutations and distinct disease processes. Understanding the molecular etiology underlying these overlapping clinical disorders will require complementary research across many disciplines, building on methodological advances such as transcriptome analysis in developing brain. We see two key areas of interest. The first will be the application of network-based methods to investigate neural mechanisms and molecular pathways. The second will be to investigate individual genes, or mechanisms in model systems.

It is tempting to look at the current data and see recurrent themes such as involvement of synaptic plasticity mechanisms, or the convergence across studies on a subset of presumably critical developmental genes. We would urge caution on two fronts. First, mutations in more than a thousand genes have been implicated in NDD, particularly ID syndromes. Finding risk genes by GWAS or sequencing analysis that are already implicated in rare Mendelian NDDs is not proof of causality: some of these observations may occur by chance. Second, with the exception of ID, a large majority of the heritability of these disorders is unexplained.

As of now we have confirmed a few "known knowns", identified more "known unknowns" but if we want to systematically examine the data, we are still mostly faced with "unknown unknowns." Compared even to other common disorders or traits (e.g., height, lipid levels, diabetes) where larger GWAS analyses have been reported, the picture is far from complete. For rare variants, the number of confirmed loci remains low and, with the exception of some of the CNVs, causality is yet to be established for individual mutations or genes. On a more positive note, ASD sequencing data suggests that proteins that are encoded by genes that harbor nonsense or missense mutations show a higher than expected level of connectivity as indexed by protein–protein interaction screens (Neale et al., 2012). In our view, larger sample sizes, with better estimates of risk, and the predicted increase in confirmed risk loci that this should bring will allow progress similar to that made in other common disorders (Corvin, 2013). For those interested in the analytical approaches available, these have been usefully reviewed elsewhere (Ramanan et al., 2012; Barabasi et al., 2011).

So what of the current evidence? Early GWAS-based pathway studies support the involvement of cell adhesion and trans-synaptic signaling in schizophrenia, bipolar disorder, and ASD (O'Dushlaine et al., 2011; Lips et al., 2012; Wang et al., 2009; Corvin, 2010). Taking a similar approach, the PGC-Cross Disorder group applied an interval-based enrichment analysis (INRICH) to their GWAS dataset of five psychiatric disorders. This found significant enrichment for a set of calcium channel activity genes with catalysis of facilitated diffusion of calcium ions through a transmembrane calcium channel. Molecular disruption of voltage-gated calcium signaling may be etiologically important across many common NDDs. This is compatible with our understanding of the etiology of epilepsy, where altered expression of calcium channel subtypes and gain-of-function mutations have been identified in calcium channel genes from epilepsy patients and in animal models of the disorder (Cain and Snutch, 2012; Noebels, 2012). This gene family is also implicated in some forms of ID, for example, the gain-of-function mutations in *CACNA1C* causing Timothy syndrome, (Splawski et al., 2004), but also mutations of other subtypes *CACNA1F* (Hope et al., 2005), *CACNA2D2* (Edvardson et al., 2013)) cause syndromes featuring ID and epilepsy.

The future of network analysis will involve more sophisticated approaches incorporating information on the expression and temporal regulation of gene function. The availability of public resources on the functional annotation of the genome (Encyclopaedia of DNA Elements (ENCODE) (http://genome.ucsc.edu/ENCODE/) and RNA sequencing (RNA-seq)-based gene expression (e.g., BrainSpan (http://www.brainspan.org) represents a tremendous advance for the field. As examples, by starting with gene expression data, but also incorporating GWAS data, Voineagu et al., (2011)

identified converging molecular abnormalities in ASD implicating transcriptional and splicing dysregulation. Network-based analyses incorporating rare genetic variants and gene expression data have identified broad gene networks for schizophrenia and ASD involving axon guidance, neuronal cell mobility, synaptic function, and chromatin remodeling (Gilman et al., 2011; Gilman et al., 2012). Broadly similar processes emerged from a recent sequencing, protein interaction, and transcriptional coexpression analysis of schizophrenia (Gulsuner et al., 2013).

An aim of network medicine is to identify critical hub genes, as these may be particularly informative in elucidating molecular etiology. From genomics, the identification of rare, highly penetrant risk mutations will be critical for the downstream functional experiments required for translational research (Karayiorgou et al., 2012). For the main disorders discussed in this review, much has been learned by studying the genes *DISC1, NRXN1, SYNE1, TCF4* or the disorder VCFS in model systems (St Clair et al., 1990; O'Roak et al., 2011; Berg and Geschwind, 2012; Blake et al., 2010; Murphy et al., 1999), including in human iPS cells (Pasca et al., 2011). This work is the subject of Chapters 10 and 11 in this volume. A recurrent criticism has been that these gene findings represent oddities that can tell us little about the larger syndromes of schizophrenia, ASD or epilepsy. With new findings, there will be more gene-based models and it will be fascinating to see whether these converge on particular molecular etiologies processes. The promise is a future for NDD diagnosis and treatment based rationally on disease mechanisms.

REFERENCES

1000 Genomes Project Consortium, Abecasis, G.R., Auton, A., Brooks, L.D., DePristo, M.A., Durbin R.M., Handsaker R.E., Kang, H.M., Marth, G.T., McVean G.A. (2012). An integrated map of genetic variation from 1,092 human genomes. Nature 491, 56–65.

Alonso, J., Angermeyer, M.C., Bernert, S., Bruffaerts, R., Brugha, T.S., Bryson, H., de Girolamo, G.,

Graaf, R., Demyttenaere, K., Gasquet, I., et al. (2004). Prevalence of mental disorders in Europe: results from the European Study of the Epidemiology of Mental Disorders (ESEMeD) project. Acta Psychiatr Scand Suppl 420, 21–27.

American Psychiatric Association. (1968). Diagnostic and Statistical Manual of Mental Disorders: DSM-II, 2nd edn. Washington, DC: American Psychiatric Association.

American Psychiatric Association. (1987). Diagnostic and Statistical Manual of Mental Disorders: DSM-III-R, 3rd rev. edn. Washington, DC: American Psychiatric Association.

American Psychiatric Association. (2013). Diagnostic and Statistical Manual of Mental Disorders: DSM-V, 5th edn. Washington, DC: American Psychiatric Association.

Amir, R.E., Van den Veyver, I.B., Wan, M., Tran, C.Q., Francke, U., Zoghbi, H.Y. (1999). Rett syndrome is caused by mutations in X-linked MECP2, encoding methyl-CpG-binding protein 2. Nat Genet 23, 185–188.

Anney, R., Klei, L., Pinto, D., Almeida, J., Bacchelli, E., Baird, G., Bolshakova, N., Bolte, S., Bolton, P.F., Bourgeron, T., et al. (2012). Individual common variants exert weak effects on the risk for autism spectrum disorderspi. Hum Mol Genet 21, 4781–4792.

Asperger, H. (1944). Die autistischen Psychopathen im Kindersalter. Arch Psychiatr Nervenkrankheiten 1, 76–136.

Atladottir, H.O., Thorsen, P., Ostergaard, L., Schendel, D.E., Lemcke, S., Abdallah, M., and Parner, E.T. (2010). Maternal infection requiring hospitalization during pregnancy and autism spectrum disorders. J Autism Dev Disord 40, 1423–1430.

Bailey, A., Le Couteur, A., Gottesman, I., Bolton, P., Simonoff, E., Yuzda, E., Rutter, M. (1995). Autism as a strongly genetic disorder: evidence from a British twin study. Psychol Med 25, 63–7.

Barabasi, A.L., Gulbahce, N., and Loscalzo, J. (2011). Network medicine: a network-based approach to human disease. Nat Rev Genet 12, 56–68.

Barrett, J.C., and Cardon, L.R. (2006). Evaluating coverage of genome-wide association studies. Nat Genet 38, 659–662.

Berg, J.M., and Geschwind, D.H. (2012). Autism genetics: searching for specificity and convergence. Genome Biol 13, 247.

Berger, H. (1929). Uber das Elektrenkephalogramm des Menschen. Archiv Psychiat Nervenkr 87, 527–570.

Berkovic, S.F., Howell, R.A., Hay, D.A., Hopper, J.L. (1998). Epilepsies in twins: genetics of the major epilepsy syndromes Ann Neurol 43, 435–45.

Biederman, J., Milberger, S., Faraone, S.V., Kiely, K., Guite, J., Mick, E., Ablon, S., Warburton, R., and Reed, E. (1995a). Family-environment risk factors for attention-deficit hyperactivity disorder. A test of Rutter's indicators of adversity. Arch Gen Psychiatry 52, 464–470.

Biederman, J., Milberger, S., Faraone, S.V., Kiely, K., Guite, J., Mick, E., Ablon, J.S., Warburton, R., Reed, E., and Davis, S.G. (1995b). Impact of adversity on functioning and comorbidity in children with attention-deficit hyperactivity disorder. J Am Acad Child Adolesc Psychiatry 34, 1495–1503.

Blackwood, D.H., Fordyce, A., Walker, M.T., St Clair, D.M., Porteous, D.J., and Muir, W.J. (2001). Schizophrenia and affective disorders--cosegregation with a translocation at chromosome 1q42 that directly disrupts brain-expressed genes: clinical and P300 findings in a family. Am J Hum Genet 69, 428–433.

Blake, D.J., Forrest, M., Chapman, R.M., Tinsley, C.L., O'Donovan, M.C., and Owen, M.J. (2010). TCF4, schizophrenia, and Pitt-Hopkins Syndrome. Schizophr Bull 36, 443–447.

Bleuler, E. (1911). Dementia Praecox oder Gruppe der Schizophrenien. Leipzig: Franz Deuticke.

Brown, A.S., Begg, M.D., Gravenstein, S., Schaefer, C.A., Wyatt, R.J., Bresnahan, M., Babulas, V.P., and Susser, E.S. (2004). Serologic evidence of prenatal influenza in the etiology of schizophrenia. Arch Gen Psychiatry 61, 774–780.

Brown, A.S., Cohen, P., Harkavy-Friedman, J., Babulas, V., Malaspina, D., Gorman, J.M., and Susser, E.S. (2001). A.E. Bennett Research Award. Prenatal rubella, premorbid abnormalities, and adult schizophrenia. Biol Psychiatry 49, 473–486.

Cain, S.M., and Snutch, T.P. (2012). Voltage-gated calcium channels in epilepsy. In: J.L. Noebels, M. Avoli, M.A. Rogawski, R.W. Olsen, and A.V. Delgado-Escueta, eds. Jasper's Basic Mechanisms of the Epilepsies. Bethesda, MD).

Canetta, S.E., and Brown, A.S. (2012). Prenatal infection, maternal immune activation, and risk for schizophrenia. Transl Neurosci 3, 320–327.

Cannon, M., Jones, P.B., and Murray, R.M. (2002). Obstetric complications and schizophrenia: historical and meta-analytic review. Am J Psychiatry 159, 1080–1092.

Cantor-Graae, E., and Selten, J.P. (2005). Schizophrenia and migration: a meta-analysis and review. Am J Psychiatry 162, 12–24.

Cardno, A.G., Gottesman, I.I. (2000). Twin studies of schizophrenia: from bow-and-arrow concordances to star wars Mx and functional genomics. Am J Med Genet 97, 12–7.

Chabchoub, E., Vermeesch, J.R., de Ravel, T., de Cock, P., and Fryns, J.P. (2008). The facial dysmorphy in the newly recognised microdeletion 2p15-p16.1 refined to a 570 kb region in 2p15. J Med Genet 45, 189–192.

Chou, I.C., Chang, Y.T., Chin, Z.N., Muo, C.H., Sung, F.C., Kuo, H.T., Tsai, C.H., and Kao, C.H. (2013). Correlation between epilepsy and attention deficit hyperactivity disorder: a population-based cohort study. PLoS One 8, e57926.

Church, S.M., Cotter, D., Bramon, E., and Murray, R.M. (2002). Does schizophrenia result from developmental or degenerative processes? J Neural Transm Suppl, 129–147.

Clarke, M.C., Harley, M., and Cannon, M. (2006). The role of obstetric events in schizophrenia. Schizophr Bull 32, 3–8.

Clarke, M.C., Tanskanen, A., Huttunen, M.O., Clancy, M., Cotter, D.R., and Cannon, M. (2012). Evidence for shared susceptibility to epilepsy and psychosis: a population-based family study. Biol Psychiatry 71, 836–839.

Clouston, T.S. (1891). Neuroses of Development: The Morrison Lectures for 1890. Edinburgh, Scotland: Oliver & Boyd.

Cooper, G.M., Coe, B.P., Girirajan, S., Rosenfeld, J.A., Vu, T.H., Baker, C., Williams, C., Stalker, H., Hamid, R., Hannig, V., et al. (2011). A copy number variation morbidity map of developmental delay. Nat Genet 43, 838–846.

Corvin, A. (2013). Schizophrenia at a genetics crossroads: where to now? Schizophr Bull 39, 490–495.

Corvin, A., Craddock, N., and Sullivan, P.F. (2010). Genome-wide association studies: a primer. Psychol Med 40, 1063–1077.

Corvin, A.P. (2010). Neuronal cell adhesion genes: key players in risk for schizophrenia, bipolar disorder and other neurodevelopmental brain disorders? Cell Adh Migr 4, 511–514.

Corvin, A.P. (2011). Two patients walk into a clinic … a genomics perspective on the future of schizophrenia. BMC Biol 9, 77.

Crichton, A.S. (1798). An Inquiry into the Nature and Origin of Mental Derangement. Comprehending a concise system of the physiology and pathology of the human mind. And a history of the passions and their effects. [With an appendix entitled: "Medical Aphorisms, on melancholy, and various other diseases connected with it", by Johann E. Greding.] London: T. Cadell; W. Davies.

Cross-Disorder Group of the Psychiatric Genomics Consortium, Lee, S.H., Ripke, S., Neale, B.M., Faraone, S.V., Purcell, S.M., Perlis, R.H., Mowry, B.J., Thapar, A., Goddard, M.E., et al. (2013). Genetic relationship between five psychiatric disorders estimated from genome-wide SNPs. Nat Genet 45, 984–994.

Cullen, W. (1769). Nosology: A Systematic Arrangement of Diseases. Edinburgh, Scotland: C Stewart and Co.

Daniels, J.L., Forssen, U., Hultman, C.M., Cnattingius, S., Savitz, D.A., Feychting, M., and Sparen, P. (2008). Parental psychiatric disorders associated with autism spectrum disorders in the offspring. Pediatrics 121, 1357–1362.

de Ligt, J., Willemsen, M.H., van Bon, B.W., Kleefstra, T., Yntema, H.G., Kroes, T., Vulto-van Silfhout, A.T., Koolen, D.A., de Vries, P., Gilissen, C. et al. (2012). Diagnostic exome sequencing in persons with severe intellectual disability. N Engl J Med 367, 1921–1929.

Davies, G., Welham, J., Chant, D., Torrey, E.F., and McGrath, J. (2003). A systematic review and meta-analysis of Northern Hemisphere season of birth studies in schizophrenia. Schizophr Bull 29, 587–593.

Dykens, E.M. and Lense, M. (2011). Intellectual disabilities and autism spectrum disorder: a cautionary note. In: D. Amaral, G. Dawson, and D. Geschwind, eds. Autism Spectrum Disorders. Oxford University Press, pp. 261–269.

Edvardson, S., Oz, S., Abulhijaa, F.A., Taher, F.B., Shaag, A., Zenvirt, S., Dascal, N., and Elpeleg, O. (2013). Early infantile epileptic encephalopathy associated with a high voltage gated calcium channelopathy. J Med Genet 50, 118–123.

EPICURE Consortium, EMINet Consortium, Steffens, M., Leu, C., Ruppert, A.K., Zara, F., Striano, P., Robbiano, A., Capovilla, G., Tinuper, P., et al. (2012). Genome-wide association analysis of genetic generalized epilepsies implicates suscepti-bility loci at 1q43, 2p16.1, 2q22.3 and 17q21.32. Hum Mol Genet 21, 5359–5372.

Eyles, D.W. (2010). Vitamin D and autism: does skin colour modify risk? Acta Paediatr 99, 645–647.

Faraone, S.V., Perlis, R.H., Doyle, A.E., Smoller, J.W., Goralnick, J.J., Holmgren, M.A., Sklar, P. (2005). Molecular genetics of attention-deficit hyperactivity disorder. Biol Psychiatry 57, 1313–1323.

Gardener, H., Spiegelman, D., and Buka, S.L. (2009). Prenatal risk factors for autism: comprehensive meta-analysis. Br J Psychiatry 195, 7–14.

Geddes, J. (1999). Prenatal and perinatal and perinatal risk factors for early onset schizophrenia, affective psychosis, and reactive psychosis. BMJ 318, 426.

Gilman, S.R., Chang, J., Xu, B., Bawa, T.S., Gogos, J.A., Karayiorgou, M., and Vitkup, D. (2012). Diverse types of genetic variation converge on functional gene networks involved in schizophre-nia. Nat Neurosci 15, 1723–1728.

Gilman, S.R., Iossifov, I., Levy, D., Ronemus, M., Wigler, M., and Vitkup, D. (2011). Rare de novo variants associated with autism implicate a large functional network of genes involved in formation and function of synapses. Neuron 70, 898–907.

Girard, S.L., Dion, P.A., and Rouleau, G.A. (2012). Schizophrenia genetics: putting all the pieces together. Curr Neurol Neurosci Rep 12, 261–266.

Glass, H.C., Glidden, D., Jeremy, R.J., Barkovich, A.J., Ferriero, D.M., and Miller, S.P. (2009). Clin-ical neonatal seizures are independently asso-ciated with outcome in infants at risk for hypoxic-ischemic brain injury. J Pediatr 155, 318–323.

Gothelf, D., Presburger, G., Levy, D., Nahmani, A., Burg, M., Berant, M., Blieden, L.C., Finkel-stein, Y., Frisch, A., Apter, A., et al. (2004). Genetic, developmental, and physical factors asso-ciated with attention deficit hyperactivity disor-der in patients with velocardiofacial syndrome. Am J Med Genet B Neuropsychiatr Genet 126B, 116–121.

Grant, W.B., and Soles, C.M. (2009). Epidemiologic evidence supporting the role of maternal vitamin D deficiency as a risk factor for the development of infantile autism. Dermatoendocrinol 1, 223–228.

Green, E.K., Grozeva, D., Forty, L., Gordon-Smith, K., Russell, E., Farmer, A., Hamshere, M., Jones, I.R., Jones, L., McGuffin, P., et al. (2013). Asso-ciation at SYNE1 in both bipolar disorder and recurrent major depression. Mol Psychiatry 18, 614–617.

Gulsuner, S., Walsh, T., Watts, A.C., Lee, M.K., Thornton, A.M., Casadei, S., Rippey, C., Shahin, H., Nimgaonkar, V.L., Go, R.C., et al. (2013). Spa-tial and temporal mapping of de novo mutations in schizophrenia to a fetal prefrontal cortical net-work. Cell 154, 518–529.

Hemmings, C.P., Gravestock, S., Pickard, M., and Bouras, N. (2006). Psychiatric symptoms and problem behaviours in people with intellectual dis-abilities. J Intellect Disabil Res 50, 269–276.

Hope, C.I., Sharp, D.M., Hemara-Wahanui, A., Siss-ingh, J.I., Lundon, P., Mitchell, E.A., Maw, M.A., and Clover, G.M. (2005). Clinical manifestations of a unique X-linked retinal disorder in a large New Zealand family with a novel mutation in CACNA1F, the gene responsible for CSNB2. Clin Experiment Ophthalmol 33, 129–136.

Howlin, P., Goode, S., Hutton, J., and Rutter, M. (2004). Adult outcome for children with autism. J Child Psychol Psychiatry 45, 212–229.

Hughlings Jackson, J. (1870). A study of convulsions. St Andrews medical graduates. Association Trans-act 1869, 162–204.

Humble, M.B., Gustafsson, S., and Bejerot, S. (2010). Low serum levels of 25-hydroxyvitamin D (25-OHD) among psychiatric out-patients in Swe-den: relations with season, age, ethnic origin and psychiatric diagnosis. J Steroid Biochem Mol Biol 121, 467–470.

Ingraham, L.J., Kety, S.S. (2000). Adoption studies of schizophrenia. Am J Med Genet 97, 18–22.

Institoris, H., Sprenger, J.O., and Summers, M. (1978). The Malleus maleficarum of Heinrich Kramer and James Sprenger. [S.l.], Dover.

International Schizophrenia Consortium, Purcell, S.M., Wray, N.R., Stone, J.L., Visscher, P.M., O'Donovan, M.C., Sullivan, P.F., and Sklar, P. (2009). Common polygenic variation contributes to risk of schizophrenia and bipolar disorder. Nature 460, 748–752.

Jamain, S., Quach, H., Betancur, C., Rastam, M., Col-ineaux, C., Gillberg, I.C., Soderstrom, H., Giros, B., Leboyer, M., Gillberg, C., et al. (2003). Muta-tions of the X-linked genes encoding neuroligins NLGN3 and NLGN4 are associated with autism. Nat Genet 34, 27–29.

Johnson, M.R., and Shorvon, S.D. (2011). Heredity in epilepsy: neurodevelopment, comorbidity, and the neurological trait. Epilepsy Behav 22, 421–427.

Kanner, L. (1943). Autistic disturbances of affective contact. Nervous Child 2, 217–250.

Karayiorgou, M., Flint, J., Gogos, J.A., Malenka, R.C., Genetic and Neural Complexity in Psychiatry 2011 Working Group. (2012). The best of times, the worst of times for psychiatric disease. Nat Neurosci 15, 811–812.

Kendler, K.S., McGuire, M., Gruenberg, A.M., O'Hare, A., Spellman, M., and Walsh, D. (1993a). The Roscommon Family Study. I. Methods, diagnosis of probands, and risk of schizophrenia in relatives. Arch Gen Psychiatry 50, 527–540.

Kendler, K.S., McGuire, M., Gruenberg, A.M., O'Hare, A., Spellman, M., and Walsh, D. (1993b). The Roscommon Family Study. III. Schizophrenia-related personality disorders in relatives. Arch Gen Psychiatry 50, 781–788.

Kendler, K.S., McGuire, M., Gruenberg, A.M., Spellman, M., O'Hare, A., and Walsh, D. (1993c). The Roscommon Family Study. II. The risk of nonschizophrenic nonaffective psychoses in relatives. Arch Gen Psychiatry 50, 645–652.

Kong, A., Frigge, M.L., Masson, G., Besenbacher, S., Sulem, P., Magnusson, G., Gudjonsson, S.A., Sigurdsson, A., Jonasdottir, A., Wong, W.S., et al. (2012). Rate of de novo mutations and the importance of father's age to disease risk. Nature 488, 471–475.

Kraepelin, E. (1893) Psychiatrie. Ein Lehrbuch für Studirende und Aerzte. Leipzig: Johann Ambrosius Barth.

Kraepelin, E. (1919). Dementia Praecox and Paraphrenia. Edinburgh: E & S Livingstone.

Kremer, E.J., Pritchard, M., Lynch, M., Yu, S., Holman, K., Baker, E., Warren, S.T., Schlessinger, D., Sutherland, G.R., Richards, R.I. (1991). Mapping of DNA instability at the fragile X to a trinucleotide repeat sequence p(CCG)n. Science 252, 1711–1714.

Lauritsen, M., and Ewald, H. (2001). The genetics of autism. Acta Psychiatr Scand 103, 411–427.

Lee, S.H., DeCandia T.R., Ripke S., Yang J., Schizophrenia Psychiatric Genome-Wide Association Study Consortium (PGC-SCZ), International Schizophrenia Consortium (ISC), Molecular Genetics of Schizophrenia Collaboration (MGS), Sullivan, P.F., Goddard, M.E., Keller, M.C., Visscher, P.M., Wray, N.R. (2012). Estimating the proportion of variation in susceptibility to schizophrenia captured by common SNPs. Nat Genet 44, 247–250.

Lichtenstein, P., Yip, B.H., Bjork, C., Pawitan, Y., Cannon, T.D., Sullivan, P.F., and Hultman, C.M. (2009). Common genetic determinants of schizophrenia and bipolar disorder in Swedish families: a population-based study. Lancet 373, 234–239.

Lichtenstein, P., Carlström, E., Råstam, M., Gillberg, C., Anckarsäter, H. (2010). The genetics of autism spectrum disorders and related neuropsychiatric disorders in childhood. Am J Psychiatry 167, 1357–1363.

Lim, J., Hao, T., Shaw, C., Patel, A.J., Szabó, G., Rual, J.F., Fisk, C.J., Li, N., Smolyar, A., Hill, D.E. et al. (2006). A protein-protein interaction network for human inherited ataxias and disorders of Purkinje cell degeneration. Cell 125, 801–814.

Lionel, A.C., Vaags, A.K., Sato, D., Gazzellone, M.J., Mitchell, E.B., Chen, H.Y., Costain, G., Walker, S., Egger, G., Thiruvahindrapuram, B., et al. (2013). Rare exonic deletions implicate the synaptic organizer Gephyrin (GPHN) in risk for autism, schizophrenia and seizures. Hum Mol Genet 22, 2055–2066.

Lips, E.S., Cornelisse, L.N., Toonen, R.F., Min, J.L., Hultman, C.M., Holmans, P.A., O'Donovan, M.C., Purcell, S.M., Smit, A.B., Verhage, M., et al. (2012). Functional gene group analysis identifies synaptic gene groups as risk factor for schizophrenia. Mol Psychiatry 17, 996–1006.

McGrath, J., Saha, S., Welham, J., El Saadi, O., MacCauley, C., and Chant, D. (2004). A systematic review of the incidence of schizophrenia: the distribution of rates and the influence of sex, urbanicity, migrant status and methodology. BMC Med 2, 13

McGrath, J.J., and Welham, J.L. (1999). Season of birth and schizophrenia: a systematic review and meta-analysis of data from the Southern Hemisphere. Schizophr Res 35, 237–242.

Moore, S., Kelleher, E., and Corvin, A. (2011). The shock of the new: progress in schizophrenia genomics. Curr Genomics 12, 516–524.

Morel, B.A. (1857). Traité des dégénérescence physiques, intellectuelles, et morales de l'espèce humaine. Paris: J.B. Balliere.

Morgan, V.A., Croft, M.L., Valuri, G.M., Zubrick, S.R., Bower, C., McNeil, T.F., and Jablensky, A.V. (2012). Intellectual disability and other neuropsychiatric outcomes in high-risk children of mothers with schizophrenia, bipolar disorder and unipolar major depression. Br J Psychiatry 200, 282–289.

Morgan, V.A., Leonard, H., Bourke, J., and Jablensky, A. (2008). Intellectual disability co-occurring with schizophrenia and other psychiatric illness: population-based study. Br J Psychiatry 193, 364–372.

Mortensen, P.B., Norgaard-Pedersen, B., Waltoft, B.L., Sorensen, T.L., Hougaard, D., and Yolken, R.H. (2007). Early infections of Toxoplasma gondii and the later development of schizophrenia. Schizophr Bull 33, 741–744.

Murphy, K.C., Jones, L.A., and Owen, M.J. (1999). High rates of schizophrenia in adults with velo-cardio-facial syndrome. Arch Gen Psychiatry 56, 940–945.

Najmabadi, H., Hu, H., Garshasbi, M., Zemojtel, T., Abedini, S.S., Chen, W., Hosseini, M., Behjati, F., Haas, S., Jamali, P., et al. (2011). Deep sequencing reveals 50 novel genes for recessive cognitive disorders. Nature 478, 57–63.

Neale, B.M., Kou, Y., Liu, L., Ma'ayan, A., Samocha, K.E., Sabo, A., Lin, C.F., Stevens, C., Wang, L.S., Makarov, V., et al. (2012). Patterns and rates of exonic de novo mutations in autism spectrum disorders. Nature 485, 242–245.

Neumann H. (1859). Lehrbuch der Psychiatrie. Erlangen.

Noebels, J.L. (2012). The voltage-gated calcium channel and absence epilepsy. In J.L. Noebels, M. Avoli, M.A. Rogawski, R.W. Olsen, and A.V. Delgado-Escueta, eds. Jasper's Basic Mechanisms of the Epilepsies. Bethesda, MD.

O'Donovan, M.C., Craddock, N., Norton, N., Williams, H., Peirce, T., Moskvina, V., Nikolov, I., Hamshere, M., Carroll, L., Georgieva, L., et al. (2008). Identification of loci associated with schizophrenia by genome-wide association and follow-up. Nat Genet 40, 1053–1055.

O'Dushlaine, C., Kenny, E., Heron, E., Donohoe, G., Gill, M., Morris, D., International Schizophrenia Consortium and Corvin, A. (2011). Molecular pathways involved in neuronal cell adhesion and membrane scaffolding contribute to schizophrenia and bipolar disorder susceptibility. Mol Psychiatry 16, 286–292.

O'Roak, B.J., Deriziotis, P., Lee, C., Vives, L., Schwartz, J.J., Girirajan, S., Karakoc, E., Mackenzie, A.P., Ng, S.B., Baker, C., et al. (2011). Exome sequencing in sporadic autism spectrum disorders identifies severe de novo mutations. Nat Genet 43, 585–589.

O'Roak, B.J., Vives, L., Girirajan, S., Karakoc, E., Krumm, N., Coe, B.P., Levy, R., Ko, A., Lee, C., Smith, J.D., et al. (2012). Sporadic autism exomes reveal a highly interconnected protein network of de novo mutations. Nature 485, 246–250.

Owen, M.J. (2012). Implications of genetic findings for understanding schizophrenia. Schizophr Bull 38, 904–907.

Pasca, S.P., Portmann, T., Voineagu, I., Yazawa, M., Shcheglovitov, A., Pasca, A.M., Cord, B., Palmer, T.D., Chikahisa, S., Nishino, S., et al. (2011). Using iPSC-derived neurons to uncover cellular phenotypes associated with Timothy syndrome. Nat Med 17, 1657–1662.

Penrose, L.S. (1938). A Clinical and Genetic Study of 1280 Cases of Mental Defect. London.

Pinel, P. (1801). Traité médico-philosophique sur l'aliénation mentale ou La manie. Paris: Richard, Caille et Ravier.

Pinto, D., Pagnamenta, A.T., Klei, L., Anney, R., Merico, D., Regan, R., Conroy, J., Magalhaes, T.R., Correia, C., Abrahams, B.S., et al. (2010). Functional impact of global rare copy number variation in autism spectrum disorders. Nature 466, 368–372.

Piven, J., Palmer, P., Jacobi, D., Childress, D., and Arndt, S. (1997). Broader autism phenotype: evidence from a family history study of multiple-incidence autism families. Am J Psychiatry 154, 185–190.

Psychiatric GWAS Consortium Bipolar Disorder Working Group. (2011). Large-scale genome-wide association analysis of bipolar disorder identifies a new susceptibility locus near ODZ4. Nat Genet 43, 977–983.

Qin, P., Xu, H., Laursen, T.M., Vestergaard, M., and Mortensen, P.B. (2005). Risk for schizophrenia and schizophrenia-like psychosis among patients with epilepsy: population based cohort study. BMJ 331, 23.

Ramanan, V.K., Shen, L., Moore, J.H., and Saykin, A.J. (2012). Pathway analysis of genomic data: concepts, methods, and prospects for future development. Trends Genet 28, 323–332.

Reiss, A.L. (2009). Childhood developmental disorders: an academic and clinical convergence point for psychiatry, neurology, psychology and pediatrics. J Child Psychol Psychiatry 50, 87–98.

Remington, J.S., Klein, J.O., Wilson, G.B., Baker, C.J. (2006). Infectious Diseases of the Fetus and Newborn Infant. Philadelphia: Elsevier Saunders.

Rommelse, N.N., Altink, M.E., Fliers, E.A., Martin, N.C., Buschgens, C.J., Hartman, C.A., Buitelaar, J.K., Faraone, S.V., Sergeant, J.A., and Oosterlaan, J. (2009). Comorbid problems in ADHD: degree of association, shared endophenotypes, and formation of distinct subtypes. Implications for a future DSM. J Abnorm Child Psychol 37, 793–804.

Ronald, A., Simonoff, E., Kuntsi, J., Asherson, P., and Plomin, R. (2008). Evidence for overlapping genetic influences on autistic and ADHD behaviours in a community twin sample. J Child Psychol Psychiatry 49,535–542.

Roth, C., Magnus, P., Schjolberg, S., Stoltenberg, C., Suren, P., McKeague, I.W., Davey Smith, G., Reichborn-Kjennerud, T., and Susser, E. (2011). Folic acid supplements in pregnancy and severe language delay in children. JAMA 306, 1566–1573.

Sanders, S.J., Murtha, M.T., Gupta, A.R., Murdoch, J.D., Raubeson, M.J., Willsey, A.J., Ercan-Sencicek, A.G., DiLullo, N.M., Parikshak, N.N., Stein, J.L., et al. (2012). De novo mutations revealed by whole-exome sequencing are strongly associated with autism. Nature 485, 237–241.

Schizophrenia Psychiatric Genome-Wide Association Study (GWAS) Consortium. (2011). Genome-wide association study identifies five new schizophrenia loci. Nat Genet 43, 969–976.

Shenton, M.E., Whitford, T.J., and Kubicki, M. (2010). Structural neuroimaging in schizophrenia: from methods to insights to treatments. Dialogues Clin Neurosci 12, 317–332.

Spence, S.J., and Schneider, M.T. (2009). The role of epilepsy and epileptiform EEGs in autism spectrum disorders. Pediatr Res 65, 599–560.

Splawski, I., Timothy, K.W., Sharpe, L.M., Decher, N., Kumar, P., Bloise, R., Napolitano, C., Schwartz, P.J., Joseph, R.M., Condouris, K., et al. (2004). Ca(V)1.2 calcium channel dysfunction causes a multisystem disorder including arrhythmia and autism. Cell 119, 19–31.

Sprich, S., Biederman, J., Crawford, M.H., Mundy, E., Faraone, S.V. (2000). Adoptive and biological families of children and adolescents with ADHD. J Am Acad Child Adolesc Psychiatry 39, 1432–1437.

St Clair, D., Blackwood, D., Muir, W., Carothers, A., Walker, M., Spowart, G., Gosden, C., and Evans, H.J. (1990). Association within a family of a balanced autosomal translocation with major mental illness. Lancet 336, 13–16.

St Clair, D., Xu, M., Wang, P., Yu, Y., Fang, Y., Zhang, F., Zheng, X., Gu, N., Feng, G., Sham, P., et al. (2005). Rates of adult schizophrenia following prenatal exposure to the Chinese famine of 1959–1961. JAMA 294, 557–562.

Steinberg, S., de Jong, S., Andreassen, O.A., Werge, T., Borglum, A.D., Mors, O., Mortensen, P.B., Gustafsson, O., Costas, J., Pietilainen, O.P., et al. (2011a). Common variants at VRK2 and TCF4 conferring risk of schizophrenia. Hum Mol Genet 20, 4076–4081.

Steinberg, S., Mors, O., Borglum, A.D., Gustafsson, O., Werge, T., Mortensen, P.B., Andreassen, O.A., Sigurdsson, E., Thorgeirsson, T.E., Bottcher, Y., et al. (2011b). Expanding the range of ZNF804A variants conferring risk of psychosis. Mol Psychiatry 16, 59–66.

Stergiakouli, E., Hamshere, M., Holmans, P., Langley, K., Zaharieva, I., Hawi, Z., Kent, L., Gill, M., Williams, N., Owen, M.J., et al. (2012). Investigating the contribution of common genetic variants to the risk and pathogenesis of ADHD. Am J Psychiatry 169, 186–194.

Still, G.F. (1902). Some abnormal psychical conditions in children: the Goulstonian lectures. Lancet 1, 1008–1012.

Sullivan, P.F., Daly, M.J., O'Donovan, M. (2012a). Genetic architectures of psychiatric disorders: the emerging picture and its implications. Nat Rev Genet 13, 537–551.

Sullivan, P.F., Magnusson, C., Reichenberg, A., Boman, M., Dalman, C., Davidson, M., Fruchter, E., Hultman, C.M., Lundberg, M., Langstrom, N., et al. (2012b). Family history of schizophrenia and bipolar disorder as risk factors for autism. Arch Gen Psychiatry 69, 1099–1103.

Suren, P., Roth, C., Bresnahan, M., Haugen, M., Hornig, M., Hirtz, D., Lie, K.K., Lipkin, W.I., Magnus, P., Reichborn-Kjennerud, T., et al. (2013). Association between maternal use of folic acid supplements and risk of autism spectrum disorders in children. JAMA 309, 570–577.

Susser, E.S., and Lin, S.P. (1992). Schizophrenia after prenatal exposure to the Dutch Hunger Winter of 1944–1945. Arch Gen Psychiatry 49, 983–988.

Voineagu, I., Wang, X., Johnston, P., Lowe, J.K., Tian, Y., Horvath, S., Mill, J., Cantor, R.M., Blencowe, B.J., and Geschwind, D.H. (2011). Transcriptomic analysis of autistic brain reveals convergent molecular pathology. Nature 474, 380–384.

Wang, K., Zhang, H., Ma, D., Bucan, M., Glessner, J.T., Abrahams, B.S., Salyakina, D., Imielinski, M., Bradfield, J.P., Sleiman, P.M., et al. (2009). Common genetic variants on 5p14.1 associate with autism spectrum disorders. Nature 459, 528–533.

Weikard M.A. (1775). Der Philosophische Arzt. Frankfurt.

Whitaker, S., Read, S. (2006). The prevalence of psychiatric disorders among people with intellectual disabilities: An analysis of the literature. J Appl ResIntellect Disabil 19, 330–345.

Willcutt, E.G., Pennington, B.F., Chhabildas, N.A., Friedman, M.C., and Alexander, J. (1999). Psychiatric comorbidity associated with DSM-IV ADHD in a nonreferred sample of twins. J Am Acad Child Adolesc Psychiatry 38, 1355–1362.

Xu, B., Ionita-Laza, I., Roos, J.L., Boone, B., Woodrick, S., Sun, Y., Levy, S., Gogos, J.A., and Karayiorgou, M. (2012). De novo gene mutations highlight patterns of genetic and neural complexity in schizophrenia. Nat Genet 44, 1365–1369.

Yeargin-Allsopp, M. (2008). The prevalence and characteristics of autism spectrum disorders in the ALSPAC cohort. Dev Med Child Neurol 50, 646.

Yu, T.W., Chahrour, M.H., Coulter, M.E., Jiralerspong, S., Okamura-Ikeda, K., Ataman, B., Schmitz-Abe, K., Harmin, D.A., Adli, M., Malik, A.N., et al. (2013). Using whole-exome sequencing to identify inherited causes of autism. Neuron 77, 259–273.

Zigler, E. (1967). Familial mental retardation: a continuing dilemma. Science 155, 292–298.

3

THE MUTATIONAL SPECTRUM OF NEURODEVELOPMENTAL DISORDERS

Nancy D. Merner,[1,2] Patrick A. Dion,[3,4] and Guy A. Rouleau[4]

[1]CHUM Research Center, Université de Montréal, Montréal, Québec, Canada
[2]Department of Drug Discovery and Development, Harrison School of Pharmacy, Auburn University, Auburn, AL, USA
[3]Department of Pathology and Cellular Biology, Université de Montréal, Montréal, Québec, Canada
[4]Montreal Neurological Institute, McGill University, Montréal, Québec Canada

3.1 INTRODUCTION

Neurodevelopmental disorder is an umbrella term that groups together a wide range of diseases, all of which involve the impaired growth and development of the brain, and are typically associated with cognitive, neurological, or psychiatric dysfunction. Common disorders such as intellectual disability (ID), autism spectrum disorder (ASD), schizophrenia, and epilepsy belong to that group of diseases; and, even though each one has its own clinical definition, some of their clinical and genetic underpinnings strongly overlap (Coe et al., 2012; Mitchell, 2011). The mutations causing or increasing risk to such diseases appear to affect a broad range of cellular mechanisms (regulation of gene expression, splicing, protein localization/translation/turnover, synaptic transmission, cell signaling, maintenance of the cytoskeleton architecture, and cell adhesion), which are believed to converge at some point during the development of the nervous system and disrupt the structure, function, and/or plasticity of neuronal networks (Pescosolido et al., 2012). Overall, the genetic architecture of these neurodevelopmental disorders is complex and has been considered an enigma for many years. This chapter will discuss our current knowledge of the neurodevelopmental mutational spectrum. It will first touch on the initial insights that were gathered from chromosomal analyses and the detection of copy number variants (CNVs), both inherited and *de novo*, and how our knowledge

The Genetics of Neurodevelopmental Disorders, First Edition. Edited by Kevin J. Mitchell.
© 2015 John Wiley & Sons, Inc. Published 2015 by John Wiley & Sons, Inc.

has expanded with advances in technology. A discussion of rare sequence variations will then follow, which will begin with the exploration of the X chromosome due to the early observations that males are significantly more affected than females. How neurodevelopmental disorders can be attributed to recessive and dominant variants is also discussed as well as how the discovery of such variants has been revolutionized by recent sequencing technology advances, which facilitated the detection of an extremely important cause of neurodevelopmental disorders, *de novo* mutations. Furthermore, it will also be acknowledged how these new sequencing technologies have given us insight on rates of mutation, paternal effects, and evolution. Finally, this chapter will close with a comparison of the two major theories of genetic causes of neurodevelopmental disorders, the common disease/common variant (CD/CV) and the common disease/rare variant (CD/RV) theories, with the evidence that has been gathered to support or refute each theory.

3.2 RARE CNVs CONTRIBUTE TO RISK OF NEURODEVELOPMENTAL DISORDERS

A CNV is a deletion or duplication of a stretch of DNA as compared to the human reference genome (Fig. 3.1a). These types of variations can involve an entire chromosome (in the case of trisomies or monosomies), or they can range in size from a kilobase (Kb) to megabases (Mb), for which, one or several genes can be affected. The human genome is deemed to be relatively tolerant to CNVs; in fact, any individual genome has a number of common CNVs, which are generally considered benign (Redon et al., 2006; Sebat et al., 2004). However, rare CNVs have been identified as risk factors for neurodevelopmental disorders. In the case of ID, some were reported over 40 years ago when trisomy 21 was established to cause Down's syndrome in 1959 (Lejeune et al., 1959). Advances in cytogenetic chromosome-banding technologies

led to the recognition that individuals with the same syndromic form of ID had deletions in the same chromosomal regions, for instance, Prader–Willi syndrome (deletion of 15q11-q13) (Butler et al., 1986), Smith–Magenis syndrome (deletion of 17p12) (Smith et al., 1986) and Williams-Beuren syndrome (deletion of 7q11.23) (Perez Jurado et al., 1996). Furthermore, by using fluorescence *in-situ* hybridization (FISH), and more recently comparative genomic hybridization (CGH) arrays, the most common causes of moderate to severe ID in individuals who are not diagnosed with a recognizable syndrome, have now been determined to be subtelomeric deletions and duplications (Ballif et al., 2007; Knight et al., 1999; Ravnan et al., 2006). Since the development of CGH arrays and SNP genotyping assays (which provides a much higher resolution than cytogenetic techniques), the diagnostic yield of CNV detection in ID cases is at least twofold higher (de Vries et al., 2005), and it has led to novel discoveries such as the identification of the microdeletion 17q21.31 as a cause of ID (Koolen et al., 2006; Sharp et al., 2006; Shaw-Smith et al., 2006).

A thorough review written by Christopher Gillberg in 1998 compiled all the preliminary reports of chromosomal anomalies in ASD; strikingly, all but two chromosomes (chromosomes 14 and 20) were reported to have some type of abnormality (Gillberg, 1998). Gillberg noted that the genes on chromosome 15, as well as the sex chromosomes, must play an important role in autism due to the shared number of anomalies recorded; specifically, he acknowledged that duplications of 15q11-13 were commonly reported in ASD cases (Gillberg, 1998). It is currently recognized that 1–3% of individuals with ASD have a maternal duplication of this region (Hogart et al., 2010), and overall it is deemed that approximately 5% of ASD cases have cytogenetic rearrangements (Folstein and Rosen-Sheidley, 2001; Jacquemont et al., 2006). Furthermore, ASD cases have been recognized to carry a higher global burden of rare genic CNVs compared to controls (1.19-fold increase), and when considering loci previously implicated in either ASD and/or ID, the burden was even more apparent (1.69-fold increase) (Pinto et al., 2010).

Rare recurrent CNVs have been associated with a range of neurodevelopmental phenotypic features and severity. For instance, microdeletions of chromosome 1q21.1 have been associated with ID cases that manifest various degrees of severity, with some affected individuals presenting additional congenital anomalies such as cataracts and congenital heart disease (Brunetti-Pierri et al., 2008; Christiansen et al., 2004; Mefford et al., 2008). Interestingly, this microdeletion is often reported to have been inherited from an unaffected or a mildly affected parent. Moreover, this microdeletion has also been reported to be a risk factor in schizophrenia (International-Schizophrenia-Consortium, 2008; Stefansson et al., 2008); it appears to be a rare, recurrent risk variant that has occurred independently in multiple founders and is subject to negative selection (Stefansson et al., 2008). Interesting as well, is the fact that duplications of the same region have also been associated with mild to moderate ID and ASD (Brunetti-Pierri et al., 2008; Mefford et al., 2008). CNVs at chromosome 16p13.11 provide another excellent example of the underlying diversity of clinical presentation that this form of genetic variation can be associated with. Deletions of this chromosomal region have been associated with ID and ASD (Ullmann et al., 2007) as well as epilepsy (de Kovel et al., 2010; Heinzen et al., 2010), and duplications have been associated with ID (Mefford et al., 2009; Ullmann et al., 2007), ASD (Ullmann et al., 2007), and schizophrenia (Kirov et al., 2009). Overall, such instances reinforce the fundamental link between the various neurodevelopmental disorders.

For decades, the cytogenetic community has recorded the presence of *de novo* CNVs in neurodevelopmental disorders (Fig. 3.1a and c). For instance, in 1992, by karyotyping a boy who was diagnosed with autism and moderate mental retardation as well as his unaffected parents, a complex chromosome rearrangement (a translocation of portions of chromosome 1p22 and 7q onto chromosome 21q) was detected in the boy, while his parents were determined to have normal karyotypes (Lopreiato and Wulfsberg, 1992). Another early example was published in 1994, when a 13-year old autistic boy was determined to have a deletion of chromosome 17p11.2 that was not present in his parents (Vostanis et al., 1994). It was not, however, until the more recent introduction of array technologies that their true significance was recognized – *de novo* CNVs have been significantly associated with autism and schizophrenia, and are particularly more frequent in sporadic cases (International-Schizophrenia-Consortium, 2008; Sanders et al., 2011; Sebat et al., 2007; Stefansson et al., 2008; Xu et al., 2008). *De novo* CNVs larger than 100 kb are not common in the general population with a predicted mutation rate of $\mu = 1.2 \times 10^{-2}$ CNVs per genome per transmission (Itsara et al., 2010); however, they are observed in approximately 10% of patients with sporadic schizophrenia (Xu et al., 2008), autism (Marshall et al., 2008; Sebat et al., 2007), and ID (Koolen et al., 2009; Vissers et al., 2010b). Furthermore, two or more of these *de novo* events have been detected in affected individuals (Marshall et al., 2008). Interesting as well, large *de novo* CNVs are found more frequently in females affected with ASD compared to affected males (11.7% and 7.4%, respectively). Considering that there is a strong gender bias, with a much higher incidence of ASD in males than in females, and large *de novo* CNVs generally comprise more genes and are more harmful, this observation suggests that females have more resistance to genetic causes of autism, and perhaps there are fewer target genes that trigger ASDs in females compared to males (Levy et al., 2011). Many *de novo* CNVs are detected exclusively in patients, which is a strong argument toward pathogenicity. *De novo* mutations represent the most extreme type of rare mutations, and in general, are more deleterious than inherited variations because they have not been subject to evolutionary selection (Veltman and

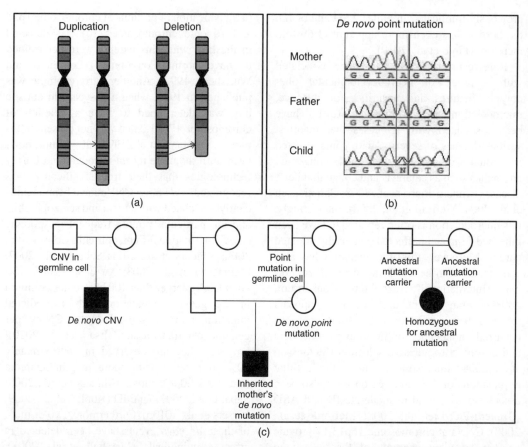

Fig. 3.1 *Overview of genetic causes of neurodevelopmental disorders.* (a) Examples of CNVs, (b) Sequence traces of DNA extracted from blood cells that detect a *de novo* mutation in the affected child of this trio, (c) Different circumstances where genetic mutations (that increase risk of a neurodevelopmental disorder) are introduced into or segregate in a pedigree. *(See insert for color representation of this figure.)*

Brunner, 2012). These facts are being considered when assessing their interpretation in disease diagnosis (Koolen et al., 2009). Additionally, when rare *de novo* CNVs in autism were grouped together to be studied using a method referred to as network-based analysis of genetic associations (NETBAG), which enabled its authors to identify a large biological network of autism genes, the network revealed itself to be related to synapse development, axon targeting, and neuron motility (Gilman et al., 2011). Such an enrichment of CNVs affecting neuronal synaptic genes had been previously proposed by others (Marshall et al., 2008).

3.3 RARE CODING VARIANTS IN SINGLE GENES THAT CAUSE NEURODEVELOPMENTAL DISORDERS

3.3.1 The Identification of X-linked Genes

The observations that ID is significantly more common in males than in females, and that it segregates in many families with an X-linked pattern, provided some of the first compelling evidence that X-linked gene defects make an important contribution to the causation of ID (Lehrke, 1972; Lehrke, 1974). Currently, X-linked ID (XLID) accounts for 5–10% of intellectual disability in males, and mutations in over 100 X-linked genes have been associated with at least 80 XLID syndromes and 35 nonsyndromic forms of XLID (Lubs et al., 2012). Additionally, approximately 30 XLID syndromes and 45 families with nonsyndromic XLID have been regionally mapped to the X chromosome but no causative gene has yet been identified. Furthermore, over 40 ID syndromes with suspected X-linked inheritance remain to be genetically mapped. To put all this in perspective, less than 400 autosomal ID genes have been identified (Lubs et al., 2012), thus this striking number of X-linked ID genes has been suggested to be the result of the relative concentration of genes that influence intelligence on the X chromosome (Gecz et al., 2009). However, this observation could also be due to the fact that recessive alleles are much more recognizable on the X chromosome, whereas on autosomes the effects of such alleles are often the result of inbreeding.

The first report of ID being linked to the X chromosome was made in 1969 (Lubs, 1969), and the discovery of the first X-linked ID gene was made in 1983 when *HPRT* mutations were determined to cause the Lesch–Nyhan syndrome (Jolly et al., 1983). Despite the early advances made using cytogenetic approaches, only a little over 30 genes were identified through cytogenetics. The combination of family-based linkage studies and screening of candidate genes subsequently proved to be a more productive approach for the discovery of ID X-linked genes; the increasing ease of sequencing accelerated the pace of X-linked gene identification by this route after 2003 (Lubs et al., 2012).

Similarly to ID, and as mentioned earlier, there is an excess of males diagnosed with autism in comparison to females. This excess is estimated to be fourfold (Skuse, 2000). However, identifying genes on the X chromosomes that increase risk to autism has not been so rewarding. The first hints toward the involvement of X chromosome genes in autism came from a cytogenetic study that reported *de novo* chromosomal deletions at Xp22.3 in three autistic individuals (recognized as the first X-linked autism susceptibility locus – *AUTSX1*

[OMIM 300425]) (Thomas et al., 1999), and two independent genome scans that demonstrated increased allele sharing for markers at Xq13-q21 in affected sib-pairs (*AUTSX2*) [OMIM: 300495] (Auranen et al., 2002; Shao et al., 2002). This was followed by the identification of mutations in *neuroligin 3* (*NLGN3*) [OMIM 300336] and *neuroligin 4* (*NLGN4*) [OMIM 300427] in autistic siblings in 2003 (Jamain et al., 2003). Interestingly, *NLGN3* is located at Xq13 within *AUTSX2*, and *NLGN4* is within the Xp22.3 deleted interval (*AUTSX1*). Unfortunately, these appear to be rare causes of autism since screening efforts in additional cohorts did not detect additional mutations (Blasi et al., 2006; Gauthier et al., 2005; Vincent et al., 2004; Ylisaukko-oja et al., 2005). Rare mutations that increase risk to autism have, however, been identified in other X chromosome genes including *RPL10* (*AUTSX5*) [OMIM 300847] (Klauck et al., 2006) and *TMLHE* (*AUTSX6*) [OMIM 300872] (Celestino-Soper et al., 2011); additionally, mutations have been detected in genes such as *MECP2* [OMIM 300005] (Lam et al., 2000) and *SLC6A8* [OMIM 300036] (Salomons et al., 2001) that cause both ID and autism. Overall, through this example, it is important to acknowledge that the different biological and environmental factors that underlie the sex differences in autism remain unclear. Noteworthy, from another genetic standpoint, even male-biased penetrance of autosomal genes has been reported (Tropeano et al., 2013).

3.3.2 The Contribution of Recessive Variants

Despite the genetic complexity of neurodevelopmental disorders, things can be simplified when studying consanguineous families and/or isolated populations where all affected individuals may share the same ancestral mutation(s) (Fig. 3.1c). Of course, such cases are rare and identifying such families is difficult. However, once identified, such families often lead to the discoveries of autosomal recessive forms of disease-causative genes through a homozygosity mapping approach. In 2002, the first autosomal recessive nonsyndromic mental retardation locus (*MRT1* [OMIM 249500]) and causative gene was identified using such an approach (Molinari et al., 2002). A homozygous truncating mutation in *PRSS12* [OMIM 606709] encoding neurotrypsin, a secreted protein that functions in synapse maturation and neural plasticity, was determine to be the cause of nonsyndromic ID in a consanguineous Algerian family. Four affected (all with cognitive impairment and an IQ below 50) and four unaffected children who were born to first cousin parents were investigated. A genome-wide screen that used 400 microsatellite markers identified only one region of shared homozygosity between the four affected siblings on chromosome 4q24–q25. Fine mapping reduced the genetic interval to a 14 Mb region between markers *D4S1570* and *D4S1575* (Z max = 3.33, at $\theta = 0$ at *D4S407* locus), which encompassed 29 genes of known function. *PRSS12*, was selected as one of the best positional and functional candidate genes, and, after screening, a homozygous four base pair (bp) deletion in exon 7 that resulted in a frameshift and a premature stop codon 147 nucleotides downstream of the deletion, was detected in the affected children. The parents were heterozygous for the deletion (Molinari et al., 2002). To date, at least 30 different MRT loci have been identified using similar approaches, and the causative gene identified in 12 of these loci (OMIM®, 2013).

Segregation analyses have traditionally supported a role for autosomal recessive genes in ASD (Ritvo et al., 1985). A large-scale autism homozygosity mapping project that was undertaken in 2008 used 104 consanguineous families in order to identify recessive loci and genes in ASDs (Morrow et al., 2008). Morrow et al. showed that individuals with related parents are more likely to have inherited causes of autism (which are most likely autosomal and recessive), and suggested that such families can provide linkage evidence when in pursuit to identify mutant genes. Runs of homozygosity (ROH) were identified in a number of families, indicating that potential autism loci were identified in this study; however, the authors stated that the large size of the linked loci prohibited

systematic gene sequencing, thus such variants remain to be identified. However, through CNV analysis, large, inherited, homozygous deletions were detected in some of the identified loci that authors suggested were likely mutations (Morrow et al., 2008). On a different note, additional support for a recessive model in autism was highlighted in an early genome-wide linkage analysis, in which a significant maximum multipoint heterogeneity LOD score of 3.0 was obtained for a marker on chromosome 13 (*D13S800*) under the recessive model; this study examined 75 affected sib-pairs that were collected by the Collaborative Linkage Study of Autism (Barrett et al., 1999). More recent studies have used exome sequencing to investigate recessive genetic causes of autism (Lim et al., 2013; Yu et al., 2013). Yu et al. studied a cohort of consanguineous families and were able to identify several causative recessive mutations. In fact, many of the mutations identified represented partial loss of function in genes where null mutations cause distinctive Mendelian disorders, such as *AMT* [OMIM 238310], *PEX7* [OMIM 601757], and so on (Yu et al., 2013). Lim et al. used exome sequencing data of 933 cases and 869 controls to identify genes with homozygous or compound heterozygous loss-of-function variants. In autosomal genes with low rates of loss-of-function variation ($\leq$ 5% frequency), the authors reported a 2-fold increase in complete knockouts in cases, and estimated these events to contribute to 3% of ASD risk (Lim et al., 2013).

A recessive model has also been suggested to be liable for some cases of genetic susceptibility of schizophrenia. For instance, using a whole-genome homozygosity association methodology, a set of nine ROHs have been determined to be significantly more common in schizophrenia cases than in controls (Lencz et al., 2007). Interestingly, four of the nine "risk ROHs" contained or neighbored genes previously associated with schizophrenia. Moreover, several of these risk ROHs were extremely rare in healthy individuals, suggesting that relatively high penetrance, recessive effects may explain a fraction of the genetic burden for schizophrenia (Lencz et al., 2007). More recent publications further discuss the genetic architecture of schizophrenia and provide evidence that recessively acting variants contribute to the risk of the disease (Curtis, 2013; Mitchell and Porteous, 2011).

3.3.3 Autosomal Dominant Inheritance

When trying to identify highly penetrant autosomal dominant variants that cause or increase risk to neurodevelopmental disorders, one of the greatest hurdles has been the genetic and clinical heterogeneity. The easiest way around this was to focus on a particular endophenotype (e.g., syndromic forms of ID) under which affected individuals could be grouped together and analyzed based on dysmorphic features that are shared and distinct. A successful example of this approach was the identification of *ZEB2* [OMIM 605802] mutations causing Mowat–Wilson syndrome [OMIM 235730], a unique form of Hirschsprung disease (Wakamatsu et al., 2001). In 2001, Nagaya and his colleagues had collected more than 200 individuals diagnosed with Hirschsprung disease but among them, five cases presented similar and unique clinical features including microcephaly, mental retardation, epilepsy and characteristic facial features. They were thus grouped together for gene discovery efforts assuming genetic homogeneity. One of the cases was determined to have a 5 Mb cytogenetic deletion on 2q22, flanked by *D2S129* and *D2S151*. Considering that deleted interval as the disease region, positional gene screening was carried out in the four remaining affected individuals. Two nonsense mutations and a 4-bp deletion were detected in the *ZEB2* gene in three of the patients. One patient did not have a coding variant in this gene, thus the authors suggested that a noncoding *ZEB2* variant could be the cause of disease or another gene. All detected *ZEB2* mutations were *de novo*.

It is also important to consider that in severe cases of neurodevelopmental disorders, autosomal dominant pedigrees are unlikely to appear in the population since the causative mutation will most likely be reproductive lethal. The prevalence of autosomal dominant diseased genes is therefore dependent on the new mutation rate. Thus, genes that cause autosomal dominant forms of neurodevelopmental disorders should have high rates of *de novo* mutations that give rise to "sporadic" cases of disease (Fig. 3.1b and c). This was in fact demonstrated in the aforementioned example of *de novo ZEB2* mutations causing Mowat–Wilson syndrome.

Currently, we are observing a rapid change of focus in *de novo* variant research. Cytogenetically detectable chromosomal anomalies were the first recognized form of *de novo* variants, then, with the introduction of array technologies, smaller *de novo* CNVs called microdeletions and duplications could be identified. More recently, the appearance of high-throughput sequencing platforms that are able to generate whole-exome or whole-genome unbiased sequence information, has made it relatively "easy" to detect *de novo* SNVs (single nucleotide variants) by screening affected individuals and their unaffected parents (Veltman and Brunner, 2012). Exome sequencing has been successful in identifying rare *de novo* mutations for rare syndromic forms of ID, including *SETBP1* [OMIM 611060] mutations that cause Schinzel–Giedion syndrome [OMIM 269150] (Hoischen et al., 2010), *MLL2* [OMIM 602113] mutations that cause Kabuki syndrome [OMIM 147920] (Ng et al., 2010), as well as mutations in *ASXL1* [OMIM 612990] that cause Bohring–Opitz syndrome [OMIM 605039] (Hoischen et al., 2011). Additionally, *de novo* mutations in *ANKRD11* [OMIM 611192] have been determined to cause KBG syndrome [OMIM 148050] through exome sequencing (Sirmaci et al., 2011). Interestingly, KBG syndrome can be mild and, in this form, has been reported to segregate in families. Sirmaci et al. also described an *ANKRD11* variant that segregated with the disease in an affected family. This observation highlights the importance of the fitness effect of specific mutations – in this case, the mutation was not reproductively lethal (had a higher fitness effect) thus an autosomal dominant pedigree was identified.

Thus, the proportion of cases (for a particular autosomal disorder) that are due to *de novo* mutations is higher when the mutations have a strong negative effect on fitness. Furthermore, *de novo* mutations in two genes, *ACTB* [OMIM 102630] and *ACTG1* [OMIM 102560], have been reported to cause Baraitser-Winter syndrome (Riviere et al., 2012), and *de novo* mutations in six genes that encode SWI/SNF subunits were determined to cause Coffin–Siris syndrome (Santen et al., 2012; Tsurusaki et al., 2012). These discoveries are great examples of the effect of mutational target size and disease frequency. Diseases that are caused by *de novo* mutations in a number of genes are more frequent in the population than diseases that have a small mutational target size (when only one gene is involved). Schinzel–Giedion syndrome represents an extreme example of small target size, where *de novo* mutations cluster in a stretch of only 11 nucleotides (Hoischen et al., 2010); consequently it is an extremely rare syndrome.

The genetic heterogeneity of the more common neurodevelopmental disorders has made grouping such cases for genetic analysis a less likely successful approach of gene discovery. Since the late 1990s, numerous teams assembled cohorts containing thousands of such cases (and their relatives) to conduct genome-wide linkage analyses and identify novel susceptibility genes. The first genome-wide search for autism susceptibility loci was performed on 87 affected sib-pairs and 12 non-sib affected relative-pairs, from families identified by an international consortium, which reported one significant signal. Using a subset of 56 affected UK sib-pairs, a maximum multipoint lod score (MLS) of 3.55 was obtained on a region of chromosome 7q near markers *D7S530* and *D7S684*, and an MLS of 2.53 was obtained when all 87 affected sib-pairs were considered (International-Molecular-Genetic-Study-of-Autism-Consortium, 1998). It should, however, be pointed out that two of the following published genome-wide scans failed to establish genome-wide significant lod scores for any of these previously identified loci (Philippe et al., 1999; Risch et al., 1999); an indication of the genetic heterogeneity likely

underlying autism. As this form of studies progressed, several other loci were replicated in a significant manner (e.g., 2q, 5, 7q, 15q, and 16p) (Li et al., 2012); although the identity of the autism genes located within these loci still remains to be established.

Identifying *de novo* SNVs that increase risk of disease is a way to overcome autosomal dominant gene identification barriers for common neurodevelopmental disorders (Fig. 3.1b and c). The *de novo* model of complex neurodevelopmental genetic disease entails the search for single variants of large effect, which essentially considers these disorders monogenic. Although, of course, it is important to note that the phenotype displayed by a particular variant is influenced by an individual's genetic background. The extreme genetic heterogeneity of the common neurodevelopmental disorders has, however, hindered the identification of causative *de novo* SNVs; both the detection and functional interpretation of these variants has been complicated. Before exome sequencing eased the identification of such variants, the Rouleau laboratory initiated a project entitled Synapse to Disease (S2D) in order to identify genes that cause or predispose to numerous disorders of brain development (including schizophrenia, autism, and ID) based on two main hypotheses: 1) that disorders of brain development are often the result of *de novo* SNVs and 2) that these new mutations take place in genes involved in the synapse. One of the first tasks of the S2D team was to review the literature in order to identify the genes that play a role at the synapse; approximately 5,000 genes were found to meet the criteria for "synapticity." Ultimately, 401 of those synaptic genes were selected and screened for mutations through Sanger sequencing.

The first gene identification publication that came out of the S2D project reported the novel discovery of *de novo* *SYNGAP1* [OMIM 603384] mutations that cause nonsyndromic ID (Hamdan et al., 2009). After sequencing *SYNGAP1*, which encodes a ras GTPase-activating protein that is critical for cognition and synapse function, in 94 individuals with nonsyndromic mental retardation, three *de novo* truncating mutations were detected in three patients. By contrast, no *de novo* or truncating mutations were detected in 190 control individuals nor 142 individuals with ASD and 143 individuals with schizophrenia (Hamdan et al., 2009). Furthermore, after screening *SHANK3* [OMIM 606230] in 285 controls and 185 schizophrenia patients with unaffected parents, two *de novo* mutations (a nonsense and a missense) were identified (Gauthier et al., 2010). The *de novo* nonsense mutation was found in three affected brothers, who account for the only children the parents had, which suggests a germ-line mosaicism. Mutations in *SHANK3* had previously been reported in autism (Durand et al., 2007), thus this discovery demonstrated a molecular genetic link between these two neurodevelopmental disorders. In another publication, after the systematic screening of the 401 selected synaptic genes, all the *de novo* SNVs that were detected in 142 individuals with ASD and 143 individuals with schizophrenia were reported (Awadalla et al., 2010), which represented the first reported large-scale sequencing study to evaluate the role of *de novo* mutations in ASD and schizophrenia. Overall, 14 *de novo* SNVs were identified, implicating genes such as *SHANK3*, *IL1RAPL1* [OMIM 300206], and *NRXN1* [OMIM 600565] in these disorders. Of note, eight of the 14 *de novo* variants were missense mutations that were predicted to alter the protein structure or function (Awadalla et al., 2010). A similar report was published for the nonsyndromic ID cohort (Hamdan et al., 2011). After sequencing 197 genes encoding glutamate receptors and a large subset of their known interacting proteins in 95 sporadic cases, 11 *de novo* mutations were detected. This included 10 potentially deleterious mutations (3 nonsense, 2 splicing, 1 frameshift, and 4 missense) and 1 neutral mutation (silent) in 8 different genes. The *de novo* truncating and/or splicing mutations in *SYN-GAP1*, *STXBP1* [OMIM 602926], and *SHANK3* were suggested to be pathogenic based on the mutation type. Functional studies were carried out on the missense mutations found in *KIF1A* [OMIM 601255], *GRIN1* [OMIM 138249], *CACNG2* [OMIM 602911], and *EPB41L1*

[OMIM 602879] and the results suggest that they may be pathogenic as well. Importantly, none of these mutations or any other *de novo* variant were identified in these synaptic genes in 285 healthy controls. Overall, all of these publications provide support for the theory that severe *de novo* SNVs are involved in the pathogenesis of common neurodevelopmental disorders.

A more unbiased approach to understanding the role of *de novo* SNVs in common neurodevelopmental disorders can be taken using next-generation sequencing. A number of pilot studies were recently carried out in order to more rapidly screen for such variations; the first publication of this type involved a family-trio exome sequencing approach of 10 individuals with sporadic ID and their unaffected parents (Vissers et al., 2010a). Vissers and colleagues attempted to identify *de novo* variants that increase risk to ID by filtering through the individual exome variant lists and focusing on *de novo* variants that were predicted to be deleterious through bioinformatics analyses and were not detected in controls. Nine nonsynonymous *de novo* variants were detected in seven of the ten ID cases, and two *de novo* nonsense mutations were detected in two previously associated ID genes, *RAB39B* [OMIM 300774] and *SYNGAP1* (Vissers et al., 2010a). Whether the *de novo* nonsynonymous variants are pathogenic remains to be elucidated; however, at least four of these variants are in genes that can affect brain function and/or structure. This small study demonstrated that *de novo* SNVs likely play an important role in nonsyndromic ID.

Similar approaches were taken to study the importance of *de novo* SNVs in sporadic forms of schizophrenia; in fact, back to back papers that were published in the summer of 2011 both provided evidence to support a *de novo* mutation paradigm for schizophrenia. The Rouleau group (Girard et al.) sequenced the exomes of 14 schizophrenia probands and their unaffected parents, and identified 15 *de novo* SNVs in eight probands. It was demonstrated that the rate of *de novo* mutation in this schizophrenia cohort was significantly higher than the general *de novo* mutation rates that were previously reported. Additionally, four of the 15 *de novo* SNVs were nonsense mutations, which was also acknowledged to be more than what is expected to occur by chance (Girard et al., 2011). Ultimately, this publication was one of the first to highlight the likelihood that *de novo* SNVs contribute to the heritability of schizophrenia, and provided a list of potentially disrupted genes that lead to the pathogenesis. Similar and supportive conclusions were gathered by an independent study that determined that there was a large excess of nonsynonymous *de novo* changes in schizophrenia cases compared to rare inherited variants (Xu et al., 2011). Xu et al. set out to examine the possibility that rare *de novo* protein-altering variants contribute to the risk of schizophrenia through exome sequencing. They investigated the exomes of 53 sporadic cases, 22 controls, and their parents, and discovered 40 *de novo* mutations in 27 schizophrenia cases that affected 40 different genes. This list of candidate schizophrenia genes included extremely promising examples, such as *DGCR2* [OMIM 600594], which is located in the microdeletion region 22q11.2 and has already been determined to predispose to schizophrenia. These pilot studies have certainly laid a foundation that rare variants likely predispose to schizophrenia (particularly rare *de novo* mutations as a cause of sporadic forms of the disease) (Girard et al., 2011; Xu et al., 2011), and further investigations continue to draw the same conclusions (Need et al., 2012; Xu et al., 2012).

The impact that *de novo* SNVs have on sporadic forms of ASD has been greatly explored. The first study was carried out by O'Roak et al. who sequenced the exomes of 20 sporadic cases of ASD and their parents (O'Roak et al., 2011). Twenty-one *de novo* variants were reported, 11 of those were protein-altering. The authors highlighted four protein-altering variants and suggested that they had the highest potential to be causative since they were identified in more severely affected individuals and were detected in genes that were all previously associated with neurodevelopmental disorders: *FOXP1* [OMIM 605515], *GRIN2B* [OMIM 138252], *SCN1A*

[OMIM 182389], and *LAMC3* [OMIM 604349]. The conclusions drawn from this preliminary paper were as follows: (1) Family-trio exome sequencing is a powerful way to identify ASD candidate genes, and (2) *de novo* mutations may contribute significantly to the genetic risk of ASD (O'Roak et al., 2011). At least four larger exome sequencing studies quickly followed the publication of the pilot study in order to further investigate the role of rare *de novo* mutations in ASD (Iossifov et al., 2012; Neale et al., 2012; O'Roak et al., 2012b; Sanders et al., 2012). It is, however, to be pointed out that three of those four studies selected their families (affected child with unaffected parents and, in some cases, an unaffected sibling) from the same cohort, the Simon Simplex Collection (SSC), so there is some overlap between these publications. The first and the largest study involved the exome sequencing of 343 families from the SSC cohort; each family had only one child with ASD and at least one unaffected sibling (Iossifov et al., 2012). The authors did not observe a significant difference in the overall number of *de novo* missense mutations in affected versus unaffected children; however, they did observe that nonsense, splice site, and frame shift mutations were twice as frequent in affected individuals. Furthermore, the genes most heavily disrupted by such mutations were associated with the fragile X protein, which was suggested to emphasize the link between autism and synaptic plasticity. Finally and interestingly, the *de novo* mutations detected in this study were determined to be mainly derived from the paternal line in an age-dependent manner (Iossifov et al., 2012). The second ASD exome sequencing publication of O'Roak and colleagues also noticed the same paternal effects, after analyzing the exomes of an additional 189 trios, the 20 trios they originally studied (O'Roak et al., 2011), and 50 unaffected siblings (O'Roak et al., 2012b). Nevertheless, these observations are consistent with the modestly increased risk of ASD for children with older fathers. Sanders et al. also set out to identify the contribution of *de novo* SNVs in ASD (Sanders et al., 2012). They selected 238 families from the SSC cohort, which included 200 phenotypically discordant sibling pairs, and also came to the same conclusion as Iossifov et al., that highly disruptive (nonsense and splice site) *de novo* mutations are associated with ASD, particularly in brain-expressed genes. Additionally, by comparing mutation rates of unaffected individuals at the same locus, the authors were able to demonstrate that, within the same gene, multiple independent *de novo* SNVs among unrelated affected individuals can be an indication of risk alleles and can be a reliable means for identifying ASD genes (Sanders et al., 2012). Neale and colleagues, who were the only group not to use the SSC cohort, studied 175 trios and reported *de novo* missense or nonsense variants in less than 50% of their cases. However, the authors did note a slightly higher mutation rate among affected individuals (compared to previously predicted rates); plus, based on protein–protein interaction screens, the *de novo* variants that were detected in affected individuals, were in genes that showed a high degree of connectivity between themselves and known ASD genes (Neale et al., 2012). Overall, these four larger exome sequencing studies indicated that ASD is very genetically heterogeneous and that spontaneous mutations in a large number of genes can increase risk of disease. The detected number of *de novo* variants per individual differed in each publication. There was a range of 0.77–1.19 and 0.63 and 1.00 *de novo* SNVs identified per affected and unaffected individuals, respectively. These differences can possibly be explained by differences in exome capture assays, sequencing methods, alignment and variant calling software as well as data filtering steps. The rate of *de novo* mutation in affected individuals was consistently higher, however. These observations provide further insight toward the role of rare *de novo* variants in neurodevelopmental disorders, in general, but ultimately, the true interpretation of their role is still in its infancy and will require significant effort to determine their overall effect on phenotype.

3.4 THE RATE OF HUMAN MUTATION, PATERNAL-AGE AFFECT AND EVOLUTION

It has become increasingly easier to estimate the rate of spontaneous mutation (at the nucleotide level) since the introduction of high-throughput sequencing platforms. Recent sequencing data indicates that a newborn's genome, on average, has approximately 60 *de novo* variations (corresponding to an average *de novo* mutation rate of 1.20×10^{-8} per nucleotide per generation) (Kong et al., 2012). That number, however, is influenced by the paternal age at conception. It has been shown that a 20-year old father will transmit, on average, 25 new variations to his child, whereas a 40-year old father will transmit, on average, 65 new variations (Kong et al., 2012); thus, this suggests that a male's germ-line genome will acquire approximately two additional new variants with each additional year of age. Interestingly, the number of *de novo* SNVs transmitted by a mother is approximately 15; a number that is consistent despite age. Currently, it is difficult to precisely determine the effects of all these mutations; they could be individually mild or severe, or, all together, they could have a substantial effect on an individual's health.

It appears that neurodevelopmental disorders, in general, are particularly vulnerable to the paternal-age effect (Saha et al., 2009), a notion that has been further corroborated through the recent ASD exome sequencing projects (Iossifov et al., 2012; O'Roak et al., 2012b). The fact that more genes are expressed in the brain than any other organ, suggests that genes that are important for proper brain function will be affected the most by these deleterious spontaneous mutations (Kondrashov, 2012). More specifically, ASD alone is estimated to have around 300 target loci (Levy et al., 2011). Thus, from an evolutionary perspective, a polygenic mutation-selection balance model best fits neurodevelopmental disorders; which suggests that many loci affect a trait, and the trait's genetic variation increases with the introduction of new, harmful mutations in each generation (Fig. 3.1c). Furthermore, once these rare, fitness-reducing mutations are introduced into the gene pool, it can take a while before they actually work their way out (which, of course, depends on the severity of each new mutation) (Keller and Miller, 2006). This model can explain why so many individuals are affected with debilitating neurodevelopmental disorders despite the efforts of natural selection and its exquisite machinery, which aim to eliminate such mutations.

3.5 THE RARE VERSUS COMMON VARIANT DEBATE FOR NEURODEVELOPMENTAL DISORDERS

The evolutionary theory predicts that disease alleles should be rare. Supporting this notion are recent empirical population genetic data, which demonstrate that selection keeps deleterious variants or fitness-reducing alleles at a low frequency (Lindblad-Toh et al., 2011; Zhu et al., 2011); additionally, many rare familial disorders with simple genetic architectures are known to be caused by rare alleles of large effect that have been identified through traditional gene discovery approaches (OMIM®, 2013). In stating that, rare disease-causing alleles have long been identified to cause syndromic forms of ID (Amir et al., 1999; Kremer et al., 1991) and epilepsy (Escayg et al., 2000; Wallace et al., 1998), which has represented a good model for gene discovery for these rarer neurodevelopmental genetic syndromes. Furthermore, rare deleterious variants are even reported to predispose to more common and complex neurodevelopmental disorders such as autism (Jamain et al., 2003) and schizophrenia (Millar et al., 2000). However, after the 2005 publication of the International Human HapMap Project, which reported that the human genome is structured into general haplotype blocks for which the containing common genetic variants are in linkage disequilibrium (International-Hapmap-Consortium, 2005), association studies became a popular method to study common diseases (Hardy and Singleton, 2009). This was the start to the CD/CV theory;

thus, common, low-risk variants that confer only a small risk of disease were aimed to be identified for many complex disorders, including neurodevelopmental disorders. The CD/CV theory has been put to the test with the growing number of genome-wide association studies (GWASs) that have been conducted for neurodevelopmental disorders; these studies made it possible to statistically compare the frequencies of multiple alleles (single nucleotide polymorphisms or SNPs) across large cohorts of cases and controls.

In 2009, one of the first attempts to study the CD/CV model in schizophrenia, for example, was reported by Purcell et al., where the genotyping of the International Schizophrenia Consortium (ISC) case-control cohort (3,322 cases and 3,587 controls) was carried out using approximately one million SNPs (Purcell et al., 2009). The most associated genotyped SNP ($p = 3.4 \times 10^{-7}$) was located in the first intron of *myosin XVIIIB* (*MYO18B*) on chromosome 22, and the second strongest association comprised more than 450 SNPs on chromosome 6p, which spanned the major histocompatibility complex (MHC). Furthermore, the best imputed SNP that reached genome-wide significance ($p = 4.79 \times 10^{-8}$) was also in the MHC (Purcell et al., 2009). Interestingly, Shi et al. also reported the association of an SNP within the MHC with schizophrenia; however, this significant association was only detectable after a meta-analysis was carried out using the datasets obtained from three different cohorts: the Molecular Genetics of Schizophrenia (MGS), ISC (the same cohort used in the aforementioned study that independently reported an association with MHC SNPs) and SGENE, since the initial GWAS that was performed solely on the MGS case-control samples achieved no genome-wide statistical significance (Shi et al., 2009). Moreover, a third study, which again used overlapping datasets (including the MGS and ISC), as well as 2,663 and 13,498 additional cases and controls, respectively, from eight European locations, reported an association with the MHC after a meta-analysis (Stefansson et al., 2009). This study also reported associations with a marker located upstream of the *neurogranin* gene (*NRGN*) [OMIM 602350] on 11q24.2, and a marker within intron four of *transcription factor 4 (TCF4)* [OMIM 602272] on 18q21.2 (Stefansson et al., 2009). Overall, these GWAS failed to identify a large number of loci strongly associated with schizophrenia. This is an outcome in disagreement with the polygenic CV/CD theory in schizophrenia, but something that is not entirely unexpected given the decreased reproductive fitness associated with this disease; taken together these observations suggest that rare alleles of large to moderate effect increase risk to schizophrenia and undergo negative selection (Svensson et al., 2007) (Craddock et al., 2007; McClellan et al., 2007). In fact, Purcell and colleagues acknowledged that their results do not exclude important contributions of rare variants for schizophrenia (Purcell et al., 2009). Moreover, Need et al. demonstrated that there was actually a lack of statistically significant findings about the risk contribution of common variants in schizophrenia, even moderately (Need et al., 2009); which essentially suggest that no common variants confer risk to schizophrenia. However, some researchers remain convinced that schizophrenia is mainly caused by common alleles that increase risk moderately (Lee et al., 2012). Altogether, the portrait of schizophrenia genetics will likely become clearer as deeper genotyping and/or sequencing studies are conducted on larger cohorts, and when the combined effects of rare and common variants can be efficiently determined. Similarly, the initial GWAS attempts for autism (Wang et al., 2009; Weiss et al., 2009), and epilepsy (Kasperaviciute et al., 2010) had only modest success as well. In fact, the second stage of the Autism Genome Project genome-wide association study, which included 2705 families, did not identify any significant associations upon evaluating the association of over a million SNPs individually and all together (Anney et al., 2012). Therefore, ultimately, it appears that common variants do not account for as much of the heritability of neurodevelopmental disorders as first thought.

3.6 THE EMERGING PORTRAIT

Over the last ten years, significant genetic advances have been made that have provided insight toward the genetic architecture of neurodevelopmental disorders; we now know that this polygenic group of disorders are attributed to rare CNVs as well as common and rare SNVs. The overall picture, however, still remains fairly abstract since it is the combination of these different alleles that affect phenotype, and it will be a challenge to truly determine how risk alleles collectively contribute to disease. Presently, we can learn from the most recent studies and improve on such methods. Studying larger cohorts will give insight to additional common variants that may be associated with disease as well as provide more opportunities to identify additional *de novo* variants at the same locus, which Sanders et al. have already shown can be a great indication of a causative gene. Once a gene (or list of genes) is highlighted as potentially disease causing, target screening larger cohorts can truly identify recurrently mutated genes (O'Roak et al., 2012b). High-throughput sequencing advances hold the key to unlocking the remaining genetic mysteries of neurodevelopmental disorders. Even in its infancy, it has provided so many answers about rates of mutations, paternal-age affect, and the types of genes and mutations that are involved in these disorders. It will be interesting to see what the future has in store.

REFERENCES

Amir, R.E., Van den Veyver, I.B., Wan, M., Tran, C.Q., Francke, U., and Zoghbi, H.Y. (1999). Rett syndrome is caused by mutations in X-linked MECP2, encoding methyl-CpG-binding protein 2. Nat Genet 23, 185–188.

Anney, R., Klei, L., Pinto, D., Almeida, J., Bacchelli, E., Baird, G., Bolshakova, N., Bolte, S., Bolton, P.F., Bourgeron, T., et al. (2012). Individual common variants exert weak effects on the risk for autism spectrum disorderspi. Hum Mol Genet 21, 4781–4792.

Auranen, M., Vanhala, R., Varilo, T., Ayers, K., Kempas, E., Ylisaukko-Oja, T., Sinsheimer, J.S., Peltonen, L., and Jarvela, I. (2002). A genomewide screen for autism-spectrum disorders: evidence for a major susceptibility locus on chromosome 3q25-27. Am J Hum Genet 71, 777–790.

Awadalla, P., Gauthier, J., Myers, R.A., Casals, F., Hamdan, F.F., Griffing, A.R., Cote, M., Henrion, E., Spiegelman, D., Tarabeux, J., et al. (2010). Direct measure of the de novo mutation rate in autism and schizophrenia cohorts. Am J Hum Genet 87, 316–324.

Ballif, B.C., Sulpizio, S.G., Lloyd, R.M., Minier, S.L., Theisen, A., Bejjani, B.A., and Shaffer, L.G. (2007). The clinical utility of enhanced subtelomeric coverage in array CGH. Am J Med Genet A 143A, 1850–1857.

Barrett, S., Beck, J.C., Bernier, R., Bisson, E., Braun, T.A., Casavant, T.L., Childress, D., Folstein, S.E., Garcia, M., Gardiner, M.B., et al. (1999). An autosomal genomic screen for autism. Collaborative linkage study of autism. Am J Med Genet 88, 609–615.

Blasi, F., Bacchelli, E., Pesaresi, G., Carone, S., Bailey, A.J., and Maestrini, E. (2006). Absence of coding mutations in the X-linked genes neuroligin 3 and neuroligin 4 in individuals with autism from the IMGSAC collection. Am J Med Genet B Neuropsychiatr Genet 141B, 220–221.

Brunetti-Pierri, N., Berg, J.S., Scaglia, F., Belmont, J., Bacino, C.A., Sahoo, T., Lalani, S.R., Graham, B., Lee, B., Shinawi, M., et al. (2008). Recurrent reciprocal 1q21.1 deletions and duplications associated with microcephaly or macrocephaly and developmental and behavioral abnormalities. Nat Genet 40, 1466–1471.

Butler, M.G., Meaney, F.J., and Palmer, C.G. (1986). Clinical and cytogenetic survey of 39 individuals with Prader-Labhart-Willi syndrome. Am J Med Genet 23, 793–809.

Celestino-Soper, P.B., Shaw, C.A., Sanders, S.J., Li, J., Murtha, M.T., Ercan-Sencicek, A.G., Davis, L., Thomson, S., Gambin, T., Chinault, A.C., et al. (2011). Use of array CGH to detect exonic copy number variants throughout the genome in autism families detects a novel deletion in TMLHE. Hum Mol Genet 20, 4360–4370.

Christiansen, J., Dyck, J.D., Elyas, B.G., Lilley, M., Bamforth, J.S., Hicks, M., Sprysak, K.A., Tomaszewski, R., Haase, S.M., Vicen-Wyhony,

L.M., et al. (2004). Chromosome 1q21.1 contiguous gene deletion is associated with congenital heart disease. Circ Res 94, 1429–1435.

Coe, B.P., Girirajan, S., and Eichler, E.E. (2012). The genetic variability and commonality of neurodevelopmental disease. Am J Med Genet C Semin Med Genet 160C, 118–129.

Craddock, N., O'Donovan, M.C., and Owen, M.J. (2007). Phenotypic and genetic complexity of psychosis. Invited commentary on … Schizophrenia: a common disease caused by multiple rare alleles. Br J Psychiatry 190, 200–203.

Curtis, D. (2013). Consideration of plausible genetic architectures for schizophrenia and implications for analytic approaches in the era of next generation sequencing. Psychiatr Genet 23, 1–10.

de Kovel, C.G., Trucks, H., Helbig, I., Mefford, H.C., Baker, C., Leu, C., Kluck, C., Muhle, H., von Spiczak, S., Ostertag, P., et al. (2010). Recurrent microdeletions at 15q11.2 and 16p13.11 predispose to idiopathic generalized epilepsies. Brain 133, 23–32.

de Vries, B.B., Pfundt, R., Leisink, M., Koolen, D.A., Vissers, L.E., Janssen, I.M., Reijmersdal, S., Nillesen, W.M., Huys, E.H., Leeuw, N., et al. (2005). Diagnostic genome profiling in mental retardation. Am J Hum Genet 77, 606–616.

Durand, C.M., Betancur, C., Boeckers, T.M., Bockmann, J., Chaste, P., Fauchereau, F., Nygren, G., Rastam, M., Gillberg, I.C., Anckarsater, H., et al. (2007). Mutations in the gene encoding the synaptic scaffolding protein SHANK3 are associated with autism spectrum disorders. Nat Genet 39, 25–27.

Escayg, A., MacDonald, B.T., Meisler, M.H., Baulac, S., Huberfeld, G., An-Gourfinkel, I., Brice, A., LeGuern, E., Moulard, B., Chaigne, D., et al. (2000). Mutations of SCN1A, encoding a neuronal sodium channel, in two families with GEFS + 2. Nat Genet 24, 343–345.

Folstein, S.E., and Rosen-Sheidley, B. (2001). Genetics of autism: complex aetiology for a heterogeneous disorder. Nat Rev Genet 2, 943–955.

Gauthier, J., Bonnel, A., St-Onge, J., Karemera, L., Laurent, S., Mottron, L., Fombonne, E., Joober, R., and Rouleau, G.A. (2005). NLGN3/NLGN4 gene mutations are not responsible for autism in the Quebec population. Am J Med Genet B Neuropsychiatr Genet 132B, 74–75.

Gauthier, J., Champagne, N., Lafreniere, R.G., Xiong, L., Spiegelman, D., Brustein, E., Lapointe, M., Peng, H., Cote, M., Noreau, A., et al. (2010). De novo mutations in the gene encoding the synaptic scaffolding protein SHANK3 in patients ascertained for schizophrenia. Proc Natl Acad Sci U S A 107, 7863–7868.

Gecz, J., Shoubridge, C., and Corbett, M. (2009). The genetic landscape of intellectual disability arising from chromosome X. Trends Genet 25, 308–316.

Gillberg, C. (1998). Chromosomal disorders and autism. J Autism Dev Disord 28, 415–425.

Gilman, S.R., Iossifov, I., Levy, D., Ronemus, M., Wigler, M., and Vitkup, D. (2011). Rare de novo variants associated with autism implicate a large functional network of genes involved in formation and function of synapses. Neuron 70, 898–907.

Girard, S.L., Gauthier, J., Noreau, A., Xiong, L., Zhou, S., Jouan, L., Dionne-Laporte, A., Spiegelman, D., Henrion, E., Diallo, O., et al. (2011). Increased exonic de novo mutation rate in individuals with schizophrenia. Nat Genet 43, 860–863.

Hamdan, F.F., Gauthier, J., Araki, Y., Lin, D.T., Yoshizawa, Y., Higashi, K., Park, A.R., Spiegelman, D., Dobrzeniecka, S., Piton, A., et al. (2011). Excess of de novo deleterious mutations in genes associated with glutamatergic systems in nonsyndromic intellectual disability. Am J Hum Genet 88, 306–316.

Hamdan, F.F., Gauthier, J., Spiegelman, D., Noreau, A., Yang, Y., Pellerin, S., Dobrzeniecka, S., Cote, M., Perreau-Linck, E., Carmant, L., et al. (2009). Mutations in SYNGAP1 in autosomal nonsyndromic mental retardation. N Engl J Med 360, 599–605.

Hardy, J., and Singleton, A. (2009). Genomewide association studies and human disease. N Engl J Med 360, 1759–1768.

Heinzen, E.L., Radtke, R.A., Urban, T.J., Cavalleri, G.L., Depondt, C., Need, A.C., Walley, N.M., Nicoletti, P., Ge, D., Catarino, C.B., et al. (2010). Rare deletions at 16p13.11 predispose to a diverse spectrum of sporadic epilepsy syndromes. Am J Hum Genet 86, 707–718.

Hogart, A., Wu, D., LaSalle, J.M., and Schanen, N.C. (2010). The comorbidity of autism with the genomic disorders of chromosome 15q11.2-q13. Neurobiol Dis 38, 181–191.

Hoischen, A., van Bon, B.W., Gilissen, C., Arts, P., van Lier, B., Steehouwer, M., de Vries, P., de Reuver, R., Wieskamp, N., Mortier, G., et al. (2010). De novo mutations of SETBP1 cause Schinzel-Giedion syndrome. Nat Genet 42, 483–485.

Hoischen, A., van Bon, B.W., Rodriguez-Santiago, B., Gilissen, C., Vissers, L.E., de Vries, P., Janssen, I., van Lier, B., Hastings, R., Smithson, S.F., et al. (2011). De novo nonsense mutations in ASXL1 cause Bohring-Opitz syndrome. Nat Genet 43, 729–731.

International-Hapmap-Consortium. (2005). A haplotype map of the human genome. Nature 437, 1299–1320.

International-Molecular-Genetic-Study-of-Autism-Consortium. (1998). A full genome screen for autism with evidence for linkage to a region on chromosome 7q. International Molecular Genetic Study of Autism Consortium. Hum Mol Genet 7, 571–578.

International-Schizophrenia-Consortium. (2008). Rare chromosomal deletions and duplications increase risk of schizophrenia. Nature 455, 237–241.

Iossifov, I., Ronemus, M., Levy, D., Wang, Z., Hakker, I., Rosenbaum, J., Yamrom, B., Lee, Y.H., Narzisi, G., Leotta, A., et al. (2012). De novo gene disruptions in children on the autistic spectrum. Neuron 74, 285–299.

Itsara, A., Wu, H., Smith, J.D., Nickerson, D.A., Romieu, I., London, S.J., and Eichler, E.E. (2010). De novo rates and selection of large copy number variation. Genome Res 20, 1469–1481.

Jacquemont, M.L., Sanlaville, D., Redon, R., Raoul, O., Cormier-Daire, V., Lyonnet, S., Amiel, J., Le Merrer, M., Heron, D., de Blois, M.C., et al. (2006). Array-based comparative genomic hybridisation identifies high frequency of cryptic chromosomal rearrangements in patients with syndromic autism spectrum disorders. J Med Genet 43, 843–849.

Jamain, S., Quach, H., Betancur, C., Rastam, M., Colineaux, C., Gillberg, I.C., Soderstrom, H., Giros, B., Leboyer, M., Gillberg, C., et al. (2003). Mutations of the X-linked genes encoding neuroligins NLGN3 and NLGN4 are associated with autism. Nat Genet 34, 27–29.

Jolly, D.J., Okayama, H., Berg, P., Esty, A.C., Filpula, D., Bohlen, P., Johnson, G.G., Shively, J.E., Hunkapillar, T., and Friedmann, T. (1983). Isolation and characterization of a full-length expressible cDNA for human hypoxanthine phosphoribosyl transferase. Proc Natl Acad Sci USA 80, 477–481.

Kasperaviciute, D., Catarino, C.B., Heinzen, E.L., Depondt, C., Cavalleri, G.L., Caboclo, L.O., Tate, S.K., Jamnadas-Khoda, J., Chinthapalli, K., Clayton, L.M., et al. (2010). Common genetic variation and susceptibility to partial epilepsies: a genome-wide association study. Brain 133, 2136–2147.

Keller, M.C., and Miller, G. (2006). Resolving the paradox of common, harmful, heritable mental disorders: which evolutionary genetic models work best? Behav Brain Sci 29, 385–404; discussion 405–352.

Kirov, G., Grozeva, D., Norton, N., Ivanov, D., Mantripragada, K.K., Holmans, P., Craddock, N., Owen, M.J., and O'Donovan, M.C. (2009). Support for the involvement of large copy number variants in the pathogenesis of schizophrenia. Hum Mol Genet 18, 1497–1503.

Klauck, S.M., Felder, B., Kolb-Kokocinski, A., Schuster, C., Chiocchetti, A., Schupp, I., Wellenreuther, R., Schmotzer, G., Poustka, F., Breitenbach-Koller, L., et al. (2006). Mutations in the ribosomal protein gene RPL10 suggest a novel modulating disease mechanism for autism. Mol Psychiatry 11, 1073–1084.

Knight, S.J., Regan, R., Nicod, A., Horsley, S.W., Kearney, L., Homfray, T., Winter, R.M., Bolton, P., and Flint, J. (1999). Subtle chromosomal rearrangements in children with unexplained mental retardation. Lancet 354, 1676–1681.

Kondrashov, A. (2012). Genetics: The rate of human mutation. Nature 488, 467–468.

Kong, A., Frigge, M.L., Masson, G., Besenbacher, S., Sulem, P., Magnusson, G., Gudjonsson, S.A., Sigurdsson, A., Jonasdottir, A., Wong, W.S., et al. (2012). Rate of de novo mutations and the importance of father's age to disease risk. Nature 488, 471–475.

Koolen, D.A., Pfundt, R., de Leeuw, N., Hehir-Kwa, J.Y., Nillesen, W.M., Neefs, I., Scheltinga, I., Sistermans, E., Smeets, D., Brunner, H.G., et al. (2009). Genomic microarrays in mental retardation: a practical workflow for diagnostic applications. Hum Mutat 30, 283–292.

Koolen, D.A., Vissers, L.E., Pfundt, R., de Leeuw, N., Knight, S.J., Regan, R., Kooy, R.F., Reyniers, E., Romano, C., Fichera, M., et al. (2006). A new chromosome 17q21.31 microdeletion syndrome associated with a common inversion polymorphism. Nat Genet 38, 999–1001.

Kremer, E.J., Pritchard, M., Lynch, M., Yu, S., Holman, K., Baker, E., Warren, S.T., Schlessinger, D., Sutherland, G.R., and Richards, R.I. (1991). Mapping of DNA instability at the fragile X to a trinucleotide repeat sequence p(CCG)n. Science 252, 1711–1714.

Lam, C.W., Yeung, W.L., Ko, C.H., Poon, P.M., Tong, S.F., Chan, K.Y., Lo, I.F., Chan, L.Y., Hui, J., Wong, V., et al. (2000). Spectrum of mutations in the MECP2 gene in patients with infantile autism and Rett syndrome. J Med Genet 37, E41.

Lee, S.H., DeCandia, T.R., Ripke, S., Yang, J., Sullivan, P.F., Goddard, M.E., Keller, M.C., Visscher, P.M., and Wray, N.R. (2012). Estimating the proportion of variation in susceptibility to schizophrenia captured by common SNPs. Nat Genet 44, 247–250.

Lehrke, R. (1972). Theory of X-linkage of major intellectual traits. Am J Ment Defic 76, 611–619.

Lehrke, R.G. (1974). X-linked mental retardation and verbal disability. Birth Defects Orig Artic Ser 10, 1–100.

Lejeune, J., Gautier, M., and Turpin, R. (1959). [Study of somatic chromosomes from 9 mongoloid children]. C R Hebd Seances Acad Sci 248, 1721–1722.

Lencz, T., Lambert, C., DeRosse, P., Burdick, K.E., Morgan, T.V., Kane, J.M., Kucherlapati, R., and Malhotra, A.K. (2007). Runs of homozygosity reveal highly penetrant recessive loci in schizophrenia. Proc Natl Acad Sci U S A 104, 19942–19947.

Levy, D., Ronemus, M., Yamrom, B., Lee, Y.H., Leotta, A., Kendall, J., Marks, S., Lakshmi, B., Pai, D., Ye, K., et al. (2011). Rare de novo and transmitted copy-number variation in autistic spectrum disorders. Neuron 70, 886–897.

Li, X., Zou, H., and Brown, W.T. (2012). Genes associated with autism spectrum disorder. Brain Res Bull 88, 543–552.

Lim, E.T., Raychaudhuri, S., Sanders, S.J., Stevens, C., Sabo, A., MacArthur, D.G., Neale, B.M., Kirby, A., Ruderfer, D.M., Fromer, M., et al. (2013). Rare complete knockouts in humans: population distribution and significant role in autism spectrum disorders. Neuron 77, 235–242.

Lindblad-Toh, K., Garber, M., Zuk, O., Lin, M.F., Parker, B.J., Washietl, S., Kheradpour, P., Ernst,

J., Jordan, G., Mauceli, E., et al. (2011). A high-resolution map of human evolutionary constraint using 29 mammals. Nature 478, 476–482.

Lopreiato, J.O., and Wulfsberg, E.A. (1992). A complex chromosome rearrangement in a boy with autism. J Dev Behav Pediatr 13, 281–283.

Lubs, H.A. (1969). A marker X chromosome. Am J Hum Genet 21, 231–244.

Lubs, H.A., Stevenson, R.E., and Schwartz, C.E. (2012). Fragile X and X-linked intellectual disability: four decades of discovery. Am J Hum Genet 90, 579–590.

Marshall, C.R., Noor, A., Vincent, J.B., Lionel, A.C., Feuk, L., Skaug, J., Shago, M., Moessner, R., Pinto, D., Ren, Y., et al. (2008). Structural variation of chromosomes in autism spectrum disorder. Am J Hum Genet 82, 477–488.

McClellan, J.M., Susser, E., and King, M.C. (2007). Schizophrenia: a common disease caused by multiple rare alleles. Br J Psychiatry 190, 194–199.

Mefford, H.C., Cooper, G.M., Zerr, T., Smith, J.D., Baker, C., Shafer, N., Thorland, E.C., Skinner, C., Schwartz, C.E., Nickerson, D.A., et al. (2009). A method for rapid, targeted CNV genotyping identifies rare variants associated with neurocognitive disease. Genome Res 19, 1579–1585.

Mefford, H.C., Sharp, A.J., Baker, C., Itsara, A., Jiang, Z., Buysse, K., Huang, S., Maloney, V.K., Crolla, J.A., Baralle, D., et al. (2008). Recurrent rearrangements of chromosome 1q21.1 and variable pediatric phenotypes. N Engl J Med 359, 1685–1699.

Millar, J.K., Wilson-Annan, J.C., Anderson, S., Christie, S., Taylor, M.S., Semple, C.A., Devon, R.S., St Clair, D.M., Muir, W.J., Blackwood, D.H., et al. (2000). Disruption of two novel genes by a translocation co-segregating with schizophrenia. Hum Mol Genet 9, 1415–1423.

Mitchell, K.J. (2011). The genetics of neurodevelopmental disease. Curr Opin Neurobiol 21, 197–203.

Mitchell, K.J., and Porteous, D.J. (2011). Rethinking the genetic architecture of schizophrenia. Psychol Med 41, 19–32.

Molinari, F., Rio, M., Meskenaite, V., Encha-Razavi, F., Auge, J., Bacq, D., Briault, S., Vekemans, M., Munnich, A., Attie-Bitach, T., et al. (2002). Truncating neurotrypsin mutation in autosomal recessive nonsyndromic mental retardation. Science 298, 1779–1781.

Morrow, E.M., Yoo, S.Y., Flavell, S.W., Kim, T.K., Lin, Y., Hill, R.S., Mukaddes, N.M., Balkhy, S., Gascon, G., Hashmi, A., et al. (2008). Identifying autism loci and genes by tracing recent shared ancestry. Science 321, 218–223.

Neale, B.M., Kou, Y., Liu, L., Ma'ayan, A., Samocha, K.E., Sabo, A., Lin, C.F., Stevens, C., Wang, L.S., Makarov, V., et al. (2012). Patterns and rates of exonic de novo mutations in autism spectrum disorders. Nature 485, 242–245.

Need, A.C., Ge, D., Weale, M.E., Maia, J., Feng, S., Heinzen, E.L., Shianna, K.V., Yoon, W., Kasperaviciute, D., Gennarelli, M., et al. (2009). A genome-wide investigation of SNPs and CNVs in schizophrenia. PLoS Genet 5, e1000373.

Need, A.C., McEvoy, J.P., Gennarelli, M., Heinzen, E.L., Ge, D., Maia, J.M., Shianna, K.V., He, M., Cirulli, E.T., Gumbs, C.E., et al. (2012). Exome sequencing followed by large-scale genotyping suggests a limited role for moderately rare risk factors of strong effect in schizophrenia. Am J Hum Genet 91, 303–312.

Ng, S.B., Bigham, A.W., Buckingham, K.J., Hannibal, M.C., McMillin, M.J., Gildersleeve, H.I., Beck, A.E., Tabor, H.K., Cooper, G.M., Mefford, H.C., et al. (2010). Exome sequencing identifies MLL2 mutations as a cause of Kabuki syndrome. Nat Genet 42, 790–793.

O'Roak, B.J., Deriziotis, P., Lee, C., Vives, L., Schwartz, J.J., Girirajan, S., Karakoc, E., Mackenzie, A.P., Ng, S.B., Baker, C., et al. (2011). Exome sequencing in sporadic autism spectrum disorders identifies severe de novo mutations. Nat Genet 43, 585–589.

O'Roak, B.J., Vives, L., Fu, W., Egertson, J.D., Stanaway, I.B., Phelps, I.G., Carvill, G., Kumar, A., Lee, C., Ankenman, K., et al. (2012). Multiplex targeted sequencing identifies recurrently mutated genes in autism spectrum disorders. Science 338, 1619–1622.

O'Roak, B.J., Vives, L., Girirajan, S., Karakoc, E., Krumm, N., Coe, B.P., Levy, R., Ko, A., Lee, C., Smith, J.D., et al. (2012). Sporadic autism exomes reveal a highly interconnected protein network of de novo mutations. Nature 485, 246–250.

OMIM® (2013). Online Mendelian Inheritance in Man. McKusick-Nathans Institute of Genetic Medicine, Johns Hopkins University, Baltimore, MD.

Perez Jurado, L.A., Peoples, R., Kaplan, P., Hamel, B.C., and Francke, U. (1996). Molecular definition of the chromosome 7 deletion in Williams syndrome and parent-of-origin effects on growth. Am J Hum Genet 59, 781–792.

Pescosolido, M.F., Yang, U., Sabbagh, M., and Morrow, E.M. (2012). Lighting a path: genetic studies pinpoint neurodevelopmental mechanisms in autism and related disorders. Dialogues Clin Neurosci 14, 239–252.

Philippe, A., Martinez, M., Guilloud-Bataille, M., Gillberg, C., Rastam, M., Sponheim, E., Coleman, M., Zappella, M., Aschauer, H., Van Maldergem, L., et al. (1999). Genome-wide scan for autism susceptibility genes. Paris Autism Research International Sibpair Study. Hum Mol Genet 8, 805–812.

Pinto, D., Pagnamenta, A.T., Klei, L., Anney, R., Merico, D., Regan, R., Conroy, J., Magalhaes, T.R., Correia, C., Abrahams, B.S., et al. (2010). Functional impact of global rare copy number variation in autism spectrum disorders. Nature 466, 368–372.

Purcell, S.M., Wray, N.R., Stone, J.L., Visscher, P.M., O'Donovan, M.C., Sullivan, P.F., and Sklar, P. (2009). Common polygenic variation contributes to risk of schizophrenia and bipolar disorder. Nature 460, 748–752.

Ravnan, J.B., Tepperberg, J.H., Papenhausen, P., Lamb, A.N., Hedrick, J., Eash, D., Ledbetter, D.H., and Martin, C.L. (2006). Subtelomere FISH analysis of 11 688 cases: an evaluation of the frequency and pattern of subtelomere rearrangements in individuals with developmental disabilities. J Med Genet 43, 478–489.

Redon, R., Ishikawa, S., Fitch, K.R., Feuk, L., Perry, G.H., Andrews, T.D., Fiegler, H., Shapero, M.H., Carson, A.R., Chen, W., et al. (2006). Global variation in copy number in the human genome. Nature 444, 444–454.

Risch, N., Spiker, D., Lotspeich, L., Nouri, N., Hinds, D., Hallmayer, J., Kalaydjieva, L., McCague, P., Dimiceli, S., Pitts, T., et al. (1999). A genomic screen of autism: evidence for a multilocus etiology. Am J Hum Genet 65, 493–507.

Ritvo, E.R., Spence, M.A., Freeman, B.J., Mason-Brothers, A., Mo, A., and Marazita, M.L. (1985). Evidence for autosomal recessive inheritance in 46 families with multiple incidences of autism. Am J Psychiatry 142, 187–192.

Riviere, J.B., van Bon, B.W., Hoischen, A., Kholmanskikh, S.S., O'Roak, B.J., Gilissen, C., Gijsen, S., Sullivan, C.T., Christian, S.L., Abdul-Rahman,

O.A., et al. (2012). De novo mutations in the actin genes ACTB and ACTG1 cause Baraitser-Winter syndrome. Nat Genet 44, 440–444.

Saha, S., Barnett, A.G., Foldi, C., Burne, T.H., Eyles, D.W., Buka, S.L., and McGrath, J.J. (2009). Advanced paternal age is associated with impaired neurocognitive outcomes during infancy and childhood. PLoS Med 6, e40.

Salomons, G.S., van Dooren, S.J., Verhoeven, N.M., Cecil, K.M., Ball, W.S., Degrauw, T.J., and Jakobs, C. (2001). X-linked creatine-transporter gene (SLC6A8) defect: a new creatine-deficiency syndrome. Am J Hum Genet 68, 1497–1500.

Sanders, S.J., Ercan-Sencicek, A.G., Hus, V., Luo, R., Murtha, M.T., Moreno-De-Luca, D., Chu, S.H., Moreau, M.P., Gupta, A.R., Thomson, S.A., et al. (2011). Multiple recurrent de novo CNVs, including duplications of the 7q11.23 Williams syndrome region, are strongly associated with autism. Neuron 70, 863–885.

Sanders, S.J., Murtha, M.T., Gupta, A.R., Murdoch, J.D., Raubeson, M.J., Willsey, A.J., Ercan-Sencicek, A.G., DiLullo, N.M., Parikshak, N.N., Stein, J.L., et al. (2012). De novo mutations revealed by whole-exome sequencing are strongly associated with autism. Nature 485, 237–241.

Santen, G.W., Aten, E., Sun, Y., Almomani, R., Gilissen, C., Nielsen, M., Kant, S.G., Snoeck, I.N., Peeters, E.A., Hilhorst-Hofstee, Y., et al. (2012). Mutations in SWI/SNF chromatin remodeling complex gene ARID1B cause Coffin-Siris syndrome. Nat Genet 44, 379–380.

Sebat, J., Lakshmi, B., Malhotra, D., Troge, J., Lese-Martin, C., Walsh, T., Yamrom, B., Yoon, S., Krasnitz, A., Kendall, J., et al. (2007). Strong association of de novo copy number mutations with autism. Science 316, 445–449.

Sebat, J., Lakshmi, B., Troge, J., Alexander, J., Young, J., Lundin, P., Maner, S., Massa, H., Walker, M., Chi, M., et al. (2004). Large-scale copy number polymorphism in the human genome. Science 305, 525–528.

Shao, Y., Wolpert, C.M., Raiford, K.L., Menold, M.M., Donnelly, S.L., Ravan, S.A., Bass, M.P., McClain, C., von Wendt, L., Vance, J.M., et al. (2002). Genomic screen and follow-up analysis for autistic disorder. Am J Med Genet 114, 99–105.

Sharp, A.J., Hansen, S., Selzer, R.R., Cheng, Z., Regan, R., Hurst, J.A., Stewart, H., Price, S.M., Blair, E., Hennekam, R.C., et al. (2006). Discovery of previously unidentified genomic disorders from the duplication architecture of the human genome. Nat Genet 38, 1038–1042.

Shaw-Smith, C., Pittman, A.M., Willatt, L., Martin, H., Rickman, L., Gribble, S., Curley, R., Cumming, S., Dunn, C., Kalaitzopoulos, D., et al. (2006). Microdeletion encompassing MAPT at chromosome 17q21.3 is associated with developmental delay and learning disability. Nat Genet 38, 1032–1037.

Shi, J., Levinson, D.F., Duan, J., Sanders, A.R., Zheng, Y., Pe'er, I., Dudbridge, F., Holmans, P.A., Whittemore, A.S., Mowry, B.J., et al. (2009). Common variants on chromosome 6p22.1 are associated with schizophrenia. Nature 460, 753–757.

Sirmaci, A., Spiliopoulos, M., Brancati, F., Powell, E., Duman, D., Abrams, A., Bademci, G., Agolini, E., Guo, S., Konuk, B., et al. (2011). Mutations in ANKRD11 cause KBG syndrome, characterized by intellectual disability, skeletal malformations, and macrodontia. Am J Hum Genet 89, 289–294.

Skuse, D.H. (2000). Imprinting, the X-chromosome, and the male brain: explaining sex differences in the liability to autism. Pediatr Res 47, 9–16.

Smith, A.C., McGavran, L., Robinson, J., Waldstein, G., Macfarlane, J., Zonona, J., Reiss, J., Lahr, M., Allen, L., and Magenis, E. (1986). Interstitial deletion of (17)(p11.2p11.2) in nine patients. Am J Med Genet 24, 393–414.

Stefansson, H., Ophoff, R.A., Steinberg, S., Andreassen, O.A., Cichon, S., Rujescu, D., Werge, T., Pietilainen, O.P., Mors, O., Mortensen, P.B., et al. (2009). Common variants conferring risk of schizophrenia. Nature 460, 744–747.

Stefansson, H., Rujescu, D., Cichon, S., Pietilainen, O.P., Ingason, A., Steinberg, S., Fossdal, R., Sigurdsson, E., Sigmundsson, T., Buizer-Voskamp, J.E., et al. (2008). Large recurrent microdeletions associated with schizophrenia. Nature 455, 232–236.

Svensson, A.C., Lichtenstein, P., Sandin, S., and Hultman, C.M. (2007). Fertility of first-degree relatives of patients with schizophrenia: a three generation perspective. Schizophr Res 91, 238–245.

Thomas, N.S., Sharp, A.J., Browne, C.E., Skuse, D., Hardie, C., and Dennis, N.R. (1999). Xp deletions associated with autism in three females. Hum Genet 104, 43–48.

Tropeano, M., Ahn, J.W., Dobson, R.J., Breen, G., Rucker, J., Dixit, A., Pal, D.K., McGuffin, P.,

Farmer, A., White, P.S., et al. (2013). Male-biased autosomal effect of 16p13.11 copy number variation in neurodevelopmental disorders. PLoS One 8, e61365.

Tsurusaki, Y., Okamoto, N., Ohashi, H., Kosho, T., Imai, Y., Hibi-Ko, Y., Kaname, T., Naritomi, K., Kawame, H., Wakui, K., et al. (2012). Mutations affecting components of the SWI/SNF complex cause Coffin-Siris syndrome. Nat Genet 44, 376–378.

Ullmann, R., Turner, G., Kirchhoff, M., Chen, W., Tonge, B., Rosenberg, C., Field, M., Vianna-Morante, A.M., Christie, L., Krepischi-Santos, A.C., et al. (2007). Array CGH identifies reciprocal 16p13.1 duplications and deletions that predispose to autism and/or mental retardation. Hum Mutat 28, 674–682.

Veltman, J.A., and Brunner, H.G. (2012). De novo mutations in human genetic disease. Nat Rev Genet 13, 565–575.

Vincent, J.B., Kolozsvari, D., Roberts, W.S., Bolton, P.F., Gurling, H.M., and Scherer, S.W. (2004). Mutation screening of X-chromosomal neuroligin genes: no mutations in 196 autism probands. Am J Med Genet B Neuropsychiatr Genet 129B, 82–84.

Vissers, L.E., de Ligt, J., Gilissen, C., Janssen, I., Steehouwer, M., de Vries, P., van Lier, B., Arts, P., Wieskamp, N., del Rosario, M., et al. (2010a). A de novo paradigm for mental retardation. Nat Genet 42, 1109–1112.

Vissers, L.E., de Vries, B.B., and Veltman, J.A. (2010b). Genomic microarrays in mental retardation: from copy number variation to gene, from research to diagnosis. J Med Genet 47, 289–297.

Vostanis, P., Harrington, R., Prendergast, M., and Farndon, P. (1994). Case reports of autism with interstitial deletion of chromosome 17 (p11.2 p11.2) and monosomy of chromosome 5 (5pter-->5p15.3). Psychiatr Genet 4, 109–111.

Wakamatsu, N., Yamada, Y., Yamada, K., Ono, T., Nomura, N., Taniguchi, H., Kitoh, H., Mutoh, N., Yamanaka, T., Mushiake, K., et al. (2001). Mutations in SIP1, encoding Smad interacting protein-1, cause a form of Hirschsprung disease. Nat Genet 27, 369–370.

Wallace, R.H., Wang, D.W., Singh, R., Scheffer, I.E., George, A.L., Jr., Phillips, H.A., Saar, K., Reis, A., Johnson, E.W., Sutherland, G.R., et al. (1998). Febrile seizures and generalized epilepsy associated with a mutation in the Na + -channel beta1 subunit gene SCN1B. Nat Genet 19, 366–370.

Wang, K., Zhang, H., Ma, D., Bucan, M., Glessner, J.T., Abrahams, B.S., Salyakina, D., Imielinski, M., Bradfield, J.P., Sleiman, P.M., et al. (2009). Common genetic variants on 5p14.1 associate with autism spectrum disorders. Nature 459, 528–533.

Weiss, L.A., Arking, D.E., Daly, M.J., and Chakravarti, A. (2009). A genome-wide linkage and association scan reveals novel loci for autism. Nature 461, 802–808.

Xu, B., Ionita-Laza, I., Roos, J.L., Boone, B., Woodrick, S., Sun, Y., Levy, S., Gogos, J.A., and Karayiorgou, M. (2012). De novo gene mutations highlight patterns of genetic and neural complexity in schizophrenia. Nat Genet 44, 1365–1369.

Xu, B., Roos, J.L., Dexheimer, P., Boone, B., Plummer, B., Levy, S., Gogos, J.A., and Karayiorgou, M. (2011). Exome sequencing supports a de novo mutational paradigm for schizophrenia. Nat Genet 43, 864–868.

Xu, B., Roos, J.L., Levy, S., van Rensburg, E.J., Gogos, J.A., and Karayiorgou, M. (2008). Strong association of de novo copy number mutations with sporadic schizophrenia. Nat Genet 40, 880–885.

Ylisaukko-oja, T., Rehnstrom, K., Auranen, M., Vanhala, R., Alen, R., Kempas, E., Ellonen, P., Turunen, J.A., Makkonen, I., Riikonen, R., et al. (2005). Analysis of four neuroligin genes as candidates for autism. Eur J Hum Genet 13, 1285–1292.

Yu, T.W., Chahrour, M.H., Coulter, M.E., Jiralerspong, S., Okamura-Ikeda, K., Ataman, B., Schmitz-Abe, K., Harmin, D.A., Adli, M., Malik, A.N., et al. (2013). Using whole-exome sequencing to identify inherited causes of autism. Neuron 77, 259–273.

Zhu, Q., Ge, D., Maia, J.M., Zhu, M., Petrovski, S., Dickson, S.P., Heinzen, E.L., Shianna, K.V., and Goldstein, D.B. (2011). A genome-wide comparison of the functional properties of rare and common genetic variants in humans. Am J Hum Genet 88, 458–468.

4

THE ROLE OF GENETIC INTERACTIONS IN NEURODEVELOPMENTAL DISORDERS

Jason H. Moore[1] and Kevin J. Mitchell[2]

[1]*Institute for Quantitative Biomedical Sciences, Departments of Genetics and Community and Family Medicine, Geisel School of Medicine, Dartmouth College, Hanover, NH, USA*
[2]*Smurfit Institute of Genetics and Institute of Neuroscience, Trinity College Dublin, Dublin 2, Ireland*

4.1 INTRODUCTION

Genetic architecture has been defined as the number of genes or loci that influence a trait, the variation at those loci and the relationship between genotype and phenotype. Although we can now measure much of the genetic variation in human populations, we understand very little about the total number of genetic risk factors for most common neurologic and psychiatric disorders and even less about how their variants map to phenotypic variation. The goal of this chapter is to review genetic interaction, or epistasis, as one of many phenomena that can give rise to complex genotype–phenotype maps for common human diseases. We will define epistasis at the individual and population levels,

provide some arguments for why it is likely to be ubiquitous for common human diseases and then present some case studies that have addressed the role of epistasis in neurodevelopmental diseases.

William Bateson first described epistasis in 1907 to explain deviations from Mendelian inheritance (Bateson, 1907). The term literally means "standing upon," and Bateson used it to describe characters that were layered on top of other characters thereby masking their expression. The *epi*static characters had to be removed before the underlying *hypo*static characters could be revealed (Bateson, 1907). The commonly used definition of epistasis – an allele at one locus masks the expression of an allele at another locus – reflects this original definition (Griffiths et al., 2007). Eye color determination in *Drosophila* provides a classic example. The genes *scarlet*, *brown*, and *white*, play major roles in a simplified model of *Drosophila* eye pigmentation. Eye pigmentation in *Drosophila* requires the synthesis and deposition of both drosopterins, red pigments synthesized from GTP, and ommochromes, brown pigments synthesized from tryptophan. A mutation in *brown* prevents production of the bright red pigment resulting in a fly with brown eyes, and a mutation in *scarlet* prevents production of the brown pigment resulting in a fly with bright red eyes. In a fly with a mutation in the *white* gene, neither of the pigments can be produced and thus the fly will have white eyes regardless of the genotype at the *brown* or *scarlet* loci. In this example, the *white* gene is epistatic to *brown* and *scarlet*. A mutant genotype at the *white* locus masks the genotypes at the other loci. This is an example of epistasis at the individual level where there is a clear biological mechanism.

Even before the advent of genomic and proteomic technologies, there was evidence that epistasis is ubiquitous in model organisms. Gene–gene interactions are well established as integral to gene regulation, signal transduction, biochemical networks, and homeostatic, developmental, and physiological pathways (Moore, 2003). However, with the rapid development of high-throughput technologies, it has become obvious how widespread epistatic interactions are. For example, Fedorowicz et al. described epistatic interactions between loci that affect olfactory behavior in *Drosophila* (Fedorowicz et al., 1998). This study was based on crosses of 12 lines derived from a common isogenic background that differed in the location of P-element insertions, each of which has homozygous effects on olfactory behavior. Eight of the 12 insertion variants defined an interactive network of genes that significantly impact the olfactory phenotype. A subsequent study that investigated the same insertions, using transcriptional profiling (Anholt et al., 2003), showed that a total of 530 genes were significantly co-regulated with one or more of these olfactory mutations. This experiment shows first that epistasis is common, and second that easily detectable

epistatic interactions involve 10 to 100 of genes. More recent studies have shown widespread epistasis in *Drosophila* (Huang et al., 2012) and *C. elegans* (Bloom et al., 2013), for example. These kinds of studies have been recently reviewed (Mackay, 2014) and connected to human health (Mackay and Moore, 2014).

Epistatic interactions between specific experimentally induced mutations are commonplace in model organisms and often indicate related functions of the encoded gene products; indeed, they are the basis of genetic suppressor and enhancer screens that have been used to work out biochemical pathways with great success (St Johnston, 2002). It could be argued, however, that interactions between such mutations do not reflect the genetic architecture of quantitative traits in natural populations. One way to address that is to attempt to decompose the variants contributing to trait variance between specific strains and determine whether these interact additively or epistatically.

Chromosome substitution strains have been employed precisely for this kind of experiment in mice and provide clear evidence for widespread, strong, and highly unpredictable epistatic interactions, particularly for behavioral traits (Spiezio et al., 2012). Inbred strains of mice can show large differences in behavioral traits, such as anxiety and activity levels. By generating lines of mice that carry only a single chromosome from one strain, on the genetic background of the other, it is possible to determine which chromosomes carry loci that contribute to the phenotypic difference between the strains (Singer et al., 2004). In general, loci on anywhere between five and ten chromosomes may be apparent. The surprise is that their individual effects tend to be much larger than would be expected from their effect in aggregate (the sum of the parts may be paradoxically greater than the whole!) (Gale et al., 2009; Shao et al., 2008; Spiezio et al., 2012). Some individual loci when moved to the other strain can even yield phenotypes outside the range of either parental strain. Epistatic interactions are thus not just important for mutations of large effect in the laboratory but pervasive in nature and are highly complex and unpredictable.

Since Bateson, there have been many different and evolving definitions of epistasis or gene–gene interaction. For example, Fisher defined epistasis in a statistical manner as an explanation for deviation from additivity in a linear model (Fisher, 1918). This nonadditivity of genetic effects measured mathematically from population-level data is different than the more biological definition of epistasis from Bateson that occurs at the individual level. We have previously made the distinction between Bateson's biological epistasis and Fisher's statistical epistasis (Moore and Williams, 2005). This distinction is important to keep in mind when thinking about the genetic architecture of common human diseases because biological epistasis happens at the cellular level in an individual while statistical epistasis is a pattern of genotype to phenotype relationships that results from genetic variation in a human population. This distinction becomes important when attempting to draw a biological conclusion from a statistical model that describes a genetic association. Moore and Williams (2005) and Phillips (2008) have discussed the idea that more modern definitions of epistasis may be needed in light of our new knowledge about gene networks and biological systems. However, the classic definitions provided by Bateson and Fisher still provide a good starting point for thinking about gene–gene interactions.

To illustrate the concept of statistical epistasis, consider the following simple example of epistasis in the form of a penetrance function. Penetrance is simply the probability (P) of disease (D) given a particular combination of genotypes (G) that was inherited (i.e., P[D|G]). Let's assume for two SNPs labeled A and B that genotypes AA, aa, BB, and bb have population frequencies of 0.25 while genotypes Aa and Bb have frequencies of 0.5. Let us also assume that individuals have a very high risk of disease if they inherit Aa or Bb but not both (i.e., the exclusive OR or XOR logic function). What makes this model interesting is that disease risk is entirely dependent on the particular

combination of genotypes inherited at more than one locus. The penetrance for each individual genotype in this model is all the same and is computed by summing the products of the genotype frequencies and penetrance values. Heritability can be calculated as outlined by Culverhouse et al. (2002). Thus, in this model, there is no difference in disease risk for each single-locus genotype as specified by penetrance values. This model is labeled M170 by Li and Reich in their categorization of genetic models involving two SNPs and is an example of a pattern that is not separable by a simple linear function (Li and Reich, 2000). This model is a special case where all of the heritability is due to epistasis or nonlinear gene–gene interaction. Methods and software for simulating epistasis data from penetrance function models have been recently developed (Urbanowicz et al., 2012a, 2012b).

4.2　WHY SHOULD EPISTASIS BE COMMON?

A central question of genetic architecture is the expected frequency of different kinds of genetic effects. We have previously hypothesized that epistasis is likely to be a ubiquitous component of the genetic architecture of common human diseases (Moore, 2003). There are several reasons for this. First, as noted earlier, epistasis is not a new idea and remains a common phenomenon in the biological literature. Second, the ubiquity of biomolecular interactions in gene regulation and biochemical and metabolic systems suggests that the relationship between DNA sequence variations and biological end points is likely to involve interactions of multiple gene products. Third, positive results from studies of SNPs typically do not replicate across independent samples. Fourth, and perhaps most importantly, epistasis is commonly found when properly investigated. These four reasons suggest that epistasis may be ubiquitous in human biology, but do not provide an explanation for why. For that, we turn to evolutionary biology for a theory that may provide a compelling mechanism for epistasis.

Canalization is an idea introduced by Waddington to explain the buffering of phenotypes to genetic and environmental perturbations (Waddington, 1942). Evolutionary biologists have described canalization as stabilizing selection that ensures that systems evolve to a robust level (Gibson, 2009). In other words, evolution seeks to keep our blood pressure, glucose levels, and other important physiological and metabolic systems in a healthy range, while insuring that these measures are resistant to most genetic and environmental perturbations. Deviations from these healthy ranges are often categorized as diseases such as hypertension and diabetes. One way evolution has succeeded in developing robust systems is through evolving redundant gene networks that are resistant to fluctuations, both genetic, and environmental. This may explain why epistasis is so ubiquitous within the context of human disease. What we observe as disease may be the result of the accumulation of multiple mutations in different parts of a gene network that are needed to perturb a robust system from its evolved range. This may explain why most single variants explain very little of the risk for any given common disease. If this is true, it is essential to look for combinations of genetic variations in human populations as a way to capture the patterns of variation across networks that are needed to move individuals into unhealthy or disease phenotypes such as autism. In essence, evolution moves a population to a state where the vast majority of people are healthy, and this is often accomplished through complex networks that involve substantial epistasis. Epistasis as a robust gene network phenomenon has recently been discussed by Tyler et al. (2009). Epistasis among regulatory variants has recently been discussed by Cowper-Sal.Lari et al. (2011).

Assuming that canalization has shaped human biology throughout history, one may ask why we see independent main effects in genetic association studies at all. Gibson suggests that human migration and recent bottlenecks may allow hidden or cryptic genetic variation to emerge as genetic risk factors (Gibson, 2009). Our recent evolutionary history may explain

why genetic architecture is likely to be a mix of different types of genetic effects including epistasis, gene–environment interactions and locus heterogeneity. Unfortunately, canalization is very difficult to determine experimentally. Nevertheless, it provides an important foundation to begin thinking about why the genetic architecture of common diseases is so complex. Gibson offers a few strategies for identifying the hallmarks of canalization (Gibson, 2009).

4.3 DETECTING EPISTASIS IN GENETIC ASSOCIATION STUDIES

Despite the fact that epistasis is likely to play an important role in the genetic architecture of common diseases it has not been widely studied. There are several reasons for this. First, epistasis is difficult to detect using standard parametric statistical methods such as linear and logistic regression because of reduced power (Lewontin, 1974, 2006; Wahlsten, 1990). Second, it is common to only fit interaction terms in a linear model when the genetic variants have a significant independent effect. This can prevent the identification of epistatic effects for which there is no genetic variant with lower-order effects. Third, epistasis modeling naturally requires looking at combinations of genetic variants that can be a computational burden in genome-wide association studies (Moore et al., 2010). Finally, models of multiple genetic variants can be difficult to interpret. Thus, epistasis modeling requires special skills in machine learning and computational optimization (McKinney et al., 2006) as well as high-performance computing (Greene et al., 2010a; Sinnott-Armstrong et al., 2009). This can be a difficult barrier to overcome for geneticists and epidemiologists without specialized training or expertise in computer science.

A general finding from GWAS of quantitative traits, such as height or body-mass index, is that there is little or no evidence for epistatic interactions at the statistical level (Lango Allen et al., 2010; Speliotes et al., 2010). Multiple SNPs have been associated with each of these traits and it is possible to assess how many "+" alleles (associated with an increase in the trait) versus "−" alleles each individual has and plot this load against the value of the trait. This relationship is remarkably linear; each "+" allele is associated with the same small average increase in the trait, across the range of "+" allele load − that is, the statistical effect of adding one more allele does not increase at the extreme levels of load. While it is true that the identified SNPs explain only a fraction of the overall genetic variance affecting the trait and only over a limited, central portion of the phenotypic range, some nonlinearity might nevertheless have been expected if biological epistasis is really so ubiquitous and important.

In fact, this expectation is not necessarily valid. Epistatic pairwise interactions between a large number of loci, all occurring at once, are actually predicted to obscure each other and generate a statistically additive, linear relationship between the trait and the load of alleles affecting it across the population (Hill et al., 2008). The absence of a statistical signature of epistasis at the population level using traditional GWAS analyses thus does not rule out important epistatic effects in individuals. If such biological epistatic interactions do exist (which seems likely for behavioral traits and for alleles affecting risk of neurodevelopmental disorders), they will place sharp limits on the ability to predict individual risk based purely on additive, population-wide statistical signals (Bao et al., 2013; Evans et al., 2009).

Although the challenges listed earlier are significant, progress has been made over the last 10–15 years in developing bioinformatics methods and software to specifically detect and characterize epistasis. Several recent reviews highlight the need for new bioinformatics methods (Moore et al., 2010; Thornton-Wells et al., 2004) and discuss and compare different strategies for detecting statistical epistasis (Cordell, 2009). We briefly review one of these novel methods, multifactor dimensionality reduction (MDR).

MDR was developed as a nonparametric (i.e., no parameters are estimated) and genetic model-free (i.e., no genetic model is assumed) data mining and machine learning strategy for identifying combinations of discrete genetic and environmental factors that are predictive of a discrete clinical end point (Hahn and Moore, 2004; Hahn et al., 2003; Moore, 2004; Moore et al., 2006; Ritchie et al., 2001, 2003; Velez et al., 2007). Unlike most other methods, MDR was designed to detect interactions in the absence of detectable main effects and thus complements statistical approaches such as logistic regression and machine learning methods such as random forests and neural networks. At the heart of the MDR approach is a feature or attribute construction algorithm that creates a new variable or attribute by pooling genotypes from multiple SNPs (Moore et al., 2006). The general process of defining a new attribute as a function of two or more other attributes is referred to as constructive induction, or attribute construction, and was first described by Michalski (1983). Constructive induction, using the MDR kernel, is accomplished in the following way. Given a threshold T, a multilocus genotype combination is considered high-risk if the ratio of cases (subjects with disease) to controls (healthy subjects) exceeds T, otherwise it is considered low-risk. Genotype combinations considered to be high-risk are labeled G_1 while those considered low-risk are labeled G_0. This process constructs a new one-dimensional attribute with values of G_0 and G_1. It is this new single variable that is assessed, using any classification method. The MDR method is based on the idea that changing the representation space of the data will make it easier for methods such as logistic regression, classification trees, or a naive Bayes classifier to detect attribute dependencies. As such, MDR significantly complements other classification method such as neural networks or decision trees. This method has been confirmed in numerous simulation studies and a user-friendly open-source MDR software package written in Java is freely available from www.epistasis.org.

The MDR method has been extended in multiple different ways. For example, several different groups have modified MDR to work with quantitative traits (Lou et al., 2007;

Mahachie John et al., 2011) or even survival data (Beretta et al., 2010; Gui et al., 2011). Several high-performance versions of MDR have been developed to help scale to genome-wide data (Bush et al., 2006; Sinnott-Armstrong et al., 2009). These will be important, especially as next-generation sequencing data become more readily available. New statistical significance testing methods have been developed to help cut down the number of permutation tests that need to be performed (Pattin et al., 2009) and to help distinguish between additive and nonadditive effects (Greene et al., 2010b). These extensions and many others have positioned MDR as a general machine learning alternative to linear and logistic regression for the detection, characterization, and interpretation of epistasis effects in genetic studies of common diseases. Indeed, Cordell has referred to MDR as a gold standard in the field (Cordell, 2009).

The MDR approach and others were developed specifically for modeling the relationship between common variants (e.g., SNPs) and common diseases. This was timely given the focus on genome-wide association studies. However, next-generation DNA sequencing is providing measured genetic variation across the human genome that also includes variants with rare alleles. An important question for future work in this area is how to incorporate rare variants into gene–gene interaction analyses. This is challenging because rare alleles might only be present in a handful of subjects creating extremely rare genotype combinations. One approach is to preprocess sequence data using methods that collapse multiple rare variants into a smaller number of variants that have more common alleles (Li and Leal, 2008). These collapsing methods are very much in the spirit of MDR and create functions of rare variants that can be included in the analysis of gene–gene interactions. Methods for combining both rare and common variants will need to be developed and evaluated using simulated data and then applied to real data as they become available through sequencing.

In addition, it will be important to apply these methods to rare neurodevelopmental diseases such as tuberous sclerosis and Fragile X syndrome where phenotypic severity is likely modified by numerous rare and common variants. Gene–gene interaction analysis methods such as MDR have been applied to a few rare diseases such as familial amyloid polyneuropathy I (Soares et al., 2005) and Hirschsprung's disease (Garcia-Barcelo et al., 2007). They may also be applied to so-called common diseases such as autism or schizophrenia, which may actually be a collection of rare diseases, raising the possibility of both epistasis and locus heterogeneity within the context of clinical heterogeneity (Thornton-Wells et al., 2004).

4.4 EPISTASIS CASE STUDIES FOR NEURODEVELOPMENTAL DISORDERS

4.4.1 Oligogenic Mechanisms in Common Neurodevelopmental Disorders

We have selected several case studies to highlight some of the epistasis concepts described here. Each of these studies highlights how epistasis can be directly or indirectly addressed in genetic studies of neurodevelopmental disorders. Although not a comprehensive review of evidence for epistasis across all neurodevelopmental disorders, these examples represent a diversity of approaches and results that we think will be useful to consider for future studies.

All of the currently known mutations associated with moderate or high risk of psychiatric disorders show both incomplete penetrance for any particular clinical diagnosis and variable expressivity. Though nongenetic factors clearly contribute to the phenotypic variance among carriers of any particular mutation, there is likely also a large contribution from genetic background. This is indicated by the fact that concordance rates for monozygotic twins for specific diagnoses, such as SZ or ASD (~50% or 80%, respectively), tend to be much higher than the penetrance levels associated with even the highest known single risk mutations (~30% risk of psychosis for 22q11.2 deletion, for example (Kirov et al., 2014)). There may be some confounding due to differences in ascertainment for twins versus unrelated mutation-carriers, but these values still suggest that the risk of disease associated with *whole-genome-types* in affected individuals is often significantly greater than the average risk associated with specific single mutations.

This implies the existence of genetic modifiers in the background, which may have no phenotypic effects in the absence of a severe mutation, or which could have some less severe clinical or subclinical manifestation alone. In theory, such modifier alleles could be either rare or common in the population and examples of both are discussed in the following section.

4.4.2 Interactions Between Rare Variants

The best characterized high-risk variants for neurodevelopmental disorders are copy number variants (CNVs) – deletions or duplication of segments of chromosomes. Many of these confer high risk for a range of clinical diagnoses (Gill, 2012; Kirov et al., 2014). Those with the highest penetrance are often found to have arisen *de novo* in the generation of sperm or eggs, rather than having been inherited. The reason for this is very simple – these disorders carry a heavy cost to evolutionary fitness by increasing mortality and drastically reducing fecundity. Mutations that predispose to them with high penetrance will tend not to be inherited as carriers tend to have far fewer offspring, on average.

For those CNVs with lower penetrance, an interesting trend has emerged. Diagnosed patients who carry such lower-risk alleles tend to also have another CNV somewhere else in the genome, at a significantly higher rate than patients who carry a more highly penetrant, *de novo* CNV (Girirajan et al., 2010, 2012). This suggests that it requires a second hit to induce frank disease in carriers of less penetrant CNVs and that ascertaining them in patients who are clinically affected enriches for such events. Similar examples of patients carrying point mutations in two or more known risk genes have also been observed, suggesting digenic or oligogenic contributions to pathogenicity (Alves et al., 2013; Chilian et al., 2013; Leblond et al., 2012; Meisler et al., 2010; Schaaf et al., 2011). Whether the interactions between mutations of relatively modest penetrance alone are additive or epistatic remains to be seen – both situations seem likely to occur.

In some cases, interactions between two mutations independently associated with disease may paradoxically reduce risk. This is illustrated by analyses of mutations in the Fragile X and tuberous sclerosis genes in mice. Mutations in either *Fmr1* or *Tsc2* genes alone can result in autism in humans and related neurophysiological and behavioral phenotypes in mice. However, these two proteins act in opposition to each other in a biochemical pathway controlling mRNA translation in response to synaptic activity. Remarkably, the deficits in synaptic biochemistry and physiology seen in either single mutant disappear when the two mutations are combined in the same mice (Auerbach et al., 2011).

Similar effects have been observed for mutations in two different ion channels, both of which cause seizures alone, but which suppress each other's effects in combination (Glasscock et al., 2007). Complex interactions of this sort may in fact be particularly common for mutations in genes encoding ion channels (Klassen et al., 2011), due to the possible counterbalancing of effects on ionic fluxes and the known plasticity of ion channel expression as a means of neuronal and circuit homeostasis (Marder and Tang, 2010).

More generally, it is important to bear in mind the possible existence of variants with protective effects (against either genetic or environmental insults), as well as ones that increase risk. Examples of such variants have been observed recently for diabetes (Flannick et al., 2014; Rees et al., 2014).

4.4.3 Interactions Between Rare and Common Variants

Specific common variants have also been found to act as modifiers of rare mutations, often at the same locus. Such variants may have little effect in a background that is otherwise wild-type at that locus (and at functionally interacting loci) but can have significant consequences on phenotypic expression of partially penetrant rare mutations. This situation is exemplified by several related conditions affecting development of the enteric nervous system, including Hirschsprung disease (Alves et al., 2013) and Bardet–Biedl syndrome (González-Del Pozo et al., 2014). Both these conditions are caused by rare mutations in a number of different genes, but both also show effects of common variants in some of the same genes. For Hirschsprung disease, mutations in 18 genes are associated with high risk of the condition. However, phenotypic expression is modified by common variants at two of these genes, RET and NRG3 – specific SNP alleles at these loci are significantly more common in patients who carry a rare mutation and are clinically affected, than in subjects carrying the same rare mutation, who are unaffected or less severely affected (Alves et al., 2013; de Pontual et al., 2007). This scenario illustrates an important general point – common SNP alleles may have very large effects, but only in those individuals who also carry a rare mutation. At the population-level, such effects might be diluted and manifest as a very small odds ratio in GWAS, if they are detectable at all.

The examples listed earlier provide clear illustrations of epistatic interactions with important consequences on phenotypic expression. These are the easiest to recognize in the context of moderately penetrant rare mutations in specific genes, though it is an open question how exclusive these relationships are. Common variants that enhance the phenotypic consequences of rare mutations across a large number of loci would presumably face stronger negative selection than ones that interact with a much smaller set. A particular exception to that rule may be the Y chromosome (or absence of an X), which seems to enhance the pathogenic effects of many different mutations affecting neurodevelopment (Chapter 1), and which obviously cannot be directly selected against.

4.4.4   Implications for Genetic Diagnosis and Prediction

The ubiquity and strength of epistatic interactions provide both challenges and opportunities for genetic diagnosis and prediction. On the one hand, if the interacting variants remain unidentified, they place limits on the predictability of phenotypes associated with single, rare mutations, even ones of large effect. These may still be recognizable as playing an important causal role in affected carriers, but prediction of illness in currently unaffected individuals will remain a matter of loose probabilities (see Chapters 1 and 13). On the other hand, the identification of more and more patients with particular rare mutations presents the opportunity to identify modifying alleles and increase predictive power associated with whole-exome or whole-genome sequencing (González-Del Pozo et al., 2014). It will be particularly interesting to examine alleles at loci identified by GWAS to determine whether common variants at such loci are associated with increased risk in carriers of rare mutations. Of course, the phenotypic effects of such rare mutations (or indeed of environmental insults) may be modified not just by one allele in the background but by the combined whole-genome-type of the individual. Aggregate scores derived from GWAS signals, based on additive models of risk will not capture the complexity of these interactions in individuals and are likely to be of limited use for prediction of risk in the clinic (Evans et al., 2009; Bao et al., 2013). Detecting and measuring such higher-order epistatic interactions will require both very large datasets of sequenced and phenotyped individuals as well as new computational methods, such as those described earlier.

REFERENCES

Alves, M.M., Sribudiani, Y., Brouwer, R.W.W., Amiel, J., Antiñolo, G., Borrego, S., Ceccherini, I., Chakravarti, A., Fernández, R.M., Garcia-Barcelo, M.-M., et al. (2013). Contribution of rare and common variants determine complex diseases-Hirschsprung disease as a model. Dev Biol 382, 320–329.

Anholt, R.R.H., Dilda, C.L., Chang, S., Fanara, J.-J., Kulkarni, N.H., Ganguly, I., Rollmann, S.M., Kamdar, K.P., and Mackay, T.F.C. (2003). The genetic architecture of odor-guided behavior in Drosophila: epistasis and the transcriptome. Nat Genet 35, 180–184.

Auerbach, B.D., Osterweil, E.K., and Bear, M.F. (2011). Mutations causing syndromic autism define an axis of synaptic pathophysiology. Nature 480, 63–68.

Bao, W., Hu, F.B., Rong, S., Rong, Y., Bowers, K., Schisterman, E.F., Liu, L., and Zhang, C. (2013). Predicting risk of type 2 diabetes mellitus with genetic risk models on the basis of established genome-wide association markers: a systematic review. Am J Epidemiol 178, 1197–1207.

Bateson, W. (1907). Facts Limiting the Theory of Heredity. Science 26, 649–660.

Beretta, L., Santaniello, A., van Riel, P.L.C.M., Coenen, M.J.H., and Scorza, R. (2010). Survival dimensionality reduction (SDR): development and clinical application of an innovative approach to detect epistasis in presence of right-censored data. BMC Bioinf 11, 416.

Bloom, J.S., Ehrenreich, I.M., Loo, W.T., Lite, T.-L.V., and Kruglyak, L. (2013). Finding the sources of missing heritability in a yeast cross. Nature 494, 234–237.

Bush, W.S., Dudek, S.M., and Ritchie, M.D. (2006). Parallel multifactor dimensionality reduction: a tool for the large-scale analysis of gene-gene interactions. Bioinformatics 22, 2173–2174.

Chilian, B., Abdollahpour, H., Bierhals, T., Haltrich, I., Fekete, G., Nagel, I., Rosenberger, G., and Kutsche, K. (2013). Dysfunction of SHANK2 and CHRNA7 in a patient with intellectual disability and language impairment supports genetic epistasis of the two loci. Clin Genet 84, 560–565.

Cordell, H.J. (2009). Detecting gene-gene interactions that underlie human diseases. Nat Rev Genet 10, 392–404.

Cowper-Sal lari R., Cole M.D., Karagas MR, Lupien M., Moore J.H. (2011). Layers of epistasis: genome-wide regulatory networks and network approaches to genome-wide association studies. Wiley Interdisc Rev Syst Biol Med. Sep–Oct; 3(5), 513–26.

Culverhouse, R., Suarez, B.K., Lin, J., and Reich, T. (2002). A perspective on epistasis: limits of models displaying no main effect. Am J Hum Genet 70, 461–471.

Evans, D.M., Visscher, P.M., and Wray, N.R. (2009). Harnessing the information contained within genome-wide association studies to improve individual prediction of complex disease risk. Hum Mol Genet 18, 3525–3531.

Fedorowicz, G.M., Fry, J.D., Anholt, R.R., and Mackay, T.F. (1998). Epistatic interactions between smell-impaired loci in Drosophila melanogaster. Genetics 148, 1885–1891.

Fisher, R.A. (1918). The Correlation Between Relatives on the Supposition of Mendelian Inheritance. Trans - R Soc Edinburgh 52, 399–433.

Flannick, J., Thorleifsson, G., Beer, N.L., Jacobs, S.B.R., Grarup, N., Burtt, N.P., Mahajan, A., Fuchsberger, C., Atzmon, G., Benediktsson, R., et al. (2014). Loss-of-function mutations in SLC30A8 protect against type 2 diabetes. Nat Genet 46, 357–363.

Gale, G.D., Yazdi, R.D., Khan, A.H., Lusis, A.J., Davis, R.C., and Smith, D.J. (2009). A genome-wide panel of congenic mice reveals widespread epistasis of behavior quantitative trait loci. Mol Psychiatry 14, 631–645.

Garcia-Barcelo, M., King, S.K., Miao, X., So, M., Holden, W.T., Moore, J.H., Sutcliffe, J.R., Hutson, J.M., and Tam, P.K.H. (2007). Application of HapMap data to the evaluation of 8 candidate genes for pediatric slow transit constipation. J Pediatr Surg 42, 666–671.

Gibson, G. (2009). Decanalization and the origin of complex disease. Nat Rev Genet 10, 134–140.

Gill, M. (2012). Developmental psychopathology: the role of structural variation in the genome. Dev Psychopathol 24, 1319–1334.

Girirajan, S., Rosenfeld, J.A., Cooper, G.M., Antonacci, F., Siswara, P., Itsara, A., Vives, L., Walsh, T., McCarthy, S.E., Baker, C., et al. (2010). A recurrent 16p12.1 microdeletion supports a two-hit model for severe developmental delay. Nat Genet 42, 203–209.

Girirajan, S., Rosenfeld, J.A., Coe, B.P., Parikh, S., Friedman, N., Goldstein, A., Filipink, R.A., McConnell, J.S., Angle, B., Meschino, W.S., et al. (2012). Phenotypic heterogeneity of genomic disorders and rare copy-number variants. N Engl J Med 367, 1321–1331.

Glasscock, E., Qian, J., Yoo, J.W., and Noebels, J.L. (2007). Masking epilepsy by combining two epilepsy genes. Nat Neurosci 10, 1554–1558.

González-Del Pozo, M., Méndez-Vidal, C., Santoyo-Lopez, J., Vela-Boza, A., Bravo-Gil, N., Rueda, A., García-Alonso, L., Vázquez-Marouschek, C., Dopazo, J., Borrego, S., et al. (2014). Deciphering intrafamilial phenotypic variability by exome sequencing in a Bardet-Biedl family. Mol Genet Genomic Med 2, 124–133.

Greene, C.S., Sinnott-Armstrong, N.A., Himmelstein, D.S., Park, P.J., Moore, J.H., and Harris, B.T. (2010a). Multifactor dimensionality reduction for graphics processing units enables genome-wide testing of epistasis in sporadic ALS. Bioinformatics 26, 694–695.

Greene, C.S., Himmelstein, D.S., Nelson, H.H., Kelsey, K.T., Williams, S.M., Andrew, A.S., Karagas, M.R., and Moore, J.H. (2010b). Enabling personal genomics with an explicit test of epistasis. Pac Symp Biocomput 327–336.

Griffiths, A.J.F., Wessler, S.R., Lewontin, R.C., and Carroll, S.B. (2007). Introduction to Genetic Analysis, 9th edn, W. H. Freeman and Company.

Gui, J., Moore, J.H., Kelsey, K.T., Marsit, C.J., Karagas, M.R., and Andrew, A.S. (2011). A novel survival multifactor dimensionality reduction method for detecting gene-gene interactions with application to bladder cancer prognosis. Hum Genet 129, 101–110.

Hahn, L.W., and Moore, J.H. (2004). Ideal discrimination of discrete clinical endpoints using multilocus genotypes. In Silico Biol 4, 183–194.

Hahn, L.W., Ritchie, M.D., and Moore, J.H. (2003). Multifactor dimensionality reduction software for detecting gene-gene and gene-environment interactions. Bioinformatics 19, 376–382.

Hill, W.G., Goddard, M.E., and Visscher, P.M. (2008). Data and theory point to mainly additive genetic variance for complex traits. PLoS Genet 4, e1000008.

Huang, W., Richards, S., Carbone, M.A., Zhu, D., Anholt, R.R.H., Ayroles, J.F., Duncan, L., Jordan, K.W., Lawrence, F., Magwire, M.M., et al. (2012). Epistasis dominates the genetic architecture of Drosophila quantitative traits. Proc Natl Acad Sci U S A 109, 15553–15559.

Kirov, G., Rees, E., Walters, J.T.R., Escott-Price, V., Georgieva, L., Richards, A.L., Chambert, K.D., Davies, G., Legge, S.E., Moran, J.L., et al. (2014). The penetrance of copy number variations for schizophrenia and developmental delay. Biol Psychiatry 75, 378–385.

Klassen, T., Davis, C., Goldman, A., Burgess, D., Chen, T., Wheeler, D., McPherson, J., Bourquin, T., Lewis, L., Villasana, D., et al. (2011). Exome sequencing of ion channel genes reveals complex profiles confounding personal risk assessment in epilepsy. Cell 145, 1036–1048.

Lango Allen, H., Estrada, K., Lettre, G., Berndt, S.I., Weedon, M.N., Rivadeneira, F., Willer, C.J., Jackson, A.U., Vedantam, S., Raychaudhuri, S., et al. (2010). Hundreds of variants clustered in genomic loci and biological pathways affect human height. Nature 467, 832–838.

Leblond, C.S., Heinrich, J., Delorme, R., Proepper, C., Betancur, C., Huguet, G., Konyukh, M., Chaste, P., Ey, E., Rastam, M., et al. (2012). Genetic and functional analyses of SHANK2 mutations suggest a multiple hit model of autism spectrum disorders. PLoS Genet 8, e1002521.

Lewontin, R.C. (1974). Annotation: the analysis of variance and the analysis of causes. Am J Hum Genet 26, 400–411.

Lewontin, R.C. (2006). Commentary: Statistical analysis or biological analysis as tools for understanding biological causes. Int J Epidemiol 35, 536–537.

Li, B., and Leal, S.M. (2008). Methods for detecting associations with rare variants for common diseases: application to analysis of sequence data. Am J Hum Genet 83, 311–321.

Li, W., and Reich, J. (2000). A complete enumeration and classification of two-locus disease models. Hum Hered 50, 334–349.

Lou, X.-Y., Chen, G.-B., Yan, L., Ma, J.Z., Zhu, J., Elston, R.C., and Li, M.D. (2007). A generalized combinatorial approach for detecting gene-by-gene and gene-by-environment interactions with application to nicotine dependence. Am J Hum Genet 80, 1125–1137.

Mackay, T.F.C. (2014). Epistasis and quantitative traits: using model organisms to study gene-gene interactions. Nat Rev Genet 15, 22–33.

Mackay, T.F., and Moore, J.H. (2014). Why epistasis is important for tackling complex human disease genetics. Genome Med 6, 42.

Mahachie John, J.M., Van Lishout, F., and Van Steen, K. (2011). Model-Based Multifactor Dimensionality Reduction to detect epistasis for quantitative traits in the presence of error-free and noisy data. Eur J Hum Genet 19, 696–703.

Marder, E., and Tang, L.S. (2010). Coordinating different homeostatic processes. Neuron 66, 161–163.

McKinney, B.A., Reif, D.M., Ritchie, M.D., and Moore, J.H. (2006). Machine learning for detecting gene-gene interactions: a review. Appl Bioinformatics 5, 77–88.

Meisler, M.H., O'Brien, J.E., and Sharkey, L.M. (2010). Sodium channel gene family: epilepsy mutations, gene interactions and modifier effects. J Physiol 588, 1841–1848.

Michalski, R.S. (1983). A theory and methodology of inductive learning. Artif Intell 20, 111–161.

Moore, J.H. (2003). The ubiquitous nature of epistasis in determining susceptibility to common human diseases. Hum Hered 56, 73–82.

Moore, J.H. (2004). Computational analysis of gene-gene interactions using multifactor dimensionality reduction. Expert Rev Mol Diagn 4, 795–803.

Moore, J.H., and Williams, S.M. (2005). Traversing the conceptual divide between biological and statistical epistasis: systems biology and a more modern synthesis. Bioessays 27, 637–646.

Moore, J.H., Gilbert, J.C., Tsai, C.-T., Chiang, F.-T., Holden, T., Barney, N., and White, B.C. (2006). A flexible computational framework for detecting, characterizing, and interpreting statistical patterns of epistasis in genetic studies of human disease susceptibility. J Theor Biol 241, 252–261.

Moore, J.H., Asselbergs, F.W., and Williams, S.M. (2010). Bioinformatics challenges for genome-wide association studies. Bioinformatics 26, 445–455.

Pattin, K.A., White, B.C., Barney, N., Gui, J., Nelson, H.H., Kelsey, K.T., Andrew, A.S., Karagas, M.R., and Moore, J.H. (2009). A computationally efficient hypothesis testing method for epistasis analysis using multifactor dimensionality reduction. Genet Epidemiol 33, 87–94.

Phillips, P.C. (2008). Epistasis--the essential role of gene interactions in the structure and evolution of genetic systems. Nat Rev Genet 9, 855–867.

De Pontual, L., Pelet, A., Clement-Ziza, M., Trochet, D., Antonarakis, S.E., Attie-Bitach, T.,

Beales, P.L., Blouin, J.-L., Dastot-Le Moal, F., Dollfus, H., et al. (2007). Epistatic interactions with a common hypomorphic RET allele in syndromic Hirschsprung disease. Hum Mutat 28, 790–796.

Rees, E., Kirov, G., Sanders, A., Walters, J.T.R., Chambert, K.D., Shi, J., Szatkiewicz, J., O'Dushlaine, C., Richards, A.L., Green, E.K., et al. (2014). Evidence that duplications of 22q11.2 protect against schizophrenia. Mol. Psychiatry 19, 37–40.

Ritchie, M.D., Hahn, L.W., Roodi, N., Bailey, L.R., Dupont, W.D., Parl, F.F., and Moore, J.H. (2001). Multifactor-dimensionality reduction reveals high-order interactions among estrogen-metabolism genes in sporadic breast cancer. Am J Hum Genet 69, 138–147.

Ritchie, M.D., Hahn, L.W., and Moore, J.H. (2003). Power of multifactor dimensionality reduction for detecting gene-gene interactions in the presence of genotyping error, missing data, phenocopy, and genetic heterogeneity. Genet Epidemiol 24, 150–157.

Schaaf, C.P., Sabo, A., Sakai, Y., Crosby, J., Muzny, D., Hawes, A., Lewis, L., Akbar, H., Varghese, R., Boerwinkle, E., et al. (2011). Oligogenic heterozygosity in individuals with high-functioning autism spectrum disorders. Hum Mol Genet 20, 3366–3375.

Shao, H., Burrage, L.C., Sinasac, D.S., Hill, A.E., Ernest, S.R., O'Brien, W., Courtland, H.-W., Jepsen, K.J., Kirby, A., Kulbokas, E.J., et al. (2008). Genetic architecture of complex traits: large phenotypic effects and pervasive epistasis. Proc Natl Acad Sci U S A 105, 19910–19914.

Singer, J.B., Hill, A.E., Burrage, L.C., Olszens, K.R., Song, J., Justice, M., O'Brien, W.E., Conti, D.V., Witte, J.S., Lander, E.S., et al. (2004). Genetic dissection of complex traits with chromosome substitution strains of mice. Science 304, 445–448.

Sinnott-Armstrong, N.A., Greene, C.S., Cancare, F., and Moore, J.H. (2009). Accelerating epistasis analysis in human genetics with consumer graphics hardware. BMC Res Notes 2, 149.

Soares, M.L., Coelho, T., Sousa, A., Batalov, S., Conceição, I., Sales-Luís, M.L., Ritchie, M.D., Williams, S.M., Nievergelt, C.M., Schork, N.J., et al. (2005). Susceptibility and modifier genes in Portuguese transthyretin V30M amyloid polyneuropathy: complexity in a single-gene disease. Hum Mol Genet 14, 543–553.

Speliotes, E.K., Willer, C.J., Berndt, S.I., Monda, K.L., Thorleifsson, G., Jackson, A.U., Lango Allen, H., Lindgren, C.M., Luan, J., Mägi, R., et al. (2010). Association analyses of 249,796 individuals reveal 18 new loci associated with body mass index. Nat Genet 42, 937–948.

Spiezio, S.H., Takada, T., Shiroishi, T., and Nadeau, J.H. (2012). Genetic divergence and the genetic architecture of complex traits in chromosome substitution strains of mice. BMC Genet 13, 38.

St Johnston, D. (2002). The art and design of genetic screens: Drosophila melanogaster. Nat Rev Genet 3, 176–188.

Thornton-Wells, T.A., Moore, J.H., and Haines, J.L. (2004). Genetics, statistics and human disease: analytical retooling for complexity. Trends Genet 20, 640–647.

Tyler, A.L., Asselbergs, F.W., Williams, S.M., and Moore, J.H. (2009). Shadows of complexity: what biological networks reveal about epistasis and pleiotropy. Bioessays 31, 220–227.

Urbanowicz, R.J., Kiralis, J., Fisher, J.M., and Moore, J.H. (2012a). Predicting the difficulty of pure, strict, epistatic models: metrics for simulated model selection. BioData Min 5, 15.

Urbanowicz, R.J., Kiralis, J., Sinnott-Armstrong, N.A., Heberling, T., Fisher, J.M., and Moore, J.H. (2012b). GAMETES: a fast, direct algorithm for generating pure, strict, epistatic models with random architectures. BioData Min 5, 16.

Velez, D.R., White, B.C., Motsinger, A.A., Bush, W.S., Ritchie, M.D., Williams, S.M., and Moore, J.H. (2007). A balanced accuracy function for epistasis modeling in imbalanced datasets using multifactor dimensionality reduction. Genet Epidemiol 31, 306–315.

Waddington, C.H. (1942). Canalization of Development and the Inheritance of Acquired Characters. Nature 150, 563–565.

Wahlsten, D. (1990). Insensitivity of the analysis of variance to heredity-environment interaction. Behav Brain Sci 13, 109–120.

5

DEVELOPMENTAL INSTABILITY, MUTATION LOAD, AND NEURODEVELOPMENTAL DISORDERS

RONALD A. YEO AND STEVEN W. GANGESTAD
Department of Psychology, University of New Mexico, Albuquerque, NM, USA

There may be no developmental task more fundamental for humans to solve than faithfully implementing the "wisdom of the genes." Captured in our shared genetic architecture is the developmental plan that over human history has been the most successful design for passing on one's genes to future generations. Ignoring this wisdom, that is, failing to accurately implement the human developmental plan, increases the risk of adverse life outcomes. This developmental challenge confronts every generation anew; it is a challenge that our species cannot solve "once and for all." For, perhaps the major hindrances to developmental fidelity – germ cell line mutations – are formed at each new conception. As detailed subsequently, we all carry mutations that first affected our parents and grandparents, and to this burden we add a few not seen before in our families, that is, *de novo* mutations. Though the very word "mutation" conjures up images of fantastic creatures from science fiction movies, the most common

consequence of mutations may well be a good deal more subtle – imprecise expression of the evolved, shared plan for human development.

Developmental Instability (DI) refers to the imprecise expression of developmental design due to perturbations of development. DI theory offers an evolutionary framework for understanding the causes and consequences of individual variation in mutation load and provides a novel perspective on central questions about neurodevelopmental variation in typically developing individuals and in individuals with neurodevelopmental disorders (NDDs), such as schizophrenia, autism, intellectual disability, and attention deficit hyperactivity disorder (Gangestad et al., 2001; Yeo et al., 2007). In our view, DI theory (1) helps us understand individual differences in resilience (or vulnerability); (2) provides novel insights into how the genetic factors that underlie NDDs persist across generations; (3) informs our understanding of the shared features across

The Genetics of Neurodevelopmental Disorders, First Edition. Edited by Kevin J. Mitchell.
© 2015 John Wiley & Sons, Inc. Published 2015 by John Wiley & Sons, Inc.

disorders, such as reduced general cognitive ability; (4) provides novel insights into how genetic factors that underlie NDDs and reduce reproductive fitness are maintained in the population; and, (5) informs our understanding of comorbidity among NDDs and the existence of important shared features across disorders, such as reduced general cognitive ability. More generally, however, this chapter attempts to place the genetics of NDDs in an evolutionary perspective.

In the following sections, we first offer a brief review of DI theory, emphasizing its deep roots in evolutionary biology. Until very recently, our ability to measure mutation load and test specific hypotheses derived from DI theory has been limited to indirect, imperfect markers. Nonetheless, an impressive body of research has emerged demonstrating its relevance for health, mate selection, and brain function. The recent revolution in genetic technology has led to the first wave of studies offering direct assessments of mutation load. We can now measure directly (though incompletely) certain types of mutations. In this chapter, we will focus mostly on a specific type of mutation – copy number variations (CNVs). These mutations have now been described in many studies and genetic considerations suggest that they may be especially important for variation in neural phenotypes. Despite many outstanding methodological issues, including the optimal procedures for identifying mutations and how best to aggregate them in measures of mutation load, exciting new results indicate the relevance of mutation load for important human phenotypes, and further, offer important suggestions as to specific developmental processes linking mutation load and adult phenotypes.

5.1 DEVELOPMENTAL INSTABILITY THEORY

The roots of DI theory lie in Waddington's writings about "canalization," the ability of an individual to produce the same phenotype despite variation in its environment or genotype (Waddington, 1942). Diverse genetic and environmental stressors introduce "noise" or imprecision into developmental pathways. Natural selection favors organisms capable of buffering the impact of the noise on an organism's observable characteristics – that is, its phenotype. Developing organisms must continually buffer themselves against such perturbations. A contemporary perspective describes DI as "the inability of a developing organism to buffer its development against random perturbations, due either to frequent, large perturbations (e.g., frequent illness, many deleterious mutations, significant oxidative stress) or to a poor buffering system (e.g., a poorly co-adapted genome)" (p.380, Van Dongen & Gangestad, 2011). As this quote makes clear, a wide variety of environmental factors, as well as genetic factors, may potentially contribute to reduced fidelity of developmental processes leading to maladaptive phenotypes. At least two different kinds of factors can lead to this infidelity: first, the perturbations themselves (including sickness and mutations); and second, a relatively general-purpose buffering system. To the extent that the latter plays an important role, imprecise expression of the evolved developmental process is not entirely unique for each type of perturbation confronting the organism. Rather, developmental precision also depends on a genetically regulated, cross-trait capacity to deal effectively with misfortune's slings and arrows. Contemporary perspectives suggest that canalization is best understood in the context of genotype-by-environment and/or genotype-by-genotype interactions (McGrath et al., 2011). Figure 5.1 provides a graphic representation of the canalization process, emphasizing the role of "expected" versus "unexpected" environmental instructions.

Historically, two types of markers have been used in most research efforts examining the causes and effects of DI. One is the presence of deviant morphological features, which in studies of humans has typically been operationalised as minor physical anomalies (MPAs). MPAs are often considered "fetal relics", that is,

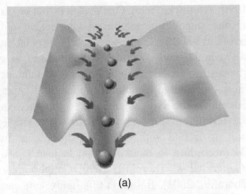

(a)

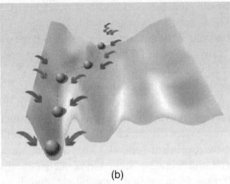

(b)

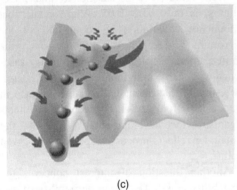

(c)

Fig. 5.1 The epigenetic landscape (from McGrath et al., 2011). The upper panel (a) shows a typical, normally developing trajectory, with expected environmental input or "developmental instructions" (red and green arrows) contributing at different times to maintain the species-typical trajectory. The middle panel (b) shows how the absence of expected instructions during early development (unbalanced arrows in the top of the figure) can lead to atypical development. The lower panel (c) shows how an adverse environmental input (large blue arrow) can also lead to decanalized, atypical development. (*See insert for color representation of this figure.*)

evidence of slowed or disrupted growth rates at the specific points in prenatal development when that feature develops. In the schizophrenia literature, MPAs such as low-set ears or a high palate are interpreted as indicators of first trimester growth abnormalities that also affect brain development (Compton & Walker, 2009). The Waldrop–Halvorsen scale (Waldrop & Halverson, 1989) is a common example of MPA assessment, though other rating scales or feature lists have been developed.

A far more commonly used marker of DI, and one having the benefit of cross-species applications, is fluctuating anatomic asymmetry (FA). Fluctuating asymmetry refers to random deviations in the symmetry of bilateral features that are, on average, symmetric at the population level. The underlying logic of FA as a measure of DI is that two sides of a bilateral feature represent independent replicates of the same developmental events. Differences between sides, then, reflect minor developmental "errors" or perturbations affecting one side and not the other (e.g., Van Dongen, 2006). In contrast to MPAs, FA of skeletal features can change across the life span, and hence, reflect cumulative DI, not DI arising solely during a discrete period (e.g., fetal life).

5.1.1 Mutations and Markers of DI

A substantial independent body of research reveals that mutations increase these markers of DI, though effects may vary across species as well as across FA of specific traits within individuals. Livshits and Kobylianski (1991) noted that diverse chromosomal abnormalities in humans are associated with increased FA. For example, Down Syndrome, caused by trisomy of chromosome, 21, is characterized by more MPAs, greater FA, diverse health problems, and very significant intellectual limitations. Møller (2002) found that radiation exposure, which is known to create mutations, increased FA in stag beetles and this impacted their mate value, though a subsequent study found no effect of radiation on FA in grasshoppers (Beasley et al., 2012). A recent study of mutations and

FA in Drosophila offered several interesting observations (Debat et al., 2009). Mutations increased FA, but the magnitude of this effect was dependent on both the specific genotype and the developmental environment (temperature stress), with mutations exerting their greatest impact in the harshest environment. In humans, relatively greater overall FA has been found to predict several features of sperm cells (reduced total number, motility, and head length; (Firman et al., 2003).

Factors associated with increased impact of mutations should also increase FA. Thus, mutations play a major role in producing the adverse consequences of inbreeding depression (Charlesworth & Charlesworth, 1999), and hence, inbreeding depression would be expected to increase FA. Inbreeding depression does just that in Drosophila melanogaster (Carter et al., 2009). Moreover, a recent study in humans reported a similar effect: a composite measure of FA was higher in high school students whose parents were first cousins than in students whose parents were unrelated (Ozener, 2010). Interestingly, evidence in humans (reviewed in Ozener, 2010) suggests that reduced environmental quality may increase the magnitude of some inbreeding depression effects. One morphometric study of human newborns, for example, found that inbreeding depression led to reduced head circumference and birth weight across socioeconomic status (SES) levels, whereas reduced body length was noted only among families of lower SES (Kulkarni & Kurian, 1990). Recent studies have also provided strong evidence for the importance of increasing paternal age for mutation load in offspring (e.g., Kong et al., 2012). One would expect that increased paternal age would be associated with increased FA, but we are aware of no reports on this issue.

5.1.2 Biometric Models of DI

A number of model-based analyses indicate that asymmetry on any given trait is a very weak indicator of underlying individual differences in DI (Van Dongen, 1998; Gangestad & Thornhill, 1999; Whitlock, 1996). One reason is that errors at one stage of development can cancel out errors at another stage, so that the association between DI and asymmetrical outcomes is a stochastic one. For skeletal features of humans (and other large vertebrates, including other primates), the typical amount of variance in the absolute value of asymmetry of a single trait associated with individual differences in DI (according to these models) is just 7–8% (Gangestad & Thornhill, 1999; Gangestad & Thornhill, 2003). Based on this figure, one can estimate that the coefficient of variation (CV; $100 \times$ standard deviation divided by mean) of DI is >20. That amount of variation is large and is consistent with DI being a fitness trait under directional selection. By contrast, the CV of a trait such as height is only about 5.

Assessment of fluctuating asymmetry of different phenotypic features permits assessment of the extent to which DI is feature-specific versus organism-general. The typical mean correlation between signed asymmetries across different features (e.g., ear height and finger lengths) is only 0.02–0.05. While small, that amount of covariation is about half of the maximum achievable (0.07–0.08), given the limited amount of variance in asymmetry associated with stable individual differences. Hence, we estimate that about half of the variance in propensities for DI for a given trait reflects organism-wide developmental processes; the remainder reflects processes specific to a given feature.

Another question of interest concerns the heritability of DI. The mean heritability of any single unsigned asymmetry is very weak – on average, about .03 (Fuller & Houle, 2002). But once again, that value is close to half (perhaps 40%) of the maximum that would be observed if 100% of the variance in DI was heritable (again, 0.07–0.08). Hence, the best guess is that perhaps 40% of the variance in DI, on average, is heritable (this is not to deny that in some instances it may be appreciably higher or lower). The estimated heritability is 0.2 for DI in fruit flies, comparable to other fitness traits in those species (Carter & Houle, 2011).

Due to the weak relationship between a specific traits' asymmetry and underlying DI, it is necessary to measure the asymmetry of multiple traits and aggregate unsigned asymmetries across these traits. In our work, we have created composites of seven to ten traits' asymmetries. Naturally, because the shared variance across these traits aggregates in a composite, composites will typically tend to tap organism-wide DI. A best estimate is that such a composite of 10 traits will possess a validity of about 0.5–0.6 for assessing underlying DI (Gangestad & Thornhill, 1999).

If a composite measure tends to tap organism-wide asymmetry, and organism-wide asymmetry is moderately heritable, then one expects a composite measure of asymmetry to possess greater heritability than single trait measures. Indeed, this expectation appears to be met. Johnson et al. (2008) measured 10 skeletal asymmetries in sets of identical and fraternal twins. On average, single traits had a heritability of 0.02–0.03. A composite of all 10 traits' asymmetries, by contrast, had a heritability of 0.30. The latter value is consistent with the majority of variance in organism-wide DI being genetic in origin.

5.1.3 DI and Neurodevelopmental Disorders

Based largely on research conducted with these two markers of DI, we proposed a two-factor DI model for NDDs (Yeo et al., 1999; Yeo et al., 1997). The first factor refers to the generalized effects of DI, of which a major determinant is hypothesized to be mutation load. A key feature of mutation theories of human phenotypic variation is their ability to account for how heritable disorders with reduced fertility are maintained in the population (Keller & Miller, 2006). Mutations at a given locus may be extremely rare, but collectively NDDs are relatively common. Hence, a successful theory must explain how an extremely diverse set of mutations, scattered across the genome, leads to a small set of clinical conditions (Gangestad & Yeo, 2006). The collective effect of mutations

contributes to developmental imprecision, that is, greater FA, more MPAs, and adverse effects on the brain. More fundamentally, these types of developmental imprecision emerge from greater sensitivity or reduced buffering to adverse genetic and environmental factors. At a mechanistic level, neurodevelopmental errors may disrupt adaptive coordination of a broad array of processes, particularly as their frequency increases. As the impact of DI is not specific to a given developmental pathway, individuals with perturbed development of one phenotypic feature may also demonstrate perturbed development of other features. Thus, high DI leads to "correlated atypicalities", or comorbidity.

The brain may be especially vulnerable to mutation load for several reasons. A large proportion of the genome contributes to its development (i.e., the "target size" of the genetic underpinnings); the relatively recent evolutionary origin of several of its features (i.e., prefrontal cortical development, prolonged childhood, intellectual ability) implies insufficient evolutionary time for the development of well-canalized neurodevelopmental trajectories; and, "tightly regulated critical windows of development [allow] few opportunities to compensate for perturbation" (p.2, McGrath et al., 2011).

The second factor posited by DI theory reflects genetic or environmental causes that are specific to particular atypical outcomes. For example, certain mutations or environmental stressors may affect only particular developmental processes and, in the context of high DI, result in specific atypical outcomes. Figure 5.2 provides a graphical representation of this two-factor approach and Fig. 5.3 illustrates the manner in which disorder-specific and the DI factor might together influence a range of phenotypes. Gene-by-gene interactions are expected, such that for individuals with high DI, lower "doses" of specific genetic liabilities are required for the development of a disorder. Specific environmental factors (e.g., infections, psychosocial stressors) may also contribute to specific outcomes, perhaps dependent on exactly when they affect the organism.

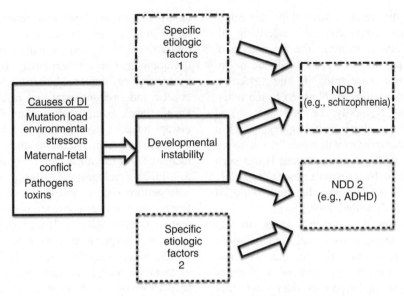

Fig. 5.2 The two-factor developmental instability (DI) model. DI is caused by a number of specific factors, most importantly, mutation load. It may contribute to neurodevelopmental variation through interaction with a host of other genetic and environmental factors. The DI component is hypothesized to be common across diverse NDDs, while different types of specific etiologic factors lead neurodevelopment along specific atypical pathways culminating in different diagnostic entities. See Yeo et al. (2007) for additional details.

5.1.4 What Motivated the Development of DI Theory of NDDs

Prior to the development of this theory of NDDs, we had done empirical work on atypical handedness, both left-handedness and extreme right-handedness (e.g., Yeo & Gangestad, 1993). Van Valen (1978) had speculated that atypical laterality, including handedness, may reflect DI and, in effect, reflect a kind of functional fluctuating asymmetry (presumably with neural underpinnings). In multiple studies, we found that atypical handedness is associated with markers of DI. A later study revealed only the association of handedness with MPAs to be robust; but the same study showed that other atypical hemispheric asymmetries of a functional sort (e.g., lateralization of certain spatial abilities) covaried with FA (Yeo et al., 1997).

Left handedness (and perhaps extreme right handedness too) is associated with a greater incidence of NDDs of various sorts. That might suggest that factors that give rise to left-handedness also give rise to NDDs. At the same time, however, left-handedness is but a very minor risk factor; the vast majority of left-handers do have diagnosable NDDs. Moreover, the NDDs with which left-handedness is associated with are themselves largely (even if not fully) independent; comorbidity is greater than expected by chance, but far from perfect. The factor shared by left-handedness and other NDDs, then, appears to have two features. First, its outcomes have a very broad bandwidth; it is associated with not just one NDD but rather is associated with many. Second, it, by itself, is not sufficient to give rise to NDDs.

We proposed the DI theory of NDDs to explain these two features. As already noted, markers of DI are weakly correlated with a great diversity of fitness-related outcomes (e.g., Van Dongen & Gangestad, 2011). Thus, we proposed DI to be the common factor typically responsible for comorbidity of NDDs and their shared features. The operation of NDD-specific other factors or their timing, we proposed, importantly affect to what extent and in what form DI gives rise to maladaptive outcomes.

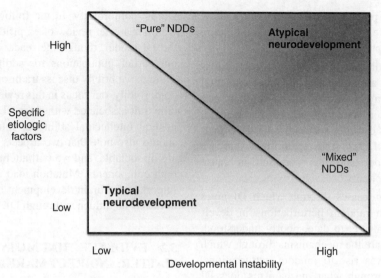

Fig. 5.3 Hypothesized relationship between developmental instability (DI) and specific etiologic factors. Different patterns of neurodevelopmental variation reflect different levels of the two etiologically important components. With high DI and low specific etiology, "mixed" clinical phenotypes are expected, expressing components of diverse disorders. With low DI and specific etiologic factors, a more "pure" form of a given disorder is expected, low in comorbidity. (*See insert for color representation of this figure.*)

We proposed that mutations are a major source of variation in DI for a reason we have already noted. Though selection eliminates deleterious mutations every generation, new mutations are generated every generation as well. At a stable equilibrium, the rate at which effects of deleterious mutations are removed by selection equals the rate at which effects of new mutations are generated. And at that equilibrium, many mutations exist and contribute to maladaptation. The fact that mutations inexorably exist, despite selection against then, partly explains why NDDs persist in populations across generations.

5.1.5   The Specification of DI Theory

Though, in our view, DI theory at its inception had a level of support (derived from the empirical and conceptual considerations mentioned earlier), it also remained relatively unspecified. For instance, consider the following.

(a) Not all deleterious mutations have their effects through disruption of developmental stability. (Indeed, we note earlier that some specific factors involved targeted effects of certain mutations.) So what sorts of mutations do have these effects, and which may not?

(b) Though it may make a good deal of theoretical sense (backed by empirical data) that mutations affect DI, factors other than mutation load may well affect DI (e.g., absence of coadapted gene complexes, toxins, pathogens). The precise extent to which DI reflects mutations remains unknown.

(c) Though we generally characterized the distinction between general and specific factors affecting disorders as discrete, the origins of phenotypic atypicality likely lie along a continuum. Some disorders may reflect predominantly generalized factors (and hence be very common outcomes of DI) and others relatively unique factors (and require very little in the way of potentiation by generalized DI). Which disorders are which type?

And, perhaps more importantly, how are we to understand this continuum conceptually?

(d) In addition, some factors (e.g., mutations affecting similar developmental pathways) may affect more than one disorder, but not all. How general, versus disorder-specific, is the DI affecting NDDs? And again, how are we to understand this variation in cause conceptually?

(e) The processes through which DI gives rise to random perturbations in development are, to date, poorly understood. What are the mechanisms through which DI gives rise to random perturbations, and through what mechanisms does DI moderate the impact of specific factors?

DI theory of NDDs is, presently, a general and provisional conceptual framework devised to explain certain observations about NDDs. Many specifics have yet to be fleshed out. When those specifics are fleshed out, we may see that some of the broad sweeping claims of DI theory require qualification. Nonetheless, DI theory is useful in that it does explain key observations, as well as guide empirical research designed to address questions regarding specificities, such as those listed earlier in this section.

As described in the following section, work on specific kinds of mutations, notably CNVs, serves to potentially flesh out DI theory in particular ways.

5.1.6   Predictions of the DI Model

The DI mutation load model offers several testable predictions. First, an increased incidence of the markers of DI should be found in each relevant disorder. Second, in each disorder, we should observe a greater incidence of known correlates of DI, such as atypical functional and anatomic brain symmetry and reduced intellectual functioning. Third, because DI increases the risk of atypical brain development in general, high DI individuals may well show features of several different NDDs – in other

words, comorbidity. In the following sections, we offer a brief review of empirical support for the DI model, though the reader is referred to our earlier publications for additional details. Though we briefly discuss traditional diagnostic comorbidity, our focus in this review is on a specific trait associated with most NDDs – reduced general intellectual ability or intelligence. We should also note that two aspects of our theory are dissociable, and we will attempt to evaluate both components. Mutation load might well be important for brain development even if it does not exert its influence through DI.

5.2   EVIDENCE THAT MUTATIONS MATTER: INDIRECT MARKERS

5.2.1   Fluctuating Asymmetry

Van Dongen and Gangestad (2011) recently reported a comprehensive meta-analysis of the health- and fitness-related correlates of FA in humans. In all, over 90 studies (most published) with nearly 300 individual outcome measures were included. The outcomes (described here in terms of lack of health or adaptation) fell into six broad domains: disease, fetal abnormalities and maternal risk factors, psychological maladaptation, hormonal sex-specific atypicality, lack of attractiveness, and lack of reproductive opportunities or poor outcomes. Overall, the analysis revealed a robust but modest association between outcomes and fluctuating asymmetry. On average, after adjusting for estimated publication bias, the correlation between outcomes and FA was about 0.1. As already noted, however, FA of single traits is only weakly associated with underlying DI. Based on a quantitative model, the best estimate of the mean correlation between outcomes and underlying DI was about 0.3 (albeit with a large confidence interval). If that value is accurate, it indicates rather impressive effects of DI. Although effects on single outcomes may be modest, effects across a wide range of very different outcomes are, on average, robust, such that the aggregate effect on health, broadly construed, is substantial.

TABLE 5.1 Estimates of average effect sizes (scaled as Pearson correlation coefficients) for associations between fluctuating asymmetry (FA), a measure of developmental instability, and selected outcomes, based on the meta-analysis of Van Dongen & Gangestad (2011).

Category	Specific outcome	Effect size	# Samples	Total N
Psychological	Schizophrenia/schizotypy	0.20	4	292
	Reduced intelligence	0.11	10	1071
Health	Infectious disease	0.09	3	504
	Other major illness	0.10	3	1337
Fetal	Fetal anomalies	0.13	5	1814
	Maternal risk factors	0.20	6	1950
Hormonal	Reproductive hormones	0.13	6	436
	Masculine/feminine features	0.09	14	1632
Attractiveness	Overall attractiveness[a]	0.03	23	2130
	Facial attractiveness[b]	0.19	14	1029
	Other forms[c]	0.15	14	701
Reproduction	Male number of partners	0.17	8	1071
	Female number of partners	0.13	4	526

Note: Estimates control for sample size and trait number, and are centered (for the full sample of effects) at 0.125. See text for full explanation.
[a]Based on body FA features only, to exclude direct effects of facial asymmetries on attractiveness.
[b]Facial FA studies only, to examine possible direct effects of facial asymmetries on attractiveness.
[c]Studies include attractiveness of scent (7), body (3), voice (2), and dance (2) in Van Dongen & Gangestad, 2011).

The meta-analysis yielded no robust differences across the six broad domains of outcomes; mean effect sizes for each were similar. More fine-grained exploratory analyses, however, suggested some outcomes of relative importance. Interestingly, one of those was schizophrenia and the related trait of schizotypy. Mean effect sizes in studies examining those outcomes were, on average, roughly double the mean effect across all outcomes. Table 5.1 provides a summary of these meta-analytic findings.

5.2.2 Inbreeding Depression

As noted earlier, the literature on inbreeding depression should also shed some light on the impact of mutation load in humans. Homozygous deleterious mutations typically exact much more than double the harm of the same mutation in a heterozygous state; inbreeding increases the number of homozygous deleterious mutations. The effect of inbreeding depression on other phenotypic features has been more frequently studied. There is abundant evidence that inbreeding depression leads to decreased

intellectual ability (e.g., Badaruddoza & Afzal, 1993). Several studies have also suggested that it leads to increased rates of schizophrenia (reviewed in Keller et al., 2012, and Mansour et al., 2010). Although many consequences of inbreeding depression have been known since the time of Darwin, the developmental processes by which this type of genetic variation leads to phenotypic variation in humans are not well understood. We assume that mutation effects are much more important than overdominance effects in inbreeding depression (Charlesworth & Charlesworth, 1999) and also that the specific mutations to be found in a sample of offspring of consanguineous marriages overlap very little. That is, the effects of inbreeding emerge from very different patterns of specific mutations across the individuals in a given study. A tremendous variety of genotypic variations thus converge on producing the same phenotype, such as increased FA or decreased general cognitive ability.

Of course, the effects of inbreeding may be in part determined by other factors. As we already noted, however, DI increases with inbreeding depression and is also associated with outcomes such as diminished cognitive ability. It is very reasonable to suspect, then, that some of the effects of inbreeding depression on phenotypic outcomes such as reduced cognitive ability are mediated through mutational effects on DI.

5.2.3 Paternal Age

Advanced paternal age effects may reflect increased mutation load, and hence, provide another indirect means to assess the impact of mutations on brain function. Mutations accumulate with age in the male, but not female germ cell line, because the precursor cells for sperm undergo 660 cell divisions by age 40 (Drake et al., 1998), greatly increasing the odds for recombination errors. Recent studies have provided surprising estimates of the magnitude of this effect (Campbell et al., 2012). Kong et al. (2012) reported that the average 20 year-old father passes on 29 de novo mutations, as compared to 69 from the average 40 year-old father. By contrast, mothers passed on an average of 14, regardless of their age. About 10% of these mutations are apt to be harmful (Kondrashov, 2012). Interestingly, some families may have higher mutation rates than others (Conrad et al., 2011).

Many studies have demonstrated associations between advanced paternal age and greater risk for NDDs, as well as reduced intelligence. A full review of this literature is beyond our scope for this chapter, but a few recent studies will be discussed for illustrative purposes. Each provided statistical control for SES and maternal age effects. A recent meta-analysis summarized six cohort studies and six case-control studies in the area of schizophrenia (Miller et al., 2011). Among the offspring of the oldest group of fathers (50 or older), the relative risk was 1.66, as compared to 1.22 in the 40–44 year-old age group and 1.00 in the 25–29 year-old age group. Reichenberg et al. (2006) noted that men 40 years or older were 5.75 times more likely to have children with Autism Spectrum Disorder than men younger than 30 years. In a very large sample of late adolescents greater paternal age

accounted for ~1% of variance in nonverbal intelligence (Malaspina et al., 2005). Analyses from the National Collaborative Perinatal Project revealed subtle cognitive impairments related to advanced paternal age on cognitive tests at ages four and seven (Saha et al., 2009). Shaw et al. (2012) explored the impact of paternal age on cortical morphology in a large sample of healthy, above average children. In a cross-sectional study, greater paternal age was associated with *increased* cortical surface in individuals up to 30 years of age, and with a decline in surface area after age 30. No effects were seen for white matter. A magnetic resonance spectroscopy (MRS) study found that advanced paternal age predicted lower brain levels of *N*-acetyl-aspartate (NAA) (Kegeles et al., 2005), a neurometabolite whose concentration positively correlates with intelligence (Jung et al., 1999). As many mutations persist for more than one generation, grandfather age (paternal and maternal) might also represent a risk factor for mutation-related phenotypic variation. Frans et al. (2013) found paternal age effects as well as paternal and maternal grandfather age effects in autism, even after controlling for family history of psychiatric disorders and parental education level. The risk accounted for by grandfathers being older than 40 years was 3%, versus 6% for fathers over 40. Though these paternal age effects are suggestive of the impact of mutations, none of the studies reviewed earlier provided a direct assessment of mutation number, size, or location. However, in mice greater paternal age has been associated with more CNVs (Wyrobek et al., 2006), a specific type of mutation discussed more fully in the following sections.

Just as with inbreeding depression, paternal age need not have effects on NDDs through mutation-driven effects on DI per se. Future research may address the extent to which offspring DI mediates the impacts of paternal age on NDDs.

In summary, we have seen that three very different approaches have provided support for the hypothesis that mutation load *in general*, that is, individually specific patterns of mutations distributed across the genome, impacts important human phenotypes, ranging from diverse health issues to intelligence to risk of NDD. In the next section, we discuss two critical issues that emerge as especially important for studies attempting direct measurements of mutations in our DNA. First, should we examine sites that code for genes, regulate genes, or both? Second, what specific kinds of genetic variations are apt to be most important for human brain development?

5.3 EVOLUTIONARY PERSPECTIVES ON MUTATIONS

Many different types of variants in the human genome have been described, and theory suggests that they may have varying functional impact. One historically important issue has been whether or not variants occur in coding versus noncoding sites. Another is the distinction between single nucleotide polymorphisms (SNPs) and CNVs. There has been quite a bit of recent research on these topics and we provide a selective review in the following sections. Most research on SNPs, however, has focused on rather common variants. Much more genetic variation is captured by rare SNPs than common SNPs (Tennessen et al., 2012), but technical limitations have precluded a full analysis of this potentially important source of genetic variation. One research strategy, based on inbreeding, involves assessment of "runs of homozygosity" (ROH) and this approach has recently provided preliminary information on the general importance of rare variants for schizophrenia and intelligence, as noted in subsequent sections.

5.3.1 The Functional Significance of Noncoding Sites

Two recent developments address how DI and risk for neurodevelopmental variation arise through mutation. First, there has been, until recently, a common assumption that 98% of the nucleotide sites in the genome are not functional

simply because they are "noncoding." They do not contain information directly affecting protein synthesis. By some views, noncoding DNA has been thought to be "junk" – of no consequence to the phenotypes of organisms. But mounting evidence indicates that noncoding DNA plays crucial roles in regulation of gene activity, epigenetic modifications of genes (e.g., imprinting), and DNA splicing and arrangement (Amaral & Mattick, 2008; Mallik & Lakhotia, 2007; Nowacki et al., 2009; Vinces et al., 2009). These functions may be especially important in more complex organisms.

Of course, evidence that *some* noncoding DNA is functional is not evidence that *all* is. Noncoding sequences are less phylogenetically conserved than are coding DNA, consistent with variation being neutral and subject to random drift (Chiaromonte et al., 2003; Lunter et al., 2006; Siepel et al., 2005). Comparative analyses (e.g., of the mouse and human genomes) suggest that perhaps 5% of the human genome is functional and subject to selection against mutations. These analyses, however, address only sequences that are similarly functional in all species compared. Some noncoding DNA may be functional in some species, not functional in others, or subject to different selection across species. Consistent with this scenario, one analysis found evidence that, as the phylogenetic distance between species narrows, the estimated proportion of functional genes increases (e.g., Smith et al., 2004). Taking these findings into account led to one estimate that ~10% of noncoding sites are functional (Ponting, 2009). The ENCODE research project (Dunham et al., 2012) recently attracted much attention with a report that 80% of noncoding DNA regions are functional (as defined by involvement in some type of biochemical interaction), though there remains much controversy regarding this estimate (Doolittle, 2013).

These developments vastly alter estimated rates of mutation. If we take the very conservative estimate that 10% of the genome is functional (a five-fold increase over 2%), the estimated total number of new mutations per functional genome is five-fold greater as well, e.g., 15 rather than 3. For an organism to be able to persist in the face of the resulting mutation load, the mean effect of these mutations on relative fitness must be much less than 2%. In fact, mutations at functional noncoding sites, though more prevalent than mutations at coding sites, may be very weakly deleterious (e.g., Smith et al., 2004). If so, these mutations will accumulate in the genome. A very substantial proportion of the total mutations at functional loci in the population may consist of very mildly deleterious mutations in noncoding DNA.

How might noncoding genes affect phenotypes? Again, the idea is that noncoding sites may possess regulatory functions. Might disruption of regulation through mutation broadly affect developmental precision and hence be particularly important to an understanding of DI? That certainly seems one possibility, though one not explicitly tested to date.

5.3.2 The Discovery of Copy Number Variations

A second important development concerns copy number variations or CNVs. It was once thought that the "normal" human genome could be defined by a shared reference genomic structure, one specifying all single nucleotide sites. In an extreme form of this view, all genetic variation between any two ("normal") individuals would consist merely of the aggregate of base differences at all 3 billion or so single nucleotide sites (e.g., A vs T, C vs G). Geneticists have long recognized the existence of exceptions – insertions, deletions, or inversion of long chromosomal segments in individual genomes. Recent discoveries, however, show that "exceptions" are anything but unusual (Iafrate et al., 2004; Sebat et al., 2004). A substantial portion of the genome is subject to "copy number variation"—differences across individuals in number of copies of a chromosomal segment at least 1000 bases long (in rare cases over 1 million bases long). Most individuals have two copies of such a sequence (one inherited from each parent), whereas others have one copy (with no copy – a

"deletion" – inherited from one parent), and yet others more than two copies. Thus far, several thousand such sequences have been found in the human genome, comprising at least 12% of it (e.g., Redon et al., 2006). Variation across individuals, then, consists not only of differences at single nucleotide sites, but also in number of copies of particular DNA strands (referred to as "structural variation"). Because CNV strands consist of many bases, CNVs may account for more total inter-individual genetic variation than single nucleotide variants combined (Beckmann et al., 2007).

CNVs originate through mutational events of sorts, but not, of course, mutations defined as single nucleotide substitutions (also known as point mutations), as treated earlier. One important cause of a new CNV is nonallelic homologous recombination (NAHR; see Bailey & Eichler, 2006; Kim et al., 2008; for a discussion of this and other processes). Through recombination, homologous chromosomes inherited from the two parents (e.g., chromosome 16 from each parent) are spliced and recombined to create new homologous chromosomes. NAHR is a mistake that occurs when a segment of DNA incorrectly matches up with a segment on the homologous chromosome during recombination, resulting in the creation of a new chromosome that contains a deletion, duplication, or inversion. Chromosomal regions containing segmental duplications (SDs) are prone to NAHR. SDs are effectively CNVs (specifically, duplications) that have gone to fixation; they are characteristic of nearly all individuals. Specific regions of the human genome are very rich in SDs. NAHR is particularly likely to occur in the presence of SDs because a long segment of DNA can readily "mismatch" with a similar DNA sequence (its duplication) on a different allele during the crossover process involved in recombination, leading to alteration in structure in the recombined chromosome. In short, duplications beget more duplications as well as deletions; duplications yield genomic instability. As expected, then, CNVs are not randomly distributed across the genome; they are 4 to 12 times more likely to appear in genomic regions rich in SDs (e.g., Iafrate et al., 2004; Sebat et al., 2004; see also Bailey & Eichler, 2006).

The rate at which mutations creating CNVs occurs is much greater than the rate at which single nucleotide mutations occurs – indeed, on average several orders of magnitude greater (perhaps 1 in 10 000; e.g., Sebat et al., 2007). CNVs (perhaps deletions more so than duplications) tend to be deleterious (Locke et al., 2006). Individuals carry a substantial number of deleterious CNVs in addition to deleterious point mutations. One study found >100 CNVs per individual, though the proportion that is deleterious remains unknown (Wong et al., 2007).

In the words of one pair of authors, psychiatry was recently hit by a "copy number variant tsunami" (Joober & Boksa, 2009). Whereas psychiatric geneticists have had difficulty identifying single nucleotide variations that robustly associate with major disorders such as schizophrenia, autism, or bipolar disorder (but see Crespi, 2008 for a review of some such variations), recent research has convincingly linked these disorders to CNVs, as we detail in the next section (at the same time, we note that the extent to which CNVs account for NDDs is still a matter of debate). One reason why CNVs may have substantial effects on psychiatric disorders is that they reflect "big" mutations (variations at many nucleotide sites). But CNVs may be especially important to psychiatric disorders for additional reasons, as discussed in the following section.

5.3.3 Segmental Duplications, CNVs, and Human Evolution

CNVs are overrepresented in regions rich in SDs (which themselves tend to be near centromeres and telomeres – toward the center and far ends of chromosomes, respectively), regions in which multiple copies of sequences of DNA are found. SDs, it is thought, were often duplications that selection favored. A duplication of a DNA sequence may bolster level of expression of a gene (or genes) contained within the segment,

and at times increased level of gene expression is favored. In addition, once a segment of DNA has been duplicated, selection may favor changes in that segment, such that it can serve functions partly distinct from the original copy (while the functions served by the original are preserved). Selection that involves a copy-paste-modify process is a common route to adaptation (e.g., Taylor & Raes, 2004).

SDs appear to have been particularly important in the evolution of the great apes and humans. A rapidly advancing science of comparative genomics finds that a burst of increased SDs occurred in the common ancestor of great apes. SD content has continued to expand in chimpanzee and human genomes (Marques-Bonet et al., 2009). Though comprising only about 5% of the human genome, SDs account for more divergent evolution between chimpanzees and humans than all single base-pair changes combined. Segmental duplications near centromeres (e.g., on chromosomes 1, 9, 16) appear to be especially central to the lineage-specific expansions of the human genome. Consistent with these duplications being adaptive, SD regions are richly inhabited by signatures of positive selection for substitutions within them (perhaps reflective of a copy-paste-modify adaptive process; Bailey & Eichler, 2006).

If much of human evolution occurred through changes in SD-rich regions, these regions are likely to play critical roles in the development and expression of many traits derived in the human lineage, phenotypically distinguishing us from close relatives. Some of these unique features coevolve in response to other species or individuals. As should be expected, then, human SDs are particularly rich in genes involved in immune function, olfaction, reproduction, and systems responsive to coevolutionary processes or changes in diet. Perhaps more interesting from an evolutionary psychological perspective, SDs also appear to contain genes involved in neuronal development or expressed in neural tissues, perhaps central to human-specific cognitive features (e.g., Dumas et al., 2007; Popesco et al., 2006; Sikela, 2006).

Though substantial levels of SD have likely been selected in the recent human lineage, SDs once again carry a special cost: they predispose genomic instability and hence deleterious CNVs. The functions that these CNVs likely disrupt are facilitated by DNA in SDs, including regulation of brain development. From an emerging understanding of the evolution of the human genome, then, it is perhaps no coincidence that CNVs are important to an understanding of major psychiatric disorders (see aforementioned paragraphs). We now turn to recent studies of the impact of CNVs on NDDs and related endophenotypes.

5.4 EVIDENCE THAT MUTATIONS MATTER

The studies reviewed earlier using indirect markers of mutation load raise the possibility that similar common, deleterious effects on brain function can emerge from an individually specific array of genetic abnormalities scattered across the genome. A limited number of phenotypic abnormalities may thus emerge from extraordinarily heterogenous genotypes. CNV studies identifying single, rare, large genetic variants emphasize a different type of genetic etiology. A minority of cases (perhaps as high as 7–20% for Autism Spectrum Disorder; Schaaf & Zoghbi, 2011) can be directly attributed to such anomalies. Though providing critical insights regarding the neurodevelopmental pathways affected in different disorders, as well as clinically important genetic information for families, such studies are limited in their ability to offer a general model of genetic influence. In moving toward more widely applicable models, researchers confront critical questions regarding genetic heterogeneity (Mitchell, 2012), polygenic causality (e.g., Fanous & Kendler, 2005; Van Os et al., 2009) and genetic interactions/background effects (Chandler et al., 2013).

Several excellent articles provide comprehensive reviews of the importance of large, rare CNVs (Cooper et al., 2011; Girirajan et al., 2012; Morrow, 2010; Vorstman & Ophoff, 2013). While the distinction between high-impact, rare variants and smaller, more common CNVs is somewhat artificial (Vorstman & Ophoff, 2013), the study of the latter is less common and presents unique methodological and theoretical challenges. Our review will focus mostly on these sorts of CNVs, often termed copy number polymorphisms (CNPs). Following Korn et al. (2008), the term CNP will be used to refer to CNVs that segregate at greater than 1% frequency in the population. While some may be quite frequent and benign, others may be relatively "uncommon" and potentially more influential. Because our interest is specifically in models of mutation load, we will focus on studies of overall CNP burden. Recognizing that the population frequency of CNPs is inversely related to the magnitude of their adverse effects, CNP studies tend to focus on "middle ground" genetic variations, that is, those that are smaller and more common than the extremely rare, highly penetrant CNVs linked with schizophrenia and autism, yet larger and less common than the SNP variations captured in GWAS studies. Girirajan et al. (2011) described some other important differences between the large, rare CNVs and CNPs. CNPs are especially enriched in SDs and may have been important in human evolution, as detailed earlier. Genes captured within these CNPs are also enriched for immune and environmental response pathways, suggesting that they are "candidates for local, adaptive, selection in human populations" (p.214). Research on overall mutation burden may be more affected by variation in genetic technology than detection of large CNVs. Arrays of greater sampling density (i.e., newer ones) detect many more small CNPs, an issue complicating comparison of different studies. Indeed, the total number of rare or uncommon deletions per individual reported across studies of schizophrenia varies by a couple of orders of magnitude.

While direct identification of rare variant SNPs awaits application of technological advances, studies of ROH provide a way to examine the importance of this potentially important source of genetic variation. ROH's are stretches of consecutive homozygous genotypes emerging from recent or (more commonly) remote consanguinity, and these regions are known to harbor rare recessive mutations associated with reduced fitness (Szpiech et al., 2013). Thus, an association between ROH (i.e., greater numbers of ROH regions or a greater proportion of the genome characterized by ROH) with adverse phenotypic outcomes implicates the overall importance of rare SNPs.

5.4.1 Intelligence

The genetic roots of intelligence have been the subject of intense study and debate for over a century. Behavior genetic studies, while limited in scope, have revealed several rather consistent findings. Intelligence is heritable (more so with advancing age), highly polygenic, and the impact of shared within-family environment declines with age (Deary, 2012). Furthermore, the behavior genetic literature distinguishes two types of intellectual deficiency (ID) that differ in terms of their genetic underpinnings, with "familial" intellectual ID reflecting polygenic contributions shared with parents, and "organic" ID reflecting large, impactful de novo mutations (Jensen, 1998). Among individuals falling below the typical cutoff IQ score of 70, the latter types are more frequent. Against this backdrop, and given the evidence for an association of intelligence with indirect markers of mutation load (e.g., Furlow et al., 1997), researchers have begun to examine the possible impact of CNVs in two ways. First, individuals with ID have been compared to controls, focusing on the impact of large, rare events. Second, individual variation in the normal range has been examined with respect to the total burden of smaller, uncommon deletions.

As would be expected from research on chromosomal abnormalities (e.g., Down Syndrome, Fragile X), many studies have demonstrated that large and rare CNVs are more common among individuals diagnosed with intellectual disability. In general, odds ratios increase with CNV size and the proportion of cases explained decreases. For example, 25.7% of children with ID have a CNV at least 400 kb in size, versus 11.5% of controls (odds ratio = 2.7) (Cooper et al., 2011). This suggests that 14.2% of ID is caused by CNVs of this size, a figure broadly consistent with earlier estimates. By contrast, 11.3% had a CNV greater than 1.5 Mb versus 6% in controls (odds ratio = 20.3). Using an array with greater sensitivity to CNVs in duplication-rich hotspots, Girirajan and colleagues (2011) examined CNVs in cases of ID with and without multiple congenital MPAs. Large CNVs (> 1 Mbp) were more common in the entire ID group (odds ratio = 13.71), and the group with anomalies had more CNVs than those without (odds ratio = 14.45). These important studies have convincingly demonstrated that rare CNVs, both deletions and duplications, account for a substantial portion of ID cases. They do not, however, inform us as to the relevance of CNVs for the 98% of the population with intelligence in the normal range, despite overwhelming evidence for substantial heritability.

Four studies have attempted to relate CNP burden to intelligence within the normal realm. Our initial study examined CNVs in a small sample ($N = 74$) of adults (mean age = 39.9) with heavy alcohol use, for whom genetic data was originally collected to predict clinical aspects of substance abuse (see Yeo et al., 2011, for methodological details). We examined CNPs occurring in 5% or less of the sample. For both uncommon deletions and duplications, we calculated the total number of CNPs, as well as the total number of base pairs included in each type of abnormality. Intelligence was assessed with the Wechsler Abbreviated Scale of Intelligence (WASI). The number of duplications and total number of base pairs captured by these duplications were unrelated to intelligence. By contrast, the total number of base pairs captured by the uncommon deletions (mean = 210,618 bp) was negatively correlated with intelligence ($r = -0.30$, $p = 0.01$) and a trend ($r = -0.21$, $p = 0.08$) was noted for the total number of uncommon deletions (mean = 10.95). Covarying clinical measures of substance abuse did not alter these findings. In contrast to these results, three new studies found no relationship between deletion burden and intellectual ability. One study found no relationship between uncommon CNPs (less than 5% frequency, greater than 20 kb length) and general cognitive ability in a sample of 800 healthy controls (McRae et al., 2013). They detected about 7.5 deletions per subject with an average length of about 63 kb. MacLeod and colleagues (MacLeod et al., 2012) combined several samples to achieve a total N of 3210. CNPs greater than 500 kb were examined, with ~ 0.05 being detected per individual. No relationship was noted between any measure of CNP and intelligence. Finally, we recently examined deletion burden in individuals with schizophrenia and healthy controls, using a frequency of 3% and size > 500 bp to define deletions. Approximately 11 deletions were seen in both groups and deletion size averaged about 10,000 base pairs. No relationship between deletions burden and general cognitive ability was noted in controls (see next section for results among patients). Though these studies varied in the details of their genetic analyses, all used valid measures of intelligence.

At this point, one conclusion seems clear: the broad measures of total deletion burden available with current methods are unrelated (or, at best, very weakly related) to general cognitive ability in individuals without ID or other serious NDD. Thus, recent attempts to move from indirect markers of mutation load, which generally reveal modest effects on intelligence, to direct measures based on genetic analysis of CNVs, have not been successful, though future studies will surely evaluate more types of genetic variants.

A recent study suggests that a greater overall burden of rare SNPs contributes to intellectual deficits among individuals with Autism Spectrum Disorder (ASD) (Gamsiz et al., 2013). A genome-wide analysis revealed greater ROH among ASD cases with IQ less than 70 as compared to their unaffected sibs, but this effect was not observed in the entire sample of ASD cases. Furthermore, among the cases with IQ less than 70, greater ROH was correlated with lower IQ but not with ASD symptom scores.

This suggests that ROH may be more closely tied to intellectual ability in this sample than with risk of ASD per se. We are not aware of any study attempting to relate ROH to intelligence in healthy controls.

5.4.2 Schizophrenia

Given its relatively high heritability and tremendous social cost, the focus on schizophrenia is not surprising. Several excellent reviews are now available, so we shall be selective in our coverage of these seminal studies. Sebat et al. (2009) reviewed the results of the first wave of studies implicating CNVs in schizophrenia. The Walsh et al. study (2008) noted that rare deletions and duplications were seen in 5% of healthy controls versus 15% of patients, and some evidence was presented that CNVs on genes had a greater effect. The International Consortium for Schizophrenia (Stone and Consortium, 2008) found a 1.15 case/control ratio for overall CNV burden, with a baseline rate in controls of 0.99 CNVs per individual. For deletions alone, the case/control rate was 1.08 with a baseline of 0.40 in controls. Need et al. (2009) also found an increased number of large deletions (> 200 Mb, 0.007 frequency in cases versus 0 in controls), but not smaller ones (500 kb – 1 Mb, 0.013 frequency in each group).

These studies suggested a causal role for large, rare CNVs in a small minority of cases, but their limited coverage of smaller CNVs greatly hampered their ability to derive conclusions about overall mutation load. Kong et al. (2012) reported that about 60 new small-scale de novo mutations occur per generation, of which six are likely to be disadvantageous. As it may take several generations to remove these mutations from the gene pool, the total individual burden far exceeds that which these studies were capable of detecting. Kirov and colleagues (2009) examined CNV burden, for rare (< 1%) deletions and duplications of various sizes. For CNVs greater than 100 kb, 0.028 were found in cases versus 0.006 in controls (ratio = 4.53); for duplications, 0.04 were found in controls and 0.024 in patients (ratio = 1.68). No group differences were noted for smaller, more common deletions or duplications. Collapsing across size categories, this study identified 0.21 total deletions and 0.32 total duplications in cases and 0.21 and 0.30, respectively, in controls. A more recent study found no group differences in the burden of CNVs occurring in genes (Ye et al., 2012), detecting a mean of 1.2 deletions per subject in the patient group and 1.4 in controls. By contrast, another recent study focusing on common and rare CNVs greater than 50 kb that affect genes found an effect for overall burden of deletions (0.71 per case, versus 64 in controls), but not duplications (Buizer-Voskamp et al., 2011). In a large Swedish sample (Bergen et al., 2012), the overall burden of rare deletions (less than 1% frequency) larger than 500 kb was greater in cases (ratio = 1.64, control mean = 0.03). Our recent report (Yeo et al., 2013) focused on deletions > 500 base pairs in size and occurring in less than 3% of our sample, yielded 11.34 deletions per patient versus 11.87 in controls, with the mean deletion length being 10,400 bp in cases versus 9988 in controls; none of these differences were significant. However, our sample size was quite low for a genetic study ($N = 79$ patients and 110 controls).

Taken as a whole, there is only mixed evidence that directly assessed CNV mutation load is greater in cases than in controls. Consistent with evidence for greater purifying selection on deletions than on duplications, there is somewhat greater evidence that deletion burden is more important than duplication burden. Nonetheless, effect sizes are small and the very small number of rare CNVs detected in most studies raises real concern about how well mutation load has been assessed and how it should be best represented (e.g., across variations in size and population frequency). There are two other weaknesses of the existing set of studies, reflecting the large sample sizes needed for most genetic studies. One is that very limited information on phenotypes is typically available beyond the diagnosis of schizophrenia. The heuristic utility of endophenotype analysis has long been noted by researchers interested in the genetics of psychopathology (Gottesman, &

Gould, 2003). Prominent examples of endophenotypes for schizophrenia include cognitive variables (intelligence, executive function, working memory), aspects of neurophysiology (e.g., sensory gating), and anatomical variables (e.g., anterior cortical gray matter volume). Another limitation consequent to the need for large sample sizes is the lack of information on early childhood environments; as noted earlier, mutation effects are most often observed in harsh or stressful environments.

We are aware of only two studies that have explored the relationship between direct measures of mutation load and endophenotypes for schizophrenia. One study examined relationships between select brain variables and several different markers of mutation load based on CNVs that affected genes (Van Scheltinga et al., 2012). After correction for multiple comparisons (critical $p = 0.003$), no effects reached significance in this study of 173 cases and 176 controls, though several interesting trends were noted. For example, the burden of deletions affecting genes was negatively related to total brain volume ($p = 0.02$). Our recent study examined the importance of uncommon deletion burden for higher cognitive functioning, select brain variables, and psychiatric symptoms (Yeo et al., 2013).

Several observations indicate the central importance of intelligence for schizophrenia. Individuals who will later develop schizophrenia have modest deficits in estimates of premorbid intelligence (effect size $d = 0.43$ in a recent meta-analysis, (Khandaker et al., 2011)) that decrease further in the prodromal period (Bilder et al., 2006). A longitudinal study found that among first episode patients, 44% showed a decline over 3 years and 56% were stable (Leeson et al., 2011). Furthermore, the association between lower intellectual ability and risk for schizophrenia in part reflects genetic covariance (Toulopoulou et al., 2008). In our study of uncommon deletion burden in schizophrenia (Yeo et al., 2013), we explored the impact of diagnosis, deletion burden, and their interaction on intelligence, as well as total gray matter volume, and ventricle size. Though patients and controls did not differ on this measure of mutation load, the interaction of diagnosis and mutation load significantly predicted two of these putative endophenotypes – intelligence and ventricle size. For each interaction, rare deletions had an adverse impact only in the patient group. Partial correlations (controlling for age, sex, and ethnicity) with general cognitive ability s were $r = -0.36$ ($p = 0.001$) for the patient group, and $r = -0.02$ (ns) for controls. Thus, as noted earlier, intellectual ability in the average range does not seem to be related to uncommon deletion burden in healthy adults. Overall ventricle volume was also related to deletion burden, though again this effect was noted only in patients. The partial correlations (controlling for age, sex, and ethnicity) with ventricle size was $r = 0.30$ ($p = 0.008$) for the patient group, and $r = 0.00$ (ns) for controls. Overall gray matter volume was not related to deletion burden in either group. However, voxel-based morphometry analysis within the patient group revealed that greater deletion burden was associated with reduced gray matter density in four clusters ($p < 0.001$, uncorrected): left anterior cingulate, left medial frontal, right inferior parietal, and right fusiform gyri (Yeo et al., unpublished observations). Finally, we examined correlations between symptom scales and deletion burden measures within the patient group. No significant relationships were observed between positive or negative symptoms and deletion burden. However, disorganized symptoms were found to correlate significantly with the number of uncommon deletions ($r = 0.25$, $p = 0.02$). Disorganized symptoms also correlated with ventricle size ($r = 0.27$, $p = 0.016$), but not with general cognitive ability.

Another endophenotype for schizophrenia is executive function (EF). Impaired executive functioning is one of the most commonly noted deficits associated with schizophrenia (Eisenberg & Berman, 2010). Executive deficits have important real-world consequences for individuals with schizophrenia. Lower executive skills predict reduced insight (Chan et al., 2012), reduced daily living skills (Puig et al., 2012),

and reduced levels of remission (Hofer et al., 2011). In the same sample as described earlier, we performed a principal components analysis of a battery of EF tests, yielding three components – verbal fluency, planning, and inhibition (Yeo et al., 2014). In a repeated measures analysis of these three components controlling for demographic variables, we examined the impact of uncommon deletions, group, and the interaction of these two variables. A significant interaction of group with uncommon deletion burden was noted, as the relationship was only observed in patients. There was no interaction of this effect with the repeated measures variable, so results are not specific to one or another EF. Thus EF, as well as general intellectual ability, appears to be influenced by uncommon deletion burden in schizophrenia, which is perhaps not too surprising given the substantial correlation between these two types of cognitive ability.

The DI model specifies two distinctly different types of genetic variation for NDDs, a general vulnerability factor (mutation load) and specific factors (undefined) strongly influencing the type of NDD. The observations that uncommon deletion burden were predictive of general cognitive ability and ventricle size only in the patient group may represent just this sort of interaction. This putative gene × genome interaction (i.e., epistasis) may complement, and act similarly to, important gene × environment interactions seen in studies of schizophrenia. For example, the neural effects of obstetric complications (McNeil et al., 2000) and both cannabis and alcohol use (Habets et al., 2011; Welch et al., 2011) are greater in individuals with a genetic liability for schizophrenia.

To summarize, large, rare CNVs, especially deletions, are more common in patients with schizophrenia, but such events probably account for a small proportion of cases. The impact of overall deletion burden, summing much more frequent but smaller CNPs across the genome, varies across studies. This likely reflects the usual suspects: method variance (especially sampling density), sample size issues, and possibly, variation in genetic background effects (Chandler et al., 2013; Johnson, 2010).

Reflecting the fact that large genetic studies may not include rich phenotype information, there is much less information available regarding the possibility that rare deletion burden may influence specific endophenotypes of schizophrenia.

Turning to the overall impact of another type of mutation, rare SNPs, two studies have examined ROH in schizophrenia. The first identified relatively common ROH's in 178 cases and 144 controls; cases had significantly more than controls (31.8 vs 28.0) (Lencz et al., 2007). Nine of 339 ROH's were individually significant in distinguishing groups, and with respect to these, 55% of controls had none versus only 19% of cases. The second study examined overall ROH in a multi-center study of 9388 cases and 12,456 controls Keller et al. (2012). Again, patients had greater overall ROH, though it accounted for only 0.1% of variance in risk. Stated another way, the odds of having schizophrenia increased about 17% with each 0.01 increase on overall homozygosity (Keller et al., 2012). These two studies suggest that rare SNPs contribute to the risk of schizophrenia, though specific rare variants have not been identified.

5.4.3   Attention Deficit Hyperactivity Disorder (ADHD)

Though not as frequently studied as schizophrenia and autism, recent evidence suggests that CNVs may also be relevant for the etiology of ADHD. In a study of 430 children with ADHD and 1156 controls, the genome-wide burden of large (> 500 kb) and rare (< 1% frequency) CNVs was greater in cases than in controls (Williams et al., 2010). More specifically, the rates of both rare deletions (0.041 per case) and rare duplications (0.115 per case) were greater than corresponding figures for controls (0.012, 0.062, respectively). Notably, among those cases with ID (IQ's < 70) both types of rare CNVs were especially elevated, though cases without ID still had excesses. In an extension of this study, researchers compared psychometric intelligence in those ADHD cases with ($N = 77$) versus without ($N = 490$) one large, rare CNV

(Langley et al., 2011). The cases with a single, large CNV had a mean IQ of 81.4 (bottom portion of the low average range) versus 85.4 in the cases without; this difference was significant at the univariate level ($p = 0.02$), though it did not meet the significance level established after corrections for multiple comparisons ($p = 0.002$). A reading test was also administered, with identical raw and corrected significance levels. The authors then limited their analyses to all cases without ID. No trend was noted for IQ (mean = 86.3 in cases with a large, rare CNV vs 87.7 in those without), though reading scores were again not significantly lower in the former group ($p = 0.02$).

In contrast to these results, two recent studies did not find evidence of an increased burden of CNVs in ADHD. Elia and colleagues (2012) noted an enrichment of CNVs affecting gene networks regulating metabotropic glutamate receptors, though no greater overall burden (see also Elia et al., 2010). Similarly, Lionel et al. (2011) identified rare de novo and inherited CNVs associated with ADHD that overlapped with CNVs increasing risk for other NDDs, but found no increased burden of any type of CNV (Lionel et al., 2011).

5.4.4   Autism

Autism was the first NDD linked to rare, large CNVs (Sebat et al., 2007). Since the appearance of this seminal study, several additional investigations have generally supported this conclusion, though specific results vary across studies. One recent review estimated that 7–20% of cases of autism might be due to such genetic anomalies (Schaaf & Zoghbi, 2011); both inherited and de novo CNVs were important, the latter more so. The Autism Genome Project (Pinto et al., 2010) found that autistic individuals had more genes influenced by CNVs than controls. Rare duplications with genes were significant only above 500 kb and rare deletions with genes were significant only in the 30–500 kb range. Sanders et al. (2011) reported an odds ratio of 3.5 for all rare CNVs, increasing to 5.6 for *de novo* events affecting multiple genes. As with schizophrenia and ADHD, these studies also provide clues as to specific loci that might be linked with critical developmental processes. Like schizophrenia and ADHD, autism occurs more often in males. Levy et al. (2011) found that female cases had a higher rate of *de novo* CNVs than males, while Gilman et al. (2011) demonstrated that greater perturbations of a genetic network governing synaptogenesis is necessary for phenotypic expression of autism in females. A study of an animal model of autistic-like traits caused by a CNV revealed that animals raised in enriched environments showed substantially reduced effects (Lacaria et al., 2012), consistent with data from inbreeding depression discussed earlier, suggesting that harsh environments may bring out mutation effects.

There is some evidence that among individuals with autism general intellectual ability might be related to variations in CNV features. In simplex autism cases (only one affected child per family), Sanders et al. (2011) found that intellectual functioning was related to the overall number of genes affected by de novo CNVs in males (a decrease of 0.42 IQ points was seen for each additional gene affected), though no such effect was noted in female cases. Coe et al. (2012) reexamined these data, including many more small CNVs down to 500 kbp. The correlation between the minimum CNV size per subject (from both deletions and duplications) was weakly but significantly negatively correlated with IQ ($N = 841$). These and related analyses suggested a "significant role for rare CNVs in phenotypic severity with both individual large CNVs and the combined effect of multiple rare CNVs leading to an increased effect size" (p.124, Coe et al., 2012).

5.4.5   The "Two-Hit" Scenario

Research on CNVs has had a major impact on our conceptualization of the genetic underpinnings of serious developmental abnormalities. While it is now well established that single, large, and rare CNVs are causally implicated in a minority of cases of schizophrenia, autism,

and intellectual disability, an important question remains about the genetic architecture of cases with these diagnoses that do not have such striking genetic abnormalities. This issue becomes more important as one considers less debilitating NDDs, such as ADHD.

The "two hit hypothesis", originally offered by Girirajan and Eichler, 2010, may extend the explanatory power of CNVs. This hypothesis was originally offered to help account for phenotypic variability among carriers of a 520 kb microdeletion on 16p12.1. About 25% of probands with this abnormality also had another large deletion or duplication, which could have been anywhere in the genome. These individuals with a second hit had more severe phenotypes, and it was hypothesized that the second hit created a "sensitized genetic background" (Girirajan & Eichler, 2010). The authors note that "in principle" the second hit could be a smaller CNV. These considerations lead to the possibility that some CNVs may be causal, while others may moderate their phenotypic impact.

A recent case report offers additional details of two-hit effects in autism. The proband, who had rather severe symptoms and also comorbid ADHD, had two notable CNVs, one inherited from his mother and one from his father. The parents were described as having only mild degrees of attentional impairment, suggesting that neither CNV was capable of producing autism on its own, but the combination was sufficient. The two-hit hypothesis has also been applied to the Velo-Cardio-Facial Syndrome (VCFS; Bassett et al., 2008), a microdeletion syndrome of 22q11.2 that is associated with a greatly elevated risk for schizophrenia. A second hit was more likely in VCFS cases with psychosis than without (Williams et al., 2013).

The most complete and recent summary of two-hit effects provided additional insights (Girirajan et al., 2012). From a sample of 32,587 children with diverse developmental abnormalities, 7.1 percent had rare CNVs in regions previously linked with clinically significant neurodevelopmental phenotypes. Of these, 8.7% (0.6% of the total sample) had a second hit that exceeded 500 kb. The second hits were more often maternally inherited, and more often noted in phenotypically variable diagnoses (e.g., autism) than syndromic disorders. Interestingly, male probands were more apt to have the former type of diagnosis, leading the authors to suggest that they might be more vulnerable to large, rare CNVs than females. The authors suggested that this might emerge from male exposure to weakly deleterious mutations on the X chromosome, implying that the sex difference in vulnerability to NDDs may represent another version of the two-hit mechanism, though other mechanisms are possible.

Conceptually, the two-hit hypothesis shares features with the DI model. Second hits modify the expression of a phenotype causally related to other genetic features. The "non-specific" genetic component of the DI model, reflecting in large part mutation load, also modifies specific phenotypes causally related to other genetic features. Additionally, the DI model hypothesizes that the non-specific component works through destabilization of canalization, rendering one vulnerable to other adverse genetic and environmental perturbations. Girirajan's original formulation pertained only to the minority of probands with a large, rare CNV, limiting application of their two-hit hypothesis to a very small proportion of individuals. In theory, the DI approach can account for more cases, as it is not based on the conjunction of very rare events. But, for a rigorous test of the model, other types of "specific" polygenic genetic influences will need to be identified.

5.5 GENERAL MECHANISMS

Our recent ability to detect large, rare CNVs has led to a better understanding of their role in NDDs: they may be causal in a minority of cases and they have phenotypically variable effects. The cumulative effects of smaller CNVs are now actively being explored, and soon technology will allow widespread assessment of rare, single nucleotide variations. All of these types of mutations will likely have both locus-specific

effects and general effects, and we suggest that the latter can best be understood as reflections of DI (Yeo et al., 2007) or decanalization (McGrath et al., 2011). The phenotypic outcomes of DI are variable across individuals, reflecting not only stochastic influences in developmental processes, but also the timing and nature of relevant genetic and environmental perturbations. Thus, DI may perhaps be considered a general risk factor for NDDs, increasing the probability that other specific etiological influences have an adverse impact on brain development. Let us consider the nature of decanalization a bit more closely.

Canalization of buffering capacity is an adaptive trait that, to paraphrase Dobzhansky, only makes sense in the light of evolution. Organisms benefit by minimizing the phenotypic impact of genetic and environmental perturbations, preserving adaptive design features. However, we know relatively little about the design features conferring this critical ability. Bergman and Siegal (2003) noted that "canalization does not require a dedicated mechanism … but instead arises as an emergent property of complex developmental-genetic networks", leading them to propose that "loss of function might be induced by … removing the function of an arbitrary gene in the network" (p.549). Reduced canalization or buffering can thus emerge from diverse mutations, increasing the odds of atypical development. Human brains may be especially vulnerable to decanalization, for several reasons, as shown in Table 5.2

There is another potential consequence to decanalization: Increased expression of previously "silent" genetic variations. Because it restricts phenotypic variation, canalization allows the accretion of unexpressed or cryptic genetic variation that can potentially lead to diverse phenotypic variations. Critically, the expression of such cryptic variation increases with environmental harshness or stress. In their comprehensive review, Jarosz and colleagues (2010) note that in a rich growth medium, over 80% of gene knockouts have no detectable effect on growth, yet "almost half of all nonessential gene deletions led to a competition disadvantage

TABLE 5.2   Reasons why the human brain may be especially vulnerable to mutations

1. A great many genes, perhaps 84% (Hawrylycz et al., 2012), are expressed in the brain, rendering it a "large target."
2. Many genes show pleiotropy, increasing the likelihood that mutations might affect brain function.
3. Genes for brain function tend to be relatively large, increasing the probability that a mutation might affect one.
4. Copy number variations occur in chromosomal regions ("hotspots") that have been important for primate brain evolution.
5. The brain has "tightly-regulated critical windows for development; thus there are few opportunities to compensate for perturbation" (p.2, McGrath et al., 2011).
6. The human brain has been subject to much recent selection pressure (for larger size, language development, etc.), providing evolution insufficient time to develop optimal buffering mechanisms.

in minimal medium" (p.191), findings reminiscent of those from inbreeding depression studies. Thus, determining the importance of genetic variation independent of variations in early environment is difficult indeed. They also note that reduced buffering leads to a range of different phenotypes dependent on genetic background. Specific mutations may exert an adverse effect only in certain environmental or genetic contexts, that is, they are "condition dependent" (Van Dyken & Wade, 2010), and this allows the accumulation of deleterious mutations in the genome by altering the mutation-selection balance. These considerations help place the neurobiological effects of mutations in an evolutionary context and demonstrate the difficulties of deriving straightforward relationships between mutations and specific phenotypes.

5.5.1   Key Challenges

Understanding the manner in which genetic variations, coupled with environmental stresses,

lead to variation in brain development is a key issue in both basic and clinical neuroscience. And while enormous progress has occurred in the past decade, based on behavior genetics, GWAS, and emerging insights regarding the importance of CNVs and rare SNP variants, the limitations of our current knowledge are striking. Aside from rather banal conclusions, such as (1) a great many SNPs, common and rare, are related to risk, (2) really large and rare CNVs are causal in a small minority of cases, and (3) genetic risk factors overlap across NDDs, the impact of the past decade of molecular genetic research has been somewhat less than transformative. From the perspective of basic research, novel theories linking genetic variation to diagnostic phenotypes have not yet emerged. From a clinical perspective, observed genetic variation in an individual cannot yet predict the most effective treatment or a patient's clinical course. Naturally, technical advances in genetic technology will soon allow a better assessment of rare SNPs and CNVs. But technical developments in genetics alone will perhaps be insufficient to meet long-term basic and clinical research agendas. As ever more genetic features are measured, ever larger samples will be needed to determine significance. Given research costs and trade-offs, this will make it *more* difficult to acquire detailed phenotypic data in the form of neuroimaging or neurocognitive assessments. Thus, conceptual or theoretical advances must accompany technological advances.

DI theory represents one attempt to bring a conceptual framework, based on evolutionary biology and psychology, to the field of NDDs. Other viewpoints, perhaps building on the two-hit hypothesis, will surely have a substantial impact. DI theory draws attention to the importance of mutation-selection balance as a way to understand the competing forces regulating the population frequency of adverse genetic influences, provides a conceptual framework that focuses on variation in brain development in general rather than disorder-specific features, and in its emphasis on the mechanism of reduced buffering draws our attention to overall mutation load, the expression of cryptic genetic variation, and the fundamentally stochastic nature of atypical brain development. At a practical and clinical level, DI theory suggests the need for targeted environmental interventions. If individuals at risk for NDDs are especially vulnerable to poor early environments or adolescent substance abuse or similar perturbations due to reduced canalization, targeting our limited mental health resources to high risk individuals in high risk environments, at the earliest age possible, may be efficacious. Identification of high risk individuals on the basis of genetic variation is a key challenge for future researchers.

REFERENCES

Amaral, P.P., and Mattick, J.S. (2008). Noncoding RNA in development. Mamm Genome 19, 454–492.

Badaruddoza, M., and Afzal, M. (1993). Inbreeding depression and intelligence quotient among north Indian children. Behav Genet 23(4), 343–347.

Bailey, J.A., and Eichler, E.E. (2006). Primate segmental duplications: Crucibles of evolution, diversity and disease. Nat Rev Genet 7, 552–564.

Bassett, A.S., Marshall, C.R., Lionel, A.C., Chow, E.W.C., and Scherer, S.W. (2008). Copy number variations and risk for schizophrenia in 22q11.2 deletion syndrome. Hum Mol Genet 17(24), 4045–4053. doi:10.1093/hmg/ddn307

Beasley, D.E., Bonisoli-Alquati, A., Welch, S.M., Møller, A.P., and Mousseau, T.A. (2012). Effects of parental radiation exposure on developmental instability in grasshoppers. J Evol Biol 25(6), 1149–1162. doi:10.1111/j.1420-9101.2012.02502.x

Beckmann, J.S., Estavill, X., and Antonarakis, S.E. (2007). Copy number variants and genetic traits: Closer to the resolution of phenotypic to genotypic variability. Nat Rev Genet 8, 639–646.

Bergen, S.E., O'Dushlaine, C.T., Ripke, S., Lee, P.H., Ruderfer, D.M., Akterin, S., Moran, J.L., et al. (2012). Genome-wide association study in a Swedish population yields support for greater CNV and MHC involvement in schizophrenia compared with bipolar disorder. Mol Psychiatry 17(9), 880–886.

Bergman, A., and Siegal, M.L. (2003). Evolutionary capacitance as a general feature of complex gene networks. Nature 424, 549–552.

Bilder, R.M., Reiter, G., Bates, J., Lencz, T., Szeszko, P., Goldman, R.S., Robinson, D., et al. (2006). Cognitive development in schizophrenia: follow-back from the first episode. J Clin Exp Neuropsychol 28(2), 270–282.

Buizer-Voskamp, J.E., Muntjewerff, J.-W., Strengman, E., Sabatti, C., Stefansson, H., Vorstman, J.a.S., and Ophoff, R.a. (2011). Genome-wide analysis shows increased frequency of copy number variation deletions in Dutch schizophrenia patients. Biol Psychiatry 70(7), 655–662.

Campbell, C.D., Chong, J.X., Malig, M., Ko, A., Dumont, B.L., Han, L., Vives, L., et al. (2012). Estimating the human mutation rate using autozygosity in a founder population. Nat Genet 44(11), 1277–1281.

Carter, A.J.R., and Houle, D. (2011). Artificial selection reveals heritable variation for developmental instability. Evolution, 65, 3558–3564.

Carter, A.J.R., Weier, T.M., and Houle, D. (2009). The effect of inbreeding on fluctuating asymmetry of wing veins in two laboratory strains of Drosophila melanogaster. Heredity 102(6), 563–572.

Chan, S.K.W., Chan, K.K.S., Lam, M.M.L., Chiu, C.P.Y., Hui, C.L.M., Wong, G.H.Y., Chang, W.C., et al. (2012). Clinical and cognitive correlates of insight in first-episode schizophrenia. Schizophr Res 135(1–3), 40–45.

Chandler, C.H., Chari, S., and Dworkin, I. (2013). Does your gene need a background check? How genetic background impacts the analysis of mutations, genes, and evolution. Trends Genet 29(6), 358–366.

Charlesworth, B., and Charlesworth, D. (1999). The genetic basis of inbreeding depression. Genet Res 74(3), 329–340.

Chiaromonte, F., Weber, R.J., Roskin, K.M., Diekhans, M., Kent, W.J., and Haussker, D. (2003). The share of genomic DNA under selection estimated from human-mouse genomic alignment. Cold Spring Harb Symp Quant Biol 68, 245–254.

Coe, B.P., Girirajan, S., and Eichler, E.E. (2012). The genetic variability and commonality of neurodevelopmental disease. Am J Med Genet, Part C 160C, 118–129.

Compton, M.T., and Walker, E.F. (2009). Physical manifestations of neurodevelopmental disruption: are minor physical anomalies part of the syndrome of schizophrenia? Schizophr Bull 35(2), 425–436.

Conrad, D.F., Keebler, J.E.M., DePristo, M.A., Lindsay, S.J., Zhang, Y., Casals, F., Idaghdour, Y., et al. (2011). Variation in genome-wide mutation rates within and between human families. Nat Genet 43(7), 712–715.

Cooper, G.M., Coe, B.P., Girirajan, S., Rosenfeld, J.a., Vu, T.H., Baker, C., Williams, C., et al. (2011). A copy number variation morbidity map of developmental delay. Nat Genet 43(9), 838–846.

Crespi, B. (2008). Genomic imprinting in the development and evolution of psychotic spectrum conditions. Biol Rev 83, 441–493.

Deary, I.J. (2012). Intelligence. Annu Rev Psychol 63(September), 453–482.

Debat, V., Debelle, A., and Dworkin, I. (2009). Plasticity, canalization, and developmental stability of the Drosophila wing: joint effects of mutations and developmental temperature. Evolution 63(11), 2864–2876.

Doolittle, W.F. (2013). Is junk DNA bunk? A critique of ENCODE. Proc Natl Acad Sci U S A 110(14), 5294–5300.

Drake, J.W., Charlesworth, B., Charlesworth, D., and Crow, J.F. (1998). Rates of spontaneous mutation. Genetics 148(4), 1667–1686.

Dumas, L., Kim, Y.H., Karimpour-Ford, A., Cox, M., Hopkinds, J., Pollack, J.R., and Sikela, J.M. (2007). Gene copy number variation spanning 60 million years of human primate evolution. Genome Res 17, 1266–1277.

Dunham, I., Kundaje, A., Aldred, S.F., Collins, P.J., Davis, C.a., Doyle, F., Epstein, C.B., et al. (2012). An integrated encyclopedia of DNA elements in the human genome. Nature 489(7414), 57–74.

Eisenberg, D.P., and Berman, K.F. (2010). Executive function, neural circuitry, and genetic mechanisms in schizophrenia. Neuropsychopharmacology 35(1), 258–277.

Elia, J, Gai, X., Xie, H.M., Perin, J.C., Geiger, E., Glessner, J.T., D'arcy, M., et al. (2010). Rare structural variants found in attention-deficit hyperactivity disorder are preferentially associated with neurodevelopmental genes. Mol Psychiatry 15(6), 637–646.

Elia, J., Glessner, J.T., Wang, K., Takahashi, N., Shtir, C.J., Hadley, D., Sleiman, P.M.a., et al. (2012).

Genome-wide copy number variation study associates metabotropic glutamate receptor gene networks with attention deficit hyperactivity disorder. Nat Genet 44(1), 78–84.

Fanous, A.H., and Kendler, K.S. (2005). Genetic heterogeneity, modifier genes, and quantitative phenotypes in psychiatric illness: searching for a framework. Mol Psychiatry 10(1), 6–13.

Firman, R.C., Simmons, L.W., Cummins, J.M., and Matson, P.L. (2003). Are body fluctuating asymmetry and the ratio of 2nd to 4th digit length reliable predictors of semen quality?. Hum Reprod 18(4), 808–812.

Frans, E.M., Sandin, S., Reichenberg, A., Langstrom, N., Lichtenstein, P., McGrath, J.J., and Hultman, C.M. (2013). Autism risk across generations: A population-based study of advancing grandpaternal and paternal Age. JAMA Psychiatry 70(5), 516–521.

Fuller, R.C., and Houle, D. (2002). Detecting genetic variation in developmental instability by artificial selection on fluctuating asymmetry. J Evol Biol 15(6), 954–960.

Furlow, F.B., Armijo-Prewitt, T., Gangestad, S.W., and Thornhill, R. (1997). Fluctuating asymmetry and psychometric intelligence. Proc Biol Sci 264(1383), 823–829.

Gamsiz, E.D., Viscidi, E.W., Frederick, A.M., Nagpal, S., Sanders, S.J., Murtha, M.T., Schmidt, M., et al. (2013). Intellectual disability is associated with increased runs of homozygosity in simplex autism. Am J Hum Genet 93(1), 103–109.

Gangestad, S.W., Bennett, K.L., and Thornhill, R. (2001). A latent variable model of developmental instability in relation to men's sexual behaviour. Proc Biol Sci 268(1477), 1677–1684.

Gangestad, S.W., and Thornhill, R. (1999). Individual differences in developmental precision and fluctuating asymmetry: a model and its implications, J Evol Biol 12, 402–416.

Gangestad, S.W., and Thornhill, R. (2003). Fluctuating asymmetry, developmental instability, and fitness: Toward a model-based interpretation. In M. Polak (eds.), Developmental instability: Causes and consequences, (pp. 62–80). Oxford University Press Cambridge, UK.

Gangestad, S.W., and Yeo, R.A. (2006). Mutations, developmental instability, and the Red Queen. Behav Brain Sci 29, 412–413.

Gilman, S.R., Iossifov, I., Levy, D., Ronemus, M., Wigler, M., and Vitkup, D. (2011). Rare de novo variants associated with autism implicate a large functional network of genes involved in formation and function of synapses. Neuron 70(5), 898–907.

Girirajan, S., Campbell, C.D., and Eichler, E.E. (2011). Human copy number variation and complex genetic disease. Annu Rev Genet 45, 203–226.

Girirajan, S., and Eichler, E.E. (2010). Phenotypic variability and genetic susceptibility to genomic disorders. Hum Mol Genet 19(R2), R176–R187.

Girirajan, S., Rosenfeld, J.A., Coe, B.P., Parikh, S., Friedman, N., Goldstein, A., Filipink, R.A., et al. (2012). Phenotypic heterogeneity of genomic disorders and rare copy-number variants. N Engl J Med 367(14), 1321–1331.

Gottesman, I.I., and Gould, T.D. (2003). Reviews and overviews the endophenotype concept in psychiatry: Etymology and strategic intentions. Am J Psychiatry 160, 636–645.

Habets, P., Marcelis, M., Gronenschild, E., Drukker, M., and Van Os, J. (2011). Reduced cortical thickness as an outcome of differential sensitivity to environmental risks in schizophrenia. Biol Psychiatry 69(5), 487–494.

Hawrylycz, M.J., Lein, E.S., Guillozet-Bongaarts, A.L., et al. (2012). An anatomically comprehensive atlas of the adult human brain transcriptome. Nature 489, 391–399.

Hofer, a., Bodner, T., Kaufmann, a., Kemmler, G., Mattarei, U., Pfaffenberger, N.M., Rettenbacher, M.a., et al. (2011). Symptomatic remission and neurocognitive functioning in patients with schizophrenia. Psychol Med 41(10), 2131–2139.

Iafrate, A.J., Feuk, L., Rivera, M.N., Listewnik, M.L., Donahoe, P.K., Qi, Y., Scherer, S.W., et al. (2004). Detection of large-scale variation in the human genome. Nat Genet 36, 949–951.

Jarosz, D.F., Taipale, M., and Lindquist, S. (2010). Protein homeostasis and the phenotypic manifestation of genetic diversity: principles and mechanisms. Annu Rev Genet 44, 189–216.

Jensen, A.R. (1998). The g factor. Westport, CT: Praeger.

Johnson, W. (2010). Understanding the genetics of intelligence: Can height help? Can corn oil? Curr Dir Psychol Sci 19(3), 177–182.

Johnson, W., Gangestad, S.W., Segal, N.L., and Bouchard, T.J. (2008). Heritability of Fluctuating Asymmetry in a Human Twin Sample: The Effect of Trait Aggregation. Am J Hum Biol 20(6), 651–658.

Joober, R., and Boksa, P. (2009). A new wave in the genetics of psychiatric disorders: J Psychiatry Neurosci 34(1), 55–60.

Jung, R.E., Brooks, W.M., Yeo, R.a., Chiulli, S.J., Weers, D.C., and Sibbitt, W.L. (1999). Biochemical markers of intelligence: a proton MR spectroscopy study of normal human brain. Proc R Soc B 266(1426), 1375–1379.

Kegeles, L.S., Shungu, D.C., Mao, X., Goetz, R., Mikell, C.B., Abi-Dargham, A., Laruelle, M., et al. (2005). Relationship of paternal age to N-acetyl-aspartate in the prefrontal cortex in schizophrenia. Schizophrenia Bulletin 31 443.

Keller, M.C., and Miller, G. (2006). Resolving the paradox of common, harmful, heritable mental disorders: which evolutionary genetic models work best? Behav Brain Sci 29(4), 385–404; discussion 405–452.

Keller, M.C., Simonson, M.A., Ripke, S., Neale, B.M., Gejman, P. V, Howrigan, D.P., Lee, S.H., et al. (2012). Runs of homozygosity implicate autozygosity as a schizophrenia risk factor. PLoS Genet 8(4), e1002656.

Khandaker, G.M., Barnett, J.H., White, I.R., and Jones, P.B. (2011). A quantitative meta-analysis of population-based studies of premorbid intelligence and schizophrenia. Schizophr Res 132(2–3), 220–227.

Kim, P.M., Lam, H.Y.K., Urban, A.E., Korbel, J.O., Affourtit, J., Grubert, F., Chen, X., et al. (2008). Analysis of copy number variants and segmental duplication in the human genome: Evidence for a change in the process of formation in recent evolutionary history. Genome Res 18, 1865–1874.

Kirov, G., Grozeva, D., Norton, N., Ivanov, D., Mantripragada, K.K., Holmans, P., Craddock, N., et al. (2009). Support for the involvement of large copy number variants in the pathogenesis of schizophrenia. Hum Mol Genet 18(8), 1497–1503.

Kondrashov, A. (2012). The rate of human mutation. Nature 488, 467–468.

Kong, A., Frigge, M.L., Masson, G., Besenbacher, S., Sulem, P., Magnusson, G., Gudjonsson, S.A., et al. (2012). Rate of de novo mutations and the importance of father's age to disease risk. Nature 488(7412), 471–475.

Korn, J.M., Kuruvilla, F.G., McCarroll, S.a., Wysoker, A., Nemesh, J., Cawley, S., Hubbell, E., et al. (2008). Integrated genotype calling and association analysis of SNPs, common copy number polymorphisms and rare CNVs. Nat Genet 40(10), 1253–1260.

Kulkarni, M.L., and Kurian, M. (1990). Consanguinity and its effect on fetal growth and development: a south Indian study. J Med Genet 27(6), 348–352.

Lacaria, M., Spencer, C., Gu, W., Paylor, R., and Lupski, J.R. (2012). Enriched rearing improves behavioral responses of an animal model for CNV-based autistic-like traits. Hum Mol Genet 21(14), 3083–3096.

Langley, K., Martin, J., Agha, S.S., Davies, C., Stergiakouli, E., Holmans, P., Williams, N., et al. (2011). Clinical and cognitive characteristics of children with attention-deficit hyperactivity disorder, with and without copy number variants. Br J Psychiatry 199(5), 398–403.

Leeson, V.C., Sharma, P., Harrison, M., Ron, M.A., Barnes, T.R.E., and Joyce, E.M. (2011). IQ trajectory, cognitive reserve, and clinical outcome following a first episode of psychosis: a 3-year longitudinal study. Schizophr Bull 37(4), 768–777.

Lencz, T., Lambert, C., DeRosse, P., Burdick, K.E., Morgan, T.V., Kane, J.M., Kucherlapati, R., et al. (2007). Runs of homozygosity reveal highly penetrant recessive loci in schizophrenia. Proc Natl Acad Sci 104(50), 19942–19947.

Levy, D., Ronemus, M., Yamrom, B., Lee, Y., Leotta, A., Kendall, J., Marks, S., et al. (2011). Rare de novo and transmitted copy-number variation in autistic spectrum disorders. Neuron 70(5), 886–897.

Lionel, A.C., Crosbie, J., Barbosa, N., Goodale, T., Thiruvahindrapuram, B., Rickaby, J., Gazzellone, M., et al. (2011). Rare copy number variation discovery and cross-disorder comparisons identify risk genes for ADHD. Sci Transl Med 3(95), 95ra75.

Livshits, G., and Kobylianski, E. (1991). Fluctuating asymmetry as a possible measure of developmental homeostasis in humans: A review. Hum Biol, 63, 441–466.

Locke, D.P., Sharp, A.J., McCarroll, S.A., McGrath, S.D., Newman, T.L., Cheng, Z., Schwartz, S., et al. (2006). Linkage disequilibrium and heritability of copy-number polymorphisms within duplicated regions of the human genome. Am J Hum Genet 79, 275–290.

Lunter, G., Ponting, C.P., and Hein, J. (2006). Genome-wide identification of human functional DNA using a neutral indel model. PLoS Comput Biol 2, 2–12.

MacLeod, A.K., Davies, G., Payton, A., Tenesa, A., Harris, S.E., Liewald, D., Ke, X., et al. (2012). Genetic copy number variation and general cognitive ability. PLoS One 7(12), e37385.

Malaspina, D., Reichenberg, A., Weiser, M., Fennig, S., Davidson, M., Harlap, S., Wolitzky, R., et al. (2005). Paternal age and intelligence: implications for age-related genomic changes in male germ cells. Psychiatr Genet 15(2), 117–125.

Mallik, M., and Lakhotia, S.C. (2007). Noncopding DNA is not "junk" but a necessity for origin and evolution of biological complexity. Proc Natl Acad Sci India Sect B 77, 43–50.

Mansour, H., Fathi, W., Klei, L., Wood, J., Chowdari, K., Watson, A., Eissa, A., et al. (2010). Consanguinity and increased risk for schizophrenia in Egypt. Schizophr Res 120(1–3), 108–112.

Marques-Bonet, T., Kidd, J.M., Ventura, M., Graves, T.a., Cheng, Z., Hillier, L.W., Jiang, Z., et al. (2009). A burst of segmental duplications in the genome of the African great ape ancestor. Nature 457(7231), 877–881.

Martin, N.S. (2009). Contributions of twin studies to understanding the etiology of complex disease. Festschrift in honor of Thomas J. Bouchard.

McGrath, J.J., Hannan, A.J., and Gibson, G. (2011). Decanalization, brain development and risk of schizophrenia. Transl Psychiatry 1(6), e14.

McNeil, T.F., Cantor-Graae, E., and Weinberger, D.R. (2000). Relationship of obstetric complications and differences in size of brain structures in monozygotic twin pairs discordant for schizophrenia. Am J Psychiatry 157(2), 203–212.

McRae, A.F., Wright, M.J., Hansell, N.K., Montgomery, G.W., and Martin, N.G. (2013). No association between general cognitive ability and rare copy number variation. Behav Genet 43, 202–207.

Miller, B., Messias, E., Miettunen, J., Alaräisänen, A., Järvelin, M.-R., Koponen, H., Räsänen, P., et al. (2011). Meta-analysis of paternal age and schizophrenia risk in male versus female offspring. Schizophr Bull 37(5), 1039–1047.

Mitchell, K.J. (2012). What is complex about complex disorders? Genome Biol 13(1), 237.

Møller, A.P. (2002). Developmental instability and sexual selection in stag beetles from Chernobyl and a control area. Ethology 204, 193–204.

Morrow, E.M. (2010). Genomic copy number variation in disorders of cognitive development. J Am Acad Child Adolesc Psychiatry 49(11), 1091–1104.

Need, A.C., Ge, D., Weale, M.E., Maia, J., Feng, S., Heinzen, E.L., Shianna, K. V., et al. (2009). A genome-wide investigation of SNPs and CNVs in schizophrenia. PLoS Genet 5(2), e1000373.

Nowacki, M., Higgins, B.P., Maquilan, G.M., Swart, E.C., Doak, T.G., and Landweber, L.F. (2009). A functional role for transposases in a large eukaryotic genome. Science 324(5929), 935–938.

Ozener, B. (2010). Effect of inbreeding depression on growth and fluctuating asymmetry in Turkish young males. Am J Hum Biol 22(4), 557–562. doi:10.1002/ajhb.21046

Pinto, D., Pagnamenta, A.T., Klei, L., Anney, R., Merico, D., Regan, R., Conroy, J., et al. (2010). Functional impact of global rare copy number variation in autism spectrum disorders. Nature 466(7304), 368–372.

Ponting, C.P. (2009). The functional repertoires of metazoan genomes. Nat Rev Genet 9, 689–698.

Popesco, M.C., MacLaaren, E.J., Hopkins, J., Dumas, L., Cox, M., Meltesen, L., McGavran, L., et al. (2006). Human lineage-specific amplification, selection, and neuronal expression of DUF1220 domains. Science 313(5791), 1304–1307.

Puig, O., Penadés, R., Baeza, I., Sánchez-Gistau, V., De la Serna, E., Fonrodona, L., Andrés-Perpiñá, S., et al. (2012). Processing speed and executive functions predict real-world everyday living skills in adolescents with early-onset schizophrenia. Eur Child Adolesc Psychiatry 21(6), 315–326.

Redon, R., Ishikawa, S., Fitch, K.R., Feuk, L., Perry, G.H., Andrews, T.D., Fiegler, H.S., et al. (2006). Global variation in copy number in the human genome. Nature 444, 444–454.

Reichenberg, A., Gross, R., Weiser, M., Bresnahan, M., Silverman, J., Harlap, S., Rabinowitz, J., et al. (2006). Advancing paternal age and autism. Arch Gen Psychiatry 63(9), 1026–1032.

Saha, S., Barnett, A.G., Foldi, C., Burne, T.H., Eyles, D.W., Buka, S.L., and McGrath, J.J. (2009). Advanced paternal age is associated with impaired neurocognitive outcomes during infancy and childhood. PLoS Med 6(3), e40.

Sanders, S.J., Ercan-Sencicek, a.G., Hus, V., Luo, R., Murtha, M.T., Moreno-De-Luca, D., Chu, S.H., et al. (2011). Multiple recurrent de novo CNVs, including duplications of the 7q11.23 Williams syndrome region, are strongly associated with autism. Neuron 70(5), 863–885.

Schaaf, C.P., and Zoghbi, H.Y. (2011). Solving the autism puzzle a few pieces at a time. Neuron 70(5), 806–808.

Sebat, J., Lakshmi, B., Malhotra, D., Troge, J., Lese, C., Walsh, T., Yamrom, B., et al. (2007). Strong association of de novo copy number mutations with autism. Science 316(5823), 445–449.

Sebat, J., Lakshmi, B., Troge, J., Alexander, J., Young, J., Lundin, P., and Al, E. (2004). Large-scale copy number polymorphism in the human genome. Science 305, 525–528.

Sebat, J., Levy, D.L., and McCarthy, S.E. (2009). Rare structural variants in schizophrenia: one disorder, multiple mutations; one mutation, multiple disorders. Trends Genet 25(12), 528–535.

Shaw, P., Gilliam, M., Malek, M., Rodriguez, N., Greenstein, D., Clasen, L., Evans, A., et al. (2012). Parental age effects on cortical morphology in offspring. Cereb Cortex 22(6), 1256–1262.

Siepel, A., Bejerano, G., Pedersen, J.S., Hinrichs, A.S., Hou, M.M., Clawson, H., Spieth, J., et al. (2005). Evolutionarily conserved elements in vertebrate, insect, worm, and year genomes. Genome Res 15, 1034–1050.

Sikela, J.M. (2006). The jewels of our genome: The search for the genomic changes underlying the evolutionarily unique capacities of the human brain. PLoS Genet 2, 646–655.

Smith, N.G.C., Brandstrom, M., and Ellegren, H. (2004). Evidence for turnover of functional noncoding DNA in mammalian genome evolution. Genomics 84, 806–813.

Stone, J.L., and Consortium, T.I.S. (2008). Rare chromosomal deletions and duplications increase risk of schizophrenia. Science 455(7210), 237–241.

Szpiech, Z.A., Xu, J., Pemberton, T.J., Peng, W., Zöllner, S., Rosenberg, N.A., and Li, J.Z. (2013). Long runs of homozygosity are enriched for deleterious variation. Am J Hum Genet 93(1), 90–102.

Taylor, J.S., and Raes, J. (2004). Duplication and divergence: the evolution of new genes and old ideas. Annu Rev Genet 38, 615–643.

Tennessen, J.a., Bigham, A.W., O'Connor, T.D., Fu, W., Kenny, E.E., Gravel, S., McGee, S., et al. (2012). Evolution and functional impact of rare coding variation from deep sequencing of human exomes. Science 337(6090), 64–69.

Toulopoulou, T., Picchioni, M., Rijsdijk, F., Hua-Hall, M., Ettinger, U., Sham, P., and Murray, R. (2008). Substantial genetic overlap between neurocognition and schizophrenia. Arch Gen Psychiatry 64(12), 1348–1355.

Van Dongen, S. (1998). How repeatable is the estimation of developmental stability by fluctuating asymmetry? Stefan van Dongen. Proc Biol Sci 265(1404), 1423–1431.

Van Dongen, S. (2006). Fluctuating asymmetry and developmental instability in evolutionary biology: Past, present, and future. J Evol Biol 19, 1727–1743.

Van Dongen, S., and Gangestad, S.W. (2011). Human fluctuating asymmetry in relation to health and quality: a meta-analysis. Evol Hum Behav 32(6), 380–398.

Van Dyken, J.D., and Wade, M.J. (2010). The genetic signature of conditional expression. Genetics 184(2), 557–570.

Van Os, J., Linscott, R.J., Myin-Germeys, I., Delespaul, P., and Krabbendam, L. (2009). A systematic review and meta-analysis of the psychosis continuum: Evidence for a psychosis proneness-persistence-impairment model of psychotic disorder. Psychol Med 39(2), 179–195.

Van Scheltinga, A.T., Bakker, S., Van Haren, N., Buizer-Voskamp, J., Boos, H., Vorstman, J., Cahn, W., et al. (2012). Association study of copy number variants with brain volume in schizophrenia patients and healthy controls. Psychiatry Res. 200(2–3), 1011–1013

Van Valen, L. (1978). The control of handedness. Behav Brain Sci 2, 230.

Vinces, M.D., Legendre, M., Caldara, M., Hagihara, M., and Verstrepen, K.J. (2009). Unstable tandem repeats in promoters confer transcriptional evolvability. Science 324, 1213.

Vorstman, J.S., and Ophoff, R.A. (2013). Genetic causes of developmental disorders. Curr Opin Neurol 26(2), 128–136.

Waddington, C. (1942). Canalization and the inheritance of acquired characters. Nature 150, 563–565.

Waldrop, M.F., and Halverson, C.F. (1989). Manual for assessing minor physical anomalies (rev. ed.). (U. Manusript, Ed.). University of Georgia: Athens.

Walsh, T., McClellan, J.M., McCarthy, S.E., Addington, A.M., Pierce, S.B., Cooper, G.M., Nord, A.S., et al. (2008). Rare structural variants disrupt multiple genes in neurodevelopmental pathways in schizophrenia. Science 320(5875), 539–43.

Welch, K.a., McIntosh, A.M., Job, D.E., Whalley, H.C., Moorhead, T.W., Hall, J., Owens, D.G.C., et al. (2011). The impact of substance use on brain structure in people at high risk of developing schizophrenia. Schizophr Bull 37(5), 1066–1076.

Whitlock, M. (1996). The heritability of fluctuating asymmetry and the genetic control of developmental stability. Proc R Soc B 263(1372), 849–853.

Williams, H.J., Monks, S., Murphy, K.C., Kirov, G.C.O.M., and Owen, M.J. (2013). Schizophrenia two-hit hypothesis in Velo-Cardio-Facial Syndrome. Am J Med Genet Part B 162, 177–182.

Williams, N.M., Zaharieva, I., Martin, A., Langley, K., Mantripragada, K., Fossdal, R., Stefansson, H., et al. (2010). Rare chromosomal deletions and duplications in attention-deficit hyperactivity disorder: a genome-wide analysis. Lancet 376(9750), 1401–1408.

Wong, K.K., DeLeeuw, R.J., Dosanjh, N.S., Kimm, L.R., Cheng, Z., Horsman, D.E., and Al, E. (2007). A comprehensive analysis of common copy-number variations in the human genome. Am J Hum Genet 80, 91–104.

Wyrobek, A.J., Eskenazi, B., Young, S., Arnheim, N., Tiemann-Boege, I., Jabs, E.W., Glaser, R.L., et al. (2006). Advancing age has differential effects on DNA damage, chromatin integrity, gene mutations, and aneuploidies in sperm. Proc Natl Acad Sci, (May), 103, 9601–9606.

Ye, T., Lipska, B.K., Tao, R., Hyde, T.M., Wang, L., Li, C., Choi, K.H., et al. (2012). Analysis of copy number variations in brain DNA from patients with schizophrenia and other psychiatric disorders. Biol Psychiatry 72(8), 651–654.

Yeo, R.A., and Gangestad, S.W. (1993). Developmental origins of variation in human hand preference. Genetica 89, 281–296.

Yeo, R.A., Gangestad, S.W., Edgar, C., and Thoma, R. (1999). The evolutionary genetic underpinnings of schizophrenia: the developmental instability model. Schizophr Res 39(3), 197–206.

Yeo, R.A., Gangestad, S.W., Liu, J., Ehrlich, S., Thoma, R.J., Pommy, J.M., Mayer, A.R., et al. (2013). The impact of copy number deletions on general cognitive ability and ventricle size in patients with schizophrenia and healthy control subjects. Biol Psychiatry 73(6), 540–545.

Yeo, R.A., Gangestad, S.W., and Thoma, R.J. (2007). Developmental instability and individual variation in brain development, Curr Dir Psychol Sci 16(5), 245–250.

Yeo, R.A., Gangestad, S.W., Thoma, R., Shaw, P., and Repa, K. (1997). Developmental instability and cerebral lateralization. Neuropsychology 11(4), 552–561.

Yeo, R.A., Gangestad, S.W., Walton, E., Ehrlich, S., Pommy, J., Turner, J.A., Liu, J., Mayer, A.R., Schulz, S.C., Ho, B.C., Bustillo, J.R., Wassink, T.H., Sponheim, S.R., and Calhoun, V.D. (2014). Genetic influences on cognitive endophenotypes in schizophrenia. Schizophrenia Research 156, 71–75.

Yeo, R.A, Gangestad, S.W., Liu, J., Calhoun, V.D., and Hutchison, K.E. (2011). Rare copy number deletions predict individual variation in intelligence. PLoS One 6(1), e16339.

6

ENVIRONMENTAL FACTORS AND GENE–ENVIRONMENT INTERACTIONS

JOHN MCGRATH[1,2]

[1]Queensland Brain Institute, The University of Queensland, St. Lucia, QLD 4072, Australia
[2]Queensland Centre for Mental Health Research, The Park Centre for Mental Health, Richlands, QLD, Australia

6.1 INTRODUCTION

The title of this book, and many of its component chapters, focus on the advances in our understanding of the genetic architecture of neurodevelopmental disorders. These discoveries have been galvanized by remarkable advances in the technical ability to capture genetic variation, and by the collaborative efforts of large groups. In addition to the input of the individuals with the clinical neurodevelopmental disorders (and their families and clinicians), these advances have drawn on the skills of statistical geneticists, chemists, engineers, mathematicians, and from the broad church of neuroscientists. Less prominent in this multidisciplinary mix has been the epidemiologist.

The science of epidemiology looks for gradients in disease-related frequency measures (e.g., incidence, prevalence, mortality, and recovery) across time and space. Based on observed gradients, candidate risk factors related to disease frequency can be generated (e.g., infection, exposure to toxins, lifestyles associated with adverse health outcomes etc.). Epidemiology is a powerful tool for generating candidate exposures, but when based solely on observational studies, and when isolated from other fields of science, it has its limitations (Davey Smith, 2001; Davey Smith and Ebrahim, 2001). Animal experiments can provide important insights into the biological plausibility of candidate exposures, and clues initially generated from observational epidemiology have led to important discoveries for basic neuroscience (McGrath and Richards, 2009). Importantly, epidemiology as a discipline is firmly grounded in population health. It tends

The Genetics of Neurodevelopmental Disorders, First Edition. Edited by Kevin J. Mitchell.
© 2015 John Wiley & Sons, Inc. Published 2015 by John Wiley & Sons, Inc.

to seek out modifiable exposures, in the hope that community-based interventions can reduce the burden of disease. Lofty goals such as the primary prevention of diseases may seem quixotic for complex neurodevelopmental disorders such as schizophrenia and autism (Brown and McGrath, 2011). However, public health interventions such as the rubella vaccine and the use of periconceptional folate supplements serve as reminders about what has been achieved in recent decades with respect to the primary prevention of neurodevelopmental disorders.

Researchers looking for genetic or non-genetic risk factors have tended to explore their respective domains independently. As a consequence, the fields of genetics and environmental epidemiology have drifted apart in their methodological thinking. The environmental risks for psychosis have generally been studied across an averaged genetic background. While large samples have provided insights into the genetic architecture of neurodevelopmental disorders, this has been studied against both an averaged environmental background and an averaged genetic background. The study of isolated populations can reduce "noise" in both domains (Holliday et al., 2009), but these studies can be handicapped by issues related to lack of power and uncertain generalizability.

The main aim of this chapter is to provide a concise outline of selected nongenetic risk factors associated with two neurodevelopmental disorders – schizophrenia and autism. These two neurodevelopmental disorders share a range of environmental risk factors (Hamlyn et al., 2013). However, the reader should remain mindful that the environmental risk factors outlined in this chapter are probably associated with a much broader range of neurodevelopmental disorders (e.g., intellectual disability, epilepsy). In addition, the chapter will outline how clues from genetics and epidemiology can be combined with respect to the disorders of interest. There are important opportunities ahead where both epidemiology and genetics can converge to catalyze discovery in the field of neurodevelopmental disorders.

6.2   HOW TO BUILD A BRAIN

The "instructions" to build a healthy brain are widely distributed – the transactional and highly contingent nature of development is not readily captured by simple dichotomies such as "genetic factors" and "environmental factors" (Chapters 7–9). Brain development requires carefully timed input from many different categories of information; (a) heritable factors related to DNA sequence and related genetic and epigenetic mechanisms, (b) expected biological factors related to optimal conditions during development and across the life span (e.g., the basic necessities of life such as oxygen concentrations and nutrients), (c) expected nurturing conditions for social and cognitive development (e.g., maternal care, the influence of family life and cultural values etc.). The absence of the expected cues can disrupt the orderly process of brain development, as key elements of brain development have evolved to be *experience-expectant* – the environment needs to provide the instructions for optimal brain development (Greenough et al., 1987). Equally, the presence of unexpected disruptive factors (e.g., genetic mutation, infections, trauma, etc.) can disrupt brain development. Removing expected environmental instructions can disrupt brain development just as "knocking out" important genes can disrupt key aspects of brain development. Just as transgenic animals can provide insight into the role of genetic factors, "knocking out" optimal sensory and cognitive stimulation results in an animal with an *environmentally edited* developmental trajectory. The potency of these environmentally mediated instructions has been demonstrated in experiments related to enriched environment versus the impoverished nature of standard rodent laboratory conditions (Nithianantharajah and Hannan, 2006). Transgenic animals engineered to express genetic variants associated with Huntington's disease have delayed onset of the disorder when a few novel objects are left in their otherwise uninteresting home cage (Nithianantharajah et al., 2008).

6.3 CAUTIONARY NOTE ON THE INTERPRETATION OF RISK FACTORS

There are many ways to compare the impact of different risk factors. As with all scientific research, consistency of findings is important. Findings that are based on systematic reviews and meta-analyses should be given more credence than isolated findings. Effect size is important – some exposures are more potent than others (e.g., asbestos exposure is more likely to cause lung cancer than cigarette smoking). The prevalence of the putative risk factor is also important, as combined with effect size, these estimates influence the population-attributable fraction. This parameter (which needs to be interpreted with some caution) is an index of how many cases could be averted if the exposure could be reduced to that found in the reference group. Because cigarette smoking tends to be more prevalent than asbestos exposure (at least in most groups), eliminating smoking will avert more cases of lung cancer than would eliminating asbestosis exposure (despite the latter having a greater effect size).

With respect to the environmental risk factors described in the following section, where the data are supported by systematic reviews or meta-analyses, these results will be preferred. In general, effect sizes for most of the exposures discussed in this chapter are modest and less than twofold. One of the most replicated findings in schizophrenia epidemiology relates to an increased risk of the disorder in those born in winter and spring – however the effect size is only 1.07 (Davies et al., 2003). For paternal age over 50 (vs 25–29 years), the risk of schizophrenia in the offspring is 1.66 (Miller et al., 2011). Compared to rural birth, urban birth is associated with an effect size of 2.37 (Vassos et al., 2012). The most potent effect sizes have been associated with migrant status, especially for dark-skinned migrants (or migrants from areas where the majority of the population is black). A systematic review and meta-analysis found that the effect size in this group (compared to native born groups in the host nations) was 4.8.

As with all population-based research, these estimates have varying degrees of imprecision, and may not always generalize to different groups or even the same group tested at different times (secular changes can influence the pattern of association). These estimates are, by necessity, averages across a population and thus reflect group- and not individual-level risk. It is thus impossible to discern whether the risk from any given factor is uniform across the population or whether some individuals are differentially sensitive to it.

Usually, the effect sizes are for persons rather than males or female offspring separately. While there are marked sex differences in the incidence of disorders such as schizophrenia and autism (McGrath et al., 2004b; Fombonne, 2005), no clear sex differences with respect to the environmental risk factors detailed as follows have been identified.

6.4 RISK FACTORS ASSOCIATED WITH NEURODEVELOPMENTAL DISORDERS

6.4.1 Prenatal Infection

The well-established links between prenatal exposure to rubella and a range of neurodevelopmental disorders have provided an informative template for how exposure to infectious agents during different critical periods of brain development can result in different phenotypes (e.g., a spectrum of outcomes including sensory deficits, intellectual handicap, epilepsy, etc.). With the re-emergence of the conceptualization of schizophrenia as a disorder of neurodevelopment in the late 1980s (Murray and Lewis, 1987; Weinberger, 1987), the impact of prenatal infection was an early favored candidate exposure. Despite some early studies that linked prenatal exposure to influenza (mostly based on ecological studies that did not directly assess exposure status), the most recent systematic review suggests that the evidence base for specificity of influenza is less convincing (Selten et al., 2010). Access to archival biological samples (e.g., prenatal sera, cord blood, and neonatal dried blood spots) has allowed the research field to assay the variable of interest at the individual level – the results from studies based on analytic epidemiology warrant greater weight compared to those based on ecological studies. To date, there is evidence to suggest that the risk of schizophrenia is elevated in those with prenatal exposure to influenza (Brown et al., 2004), rubella (Brown et al., 2000), and Toxoplasmosis gondii (Brown et al., 2005; Mortensen et al., 2007). There is mixed evidence for herpes simplex virus type 2 (HSV2) (Buka et al., 2001; Brown et al., 2006).

With respect to the association between prenatal infection and risk of autism, studies have reported an association between maternal hospitalization for infection and an increased risk of autism (Atladottir et al., 2010; Atladottir et al., 2012), and there is some evidence that maternal immune activation may be linked to autism (Libbey et al., 2005; Brown, 2012). A large cohort study from Finland has found that elevated prenatal C-reactive protein (a marker associated with immune activation) was associated with an increased risk of autism, providing further support for the links between prenatal inflammation and/or immune activation adversely impacting on brain development (Brown et al., 2014).

The biological plausibility between prenatal infection and risk of neurodevelopmental disorders has been strengthened by a convincing body of research related to prenatal immune activation (Meyer and Feldon, 2010). In these models, pregnant rodents have been exposed to noninfectious agents that mimic viruses (using artificial RNA-like constructs such as poly I:C) or bacteria (using a component of the bacterial cell wall; lipopolysaccharide). These agents stimulate the activation of innate immune cascades. The offspring of these animals display changes in neuroanatomy, neurochemistry, and behavior (Zuckerman and Weiner, 2005; Patterson, 2009; Meyer and Feldon, 2010). Recent studies have examined "two hit" animal models, with both maternal immune activation and later (peri-adolescent) stressors (Giovanoli et al.,

2013). Many of these changes are informative for schizophrenia research. Thus, the field has shifted from the expectation that a discrete set of infectious agents may be linked to schizophrenia and autism, to a broader conceptual model where the magnitude and type of maternal immune response may be the culprit (Patterson, 2002; Patterson, 2009; Patterson, 2011; Harvey and Boksa, 2012). It is becoming increasingly clear that the immune system and brain development share regulatory pathways (Boulanger and Shatz, 2004; Perry and O'Connor, 2008; Boulanger, 2009). For example, experimental models based on prenatal exposure to poly I:C implicate interleukin 6 (IL6) as a potentially key intermediary factor linking maternal immune activation and brain development (Smith et al., 2007).

It should not come as a surprise that there is cross talk between immune function and brain development – both systems are designed to extract and store information from the environment. Because acquired immunity is a more recent evolutionary innovation than complex nervous systems (e.g., Drosophila has a complex brain but no acquired immunity), it is feasible that mechanisms originally selected to facilitate central nervous system development or functioning (e.g., learning and memory) may have been later co-opted by natural selection in order to refine the molecular machinery of acquired immunity. While the links between infection, maternal immune activation, and neurodevelopmental disorders are tantalizing with respect to prevention, it is unclear if the adverse brain outcomes associated with prenatal infection are mediated by nonspecific inflammatory pathways (Miller et al., 2013) and/or placental dysfunction (O'Donnell et al., 2009), and the relative influence of innate versus acquired immunity on these processes is still unclear.

6.4.2   Prenatal Nutrition

The links between periconceptual folate supplementation and the risk of spina bifida has galvanized the field to consider nutritional candidates and a wider spectrum of neuro-developmental disorders. Studies based on catastrophic famines have found that those in utero during the events were at increased risk of developing schizophrenia and related disorders (Susser and Lin, 1992; St Clair et al., 2005). With respect to specific maternal micronutrients, homocysteine (a marker of folate of metabolism) was found to be significantly elevated in the third trimester sera from mothers of individuals with schizophrenia (Brown et al., 2007). There is also a growing body of evidence linking the use of prenatal folate use and a reduced risk of autism and autism-related outcomes (Roth et al., 2011; Suren et al., 2013).

The other candidate micronutrient linked to both schizophrenia and autism is vitamin D (McGrath et al., 2003; McGrath et al., 2004a; Cannell, 2008; Waterland, 2009). Based initially on clues from epidemiology (e.g., season of birth), there is now robust evidence from animal experiments showing that low prenatal vitamin D alters brain development (McGrath et al., 2010; Eyles et al., 2013). Based on a Danish population-based case-control study using dried blood spots ($n = 848$), an increased risk of schizophrenia was associated with low (and perhaps high) neonatal vitamin D (McGrath et al., 2010).

With respect to autism, there are no direct studies examining the association between developmental vitamin D status and risk of the clinical disorder. However studies based on birth cohorts have found that low prenatal vitamin D was associated with several autism-related phenotypes including; (a) language impairment at both age 5 and 10 years (Whitehouse et al., 2013), (b) subscores of the Autism-Spectrum Quotient (Whitehouse et al., 2012b), and (c) impaired motor and mental subscores on the Bayley Scales of Infant Development at age 14 months (Morales et al., 2012).

6.4.3 Obstetric Complications

The developing brain is vulnerable to a range of insults during development, and these are often lumped under the broad heading of obstetric complications (or pregnancy and birth complications). While biologically plausible, this group of exposures covers many different domains (e.g., toxemia, maternal diabetes, and prenatal infection) and markers of disruption (e.g., intrauterine growth restriction and antepartum hemorrhage). It can be difficult to confidently attribute some obstetric complications to fetal-versus maternally-derived exposures (e.g., both fetal genetic factors and maternal smoking may lead to intrauterine growth restriction). As is often the way in development, events can be transactional and compounding (e.g., early prenatal brain damage may lead to a "clumsy" fetus, which in turn increases the risk of delivery complications) (McNeil and Cantor-Graae, 1999).

Based on systematic reviews and meta-analyses (Geddes et al., 1999; Cannon et al., 2002), there is evidence that these exposures have a significant but modest effect in increasing the risk of later schizophrenia. Based on prospective population-based studies, Cannon et al. (2002) reported that the following specific exposures were associated with increased risk of schizophrenia; antepartum hemorrhage, gestational diabetes, rhesus incompatibility, preeclampsia, low birth weight, congenital malformations, reduced head circumference, uterine atony, asphyxia, and emergency caesarean section.

Gardener et al. (2009) summarized evidence related to pregnancy and birth complications and risk of autism in a comprehensive meta-analysis. Gestational diabetes, maternal bleeding during pregnancy and the use of medication by the mother during pregnancy were associated with increased risk of autism. There is also evidence that prenatal exposure to valproate (a medication used to treat epilepsy) may be associated with an increased risk of autism (Williams et al., 2001), and animal models based on this exposure are associated with autism-related phenotypes (Roullet et al., 2013).

6.4.4 Advanced Paternal Age

Epidemiology has provided robust evidence that the offspring of older fathers have an increased risk of schizophrenia and autism (and probably several other neurodevelopmental disorders). A meta-analysis by Miller et al. (2011) reported that offspring of fathers aged 30 or older had a significant increased risk of schizophrenia compared to fathers aged 29 or younger. The greatest increased risk was found in fathers who were 50 years or older. There was also a small but significant increase in risk for offspring of fathers aged 25 or younger (compared to those aged 25–29). Maternal age was not associated with risk of schizophrenia. There is also strong evidence that increasing paternal age is associated with an increased risk of autism. A meta-analysis by Hultman et al. (2011) reported the risk of autism in offspring increased in line with chronological age for fathers aged 30 or older compared to those aged 29 or younger. The association remained significant after controlling for maternal age and other potential risk factors for autism and remained present in families with discordant siblings. Recently, studies have also linked grandpaternal age (i.e., at the time of conception of the parent) versus risk of schizophrenia (Frans et al., 2011) and autism (Frans et al., 2013).

Recently, studies based on deep sequencing have demonstrated that the offspring of older father have more *de novo* mutations, probably as a result of more cell divisions in the male versus female germ line (Crow, 2003; Kong et al., 2012; Neale et al., 2012; Sanders et al., 2012; Sun et al., 2012; Veltman and Brunner, 2012). These findings provide a direct mechanism for the effect of increased paternal age, as cases of ASD and SZ may be linked to *de novo* mutations (Chapter 3).

Animal experiments have also shown that the offspring of older sires have altered behavior (Smith et al., 2009; Foldi et al., 2010; Foldi et al., 2011), altered brain structure (Foldi et al., 2010), and increased *de novo* copy number variants (Flatscher-Bader et al., 2011).

Commentators have noted that somatic mutations in male germ cells that modify proliferation via dysregulation of the RAS pathway can lead to within-testis expansion of mutant clonal lines (Goriely and Wilkie, 2010; Goriely

and Wilkie, 2012). First identified in association with rare paternal age-effect disorders (e.g., Apert syndrome, achondroplasia), this process is known as "selfish spermatogonial selection." This mechanism will favor propagation of germ cells carrying a particular subset of pathogenic mutations and result in an enrichment of *de novo* mutations in the offspring of older fathers that preferentially impact on particular cellular signaling pathways (Goriely et al., 2013).

Apart from paternal-age related *de novo* mutations, epigenetic changes and factors related to paternal personality and social skills (which may be associated with delayed parenthood) may also contribute to this finding. Many cultural and social factors can influence when men have their children, and in theory, this exposure is "modifiable" from a public health perspective.

6.4.5 Migrant Status

Systematic reviews have consistently shown that certain migrant groups in some countries have an increased risk of schizophrenia (McGrath et al., 2004b; Cantor-Graae and Selten, 2005). These studies, based mainly in the UK, Europe, and Scandinavia, show that both the first and the second generation migrants have an increased risk of developing schizophrenia, and systematic reviews have suggested that the effect is most pronounced in dark-skinned migrants (Cantor-Graae and Selten, 2005; Bourque et al., 2011; Dealberto, 2010).

Being the offspring of a migrant has also been associated with an increased risk of autism, but this finding does not generalize to all migrants in all nations (as is the case with schizophrenia). In particular, the offspring of dark-skinned migrants to cold countries seem to be at high risk (Eyles, 2010; Humble et al., 2010). A large study based in Stockholm county ($n = 589$ 114) found that the offspring of migrants had a significantly increased risk of low-functioning autism with comorbid intellectual disability (Magnusson et al., 2012). They noted that this risk was particularly elevated in the offspring of parents from dark skinned migrants. The authors speculated that stress, infection, and/or low vitamin D may be candidate risk factors underpinning these findings. Comparable findings have recently been reported from a study in the Netherlands ($n = 106\ 953$) (van der Ven et al., 2013). A systematic review by Dealberto (2011) reported an increase in relative risk of autism in the offspring of dark-skinned migrants. A meta-analysis by Gardener et al. (2009) also reported an increased risk of autism for children who had mothers born abroad. Again, offspring of dark skinned migrants were found to be at particularly high risk of autism.

It has been proposed that the increased risk of neurodevelopmental disorders such as schizophrenia and autism in the offspring of dark-skinned migrants could be due to developmental vitamin D deficiency (Eyles et al., 2013). Alternatively, some commentators have suggested that belonging to an obviously different ethnic minority group (e.g., dark skin) may contribute to psychosocial stress and "social defeat" (Selten and Cantor-Graae, 2005; Cantor-Graae, 2007). Stress-related mechanisms may contribute to the risk of schizophrenia in some migrant groups. However, with respect to autism, it is not clear if these stressors impact directly on infants or indirectly via parental stress. Infants and children usually experience their social milieu from the immediate family rather than the wider community. While it is feasible that mothering skills and/or prenatal stress in ethnic minority groups may contribute to offspring brain-related outcomes, a Dutch study based on age-at-migration in first generation migrants reported that migrants who arrived as infants and young children have a greater risk of later schizophrenia (compared to those who arrive as adolescents or young adults) (Veling et al., 2011). Regardless of the underlying mechanism, the migrant studies strongly implicate a gene-by-environment (GxE) interaction – certain ethnic groups (e.g., those with genes linked to dark skin, or genes linked to increased risk of migration), in certain environments (e.g., certain developed nations, or in cold climates) have an increased risk of neurodevelopmental disorders.

6.4.6 Season of Birth

Many exposures fluctuate across the season. Apart from obvious climate-related variables (e.g., temperature, photoperiod, and rainfall), other exposures can have within-year fluctuation (e.g., related to food availability, winter respiratory viruses, etc.). Over the last 90 years, it has been noted repeatedly that individuals born in winter and spring tend to have a slightly increased risk of developing schizophrenia. The effect has been confirmed in systematic reviews (McGrath and Welham, 1999; Davies et al., 2003), and varies across latitude gradients (Davies et al., 2003). Similarly, there is some (inconsistent) evidence to suggest that risk of autism fluctuates across season of birth, and that the nature of this relationship is related to latitude (Grant and Soles, 2009). A US group (Zerbo et al., 2011) examined a large sample of cases and found that when conception occurred in December, January, February (northern hemisphere winter), this was associated with a 6% increased risk of autism (compared to summer births; Odds Ratio = 1.06, 95%CI 1.02–1.10). The authors speculate that seasonally fluctuating candidate exposures such as infection, toxins, and vitamin D warrant closer inspection. The links between winter/spring birth versus schizophrenia was a primary contributor to the hypothesis that developmental vitamin D deficiency was associated with schizophrenia (McGrath, 1999).

6.4.7 Other Environmental Risk Factors

People born or raised in cities have an increased risk of developing schizophrenia. A recently published systematic review and meta-analysis found that the risk for schizophrenia at the most urban environment was estimated to be 2.37 times higher than in the most rural environment (Vassos et al., 2012). Urbanicity indexes yet-to-be-identified risk-modifying variables operating around birth and early life. However, the nature of the risk factor remains unclear (McGrath and Scott, 2006). With respect to autism, some epidemiological studies have identified an increased risk of autism in urban setting (Chen et al., 2008; Kirkbride and Jones, 2011; Rossignol and Frye, 2011); however, it is thought that differential access to care and diagnosis may explain at least part of this gradient. It is thought that an increase in the prevalence of autism diagnoses in recent years, and factors related to widening diagnostic criteria, diagnostic substitution (King and Bearman, 2009), and increased recognition of the disorder (e.g., in urban setting) may have contributed to this finding (Fombonne, 2005; King and Bearman, 2011). A systematic review of the prevalence of autism also found an association between urbanicity and the frequency of autism (Williams et al., 2006) – this may be due to better detection or due to urban-related etiological risk factors. Increased perinatal air pollution has been linked to an increased risk of autism (Becerra et al., 2013). This may be mediated by pollution-related toxins, and/or low maternal vitamin D concentrations (which is also associated with air pollution (Baiz et al., 2012).

This chapter has focused on exposures during the prenatal and early life period. However, there is consistent evidence that (a) cannabis use (especially early use as teenagers, and heavy use), and (b) exposure to trauma, are associated with an increased risk of psychosis (van Os et al., 2010). Thus, risk factors for schizophrenia are not only restricted to the prenatal period. Both of these exposures are relatively common, thus it is thought that pre-existing genetic vulnerability may be required in order to precipitate psychosis (van Os et al., 2010; Brown, 2011).

at mental health services). The recruitment of large, representative samples of cases from national registers is feasible in some nations. The Wellcome Trust Case Control Consortium used the large UK 1958 birth cohort for the "healthy control" sample in their landmark studies (Wellcome Trust Case Control, 2007). Studies related to the genetics of schizophrenia have been published that have recruited large samples based on national registers (Humphreys et al., 2011; Bergen et al., 2012; Borglum et al., 2014).

The use of these large population-based samples provides more robust estimates of population attributable fractions. There are now several large population-based birth cohorts that have been extensively and repeatedly phenotypes, as well as genotyped. In isolation, each cohort would be underpowered to explore genetic or GxE interactions for low prevalence disorders such as schizophrenia and autism. Here there are important lessons that the epidemiology research community can learn from the recent large scale collaborative networks established within the genetics community to attempt to discover (and replicate in independent samples) genetic risk factors for diseases or phenotypes of interest (Sullivan, 2010; Ripke et al., 2011; Sullivan and Psychiatric Genetics, 2012). Such large-scale collaborations are now happening in autism research, where several groups have harmonized phenotyptic variables and pooled data for the International Collaboration for Autism Registry Epidemiology (iCARE).

6.5 EPIDEMIOLOGICAL FRAMEWORKS CAN IMPROVE SAMPLING FOR GENETIC STUDIES

As mentioned in the previous section, the disciplines of epidemiology and genetics have diverged somewhat in methodology. Genetic samples have traditionally been recruited from (a) informative samples (e.g., multiplex families and isolated populations), or (b) convenient samples (e.g., cases recruited from attendance

6.6 COMBING CLUES FROM GENETICS AND EPIDEMIOLOGY

It is evident that disorders such as schizophrenia and autism are influenced by a wide range of genetic factors and environmental factors (van Os et al., 2010). Twin studies and family studies have been used to derive heritability estimates, an oft misunderstood parameter that is best equipped to capture the amount of variation in a continuous phenotype that can be explained by additive genetic factors for a given population in a given environment (Visscher et al., 2008). Mindful of issues in the application of this parameter to diseases such as schizophrenia (Mitchell and Porteous, 2011), recent twin studies clearly show the influence of shared and/or unique environmental factors in schizophrenia (Sullivan et al., 2003) and autism (Hallmayer et al., 2011). While rarely used in psychiatric genetic epidemiology, if sample size permits, it is feasible to stratify twin or family by environmental exposures of interest in order to explore the influence of the candidate exposure on heritability estimates. Another parameter related to both genetic and environmental factors is the sibling recurrence risk. The risk of schizophrenia in siblings has been examined when adjusted for the influence of proxy markers of yet-to-be-discovered environmental factors such as migrant status (it was lower in the offspring of migrants) and season of birth (no difference according to this variable) (Svensson et al., 2012).

In light of the substantial body of research published in recent years on both genetic and environmental risk factors of neurodevelopmental disorders, it is surprising that there is so little work that examines both domains in the same study. To a certain extent, this may reflect the ideological bifurcation between the two disciplines. However, the relative absence of this type of research reflects the lack of large samples with both genetic data and markers related to environmental risk factors. Technology has allowed for the collection of large scale and affordable genetic information; however, we will never to be able to systematically perform "environment-wide" association studies. That said, in cohorts with large amounts of phenotypic data, "phenome-wide" association studies (i.e., studies that simultaneously assess a large number of different environmental risk factors) are feasible (Pendergrass et al., 2011; Pendergrass et al., 2013).

In the absence of precise genetic data, epidemiology has mainly relied on crude measures such as family history (van Os et al., 2008; Binbay et al., 2012). However, it is now clear that this measure is a poor index of genetic susceptibility when assessed at the population level (Wray and Visscher, 2010). With respect to schizophrenia, this strategy has been informative with respect to exploring the association between (a) urbanicity and family history (van Os et al., 2004), (b) cannabis use and family history (Genetic Risk and Outcome in Psychosis (GROUP) Investigators, 2011) and (c) trauma exposure and family history (Wigman et al., 2012). The use of cross-twin and cross-exposure studies in nonclinical samples can also help demarcate the influence of overall genetic factors and specific candidate environmental exposures, and this has been used to demonstrate that psychotic-like experiences cosegregate with increased reactivity to stress in daily life (Lataster et al., 2009).

6.7 LINKING GENETICS AND THE ENVIRONMENT – SPECIFIC CANDIDATE STUDIES

GxE interactions is expected in our field, and it is thought that they could account for some of the "missing heritability" identified for disorders such as schizophrenia (Thomas, 2010). Disappointingly, the evidence linking specific candidate genes (i.e., single nucleotide polymorphisms (SNPs) in these gene) and specific environmental exposures has been charactered by lack of replication, diminishing effect size over time, and probable publication biases (Duncan and Keller, 2011), and there are concerns about the conceptual framework underpinning "classic" GxE interaction analyses (Zammit, 2008; Zammit et al., 2010).

Studies have examined GxE interactions in schizophrenia. The productive group of Jim van Os and colleagues have examined the links between (a) cannabis use and polymorphisms in genes involved in related dopaminergic pathways (van Winkel et al., 2008; van Winkel, 2011); and (b) variants in stress pathways and vulnerability to psychotic like experience (van Winkel et al., 2008). With respect to autism, recent clues have found a decreased risk of autism-related outcomes in the offspring of mothers who used periconceptual folate supplementation (Schmidt et al., 2012). Subsequently, studies have found that this relationship was the strongest for mothers and children with particular variants in key folate-related genes (Schmidt et al., 2012).

The value of examining the impact of single SNPs or groups of SNPs in selected pathways has been overshadowed by the highly polygenic nature of the genetic architecture for disorders such as schizophrenia (Wray and Visscher, 2010; Lee et al., 2012). Thus, the field has lowered its expectations with respect to GxE interactions based on the variants in single SNPs. Of course, it remains to be seen if rare, large-effect CNVs or point mutations are more sensitive to environmental influences. One can certainly imagine how such mutations could lead to a greater vulnerability to environmental risk factors. However, mindful of how difficult it is to confidently link rare genetic variants with disease outcomes (Gratten et al., 2013), it will be an even greater challenge to design studies with sufficient power to explore the environmental interactions on these mutations.

Epidemiologists have developed creative methods to leverage genetic discoveries. If an intermediate phenotype is in the causal pathway to a disease outcome (e.g., serum lipid profile vs cardiovascular disease), then knowledge of SNPs that predict that intermediate phenotype can be used as a proxy (or instrumental) variables. Of particular interest for observational epidemiology, variants that contribute to SNP-based instruments are (a) inherited (and thus predate the onset of the disease outcome of interest), and (b) risk alleles are randomly divided during meiotic recombination (thus, this type of research is often called Mendelian Randomization; MR)(Smith and Ebrahim, 2004). It is expected that when SNP-based instrumental variables are available that explain sufficient variance of the intermediate phenotype, these strategies may have utility in disorders such as schizophrenia and autism (Attermann et al., 2012).

6.8 LINKING GENETICS AND THE ENVIRONMENT – GENOME-WIDE APPROACHES

In recent years, there have been important methodological developments in statistical genetics. For example, SNP-derived, genome-wide metrics can capture disease risk estimates in the absence of knowing the precise nature of the individual risk alleles (e.g., number, location, etc.) (Wray et al., 2007). These methods were applied to the schizophrenia GWAS data (Purcell et al., 2009). Briefly, the method uses odds ratios estimated from the association analysis of a "discovery" sample. Subsequently, in an independent sample (the replication set), a score can be derived (i.e., a polygene profile score) based on the presence or absence of the risk allele and the effect size in the discovery set. While these scores only explain a small proportion of the variance currently, this may improve as the size of the discovery sample is increased.

Polygene profile scores allow for new types of GxE interaction studies. For example, the addition of information on environmental exposures may increase the predictive value of a polygene profile score in independent case-control samples. Based on caseness as the outcome, logistic regression models can also explore polygene profile score by environmental interaction effects. It may be feasible to explore case-only designs, and compare mean polygene profile scores in cases when stratified according to an exposure of interest (e.g., season of birth, urban birth, and neonatal vitamin D concentration). If some of the SNPs that contribute to a polygene scores are related to the exposure of interest, then stratifying the group according to the exposure may reveal nuances in the genetic architecture of these heterogeneous disorders. For example, if some of the SNPs that contribute to a polygene risk score may be involved in vitamin D metabolism, or antibody concentrations related to prenatal infection, then significant correlations between the variables of interest may emerge. Conversely, if these associations were absent (or inverted) in control-only sample, this could lend further weight to the hypothesis that some of the SNPs in the polygene score influence the response to the environmental exposure.

More recently, methods have been developed that use genome-wide similarities in genotypes between all pairs of individuals have been able to estimate the proportion of variance tagged by SNPs for quantitative traits (Yang et al., 2010) and for case-control traits (Lee et al., 2011). As with the polygene scores described earlier, if the cases could be stratified according to exposures of interest, then genome-wide similarities may be greater within these strata versus between the strata.

These techniques offer new strategies for the research community. Already, researchers are exploring links between GWAS results for schizophrenia and GWAS results related to response to candidate risk factors for schizophrenia such as the concentration of neonatal antibodies to cytomegalovirus (Borglum et al., 2014).

6.9 SUMMARY AND CONCLUSIONS

Despite the meager scientific yield and the past reliance on proxy measures of genetic susceptibility, there is some reason for optimism that future studies will be able to explore the influence of genetic and environmental factors in a meaningful fashion. Large population-based samples with detailed genetic and phenotypic data are now available, and the large genetic consortia have clearly proven the utility of these collaborative exercises. Developments in statistical genetics have provided genome-wide tools that have not yet been fully leveraged by the epidemiology research community.

Genetic studies are required to discover variants in pathways that underlie inherited susceptibility to neurodevelopmental disorders. However, from a public health perspective, unless these clues point to modifiable risk factors, they may have limited impact at the population level. Epidemiology has a particular focus on modifiable risk factors (McGrath and Lawlor, 2011), and some modifiable variables are well suited to public health intervention (e.g., nutrition and infection).

As has been detailed earlier in this book (Chapters 1 and 2), it is becoming increasingly clear that the broad class of neurodevelopmental disorders share both genetic and environmental risk factors. Public health has long recognized the value of nonspecificity of outcomes. If one exposure can be linked to several adverse health outcomes (e.g., smoking causes increased risk of lung cancer, cardiovascular disease, etc.), then interventions designed to reduce the exposure can translate to the reduction of several disease outcomes (Rose, 1992). As has been detailed earlier, neurodevelopmental disorders such as schizophrenia and autism do share modifiable environmental risk factors (Hamlyn et al., 2013). As we learn more about how these exposures interact with genetic vulnerability, future researchers may be able to "personalize" health recommendations. To reach this goal, we need to facilitate the collection of large, population-based samples enriched with genetic and phenotypic data. Finally, we need to facilitate more "intellectual collisions" between the fields of genetics and epidemiology, because now, more than ever, the two fields need to generate new strategies to unravel the risk architecture of neurodevelopmental disorders.

REFERENCES

Atladottir, H.O., Henriksen, T.B., et al. (2012). Autism after infection, febrile episodes, and antibiotic use during pregnancy: an exploratory study. Pediatrics 130(6), e1447–e1454.

Atladottir, H.O., Thorsen, P., et al. (2010). Association of hospitalization for infection in childhood with diagnosis of autism spectrum disorders: a Danish cohort study. Arch Pediatr Adolesc Med 164(5), 470–477.

Attermann, J., Obel, C., et al. (2012). Traits of ADHD and autism in girls with a twin brother: a Mendelian randomization study. Eur Child Adolesc Psychiatry 21(9), 503–509.

Baiz, N., Dargent-Molina, P., et al. (2012). Gestational exposure to urban air pollution related to a decrease in cord blood vitamin d levels. J Clin Endocrinol Metab 97(11), 4087–4095.

Becerra, T.A., Wilhelm, M., et al. (2013). Ambient Air Pollution and Autism in Los Angeles County, California Environ Health Perspect. 121(3), 380–6.

Bergen, S.E., O'Dushlaine, C.T., et al. (2012). Genome-wide association study in a Swedish population yields support for greater CNV and MHC involvement in schizophrenia compared with bipolar disorder. Mol Psychiatry 17(9), 880–886.

Binbay, T., Drukker, M., et al. (2012). Testing the psychosis continuum: differential impact of genetic and nongenetic risk factors and comorbid psychopathology across the entire spectrum of psychosis. Schizophr Bull 38(5), 992–1002.

Borglum, A.D., Demontis, D., et al. (2014). Genome-wide study of association and interaction with maternal cytomegalovirus infection suggests new schizophrenia loci. Mol Psychiatry 19(3), 325–33.

Boulanger, L.M. (2009). Immune proteins in brain development and synaptic plasticity. Neuron 64(1), 93–109.

Boulanger, L.M., and Shatz, C.J. (2004). Immune signalling in neural development, synaptic plasticity and disease. Nat Rev Neurosci 5(7), 521–531.

Bourque, F., van der Ven, E., et al. (2011). A meta-analysis of the risk for psychotic disorders among first- and second-generation immigrants. Psychol Med 41(5), 897–910.

Brown, A.S. (2011). The environment and susceptibility to schizophrenia. Prog Neurobiol 93(1), 23–58.

Brown, A.S. (2012). Epidemiologic studies of exposure to prenatal infection and risk of schizophrenia and autism. Dev Neurobiol 72(10), 1272–1276.

Brown, A.S., Begg, M.D., et al. (2004). Serologic evidence of prenatal influenza in the etiology of schizophrenia. Arch Gen Psychiatry 61(8), 774–780.

Brown, A.S., Bottiglieri, T., et al. (2007). Elevated prenatal homocysteine levels as a risk factor for schizophrenia. Arch Gen Psychiatry 64(1), 31–39.

Brown, A.S., Cohen, P., et al. (2000). Nonaffective psychosis after prenatal exposure to rubella. Am J Psychiatry 157(3), 438–443.

Brown, A.S., and McGrath, J.J. (2011). The prevention of schizophrenia. Schizophr Bull 37(2), 257–261.

Brown, A.S., Schaefer, C.A., et al. (2005). Maternal exposure to toxoplasmosis and risk of schizophrenia in adult offspring. Am J Psychiatry 162(4), 767–773.

Brown, A.S., Schaefer, C.A., et al. (2006). No evidence of relation between maternal exposure to herpes simplex virus type 2 and risk of schizophrenia? Am J Psychiatry 163(12), 2178–2180.

Brown, A.S., Sourander, A., et al. (2014). Elevated maternal C-reactive protein and autism in a national birth cohort. Mol Psychiatry 19(2), 259–64.

Buka, S.L., Tsuang, M.T., et al. (2001). Maternal Infections and Subsequent Psychosis Among Offspring. Arch Gen Psychiatry 58, 1032–1037.

Cannell, J.J. (2008). Autism and vitamin D. Med Hypotheses 70(4), 750–759.

Cannon, M., Jones, P.B., et al. (2002). Obstetric complications and schizophrenia: historical and meta-analytic review. Am J Psychiatry 159(7), 1080–1092.

Cantor-Graae, E. (2007). The contribution of social factors to the development of schizophrenia: a review of recent findings. Can J Psychiatry 52(5), 277–286.

Cantor-Graae, E., and Selten, J.P. (2005). Schizophrenia and migration: a meta-analysis and review. Am J Psychiatry 162(1), 12–24.

Chen, C.Y., Liu, C.Y., et al. (2008). Urbanicity-related variation in help-seeking and services utilization among preschool-age children with autism in Taiwan. J Autism Dev Disord 38(3), 489–497.

Crow, J.F. (2003). Development. There's something curious about paternal-age effects. Science 301(5633), 606–607.

Davey Smith, G. (2001). Reflections on the limitations to epidemiology. J Clin Epidemiol 54(4), 325–331.

Davey Smith, G., and Ebrahim, S. (2001). Epidemiology--is it time to call it a day? Int J Epidemiol 30(1), 1–11.

Davies, G., Welham, J., et al. (2003). A systematic review and meta-analysis of Northern Hemisphere season of birth studies in schizophrenia. Schizophr Bull 29(3), 587–593.

Dealberto, M.J. (2010). Ethnic origin and increased risk for schizophrenia in immigrants to recent and traditional countries of immigration. Acta Psychiatr Scand 21(5), 325–39.

Dealberto, M.J. (2011). Prevalence of autism according to maternal immigrant status and ethnic origin. Acta Psychiatr Scand 123(5), 339–348.

Duncan, L.E., and Keller, M.C. (2011). A critical review of the first 10 years of candidate gene-by-environment interaction research in psychiatry. Am J Psychiatry 168(10), 1041–1049.

Eyles, D.W. (2010). Vitamin D and autism: does skin colour modify risk? Acta Paediatr 99(5), 645–647.

Eyles, D.W., Burne, T.H., et al. (2013). Vitamin D, effects on brain development, adult brain function and the links between low levels of vitamin D and neuropsychiatric disease. Front Neuroendocrinol 34(1), 47–64.

Flatscher-Bader, T., Foldi, C.J., et al. (2011). Increased *de novo* copy number variants in the offspring of older males. Transl Psychiatry 1, e34.

Foldi, C.J., Eyles, D.W., et al. (2011). New perspectives on rodent models of advanced paternal age: relevance to autism. Front Behav Neurosci 5, 32.

Foldi, C.J., Eyles, D.W., et al. (2010). Advanced paternal age is associated with alterations in discrete behavioural domains and cortical neuroanatomy of C57BL/6J mice. Eur J Neurosci 31(3), 556–564.

Fombonne, E. (2005). Epidemiology of autistic disorder and other pervasive developmental disorders. J Clin Psychiatry 66 (Suppl 10), 3–8.

Frans, E., Sandin, S. et al. (2013). Autism risk develops across generations: a population based study of advancing grandpaternal and paternal age. JAMA Psychiatry 70(5), 516–21.

Frans, E.M., McGrath, J.J., et al. (2011). Advanced paternal and grandpaternal age and schizophrenia: a three-generation perspective. Schizophr Res 133(1–3), 120–124.

Gardener, H., Spiegelman, D., et al. (2009). Prenatal risk factors for autism: comprehensive meta-analysis. Br J Psychiatry 195(1), 7–14.

Geddes, J.R., Verdoux, H., et al. (1999). Schizophrenia and complications of pregnancy and labor: an individual patient data meta-analysis. Schizophr Bull 25(3), 413–423.

Genetic Risk and Outcome in Psychosis (GROUP) Investigators (2011). Evidence that familial liability for psychosis is expressed as differential sensitivity to cannabis: an analysis of patient-sibling and sibling-control pairs. Arch Gen Psychiatry 68(2), 138–47.

Giovanoli, S., Engler, H., et al. (2013). Stress in puberty unmasks latent neuropathological consequences of prenatal immune activation in mice. Science 339(6123), 1095–1099.

Goriely, A., McGrath, J.J., et al. (2013). "Selfish Spermatogonial Selection": A novel mechanism for the association between advanced paternal age and neurodevelopmental disorders. Am J Psychiatry 170(6), 599–608.

Goriely, A., and Wilkie, A.O.M. (2010). Missing heritability: paternal age effect mutations and selfish spermatogonia. Nat Rev Genet 11(8), 589.

Goriely, A., and Wilkie, A.O.M. (2012). Paternal age effect mutations and selfish spermatogonial selection: causes and consequences for human disease. Am J Hum Genet 90(2), 175–200.

Grant, W.B., and Soles, C.M. (2009). Epidemiologic evidence supporting the role of maternal vitamin D deficiency as a risk factor for the development of infantile autism. Derm-Endocrinol 1(4), 223–228.

Gratten, J., Visscher, P.M., et al. (2013). Interpreting the role of de novo protein-coding mutations in neuropsychiatric disease. Nat Genet 45(3), 234–238.

Greenough, W.T., Black, J.E., et al. (1987). Experience and brain development. Child Dev 58(3), 539–559.

Hallmayer, J., Cleveland, S., et al. (2011). Genetic heritability and shared environmental factors among twin pairs with autism. Arch Gen Psychiatry 68(11), 1095–1102.

Hamlyn, J., Duhig, M., et al. (2013). Modifiable risk factors for schizophrenia and autism - Shared risk factors impacting on brain development. Neurobiol Dis 53, 3–9.

Harvey, L., and Boksa, P. (2012). Prenatal and postnatal animal models of immune activation: relevance to a range of neurodevelopmental disorders. Dev Neurobiol 72(10), 1335–1348.

Holliday, E.G., Nyholt, D.R., et al. (2009). Strong evidence for a novel schizophrenia risk locus on chromosome 1p31.1 in homogeneous pedigrees from Tamil Nadu, India. Am J Psychiatry 166(2), 206–215.

Hultman, C.M., Sandin, S., et al. (2011). Advancing paternal age and risk of autism: new evidence from a population-based study and a meta-analysis of epidemiological studies. Mol Psychiatry 16(12), 1203–12.

Humble, M.B., Gustafsson, S., et al. (2010). Low serum levels of 25-hydroxyvitamin D (25-OHD) among psychiatric out-patients in Sweden: Relations with season, age, ethnic origin and psychiatric diagnosis. J Steroid Biochem Mol Biol 121(1–2), 467–70.

Humphreys, K., Grankvist, A., et al. (2011). The genetic structure of the Swedish population. PLoS One 6(8), e22547.

King, M., and Bearman, P. (2009). Diagnostic change and the increased prevalence of autism. Int J Epidemiol 38(5), 1224–1234.

King, M.D., and Bearman, P.S. (2011). Socioeconomic Status and the Increased Prevalence of Autism in California. Am Sociol Rev 76(2), 320–346.

Kirkbride, J.B., and Jones, P.B. (2011). The prevention of schizophrenia--what can we learn from eco-epidemiology? Schizophr Bull 37(2), 262–271.

Kong, A., Frigge, M.L., et al. (2012). Rate of de novo mutations and the importance of father's age to disease risk. Nature 488(7412), 471–475.

Lataster, T., Wichers, M., et al. (2009). Does reactivity to stress cosegregate with subclinical psychosis? A general population twin study. Acta Psychiatr Scand 119(1), 45–53.

Lee, S.H., DeCandia, T.R., et al. (2012). Estimating the proportion of variation in susceptibility to schizophrenia captured by common SNPs. Nat Genet 44(3), 247–250.

Lee, S.H., Wray, N.R., et al. (2011). Estimating missing heritability for disease from genome-wide association studies. Am J Hum Genet 88(3), 294–305.

Libbey, J.E., Sweeten, T.L., et al. (2005). Autistic disorder and viral infections. J Neurovirol 11(1), 1–10.

Magnusson, C., Rai, D., et al. (2012). Migration and autism spectrum disorder: population-based study. Br J Psychiatry 201, 109–115.

McGrath, J. (1999). Hypothesis: is low prenatal vitamin D a risk-modifying factor for schizophrenia? Schizophr Res 40(3), 173–177.

McGrath, J., Eyles, D., et al. (2003). Low maternal vitamin D as a risk factor for schizophrenia: a pilot study using banked sera. Schizophr Res 63, 73–78.

McGrath, J., Saari, K., et al. (2004a). Vitamin D supplementation during the first year of life and risk of schizophrenia: a Finnish birth-cohort study. Schizophr Res 67(2,3), 237–245.

McGrath, J., Saha, S., et al. (2004b). A systematic review of the incidence of schizophrenia: the distribution of rates and the influence of sex, urbanicity, migrant status and methodology. BMC Med 2(1), 13.

McGrath, J., and Scott, J. (2006). Urban birth and risk of schizophrenia: a worrying example of epidemiology where the data are stronger than the hypotheses. Epidemiol Psichiatr Soc 15(4), 243–246.

McGrath, J.J., Burne, T.H., et al. (2010). Developmental vitamin D deficiency and risk of schizophrenia: a 10-year update. Schizophr Bull 36(6), 1073–1078.

McGrath, J.J., Eyles, D.W., et al. (2010). Neonatal vitamin D status and risk of schizophrenia: a population-based case–control study. Arch Gen Psychiatry 67(9), 889–894.

McGrath, J.J., and Lawlor, D.A. (2011). The search for modifiable risk factors for schizophrenia. Am J Psychiatry 168(12), 1235–1238.

McGrath, J.J., and Richards, L.J. (2009). Why schizophrenia epidemiology needs neurobiology--and vice versa. Schizophr Bull 35(3), 577–581.

McGrath, J.J., and Welham, J.L. (1999). Season of birth and schizophrenia: a systematic review and meta-analysis of data from the Southern Hemisphere. Schizophr Res 35, 237–242.

McNeil, T.F., and Cantor-Graae, E. (1999). Does pre-existing abnormality cause labor-delivery complications in fetuses who will develop schizophrenia? Schizophr Bull 25(3), 425–435.

Meyer, U., and Feldon, J. (2010). Epidemiology-driven neurodevelopmental animal models of schizophrenia. Prog Neurobiol 90(3), 285–326.

Miller, B., Messias, E., et al. (2011). Meta-analysis of Paternal Age and Schizophrenia Risk in Male Versus Female Offspring. Schizophr Bull 37(5), 1039–1047.

Miller, B.J., Culpepper, N., et al. (2013). Prenatal inflammation and neurodevelopment in schizophrenia: a review of human studies. Prog Neuropsychopharmacol Biol Psychiatry 42, 92–100.

Mitchell, K.J., and Porteous, D.J. (2011). Rethinking the genetic architecture of schizophrenia. Psychol Med 41(1), 19–32.

Morales, E., Guxens, M., et al. (2012). Circulating 25-Hydroxyvitamin D3 in Pregnancy and Infant Neuropsychological Development. Pediatrics 130(4), e913–20.

Mortensen, P.B., Norgaard-Pedersen, B., et al. (2007). Early infections of Toxoplasma gondii and the later development of schizophrenia. Schizophr Bull 33(3), 741–744.

Murray, R.M., and Lewis, S.W. (1987). Is schizophrenia a neurodevelopmental disorder? Br Med J (Clin Res Ed) 295(6600), 681–682.

Neale, B.M., Kou, Y., et al. (2012). Patterns and rates of exonic de novo mutations in autism spectrum disorders. Nature 485(7397), 242–245.

Nithianantharajah, J., Barkus, C., et al. (2008). Gene-environment interactions modulating cognitive function and molecular correlates of synaptic plasticity in Huntington's disease transgenic mice. Neurobiol Dis 29(3), 490–504.

Nithianantharajah, J., and Hannan, A.J. (2006). Enriched environments, experience-dependent plasticity and disorders of the nervous system. Nat Rev Neurosci 7(9), 697–709.

O'Donnell, K., O'Connor, T.G., et al. (2009). Prenatal stress and neurodevelopment of the child: focus on the HPA axis and role of the placenta. Dev Neurosci 31(4), 285–292.

Patterson, P.H. (2002). Maternal infection: window on neuroimmune interactions in fetal brain development and mental illness. Curr Opin Neurobiol 12(1), 115–118.

Patterson, P.H. (2009). Immune involvement in schizophrenia and autism: etiology, pathology and animal models. Behav Brain Res 204(2), 313–321.

Patterson, P.H. (2011). Maternal infection and immune involvement in autism. Trends Mol Med 17(7), 389–394.

Pendergrass, S.A., Brown-Gentry, K., et al. (2013). Phenome-Wide Association Study (PheWAS) for Detection of Pleiotropy within the Population Architecture using Genomics and Epidemiology (PAGE) Network. PLoS Genet 9(1), e1003087.

Pendergrass, S.A., Brown-Gentry, K., et al. (2011). The use of phenome-wide association studies (PheWAS) for exploration of novel genotype-phenotype relationships and pleiotropy discovery. Genet Epidemiol 35(5), 410–422.

Perry, V.H., and O'Connor, V. (2008). C1q: the perfect complement for a synaptic feast? Nat Rev Neurosci 9(11), 807–811.

Purcell, S.M., Wray, N.R., et al. (2009). Common polygenic variation contributes to risk of schizophrenia and bipolar disorder. Nature 460(7256), 748–752.

Ripke, S., Sanders, A.R., et al. (2011). Genome-wide association study identifies five new schizophrenia loci. Nat Genet 43(10), 969–976.

Rose, G. (1992). The Strategy of Preventive Medicine. Oxford, Oxford University Press.

Rossignol, D.A., and Frye, R.E. (2011). Melatonin in autism spectrum disorders: a systematic review and meta-analysis. Dev Med Child Neurol 53(9), 783–792.

Roth, C., Magnus, P., et al. (2011). Folic acid supplements in pregnancy and severe language delay in children. JAMA 306(14), 1566–1573.

Roullet, F.I., Lai, J.K., et al. (2013). In utero exposure to valproic acid and autism - A current review of clinical and animal studies. Neurotoxicol Teratol 36, 47–56.

Sanders, S.J., Murtha, M.T., et al. (2012). De novo mutations revealed by whole-exome sequencing are strongly associated with autism. Nature 485(7397), 237–241.

Schmidt, R.J., Tancredi, D.J., et al. (2012). Maternal periconceptional folic acid intake and risk of autism spectrum disorders and developmental delay in the CHARGE (CHildhood Autism Risks from Genetics and Environment) case–control study. Am J Clin Nutr 96(1), 80–89.

Selten, J.P., and Cantor-Graae, E. (2005). Social defeat: risk factor for schizophrenia? Br J Psychiatry 187, 101–102.

Selten, J.P., Frissen, A., et al. (2010). Schizophrenia and 1957 pandemic of influenza: meta-analysis. Schizophr Bull 36(2), 219–228.

Smith, G.D., and Ebrahim, S. (2004). Mendelian randomization: prospects, potentials, and limitations. Int J Epidemiol 33(1), 30–42.

Smith, R.G., Kember, R.L., et al. (2009). Advancing paternal age is associated with deficits in social and exploratory behaviors in the offspring: a mouse model. PLoS One 4(12), e8456.

Smith, S.E., Li, J., et al. (2007). Maternal immune activation alters fetal brain development through interleukin-6. J Neurosci 27(40), 10695–10702.

St Clair, D., Xu, M., et al. (2005). Rates of adult schizophrenia following prenatal exposure to the Chinese famine of 1959–1961. JAMA 294(5), 557–562.

Sullivan, P., and Psychiatric Genetics, I. (2012). Don't give up on GWAS. Mol Psychiatry 17(1), 2–3.

Sullivan, P.F. (2010). The psychiatric GWAS consortium: big science comes to psychiatry. Neuron 68(2), 182–186.

Sullivan, P.F., Kendler, K.S., et al. (2003). Schizophrenia as a complex trait: evidence from a meta-analysis of twin studies. Arch Gen Psychiatry 60(12), 1187–1192.

Sun, J.X., Helgason, A., et al. (2012). A direct characterization of human mutation based on microsatellites. Nat Genet 44(10), 1161–1165.

Suren, P., Roth, C., et al. (2013). Association between maternal use of folic acid supplements and risk of autism spectrum disorders in children. JAMA 309(6), 570–577.

Susser, E.S., and Lin, S.P. (1992). Schizophrenia after prenatal exposure to the Dutch hunger winter of 1944–1945. Arch Gen Psychiatry 49, 938–988.

Svensson, A.C., Lichtenstein, P., et al. (2012). Familial aggregation of schizophrenia: the moderating effect of age at onset, parental immigration, paternal age and season of birth. Scand J Public Health 40(1), 43–50.

Thomas, D. (2010). Gene--environment-wide association studies: emerging approaches. Nat Rev Genet 11(4), 259–272.

van der Ven, E., Termorshuizen, F., et al. (2013). An incidence study of diagnosed autism-spectrum disorders among immigrants to the Netherlands. Acta Psychiatr Scand 128(1), 54–60.

van Os, J., Kenis, G., et al. (2010). The environment and schizophrenia. Nature 468(7321), 203–212.

van Os, J., Pedersen, C.B., et al. (2004). Confirmation of synergy between urbanicity and familial liability in the causation of psychosis. Am J Psychiatry 161(12), 2312–2314.

van Os, J., Rutten, B.P., et al. (2008). Gene-environment interactions in schizophrenia: review of epidemiological findings and future directions. Schizophr Bull 34(6), 1066–1082.

van Winkel, R. (2011). Family-based analysis of genetic variation underlying psychosis-inducing effects of cannabis: sibling analysis and proband follow-up. Arch Gen Psychiatry 68(2), 148–157.

van Winkel, R., Henquet, C., et al. (2008). Evidence that the COMT(Val158Met) polymorphism moderates sensitivity to stress in psychosis: an experience-sampling study. Am J Med Genet B Neuropsychiatr Genet 147B(1), 10–17.

Vassos, E., Pedersen, C.B., et al. (2012). Meta-analysis of the association of urbanicity with schizophrenia. Schizophr Bull 38(6), 1118–1123.

Veling, W., Hoek, H.W., et al. (2011). Age at migration and future risk of psychotic disorders among immigrants in the Netherlands: a 7-year incidence study. Am J Psychiatry 168(12), 1278–1285.

Veltman, J.A., and Brunner, H.G. (2012). De novo mutations in human genetic disease. Nat Rev Genet 13(8), 565–575.

Visscher, P.M., Hill, W.G., et al. (2008). Heritability in the genomics era--concepts and misconceptions. Nat Rev Genet 9(4), 255–266.

Waterland, R.A. (2009). Is epigenetics an important link between early life events and adult disease? Horm Res 71 (Suppl 1), 13–16.

Weinberger, D.R. (1987). Implications of normal brain development for the pathogenesis of schizophrenia. Arch Gen Psychiatry 44(7), 660–669.

Wellcome Trust Case Control, C. (2007). Genome-wide association study of 14,000 cases of seven common diseases and 3,000 shared controls. Nature 447(7145), 661–678.

Whitehouse, A.J., Holt, B.J., et al. (2013). Maternal Vitamin D Levels and the Autism Phenotype Among Offspring. J Autism Dev Disord 43(7), 1495–504.

Whitehouse, A.J., Holt, B.J., et al. (2012b). Maternal serum vitamin D levels during pregnancy and offspring neurocognitive development. Pediatrics 129(3), 485–493.

Wigman, J.T., van Winkel, R., et al. (2012). Early trauma and familial risk in the development of the extended psychosis phenotype in adolescence. Acta Psychiatr Scand 126(4), 266–273.

Williams, G., King, J., et al. (2001). Fetal valproate syndrome and autism: additional evidence of an association. Dev Med Child Neurol 43(3), 202–206.

Williams, J.G., Higgins, J.P., et al. (2006). Systematic review of prevalence studies of autism spectrum disorders. Arch Dis Child 91(1), 8–15.

Wray, N.R., Goddard, M.E., et al. (2007). Prediction of individual genetic risk to disease from genome-wide association studies. Genome Res 17(10), 1520–1528.

Wray, N.R., and Visscher, P.M. (2010). Narrowing the boundaries of the genetic architecture of schizophrenia. Schizophr Bull 36(1), 14–23.

Yang, J., Benyamin, B., et al. (2010). Common SNPs explain a large proportion of the heritability for human height. Nat Genet 42(7), 565–569.

Zammit, S. (2008). Commentary on 'The case for gene-environment interactions in psychiatry'. Curr Opin Psychiatry 21(4), 326–327.

Zammit, S., Owen, M.J., et al. (2010). Misconceptions about gene-environment interactions in psychiatry. Evid Based Ment Health 13(3), 65–8.

Zerbo, O., Iosif, A.M., et al. (2011). Month of conception and risk of autism. Epidemiology 22(4), 469–475.

Zuckerman, L., and Weiner, I. (2005). Maternal immune activation leads to behavioral and pharmacological changes in the adult offspring. J Psychiatr Res 39(3), 311–323.

7

THE GENETICS OF BRAIN MALFORMATIONS

M. Chiara Manzini[1] and Christopher A. Walsh[2]

[1]Department of Pharmacology and Physiology, and Integrative Systems Biology, The George Washington University, Washington, DC, USA

[2]Division of Genetics, The Manton Center for Orphan Disease Research and Howard Hughes Medical Institute, Boston Children's Hospital, Boston, MA, USA

7.1 INTRODUCTION

During the 40 weeks of human fetal gestation, the brain undergoes a series of complex morphogenetic and molecular processes regulating the differentiation of around 80 billion neurons and coordinating the formation of 100 trillion synaptic contacts. As the brain is formed, progenitor cells proliferate close to the ventricular surface to generate neuronal and glial cells, which will migrate to the cortical plate and differentiate to become organized and connected in a stereotypical fashion to form neuronal circuits. Brain malformations are global or regional disruption in brain development caused by the faulty completion of these developmental processes often, because of genetic mutations in the genes, regulating specific developmental steps. In the past 20 years, the identification of the genes responsible for a host of brain malformation has greatly advanced the understanding of the molecular mechanisms essential for normal brain development while informing us on the pathogenetic process in these patients. In the mid-2000s, the advent of next-generation sequencing techniques, which allow the sequencing of the entire genome of an individual, has nearly doubled the number of known cortical malformation genes providing an even deeper understanding of brain development. While malformations are radiographically evident changes often leading to early mortality and severe cognitive and physical impairment, next-generation approaches studying neuropsychiatric disorders are beginning to find hypomorphic variants in malformation genes associated with these conditions suggesting that partial disruption of key developmental mechanisms can cause a range of disorders not always obvious in standard brain imaging techniques.

The Genetics of Neurodevelopmental Disorders, First Edition. Edited by Kevin J. Mitchell.
© 2015 John Wiley & Sons, Inc. Published 2015 by John Wiley & Sons, Inc.

Barkovich et al. generated a useful clinical classification of malformations of the cortex (Barkovich et al., 2005; 2012) and of the midbrain and hindbrain (Barkovich et al., 2009) based on the general developmental process expected to be disrupted and on the genes known at the time of writing. Disorders presenting with a significantly smaller or larger brain, such as microcephaly (from the Greek, small head) or megalencephaly (large head) were classified as defects in cell proliferation leading to either a reduction or to a nonneoplastic increase in brain size. Disorders where neurons were unable to leave the germinal zone or were found in the wrong location in the cortical plate, such a periventricular nodular heterotopia, double cortex or lissencephaly (smooth brain), were classified as disorders of migration. While this correlation between a morphological defect and a specific biological process is correct and it is very useful to conceptualize the causes of these disorders, the more genes and mutations that are described, the more brain malformations tend to escape the boundaries of classification, as proliferation and migration disorders appear to coexist in the same patients or are caused by mutations in the same gene in different patients. The ever-increasing number of brain malformation genes is now pointing to specific molecular mechanisms and defining the inter-actions between different pathways. Because of the current speed of discovery, which leads to the publication of new genes on a weekly basis, and the extreme depth of the functional characterization of some of the known genes, we will not be able to discuss everything in detail. We will provide a general overview of emerging mechanistic groups and their role in brain development and disease and list additional review articles for further reading.

7.2 THE MICROCEPHALIES

Microcephaly is a disorder in which the brain is disproportionately smaller than the body and is diagnosed by measuring a head circumference more than two standard deviations lower than the population average. Primary microcephaly or microcephaly *vera* is an autosomal recessive condition only affecting the brain where the gyral pattern is often preserved upon radiolog-ical analysis, so that the brain just appears as a smaller version of a normal brain (Fig. 7.1a). Multiple other forms of microcephaly have been reported in a syndromic setting with or without cognitive deficits and seizures. Traditionally, microcephaly has been classified as a disorder of proliferation, where the neuronal progenitors produce fewer neurons leading to reduced brain growth (Barkovich et al., 2012). Similarly to many other brain malformations discussed in this chapter, microcephaly has proven to be genetically heterogeneous leading to the iden-tification of numerous genes in patients with indistinguishable phenotype. The majority of these genes have overlapping function outlining two mechanisms that control proliferation and neuronal specification: DNA repair and mitotic spindle organization by centrosomal proteins. However, additional causes of microcephaly ranging from epigenetic regulation of gene transcription to control of metabolic function revealed that multiple molecular mechanisms can be disrupted in this disorder.

7.2.1 Microcephaly and DNA Repair

Analysis of the first genetic locus for primary microcephly, MCPH1, identified mutations in a gene involved in chromosome condensation and DNA damage response, named microcephalin (*MCPH1*) (Jackson et al., 2002), revealing that the ability of the cell to repair DNA after replication is an important determinant of brain size. As cells proliferate and the genome is duplicated, errors must be detected and cor-rected, and cells with a defective genome will undergo cell cycle arrest and be removed via apoptosis. MCPH1 is involved in DNA damage response mediated via the DNA damage sensor kinase ATR and it recruits the downstream kinase Chk1 to prevent cell cycle exit. Loss of *Mcph1* in the mouse shows premature Chk1 activation and increased cell death, indicating that progenitors tend to exit earlier than normal

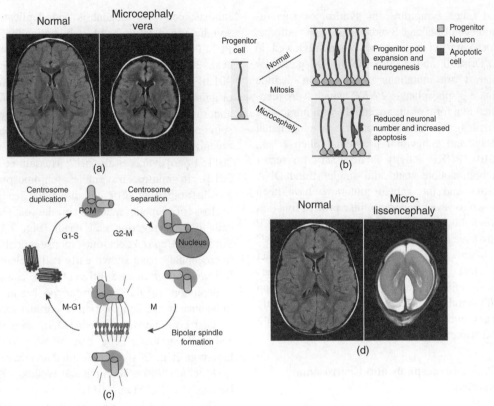

Fig. 7.1 *Neuronal proliferation in microcephaly.* (a) In microcephaly *vera* the brain is disproportionately smaller than the body, but the gyral pattern is often preserved upon radiological analysis. (b) Normal cortical expansion is regulated by the balance of progenitor proliferation and neurogenesis. In microcephaly models, several processes can affect brain size: a reduction in progenitor proliferation, neurons are generated too early reducing the number of progenitors and cell death of newly born neurons and progenitors is also observed. (c) A number of genes mutated in patients affected by microcephaly, disrupt aspects of centrosome biogenesis and function: centrosome duplication and separation or formation of a normal bipolar spindle for mitosis. (d) In severe cases, microcephaly is associated with lissencephaly (smooth brain) and fluid filled space between the skull and the brain. These additional defects could indicate problems in neuronal migration and massive cell death following initial brain expansion. *(See insert for color representation of this figure.)*

from the cells cycle and undergo premature differentiation, causing a depletion of the pool of progenitor cells (Fig. 7.1b) (Gruber et al., 2011).

Mutations in another damage response gene *CEP152* can cause either primary microcephaly (Guernsey et al., 2010) or Seckel syndrome (microcephalic primordial dwarfism), a syndrome characterized by microcephaly, short stature, intellectual disability, and characteristic facial dysmorphisms leading to a bird-like appearance (Kalay et al., 2011). Mutations in

ATR itself (O'Driscoll et al., 2003), in ATR interacting protein (*ATRIP*) (Ogi et al., 2012), and in the ATR regulator *RBBP8* (Qvist et al., 2011) also cause Seckel syndrome showing how the detection of DNA damage is necessary for both neuronal progenitor proliferation and the overall regulation of body size.

Finally, microcephaly is also usually described in mutations of numerous genes directly involved in the repair of DNA breaks in combination with immunodeficiency, growth retardation, chromosomal instability, and other symptoms, in syndromes such as Nijmegen Breakage Syndrome, Lig 4 syndrome, Cockayne syndrome, and others reviewed in (O'Driscoll and Jeggo, 2008). Of particular interest are mutations in the polynucleotide kinase 3'-phosphatase *PNKP*, which were identified in a form of microcephaly with intractable seizures of infantile onset, developmental delay, and behavioral problems (Shen et al., 2010). PNKP activity is necessary for repair of both double stand and single strand DNA breaks and the known mutations have been shown to severely compromise protein function (Reynolds et al., 2012), suggesting that PNKP may have a specific role in the brain.

Many DNA damage response genes act in close association with the centrosomes during mitosis, leading to a substantial overlap with another main category of microcephaly genes encoding for proteins associated with centrosomal organization and function.

7.2.2 Microcephaly and Centrosomal Function

Most of the other known primary microcephaly genes are associated with the centrosome, a complex structure composed of two centrioles and the pericentriolar material (PCM), an electron-dense protein-rich substance, whose primary roles are to nucleate microtubules and anchor the cytoskeleton. During mitosis, the centrosome is duplicated and secures the poles of the mitotic spindle, controlling chromosomal segregation and DNA migration to the two daughter cells (Fig. 7.1c). A wide array of centrosomal genes are mutated in primary microcephaly, *ASPM* (Bond et al., 2002), *CDK5RAP2* (Bond et al., 2005), *STIL* (Kumar et al., 2009), *WDR62* (Bilgüvar et al., 2010; Nicholas et al., 2010; Yu et al., 2010), *CEP63* (Sir et al., 2011), and *CEP135* (Hussain et al., 2012); Seckel Syndrome, pericentrin (*PCNT*) (Griffith et al., 2008), and ninein (*NIN*) (Dauber et al., 2012), or in both disorders, *CENPJ* (Bond et al., 2005; Al-Dosari et al., 2010). These genes encode proteins which are necessary for different aspects of centrosome regulation during

mitosis: centriole biogenesis and duplication, spindle organization, and stabilization of the PCM (Thornton and Woods, 2009; Bogoyevitch et al., 2012; Hussain et al., 2012; Vulprecht et al., 2012). Loss of function mutations in cell lines or animal models often lead to the formation of abnormal mitotic spindles, where the bipolar spindle morphology is replaced by a multipolar organization (Lizarraga et al., 2010, Sir et al., 2011; Bogoyevitch et al., 2012; Hussain et al., 2012). In multipolar spindles, chromosomes are distributed in different directions leading to loss of genetic material in the daughter cells likely triggering cell death (Fig. 7.1b). Similar to *Mcph1* knock-outs, mouse models of microcephaly have shown early cell cycle exit followed by premature differentiation, causing a depletion of the progenitor pool and an imbalance in the composition of cortical layers as later-born layers are reduced in thickness and cell number (Feng and Walsh, 2004a; Lizarraga et al., 2010). For detailed review, refer to (Mochida, 2009; Thornton and Woods, 2009; Bettencourt-Dias et al., 2011).

Thus, depending on the mutated gene, microcephaly could result from a variety of mechanisms including loss of progenitors and neurons due to (1) cell death of aneuploid daughter cells dividing from cells with multipolar spindles, (2) early cell cycle exit of progenitors because of mitotic defects, (3) perturbed DNA damage responses, or to a combination of all these phenomena. Mice deficient for microcephaly genes involved in either DNA repair or centrosome stability had shown widespread cell death, cell cycle arrest, and early cell cycle exit (Feng and Walsh, 2004a; Lizarraga et al., 2010; Gruber et al., 2011). In addition, invertebrate research has shown how regulation of mitotic spindle orientation and daughter centriole inheritance are implicated in cell fate decisions, suggesting that some forms of microcephaly could represent defects of neural cell fate determination (Wang et al., 2009; Januschke et al., 2011). As more of these proteins are found to interact and function together during differentiation delineating overlapping phenotypes, the better our understanding of the underlying mechanisms becomes.

7.2.3 Microcephaly and Cell Fate Specification

While mutations in genes involved in mitotic progression and DNA repair are a major determinant of microcephaly, they are not the only cause of this disorder and the identification of additional genes has revealed multiple additional mechanisms controlling brain size. As previously discussed, cell fate specification has been implicated in the pathogenesis of microcephaly by studies revealing that centrosomal organization and inheritance can also determine cell fate (Wang et al., 2009). The importance of cell fate decisions in generating and maintaining the appropriate number of neurons was supported by the discovery of mutations in the chromatin regulators ZNF335 and CHMP1A. ZNF335 is a transcriptional regulator, which associates with promoters as part of the H3K4 methyltransferase complex, a key chromatin-remodeling complex controlling gene expression. A hypomorphic missense mutation in ZNF335 was inherited in a recessive fashion in a family affected by severe lethal microcephaly (9 SD below the mean) with simplified gyral pattern and enlarged extra-axial space (Yang et al., 2012). Since brain growth drives skull expansion, the fluid filled space between the skull and the brain indicates degeneration and cell death following initial brain expansion. Znf335 knock-out mice display a more severe phenotype than the one observed in the patients with retarded growth and death in mid-gestation, and a cerebral cortex-specific conditional knock-out shows massive cortical loss, stressing the vital importance of this gene for neuronal differentiation and survival (Yang et al., 2012). Loss of Znf335 affects expression of several genes involved in neurogenesis and neuronal cell fate specification leading to both reduced proliferation and cell death of the resulting neurons (Yang et al., 2012). Similarly, mutations in CHMP1A, which interacts with the Polycomb chromatin-remodeling complex, greatly affect cerebellar development causing profound cerebellar hypoplasia

and loss of cerebellar cells (Mochida et al., 2012).

An analogous disruption in both neurogenesis and neuronal differentiation has been hypothesized for mutations in DYRK1A, a highly conserved kinase, which acts on numerous substrates involved in proliferation, dendrite extension, synapse formation, and cytoskeletal regulation (Guedj et al., 2012). Because of its location in the Down Syndrome critical region on chromosome 21, DYRK1A overexpression has been extensively studied as a possible cause of the cognitive phenotypes in trisomy 21 cases (Smith et al., 1997), but heterozygous loss of DYRK1A via translocation or de novo deletions also causes intellectual disability, seizures, ataxic gait, and microcephaly with a progressive reduction in brain size due to atrophy (Møller et al., 2008; van Bon et al., 2011). In fact, this gene was initially identified in the fly in a screen for brain growth regulators, and it was aptly called minibrain (mnb) (Tejedor et al., 1995). Heterozygous Dyrk1a-deficient mice display microcephaly associated with an increase of cortical thickness, suggesting that a migration defect may follow reduced proliferation (Fotaki et al., 2002).

Studies in mouse models indicated that vesicle trafficking is also essential for normal polarized expression of cell fate determinants within cortical progenitor cells (Chae et al., 2004) and trafficking regulators have been found mutated in syndromic cases of microcephaly. A severe form with microcephaly also characterized by migration defects is caused by mutations in ARFGEF2, which encodes for a major regulator of vesicle trafficking, BIG2 (Sheen et al., 2004). Another gene COH1, which is mutated in Cohen syndrome, where microcephaly is associated with retinal lesions and mild dysmorphic features, encodes for vesicular sorting protein 13B (VPS13B), which is predicted to regulate sorting in the Golgi (Kolehmainen et al., 2003). It is currently not known whether these genes have any roles in cell fate decisions, but vesicle trafficking also deserves further study as a regulator of neurogenesis and neuronal differentiation.

All these mutations in regulators of gene expression and intracellular signaling and trafficking have opened new avenues of investigation revealing that neuronal differentiation and survival may be as important as proliferation in the pathogenesis of microcephaly. In fact, microcephaly has also been observed in multiple syndromes where metabolic function is disrupted, as neurons are particularly sensitive to metabolic defects (Tarrant et al., 2009). A classic example is Amish lethal microcephaly (MCPHA), which has been described exclusively in the Old Order Amish population in the United States and is characterized by profound microcephaly (6–12 SD below the mean), increased levels of urinary α-ketoglutarate and lethality within the first year of life. This disorder is caused by a recessive missense mutation in *SLC25A19*, which encodes a mitochondrial carrier for thiamine pyrophosphate, a derivative of vitamin B1, which is an essential nutrient and necessary cofactor for multiple metabolic processes (Kang and Samuels, 2008; Rosenberg et al., 2002). Since the brain is one of the organs with the highest energy consumption, using up to 20% of the body energy budget, these metabolic deficiencies also have a devastating effect on neuronal differentiation and maintenance.

7.2.4 Beyond Proliferation: Phenotypic Variability in Microcephaly

The variability of molecular mechanisms leading to microcephaly has helped explain the range of phenotypes observed in the patients, but sequence analysis of known genes in larger patient cohorts has also revealed clinical differences in patients carrying mutations in the same gene. The overlapping defects caused by mutations in a single gene are best exemplified by *WDR62*, which maps to the MCPH2 locus and is the second most frequent cause of primary microcephaly. In addition to primary microcephaly, *WDR62* mutations cause reduced brain size associated with a wide spectrum of other malformations such as lissencephaly (smooth brain) and pachygyria (few gyri), as

well as polymicrogyria (many small gyri) and schizencephaly (split brain) (Bilgüvar et al., 2010; Nicholas et al., 2010; Yu et al., 2010). While loss of *WDR62* function has only been explored in cell lines to date showing a disruption in spindle polarity as described for other microcephaly genes (Bogoyevitch et al., 2012), these widespread defects suggest that this gene must have an additional role in differentiation, so that the cells which manage to escape the proliferation defect may still be impaired in their migratory capacity. Both lissencephaly and pachygyria are migration disorders, where neurons fail to reach their correct destination leading to a cortical plate where neurons from different layers are mixed together. Mutations in another centrosomal protein *NDE1* whose loss of function in the mouse leads to a reduction in brain size with preserved migration (Feng and Walsh, 2004a), in humans cause severe microlissencephaly, characterized by profound microcephaly and loss of gyration with thickened disorganized cortex (Fig. 7.1d) (Alkuraya et al., 2011). Interestingly, NDE1 is a binding partner to LIS1, whose *de novo* deletions and mutations are the principal cause of classic lissencephaly (see subsequently). LIS1 is a microtubule-binding protein closely associated with the centrosome and with the molecular motor dynein, and it is necessary for nuclear translocation during migration. Patients carrying *LIS1* mutations do not have microcephaly, suggesting that *LIS1* is primarily involved in regulation of migration, while *NDE1* has roles on both migration and cell division. A similar scenario can be imagined for *WDR62*. Thus, a malformation can be caused by a combination of events due to dysfunction of the same protein and centrosomal protein defects can lead to disruptions in both proliferation and migration.

7.3 THE LISSENCEPHALIES

The term lissencephaly derives from the Greek smooth brain and it describes a group of disorders where the normal gyral pattern of the human brain is extremely simplified or absent. It is usually accompanied by a thickened and disorganized cortical plate, which results from a defect in neuronal migration. Migrating neurons are unable to reach their normal layer location and neurons from different layers can be mixed or disorganized globally or locally. Like microcephalies, lissencephalies are also very heterogeneous, but tend to fall in two broad categories that are morphologically different upon radiological analysis: cytoskeletal defects and extracellular matrix (ECM) interaction defects.

7.3.1 Lissencephaly and Cytoskeletal Organization and Stability

The importance of the cytoskeleton in regulating neuronal migration was first revealed more than a decade ago by the discovery of mutations in *LIS1* and *DCX* in patients affected with lissencephaly (Reiner et al., 1993; Fox et al., 1998; Gleeson et al., 1998; des Portes et al., 1998). Heterozygous deletions in *LIS1*, a regulator of cytoskeletal transport, cause classical lissencephaly, where neuronal migration is severely impaired leading to a thickened disorganized cortex and smooth cortical surface (Dobyns et al., 1993; Forman et al., 2005) (Fig. 7.2a–b). *DCX* is an X-linked gene, which encodes doublecortin, a microtubule-binding protein. *DCX* mutations result in lissencephaly in males and the formation of an ectopic layer of neurons (subcortical band heterotopia or double cortex) in the white matter in females (Gleeson et al., 1998). The double cortex phenotype is particularly interesting since it is hypothesized to results from random inactivation of the X chromosome in females: cells expressing the normal *DCX* allele complete their migration successfully and cells carrying the mutated gene are delayed and fall behind, clearly showing the migration phenotype caused by *DCX* loss of function in the same patient (Fig. 7.2a–b). The identification of these genes and a multitude of follow-up functional studies have shaped our current understanding of neuronal migration. Microtubules provide a scaffold sustaining the leading process, which extends upward. The centrosome, which during migration is located above the nucleus, anchors both the leading process cytoskeleton and a cage of microtubules surrounding the nucleus. Each time the leading process moves forward, the perinuclear cage lifts the nucleus to follow in what is called nuclear translocation (for review see (Vallee and Tsai, 2006; Kerjan and Gleeson, 2007)). Both cytoskeletal stability and transport have been hypothesized as necessary for normal migration, and lissencephaly genes have been involved in both. While both LIS1 and DCX are able to stabilize microtubules (Sumigray et al., 2011; Bechstedt and Brouhard, 2012), they have also been shown to control transport along the cytoskeleton: LIS1 is a regulator of cytoplasmic dynein, the molecular motor controlling transport from the periphery toward the centrosome (Huang et al., 2012), and DCX forms a ternary complex with the kinesin 3 motor Kif1a and microtubules to regulate transport to the periphery of the cell (Liu et al., 2012). In fact, lissencephaly and other migration defects have also been found in patients carrying mutations in the dynein heavy chain gene, *DYNC1H1*, and two different kinesis, *KIF5C* and *KIF2A*, supporting an important role for molecular motors in neuronal migration (Willemsen et al., 2012; Poirier et al., 2013).

The building blocks of microtubules themselves, α and β-tubulin, have been also involved in an array of cortical malformations. Dominant missense or *de novo* mutations in multiple tubulin isoforms *TUBA1A* (Poirier et al., 2007), *TUBB2B* (Jaglin et al., 2009), *TUBB3* (Poirier et al., 2010), and *TUBB5* (Breuss et al., 2012) cause classical lissencephaly (*TUBA1A*), pachygyria (*TUBA1A*, *TUBB2B*, *TUBB3*), polymicrogyria (many small gyri; *TUBA1A*, *TUBB2B*, *TUBB3*), all with brain stem and cerebellar abnormalities, and microcephaly with basal ganglia abnormalities (*TUBB5*). Recessive mutation in *TUBA8* is found in cases of polymicrogyria with optic nerve hypoplasia (Abdollahi et al., 2009). Functional analysis of the different missense changes suggested the same disease mechanisms discussed earlier: (1) microtubule instability due to inability of the

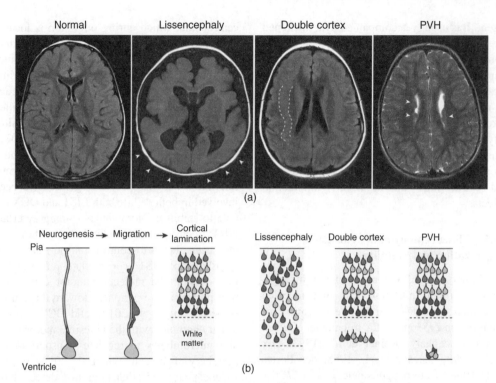

Fig. 7.2 *Neuronal migration defects lead to a range of malformations.* (a) Different types of brain malformations are characterized by defects in neuronal migration. Normal migration leads to correct lamination of the six cortical layers (schematic in b), but in classical lissencephaly. the cortex is thickened and disorganized (4-layer structure with inverted and mixed layers is shown here; see Forman et al., 2005). Doublecortin (*DCX*) mutations cause lissencephaly in males and double cortex in females, likely due to random inactivation of the X-chromosome carrying the mutated gene. Some cells migrate correctly, while other remain stuck in a disorganized band in the white matter. In some cases, neurons cannot leave the ventricular zone at all and form nodules lining the ventricles leading to periventricular nodular heterotopia (PVH). *(See insert for color representation of this figure.)*

mutated tubulin isoform to polymerize normally and (2) disruption of lateral residues necessary for binding to molecular motors or microtubule associated proteins (MAPs). The location of the mutation on the protein may dictate the phenotypic variant observed in the patients, reviewed in detail by Tischfield et al., 2011.

In addition to the migration defects, mutations in all the genes listed earlier also display axon guidance defects such as corpus callosum abnormalities and cranial nerve guidance defects. *TUBB3* mutations in particular were initially identified in a form of paralytic strabismus, congenital fibrosis of the extraocular muscles 3 (CFEOM3), resulting from hypoplasia and faulty axon guidance of the oculomotor nerves (Tischfield et al., 2010). All CFEOM3 causing mutations specifically affect binding to the kinesin KIF21A, which is itself mutated in a related disease, CFEOM1 (Yamada et al., 2003), while *TUBB3* mutations causing cortical malformations disrupt tubulin polymerization (Poirier et al., 2010). It is obvious that without correct microtubule polymerization neuronal processes will fail to grow; however, even when the cytoskeleton is stable, axonal transport appears critical for correct axon navigation through the brain, as transport defects could affect delivery of guidance receptors and cues or of other factors necessary for outgrowth.

While tubulins and associated proteins appear to have the lion's share of mutations in migration disorders, the actin cytoskeleton has also been involved. *De novo* gain-of-function mutations in the *β*- and *γ*-actin genes (*ACTB* and *ACTG1*) have been linked to anterior lissencephaly as part of Baraitser-Winter Syndrome, which is also associated with multiple dysmorphic features (Rivière et al., 2012b). Moreover, DCX has also been shown to interact with the actin cytoskeleton (Tsukada et al., 2005) and to regulate filamentous actin structures in the growing processes of developing neurons (Fu et al., 2013), supporting an important role of the actin cytoskeleton in the pathogenesis of lissencephaly. Mutations in *FLNA*, an X-linked gene, which encodes the actin binding protein FLNA cause periventricular nodular heterotopia in women, a disorder were groups of affected neurons form characteristic nodules or ribbons of cells along the ventricular surface (Fox et al., 1998) (Fig. 7.2a–b). FLNA is a molecular scaffold involved in the cross-linking of actin filaments and binding a wide array of proteins including membrane receptors and kinases in multiple signaling pathways controlling cell cycle progression, cell shape and protein–protein interactions (Feng and Walsh, 2004b). However, the mechanisms underlying the formation of heterotopic nodules and whether this disorder is due to a failure of migration initiation or a local disruption of progenitor proliferation leading to the birth of ectopic neurons at the ventricular surface are still not known. Mice deficient for *FlnA* show a phenotype more consistent with a proliferation disorder than a migration deficit (Feng et al., 2006; Lian et al., 2012). Interestingly, the other known cause of PNH are mutations in the vesicle trafficking regulator *ARFGEF2* (Sheen et al., 2004), already discussed as a cause of severe microcephaly, further stressing that defects in molecules involved in cortical malformations may affect multiple steps of differentiation. Numerous cases of PNH have been reported with no mutations in either gene, indicating that additional genes remain to be identified and possibly novel cellular mechanism underlying migration disorders.

7.3.2 Lissencephaly and Extracellular Matrix Interactions

The ECM is a lattice of proteins and proteoglycans closely surrounding cells and organs. In the brain, it is found both enveloping the neurons and deposited on the pial surface where the end feet of the neuronal progenitors are anchored in an ECM layer called the basement membrane. The discovery of mutations in multiple ECM components and regulators has revealed a vital role for cell-ECM interactions in neuronal migration and differentiation, in addition to the classic structural role of the ECM. Reelin (*RELN*) is a large secreted ECM protein released close to the pial surface by the Cajal-Retzius cells, horizontal neuronal cells located under the basement membrane during brain development and thought to be involved in early circuit establishment (Fig. 7.3a). Loss of the *RELN* gene or of its receptor *VLDLR* causes lissencephaly with cerebellar hypoplasia, a disorder where cerebellar size is profoundly reduced and the cortical plate is thickened with a few or no discernible gyri (Hong et al., 2000; Boycott et al., 2005). A unique pathological feature of *RELN* mutations is the fact that the layer organization of the cortex is inverted, so that layer VI neurons are closer to the pial surface and layer II neurons are near the white matter, revealing a specific role for this protein in cortical organization (Fig. 7.3b). The reeler mouse, which is a spontaneous *reelin* mutant first described more than sixty years ago (Falconer, 1951), accurately replicates the human phenotypes and has provided a valuable tool to study reelin function, its binding partners and receptors. However, the mechanism controlling where cortical neurons stop their migration is still a mystery.

Other groups of disorders of cell-ECM interaction are the *α*-dystroglycanopathies, which present with a varied spectrum of cortical malformations. Dystroglycan is a transmembrane glycoprotein linking the dystrophin complex to the ECM via its glycan moieties. *α*-dystroglycanopathies are characterized by muscular dystrophy often associated with an array of ocular and brain malformations, but

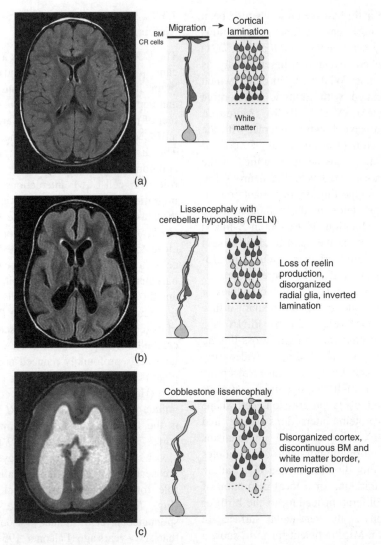

Fig. 7.3 *Neuronal migration defects caused by extracellular signals.* (a) Extracellular signals present in the basement membrane (BM) or secreted by Cajal-Retzius (CR) cells under the pial surface are necessary for normal cortical lamination. (b) Loss of reelin (RELN) signaling from the CR cells generates a characteristic inversion in cortical layers, whereby layer VI is now on top and layer I at the bottom. (c) Loss of BM and extracellular matrix signals is also important, leading to cobblestone lissencephaly and characteristic migration defects: overmigration of neurons to the pial surface and disruptions in the gray-white matter boundary. *(See insert for color representation of this figure.)*

occasional renal malformations and cardiomyopathy have also been reported. In all these tissues, the ability of the cells to interact with the basement membrane and ECM is vital for their function and/or organization leading to a multitude of defects. Recessive missense mutations have been identified in dystroglycan itself (*DAG1*) in patients with a milder muscular dystrophy phenotype (Hara et al., 2011), as null *DAG1* mutations in humans probably lead to early embryonic lethality similarly to the *Dag1*-deficient mouse (Cohn et al., 2002). In fact, one of the known *DAG1* mutations slightly reduces dystroglycan glycosylation in the patient and in a knock-in mouse model (Hara et al., 2011). The ever increasing list of genes found to be mutated in α-dystroglycanopathies all have been shown to severely reduce dystroglycan glycosylation. Seven are known glycosyltransferase enzymes (*POMT1*, *POMT2*, *POMGNT1*, *POMGNT2*, *LARGE*, *B3GALNT2*, and *B3GNT1*) and five have been shown to be predicted glycosyltransferases or other enzymes involved in dystroglycan function (*FKTN*, *FKRP*, *ISPD*, *TMEM5*, *POMK*) (Muntoni et al., 2011; Manzini et al., 2012; Roscioli et al., 2012; Willer et al., 2012; Buysse et al., 2013; Jae et al., 2013; Stevens et al., 2013). In the patients, mutations in these genes cause an array of cortical malformations ranging from cobblestone lissencephaly, a form of lissencephaly where the cortical plate is grossly disorganized and neurons overmigrate through the basement membrane onto the pial surface, to pachygyria and polymicrogyria (Fig. 7.3e). The same layering and migration defects are present in other neuronal epithelia such as the cerebellum and the retina. A major difficulty in the genetic analysis of these disorders is their extreme clinical heterogeneity, where mutations in the same gene can cause a wide spectrum of phenotypes and each phenotypic presentation in the spectrum can be caused by any one of the known genes. This variability makes the development of guidelines for genetic testing very difficult and the cost of testing each patient for more than a dozen genes can be prohibitive. In addition, the known genes explain only 50–60% of cases and genetic linkage analyses have shown that multiple additional genes are predicted to be involved, but family size has been often too small to lead to gene identification.

Innovative approaches have been used recently to circumvent these difficulties. Willer et al. (2012) developed a genetic complementation assay based on patient fibroblasts: when cells from two patients are fused, α-dystroglycan glycosylation will be restored if they carry mutations in different genes and each cell line now supplies an intact copy of the gene mutated in the other, but when both patients have mutations in the same gene glycosylation will still be reduced. By identifying multiple complementation groups, it was possible to define how many different genes were involved in the patient cohort enrolled in the study and combine patients for genetic analysis leading to the identification of *ISPD* (Willer et al., 2012). A second approach focuses on the role of the carbohydrate moieties on α-dystroglycan as pathogen receptors (Jae et al., 2013). Lassa virus can only infect cells by binding to specific glycans on α-dystroglycan and a mutagenesis screen was conducted to identify mutants that would disrupt glycan synthesis and no longer allow infection. In addition to most known dystroglycanopathy genes, several new candidates were identified leading to the discovery of mutations in *TMEM5* and *POMK* (Jae et al., 2013).

Dystroglycan is known to bind laminins in the ECM and mutations in one of its best studied ligands laminin-α2 (*LAMA2*) cause congenital muscular dystrophy with malformations in the less severe range of the dystroglycanopathy spectrum and no eye defects (Helbling-Leclerc et al., 1995). Interestingly, laminin-β1 (*LAMB1*) mutations were found to cause cobblestone lissencephaly without muscle or eye defects (Radmanesh et al., 2013), while laminin-γ3 (*LAMC3*) is involved in occipital pachygyria and polymicrogyria (Barak et al., 2011). Whether these defects are mediated via dystroglycan binding or through interactions with other receptors is not known, but these findings clearly identify a common role for laminins in cortical organization.

Other major ECM components, the collagens, are also involved in a range of malformations. Dominant collagen IV (*COL4A1*) mutations have been described in multiple cases of porencephaly, where the brain is affected by cystic lesions, schizencephaly, a malformation where the pial surface become continuous with the ventricle forming a cleft in the hemisphere (Yoneda et al., 2013), and even in two dystroglycanopathy patients (Labelle-Dumais et al., 2011). Recessive collagen XVIII (*COL18A1*) mutations cause Knobloch syndrome, which is associated with occipital cranial and cortical malformations and ocular defects. Collagen III (COL3A1) was found to be a ligand for the transmembrane glycoprotein, GPR56 (Luo et al., 2011), which is mutated in a form of polymicrogyria restricted to the frontoparietal region, bilateral frontoparietal polymicrogyria or BFPP (Piao et al., 2004). Upon radiological and histopathological analysis BFPP shows striking similarity to cobblestone cortex (Bahi-Buisson et al., 2010), but whether dystroglycan function is in any way related to GPR56 is not known. The increasing functional and clinical overlap among mutations involving ECM components and their receptors implies a common molecular mechanism, but the downstream signaling partners of many of these proteins remain relatively unexplored and may provide important insight into how the ECM controls neuronal differentiation.

7.4 THE POLYMICROGYRIAS

Polymicrogyria (PMG), which is characterized by a disruption in cortical appearance by many small gyri, is one of the most common cortical malformations and is often found in spectrum or associated with other malformations. PMG is extremely variable in appearance upon radiology and pathology and is found in multiple locations, diffuse, focal or multifocal, unilateral, bilateral, or asymmetrical (Barkovich, 2010). In addition to genetic causes, PMG has also been attributed to *in utero* events such as ischemia or cytomegalovirus infections. This extreme clinical variability and the possibility that sporadic cases may be due to nongenetic causes, had made genetic analysis of this malformation challenging and comprehensive surveys of hundred of patients indicate that PMG may actually comprise multiple different disorders (Barkovich, 2010).

In fact, while PMG has been classified as a disorder of postmigratory development, meaning that migration is thought to be normal and that some other differentiation process must generate the multiple small gyri (Barkovich

et al., 2012), the postmigratory mechanisms involved remain unidentified. The description of PMG associated with mutations in each of the categories described earlier (*WDR62*, tubulin genes, laminins, α-dystroglycanopathy genes) has also begun to shake the hypothesis of a purely postmigratory malformation.

The best characterized gene associated with PMG is *GPR56*, whose mutation causes a form of PMG restricted to the frontoparietal region of the brain, bilateral frontoparietal polymicrogyria, BFPP (Piao et al., 2004). The *Gpr56* knock-out mouse shows regions where cortical layer organization is disrupted and neurons from deeper layers are found to overmigrate to the pial surface in a fashion reminiscent of the α-dystroglycanopathy phenotype (Li et al., 2008). In α-dystroglycanopathies, these defects are thought to be primarily due to radial glial progenitors, since conditional removal of dystroglycan in radial glia replicates the cortical lamination defects, but not removal in differentiated neurons (Satz et al., 2008). In the *Gpr56* knock-out, the basal processes of the radial glia are disorganized and their end feet are not firmly anchored in the basement membrane, which is discontinuous (Li et al., 2008). Mutations in the *LAMC3* gene are associated with occipital PMG (Barak et al., 2011). Since *LAMC3* encodes for a laminin gene that is presumably part of the ECM, this form of PMG may reflect a similar defect of ECM-end foot interactions, though this has not been shown. Interestingly, a similar disruption of the radial glial scaffold was also observed in neuropathology specimens from a fetus carrying a *TUBB2* mutation causing asymmetric PMG (Jaglin et al., 2009). *TUBB2* mutations may destabilize microtubule stability and disrupt cytoskeletal support or trafficking in the basal process, leading to an analogous effect to the loss of GPR56 and α-dystroglycan, which are important for interactions with the basement membrane. In summary, radial glial instability may cause at least one form of PMG in a spectrum with cobblestone lissencephaly, and in fact, both of these malformations have been observed in the same brain (Bahi-Buisson et al., 2010).

While the appearance of BFPP and dystroglycanopathy PMG is very characteristic, other forms of PMG may have a variety of pathogenetic mechanisms. *WDR62* mutations cause both PMG and schizencephaly, which is sometimes caused by PMG so severe to cause a cleft in the hemisphere continuous with the ventricle (Bilgüvar et al., 2010; Yu et al., 2010). As discussed earlier, why *WDR62* mutations cause such a wide range of malformations from microcephaly to lissencephaly to PMG is not known, but the study of the migratory and postmigratory roles of this protein may help reveal some of the mechanisms involved. PMG localized around the Sylvian fissure (perisylvian PMG) is also sometimes found in velocardiofacial or DiGeorge syndrome, a common microdeletion syndrome associated with deletions in 22q11.2 and characterized by hypocalcemia due to parathyroid hypoplasia, cardiac defects, facial dysmorphisms, and learning or behavioral defects (Robin et al., 2006). Additional genetic causes of PMG have been reported, often in one family with no additional alleles identified, but many cases remain unexplained. Mechanistic studies may be difficult to complete in mouse models, mostly due to the fact that mice have lissencephalic brains and it may not be feasible to use them to model changes in gyrification. Neuronal differentiation during gyrus formation may be better addressed in gyrencephalic animals such as ferrets (Reillo et al., 2011), where a model of PMG may be achievable.

7.5 BRAIN OVERGROWTH AND SOMATIC MUTATIONS IN THE AKT/mTOR PATHWAY

Multiple malformations are associated with overgrowth phenotypes, where proliferation appears to be disrupted locally as in focal cortical dysplasias or more globally as in megalencephaly (large brain) and hemimegalencephaly (half large brain, Fig. 7.4a). In these patients, a variable portion of the brain is enlarged in an often disorganized manner with lamination defects, polymicrogyria, and heterotopias. These changes can be restricted to a specific brain region or a single hemisphere and while they are not tumors and do not continue to grow, they are reminiscent of neoplastic events. In cancer, a somatic mutation, a "new" mutation not inherited from the parents and localized to a certain tissue, appears to change the proliferative status of specific cell type triggering growth. Analogous somatic mutations appearing during development and affecting only the group of cells originating from the mutated progenitor had been identified in males affected by subcortical band heterotopia (SBH) or double cortex (Gleeson et al., 2000). As we have previously described, mutations in DCX, an X-linked gene, cause lissencephaly in males who have only one copy of the X chromosome and SBH in females where the mutated X undergoes random inactivation generating a portion of normal cells, which migrate normally and a portion of affected cells (Gleeson et al., 1998). However, when males with SBH were also found to carry *DCX* mutations and mutations in *LIS1*, the classical lissencephaly gene, somatic mutations were invoked to explain the less severe phenotype and the ability of some cells to migrate normally (Pilz et al., 1999). In these cases, an imbalance in the levels of the normal versus the mutant *DCX* or *LIS1* alleles was identified in the patient DNA, suggesting that the mutation was present only in portion of cells, leading to mosaicism (Gleeson et al., 2000; Poolos et al., 2002; Sicca et al., 2003).

A small amount of mosaicism in DNA derived from the blood or buccal swab indicates that the mutation originated early enough during development to be present at low level in those tissues, but may not accurately reflect the level of mosaicism in the brain. Moreover, if the mutation originated later during brain development, it may not be detectable in DNA extracted from other tissues that developed independently. Recently, the study of hemimegalencephaly and megalencephaly and the application of next-generation sequencing techniques have promoted great advances in our understanding of how to detect somatic mutations. Hemimegalencephaly is usually associated with intractable

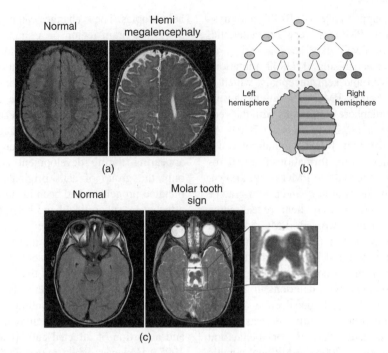

Fig. 7.4 *Overgrowth and axon guidance defects.* (a) In patients with hemimegalencephaly, one hemisphere appears normal while the other one is enlarged and often showing signs of cortical disorganization. (b) Recent studies have shown that this can be due to mutation that has originated during brain development only in a subset of cells contributing to the diseased hemisphere. When this is the case, a portion of the cells in the enlarged hemisphere carry a somatic mutation inherited from a common progenitor. (c) Ciliopathies affect multiple organs but the most common brain defect is a disruption in axonal targeting in the midbrain, which is visible radiographically and which is termed the molar tooth sign. *(See insert for color representation of this figure.)*

seizures and early resection of the affected hemisphere has proven to be an effective treatment. The tissue collected during surgery can then be tested for mutations in parallel to blood or saliva from the same individual. This approach has lead to the identification of somatic *de novo* copy-number gains and mutations in several members of the AKT/mTor signaling pathway: *AKT3, MTOR, PIK3CA,* and *PIK3RC* (Lee et al., 2012; Poduri et al., 2012; Rivière et al., 2012a). Activation of this pathway leads to an increase in proliferation and cell size and all mutations identified appear to be gain-of-function changes. Through conventional Sanger sequencing, some of these mutations were not readily identified in DNA originated from the blood, which is a common source of genomic DNA for testing, while they were quite frequent in the affected brain

tissue (Poduri et al., 2012). Deep sequencing of the affected genes in patient DNA from various origins, demonstrated that when the mutation is sequenced at high enough depth (>100,000 times), even somatic mutation frequencies of 1% could be detected, suggesting that if a small amount of mosaicism is maintained throughout the body, this may be a sensitive testing method to identify it (Rivière et al., 2012a). In addition, single cell analysis from affected tissue was able to reveal that only 30–40% of cells carried the mutation and identified that both neurons and glia were involved, suggesting that the mutation must have originated in a common progenitor and that a third of affected cells is sufficient to severely disrupt brain structure (Fig. 7.4b) (Evrony et al., 2012).

Somatic mutations delimited to a very small number of cells have also been hypothesized as a cause of focal cortical dysplasias in tuberous sclerosis (TSC), a disorder characterized by the growth of nonmalignant tumors in multiple tissues, including the brain. The brain growths, termed cortical tubers, are localized disruptions in lamination and neuronal orientation characterized by the presence of enlarged cell bodies. Heterozygous germline mutations in two upstream regulators of the mTor pathway, *TSC1* or *TSC2*, are found in the patients and analysis of the tumors or hamartomas identified an additional loss of the DNA region containing one of these genes in the tumor tissue, suggesting that a second hit is necessary to develop the growth similar to the somatic genetic instability observed in cancer progression (Sepp et al., 1996; Niida et al., 2001). Sanger sequencing efforts in tuber tissue from a small group of patients has identified multiple cases where a second missense mutation was present in the giant cells (Crino et al., 2010), but this does not appear to be the case in all hamartomas. It will be important to survey a large number of focal cortical dysplasia presentations using deep sequencing technologies to assess whether somatic changes in a small number of cells not detectable via Sanger sequencing could be involved in the pathogenesis of these malformations in patients where a second hit was not identified. Deep sequencing has been useful in explaining some of 10–15% of TSC patients who have no detectable germline mutations in *TSC1* or *TSC2*, by identifying somatic *TSC2* mutations in some of the cases (Qin et al., 2010).

7.6 THE CILIOPATHIES: SIGNALING AT THE PRIMARY CILIUM AND BRAIN DEVELOPMENT

Ciliopathies are a heterogeneous group of disorders where function of the primary cilium is affected. Cilia are present in all vertebrate cells, and are structures supported by a microtubule cytoskeleton anchored by a centriole, which in this instance is called the basal body

(Bettencourt-Dias et al., 2011). Cilia can be motile and be used for locomotion as in sperm cells or for moving fluid and particles as in the respiratory tract; or they can be immotile primary cilia, which are used for sensing extracellular signaling molecules. Ten different disorders comprise the ciliopathies and the phenotypes, which vary depending on the disease, involve multiple organs where ciliary function is necessary, such as the kidney, the liver, the skeleton, the brain, and the eye. There are more than fifty genetic loci identified to date and the genetic and clinical heterogeneity is staggering with tenuous correlation between genotype and phenotype. Because of this extreme complexity here, we will focus on the brain phenotypes found in some of these disorders and further reading on the genes and clinical findings involved can be found in (Hildebrandt et al., 2011; Sattar and Gleeson, 2011; Davis and Katsanis, 2012).

All ciliopathies are associated with intellectual disability, and brain malformations most frequently comprising axon outgrowth defects are observed in several of these disorders such as Joubert Syndrome (JBTS), Meckel–Gruber Sydrome (MKS), Bardet Biedl Syndrome (BBS), and oro-facial-digital syndrome 1 (OFD1), in combination with polydactyly, cystic kidneys, retinal degeneration or retinitis pigmentosa, and several other findings. A characteristic sign of JBTS and other ciliopathies is the molar tooth sign, a radiographic sign in the shape of a molar tooth visible on axial MRI sections immediately above the pons, caused by the inability of axons in the cerebellar peduncles to cross the midline (Fig. 7.4c) (Sattar and Gleeson, 2011). MKS, which is early neonatal lethal and the most severe disorder on this spectrum, is also associated with occipital encephalocele, a neural tube closure defect, which results in a sac-like structure protruding from the back of the skull (Gupta and Jain, 2008). Ventricular enlargement or hydrocephalus is often described in several ciliopathies and polymicrogyria has been reported in JBTS (Dixon-Salazar et al., 2004).

The primary cilium is involved in sensing multiple stimuli, mechanical, thermal, and chemical, but many of the phenotypes observed in the patients may be attributed to a disruption of signaling through the sonic hedgehog (Shh) and wingless (Wnt) pathways. Receptors for both Shh and Wnt are present at the shaft and near the base of the cilia and all proteins mutated in cliopathies are also localized to the same location and have been directly involved in Shh and/or Wnt activity regulation. Both Shh and Wnt are categorized as morphogens, signaling molecules controlling the patterning and organization of tissues and organs in the body (Davis and Katsanis, 2012). Shh, for example, regulates the polarization and asymmetry of the hand and Shh signaling defects will lead to polydactyly, where supranumerary digits are generated (te Welscher et al., 2002). In the brain, Shh and Wnt are critical for patterning the neural tube, and control neuronal proliferation and axon guidance, in particular in the developing cerebellum and hippocampus (for review see Sotelo, 2004; Pozniak and Pleasure, 2006; Borello and Pierani, 2010). Because of the multiple roles of these signaling pathways throughout development, modeling the different human phenotypes has proven complex and several open questions remain. However, multiple mouse models have been generated for almost all the known ciliopathy genes providing important insight in the pathogenesis of these disorders (reviewed in Norris and Grimes, 2012) and showing that while null mutations often result in embryonic lethality, the variable phenotypes observed in humans can be explained by reduced or partially disrupted signaling. Knock-in and hypomorphic alleles in the mouse may be better suited to study more subtle signaling changes.

The sensitivity of different organs to variation in signaling at the primary cilia was further confirmed by the discovery of transheterozygous mutations. Transheterozygous mutations where heterozygous mutations in a related disease gene contribute to the patient's phenotype have been hypothesized for multiple recessive disorders, but rarely described. Genetic studies in ciliopathies have revealed that this type of mutation could help explain the puzzling variability of the clinical phenotypes observed in the patients, where different individuals in the same family presented with findings in different organs. For example, recessive mutations in *NHPH1* usually cause nephronophthisis, a juvenile kidney disorder characterized by renal cysts and fibrosis, but additional heterozygous changes in the JBTS genes *AHI1* or *CEP290* lead to a brain phenotype more similar to JBST (Tory et al., 2007). These heterozygous changes alone may not lead to disease, but in a background of *NHPH1* loss of function, they are able to exacerbate the disease presentation, and this was confirmed by showing that adding an *Ahi1* heterozygous loss of function allele in an *Nhph1* knock-out mouse generates a neuronal phenotype not previously observed in these mice (Louie et al., 2010).

7.7 IMPLICATIONS FOR NEUROPSYCHIATRIC DISORDERS

Most of the brain malformations described here are associated with mild to severe intellectual disability and intractable seizures often leading to additional cognitive deterioration. When a major disruption in brain structure is observed, it is expected that neuronal circuits may not be able to form correctly leading to cognitive deficits, but the genes identified for brain malformations have also proven to be involved in more subtle conditions where the brain appears normal macroscopically, but cognition or behavior are altered, such as intellectual disability (ID) and autism spectrum disorder (ASD). The genetic architecture of these disorders is complex and despite extensive study, it is still confusing (see Devlin and Scherer, 2012; Sullivan et al., 2012 for review).

Among cortical malformation genes, patients with Cohen syndrome, which is associated with microcephaly, are diagnosed with ASD in more than 50% of cases (Howlin et al., 2005), and *COH1* mutations have recently been discovered in cohorts of patients that were prospectively ascertained with ASD (Yu et al., 2013). Hypomorphic mutations in known malformation genes may lead to ID and/or ASD instead of the classical presentation of the original syndrome: recessive missense mutations in the dystroglycanopathy gene *POMT1* cause a form of muscular dystrophy with ID without any cortical malformations (Van Reeuwijk et al., 2006), and mutations in *POMGNT1* were identified in ASD cases with no other associated findings (Yu et al., 2013). A clear example of phenotypic variation when gene dosage is altered, are mutations in the *DYRK1A* gene as heterozygous deletions cause microcephaly, neurodegeneration, seizures, and ID (Møller et al., 2008; van Bon et al., 2011) and gain of one copy in Down syndrome has been described as a critical candidate for ID in these patients (Smith et al., 1997). Recurrent *de novo* truncating mutations in *DYRK1A* were also identified in a large cohort of ASD patients (O'Roak et al., 2012), showing how perturbations of this gene which is critical for multiple aspects of neuronal differentiation can lead to a wide range of neuropsychiatric phenotypes. One of the most common recurrent copy-number variants (CNVs) associated with ASD and schizophrenia involves the 16p11.2 region on chromosome 16: duplications of 16p11.2 are associated with microcephaly, epilepsy, and in some cases brain malformations, while deletions are associated with mild macrocepahly, again showing the importance of gene dosage regulation for the development of brain structure and function (Weiss et al., 2008; McCarthy et al., 2009).

De novo dominant mutations and CNVs have all been described as causes of ASD, ID, and other neuropsychiatric disorders, and among the deleted or mutated genes are multiple brain malformation genes, though in some cases, the causative nature of the mutation is not always certain. As more malformation genes are identified and are considered a candidate for cognitive deficits, the list of candidate mutations will grow to better define the architecture of ID and ASD, and other neuropsychiatric conditions such as attention deficit hyperactivity disorder (ADHD), schizophrenia, bipolar disorder, and anxiety disorders, which in copy-number variant studies have been found to be caused by the same rearrangements as ASD/ID.

Studies on cortical malformation cases have also been important in understanding the etiology of dyslexia, as the analysis of individuals with PVH revealed that local changes in circuit organization affect reading ability (Chang et al., 2007). When the nodule burden is limited, PVH usually generates no cognitive defects, but comparison of reading fluency in cohorts with PVH or dyslexia showed how speed in naming objects or rapid reading tests was equally affected in both conditions compared to controls. It has been hypothesized that processing speed may be affected by the disorganization of fiber tracts observed around the nodules (Chang et al., 2007) and white matter defects have also been described in dyslexic children (Peterson and Pennington, 2012). These findings point to subtle changes in circuit formation during development leading to localized disruptions in neuronal transmission and again raise the issue of subthreshold or microscopic malformations being involved in common neuropsychiatric conditions.

7.8 WHERE DO WE GO FROM HERE?

The advent of next-generation sequencing (NGS) has spurred an explosion in gene identification for brain malformations in the past 5 years and more and more genes are being identified on a daily basis. The ultimate goal is to define a clear picture of the genetic architecture of every malformation and to be able to provide a genetic diagnosis for every patient. In disorders such as polymicrogyria, where ischemia or infection may be to blame, this may not be possible, but the identification of the causative mutations in the genetic cases will provide a better understanding of the etiology of the disorder, be it genetic or environmental. The discovery of somatic mutations in the brain, which may be present at very low level in other tissues or completely absent, generates both challenges and opportunities. Challenges because the simple genetic test from blood or buccal swab may not represent the most appropriate diagnostic route and a large amount of research needs to be conducted in defining (1) what is the sensitivity of current NGS assays to detect somatic mutations in bulk genomic DNA? And (2) how many patients are affected by this elusive type of mutation? It is possible that several focal malformations may be due to somatic mutations originated in a small number of neuronal progenitors leading to a local disruption in differentiation, and it is also possible that cognitive deficits not associated with visible malformations may be due to analogous local disruptions in synaptic activity and function in a subset of cells. While these hypotheses are intriguing, only the systematic collection of large numbers of postmortem brain and other tissue samples from affected individuals and a thorough analysis of patterns of mutation across different brain regions will be able to support or dismiss it.

This multitude of disorders and mutations show that the human brain in its exquisite complexity is very sensitive to developmental insults and that hypomorphic mutations in genes responsible for more severe multiorgan syndromes could still be responsible for milder cognitive and behavioral phenotypes. How the structural defects that are detectable radiographically are related to the cognitive deficits found in individuals with mutations in brain malformation genes and an apparently normal brain is still not known. The identification of the molecular and cellular mechanisms underlying macroscopic structural changes in the brain may be able to inform on the specific steps necessary for normal cognitive development and vice versa, leading to a better understanding of how the brain is put together at the microscopic and macroscopic level. In addition, while many cortical malformations are regionalized in their presentation (preferentially frontal or occipital), sometimes variability is observed even in different mutations in the same gene or different cases with the same mutation suggesting that additional factors, such as epigenetic modifications, must be taken into consideration when studying neurodevelopmental disorders. Despite a common genetic background, different neurons may respond differently to developmental processes, and understanding how the balance of genetic, epigenetic, and environmental influences regulates differentiation may be the key to revealing how the same mutation can lead to autism or schizophrenia or not detectably affect cognition at all.

REFERENCES

Abdollahi, M.R., Morrison, E., Sirey, T., Molnár, Z., Hayward, B.E., Carr, I.M., Springell, K., Woods, C.G., Ahmed, M., Hattingh, L., et al. (2009). Mutation of the variant alpha-tubulin TUBA8 results in polymicrogyria with optic nerve hypoplasia. Am J Hum Genet 85, 737–744.

Al-Dosari, M.S., Shaheen, R., Colak, D., and Alkuraya, F.S. (2010). Novel CENPJ mutation causes Seckel syndrome. J Med Genet 47, 411–414.

Alkuraya, F.S., Cai, X., Emery, C., Mochida, G.H., Al-Dosari, M.S., Felie, J.M., Hill, R.S., Barry, B.J., Partlow, J.N., Gascon, G.G., et al. (2011). Human mutations in NDE1 cause extreme microcephaly with lissencephaly [corrected]. Am J Hum Genet 88, 536–547.

Bahi-Buisson, N., Poirier, K., Boddaert, N., Fallet-Bianco, C., Specchio, N., Bertini, E., Caglayan, O., Lascelles, K., Elie, C., Rambaud, J., et al. (2010). GPR56-related bilateral frontoparietal polymicrogyria: further evidence for an overlap with the cobblestone complex. Brain 133, 3194–3209.

Barak, T., Kwan, K.Y., Louvi, A., Demirbilek, V., Saygı, S., Tüysüz, B., Choi, M., Boyacı, H., Doerschner, K., Zhu, Y., et al. (2011). Recessive LAMC3 mutations cause malformations of occipital cortical development. Nat Genet 43, 590–594.

Barkovich, A.J., Kuzniecky, R.I., Jackson, G.D., Guerrini, R., and Dobyns, W.B. (2005). A developmental and genetic classification for malformations of cortical development. Neurology 65, 1873–1887.

Barkovich, A.J. (2010). Current concepts of polymicrogyria. Neuroradiology 52, 479–487.

Barkovich, A.J., Guerrini, R., Kuzniecky, R.I., Jackson, G.D., and Dobyns, W.B. (2012). A developmental and genetic classification for malformations of cortical development: update 2012. Brain 135, 1348–1369.

Barkovich, A.J., Millen, K.J., and Dobyns, W.B. (2009). A developmental and genetic classification for midbrain-hindbrain malformations. Brain 132, 3199–3230.

Bechstedt, S., and Brouhard, G.J. (2012). Doublecortin recognizes the 13-protofilament microtubule cooperatively and tracks microtubule ends. Dev Cell 23, 181–192.

Bettencourt-Dias, M., Hildebrandt, F., Pellman, D., Woods, G., and Godinho, S.A. (2011). Centrosomes and cilia in human disease. Trends Genet 27, 307–315.

Bilgüvar, K., Oztürk, A.K., Louvi, A., Kwan, K.Y., Choi, M., Tatli, B., Yalnizoğlu, D., Tüysüz, B., Cağlayan, A.O., Gökben, S., et al. (2010). Whole-exome sequencing identifies recessive WDR62 mutations in severe brain malformations. Nature 467, 207–210.

Bogoyevitch, M.A., Yeap, Y.Y.C., Qu, Z., Ngoei, K.R., Yip, Y.Y., Zhao, T.T., Heng, J.I., and Ng, D.C.H. (2012). WD40-repeat protein 62 is a JNK-phosphorylated spindle pole protein required for spindle maintenance and timely mitotic progression. J Cell Sci 125, 5096–5109.

Bond, J., Roberts, E., Mochida, G.H., Hampshire, D.J., Scott, S., Askham, J.M., Springell, K., Mahadevan, M., Crow, Y.J., Markham, A.F., et al. (2002). ASPM is a major determinant of cerebral cortical size. Nat Genet 32, 316–320.

Bond, J., Roberts, E., Springell, K., Lizarraga, S.B., Lizarraga, S., Scott, S., Higgins, J., Hampshire, D.J., Morrison, E.E., Leal, G.F., et al. (2005). A centrosomal mechanism involving CDK5RAP2 and CENPJ controls brain size. Nat Genet 37, 353–355.

Borello, U., and Pierani, A. (2010). Patterning the cerebral cortex: traveling with morphogens. Curr Opin Genet Dev 20, 408–415.

Boycott, K.M., Flavelle, S., Bureau, A., Glass, H.C., Fujiwara, T.M., Wirrell, E., Davey, K., Chudley, A.E., Scott, J.N., McLeod, D.R., et al. (2005). Homozygous deletion of the very low density lipoprotein receptor gene causes autosomal recessive cerebellar hypoplasia with cerebral gyral simplification. Am J Hum Genet 77, 477–483.

Breuss, M., Heng, J.I.-T., Poirier, K., Tian, G., Jaglin, X.H., Qu, Z., Braun, A., Gstrein, T., Ngo, L., Haas, M., et al. (2012). Mutations in the β-tubulin gene TUBB5 cause microcephaly with structural brain abnormalities. Cell Rep 2, 1554–1562.

Buysse, K., Riemersma, M., Powell, G., Van Reeuwijk, J., Chitayat, D., Roscioli, T., Kamsteeg, E.-J., Van Den Elzen, C., van Beusekom, E., Blaser, S., et al. (2013). Missense mutations in β-1,3-N-acetylglucosaminyltransferase 1 (B3GNT1) cause Walker-Warburg syndrome. Hum Mol Genet.

Chae, T.H., Kim, S., Marz, K.E., Hanson, P.I., and Walsh, C.A. (2004). The hyh mutation uncovers roles for alpha Snap in apical protein localization and control of neural cell fate. Nat Genet 36, 264–270.

Chang, B.S., Katzir, T., Liu, T., Corriveau, K., Barzillai, M., Apse, K.A., Bodell, A., Hackney, D., Alsop, D., Wong, S.T., et al. (2007). A structural basis for reading fluency: white matter defects in a genetic brain malformation. Neurology 69, 2146–2154.

Cohn, R.D., Henry, M.D., Michele, D.E., Barresi, R., Saito, F., Moore, S.A., Flanagan, J.D., Skwarchuk, M.W., Robbins, M.E., Mendell, J.R., et al. (2002). Disruption of DAG1 in differentiated skeletal muscle reveals a role for dystroglycan in muscle regeneration. Cell 110, 639–648.

Crino, P.B., Aronica, E., Baltuch, G., and Nathanson, K.L. (2010). Biallelic TSC gene inactivation in tuberous sclerosis complex. Neurology 74, 1716–1723.

Dauber, A., Lafranchi, S.H., Maliga, Z., Lui, J.C., Moon, J.E., McDeed, C., Henke, K., Zonana, J., Kingman, G.A., Pers, T.H., et al. (2012). Novel microcephalic primordial dwarfism disorder associated with variants in the centrosomal protein ninein. J Clin Endocrinol Metab 97, E2140–E2151.

Davis, E.E., and Katsanis, N. (2012). The ciliopathies: a transitional model into systems biology of human genetic disease. Curr Opin Genet Dev 22, 290–303.

Devlin, B., and Scherer, S.W. (2012). Genetic architecture in autism spectrum disorder. Curr Opin Genet Dev 22, 229–237.

Dixon-Salazar, T., Silhavy, J.L., Marsh, S.E., Louie, C.M., Scott, L.C., Gururaj, A., Al-Gazali, L., Al-Tawari, A.A., Kayserili, H., Sztriha, L., et al. (2004). Mutations in the AHI1 gene, encoding jouberin, cause Joubert syndrome with cortical polymicrogyria. Am J Hum Genet 75, 979–987.

Dobyns, W.B., Reiner, O., Carrozzo, R., and Ledbetter, D.H. (1993). Lissencephaly. A human brain malformation associated with deletion of the LIS1 gene located at chromosome 17p13. JAMA 270, 2838–2842.

Evrony, G.D., Cai, X., Lee, E., Hills, L.B., Elhosary, P.C., Lehmann, H.S., Parker, J.J., Atabay, K.D., Gilmore, E.C., Poduri, A., et al. (2012). Single-neuron sequencing analysis of 11 retrotransposition and somatic mutation in the human brain. Cell 151, 483–496.

Falconer, D.S. (1951). Two new mutants, 'trembler' and "reeler," with neurological actions in the house mouse (Mus musculus L.). J Genet 50, 192–205.

Feng, Y., and Walsh, C.A. (2004a). Mitotic spindle regulation by Nde1 controls cerebral cortical size. Neuron 44, 279–293.

Feng, Y., and Walsh, C.A. (2004b). The many faces of filamin: a versatile molecular scaffold for cell motility and signalling. Nat Cell Biol 6, 1034–1038.

Feng, Y., Chen, M.H., Moskowitz, I.P., Mendonza, A.M., Vidali, L., Nakamura, F., Kwiatkowski, D.J., and Walsh, C.A. (2006). Filamin A (FLNA) is required for cell-cell contact in vascular development and cardiac morphogenesis. Proc Natl Acad Sci USA 103, 19836–19841.

Forman, M.S., Squier, W., Dobyns, W.B., Golden, J.A. (2005). Genotypically different lissencephalies show distincs pathologies. J Neuropathol Exp Neurol 64, 847–857.

Fotaki, V., Dierssen, M., Alcántara, S., Martínez, S., Martí, E., Casas, C., Visa, J., Soriano, E., Estivill, X., and Arbonés, M.L. (2002). Dyrk1A haploinsufficiency affects viability and causes developmental delay and abnormal brain morphology in mice. Mol Cell Biol 22, 6636–6647.

Fox, J.W., Lamperti, E.D., Ekşioğlu, Y.Z., Hong, S.E., Feng, Y., Graham, D.A., Scheffer, I.E., Dobyns, W.B., Hirsch, B.A., Radtke, R.A., et al. (1998). Mutations in filamin 1 prevent migration of cerebral cortical neurons in human periventricular heterotopia. Neuron 21, 1315–1325.

Fu, X., Brown, K.J., Yap, C.C., Winckler, B., Jaiswal, J.K., and Liu, J.S. (2013). Doublecortin (Dcx) family proteins regulate filamentous actin structure in developing neurons. J Neurosci 33, 709–721.

Gleeson, J.G., Allen, K.M., Fox, J.W., Lamperti, E.D., Berkovic, S., Scheffer, I., Cooper, E.C., Dobyns, W.B., Minnerath, S.R., Ross, M.E., et al. (1998). Doublecortin, a brain-specific gene mutated in human X-linked lissencephaly and double cortex syndrome, encodes a putative signaling protein. Cell 92, 63–72.

Gleeson, J.G., Minnerath, S., Kuzniecky, R.I., Dobyns, W.B., Young, I.D., Ross, M.E., and Walsh, C.A. (2000). Somatic and germline mosaic mutations in the doublecortin gene are associated with variable phenotypes. Am J Hum Genet 67, 574–581.

Griffith, E., Walker, S., Martin, C.-A., Vagnarelli, P., Stiff, T., Vernay, B., Al Sanna, N., Saggar, A., Hamel, B., Earnshaw, W.C., et al. (2008). Mutations in pericentrin cause Seckel syndrome with defective ATR-dependent DNA damage signaling. Nat Genet 40, 232–236.

Gruber, R., Zhou, Z., Sukchev, M., Joerss, T., Frappart, P.-O., and Wang, Z.-Q. (2011). MCPH1 regulates the neuroprogenitor division mode by coupling the centrosomal cycle with mitotic entry through the Chk1-Cdc25 pathway. Nature 13, 1325–1334.

Guedj, F., Pereira, P.L., Najas, S., Barallobre, M.-J., Chabert, C., Souchet, B., Sebrie, C., Verney, C., Herault, Y., Arbones, M., et al. (2012). DYRK1A: a master regulatory protein controlling brain growth. Neurobiol Dis 46, 190–203.

Guernsey, D.L., Jiang, H., Hussin, J., Arnold, M., Bouyakdan, K., Perry, S., Babineau-Sturk, T., Beis, J., Dumas, N., Evans, S.C., et al. (2010). Mutations in centrosomal protein CEP152 in primary microcephaly families linked to MCPH4. Am J Hum Genet 87, 40–51.

Gupta, P., and Jain, S. (2008). MRI in a fetus with Meckel-Gruber syndrome. Pediatr Radiol. 38, 122.

Hara, Y., Balci-Hayta, B., Yoshida-Moriguchi, T., Kanagawa, M., Beltrán-Valero De Bernabé, D., Gündeşli, H., Willer, T., Satz, J.S., Crawford, R.W., Burden, S.J., et al. (2011). A dystroglycan mutation associated with limb-girdle muscular dystrophy. N Engl J Med 364, 939–946.

Helbling-Leclerc, A., Zhang, X., Topaloglu, H., Cruaud, C., Tesson, F., Weissenbach, J., Tomé, F.M., Schwartz, K., Fardeau, M., and Tryggvason, K. (1995). Mutations in the laminin alpha 2-chain gene (LAMA2) cause merosin-deficient congenital muscular dystrophy. Nat Genet 11, 216–218.

Hildebrandt, F., Benzing, T., and Katsanis, N. (2011). Ciliopathies. N Engl J Med 364, 1533–1543.

Hong, S.E., Shugart, Y.Y., Huang, D.T., Shahwan, S.A., Grant, P.E., Hourihane, J.O., Martin, N.D., and Walsh, C.A. (2000). Autosomal recessive lissencephaly with cerebellar hypoplasia is associated with human RELN mutations. Nat Genet 26, 93–96.

Howlin, P., Karpf, J., and Turk, J. (2005). Behavioural characteristics and autistic features in individuals with Cohen Syndrome. Eur Child Adolesc Psychiatry 14, 57–64.

Huang, J., Roberts, A.J., Leschziner, A.E., and Reck-Peterson, S.L. (2012). Lis1 acts as a "clutch" between the ATPase and microtubule-binding domains of the dynein motor. Cell 150, 975–986.

Hussain, M.S., Baig, S.M., Neumann, S., Nürnberg, G., Farooq, M., Ahmad, I., Alef, T., Hennies, H.C., Technau, M., Altmüller, J., et al. (2012). A truncating mutation of CEP135 causes primary microcephaly and disturbed centrosomal function. Am J Hum Genet 90, 871–878.

Jackson, A.P., Eastwood, H., Bell, S.M., Adu, J., Toomes, C., Carr, I.M., Roberts, E., Hampshire, D.J., Crow, Y.J., Mighell, A.J., et al. (2002). Identification of microcephalin, a protein implicated in determining the size of the human brain. Am J Hum Genet 71, 136–142.

Jae, L.T., Raaben, M., Riemersma, M., van Beusekom, E., Blomen, V.A., Velds, A., Kerkhoven, R.M., Carette, J.E., Topaloglu, H., Meinecke, P., et al. (2013). Deciphering the glycosylome of dystroglycanopathies using haploid screens for Lassa virus entry. Science 340, 479–483.

Jaglin, X.H., Poirier, K., Saillour, Y., Buhler, E., Tian, G., Bahi-Buisson, N., Fallet-Bianco, C., Phan-Dinh-Tuy, F., Kong, X.P., Bomont, P., et al. (2009). Mutations in the beta-tubulin gene TUBB2B result in asymmetrical polymicrogyria. Nat Genet 41, 746–752.

Januschke, J., Llamazares, S., Reina, J., and Gonzalez, C. (2011). Drosophila neuroblasts retain the daughter centrosome. Nat Commun 2, 243.

Kalay, E., Yigit, G., Aslan, Y., Brown, K.E., Pohl, E., Bicknell, L.S., Kayserili, H., Li, Y., Tüysüz, B., Nürnberg, G., et al. (2011). CEP152 is a genome maintenance protein disrupted in Seckel syndrome. Nat Genet 43, 23–26.

Kang, J., and Samuels, D.C. (2008). The evidence that the DNC (SLC25A19) is not the mitochondrial deoxyribonucleotide carrier. Mitochondrion 8, 103–108.

Kerjan, G., and Gleeson, J.G. (2007). Genetic mechanisms underlying abnormal neuronal migration in classical lissencephaly. Trends Genet 23, 623–630.

Kolehmainen, J., Black, G.C.M., Saarinen, A., Chandler, K., Clayton-Smith, J., Träskelin, A.-L., Perveen, R., Kivitie-Kallio, S., Norio, R., Warburg, M., et al. (2003). Cohen syndrome is caused by mutations in a novel gene, COH1, encoding a transmembrane protein with a presumed role in vesicle-mediated sorting and intracellular protein transport. Am J Hum Genet 72, 1359–1369.

Kumar, A., Girimaji, S.C., Duvvari, M.R., and Blanton, S.H. (2009). Mutations in STIL, encoding a pericentriolar and centrosomal protein, cause primary microcephaly. Am J Hum Genet 84, 286–290.

Labelle-Dumais, C., Dilworth, D.J., Harrington, E.P., de Leau, M., Lyons, D., Kabaeva, Z., Manzini, M.C., Dobyns, W.B., Walsh, C.A., Michele, D.E., et al. (2011). COL4A1 mutations cause ocular dysgenesis, neuronal localization defects, and myopathy in mice and Walker-Warburg syndrome in humans. PLoS Genet 7, e1002062.

Lee, J.H., Huynh, M., Silhavy, J.L., Kim, S., Dixon-Salazar, T., Heiberg, A., Scott, E., Bafna, V., Hill, K.J., Collazo, A., et al. (2012). De novo somatic mutations in components of the PI3K-AKT3-mTOR pathway cause hemimegalencephaly. Nat Genet 44, 941–945.

Li, S., Jin, Z., Koirala, S., Bu, L., Xu, L., Hynes, R.O., Walsh, C.A., Corfas, G., and Piao, X. (2008). GPR56 regulates pial basement membrane integrity and cortical lamination. J Neurosci 28, 5817–5826.

Lian, G., Lu, J., Hu, J., Zhang, J., Cross, S.H., Ferland, R.J., and Sheen, V.L. (2012). Filamin a regulates neural progenitor proliferation and cortical size through Wee1-dependent Cdk1 phosphorylation. J Neurosci 32, 7672–7684.

Liu, J.S., Schubert, C.R., Fu, X., Fourniol, F.J., Jaiswal, J.K., Houdusse, A., Stultz, C.M., Moores, C.A., and Walsh, C.A. (2012). Molecular basis for specific regulation of neuronal kinesin-3 motors by doublecortin family proteins. Mol Cell 47, 707–721.

Lizarraga, S.B., Margossian, S.P., Harris, M.H., Campagna, D.R., Han, A.-P., Blevins, S., Mudbhary, R., Barker, J.E., Walsh, C.A., and Fleming, M.D. (2010). Cdk5rap2 regulates centrosome function and chromosome segregation in neuronal progenitors. Development 137, 1907–1917.

Louie, C.M., Caridi, G., Lopes, V.S., Brancati, F., Kispert, A., Lancaster, M.A., Schlossman, A.M., Otto, E.A., Leitges, M., Gröne, H.-J., et al. (2010). AHI1 is required for photoreceptor outer segment development and is a modifier for retinal degeneration in nephronophthisis. Nat Genet 42, 175–180.

Luo, R., Jeong, S.-J., Jin, Z., Strokes, N., Li, S., and Piao, X. (2011). G protein-coupled receptor 56 and collagen III, a receptor-ligand pair, regulates cortical development and lamination. Proc Natl Acad Sci USA 108, 12925–12930.

Manzini, M.C., Tambunan, D.E., Hill, R.S., Yu, T.W., Maynard, T.M., Heinzen, E.L., Shianna, K.V., Stevens, C.R., Partlow, J.N., Barry, B.J., et al. (2012). Exome sequencing and functional validation in zebrafish identify GTDC2 mutations as a cause of Walker-Warburg syndrome. Am J Hum Genet 91, 541–547.

McCarthy, S.E., Makarov, V., Kirov, G., Addington, A.M., McClellan, J., Yoon, S., Perkins, D.O., Dickel, D.E., Kusenda, M., Krastoshevsky, O., et al. (2009). Microduplications of 16p11.2 are associated with schizophrenia. Nat Genet 41, 1223–1227.

Mochida, G.H. (2009). Genetics and biology of microcephaly and lissencephaly. Semin Pediatr Neurol 16, 120–126.

Mochida, G.H., Ganesh, V.S., de Michelena, M.I., Dias, H., Atabay, K.D., Kathrein, K.L., Huang, H.-T., Hill, R.S., Felie, J.M., Rakiec, D., et al. (2012). CHMP1A encodes an essential regulator of BMI1-INK4A in cerebellar development. Nat Genet 44, 1260–1264.

Muntoni, F., Torelli, S., Wells, D.J., and Brown, S.C. (2011). Muscular dystrophies due to glycosylation defects. Curr Opin Neurol 24, 437–442.

Møller, R.S., Kübart, S., Hoeltzenbein, M., Heye, B., Vogel, I., Hansen, C.P., Menzel, C., Ullmann, R., Tommerup, N., Ropers, H.-H., et al. (2008). Truncation of the Down syndrome candidate gene DYRK1A in two unrelated patients with microcephaly. Am J Hum Genet 82, 1165–1170.

Nicholas, A.K., Khurshid, M., Désir, J., Carvalho, O.P., Cox, J.J., Thornton, G., Kausar, R., Ansar, M., Ahmad, W., Verloes, A., et al. (2010). WDR62 is associated with the spindle pole and is mutated in human microcephaly. Nat Genet 42, 1010–1014.

Niida, Y., Stemmer-Rachamimov, A.O., Logrip, M., Tapon, D., Perez, R., Kwiatkowski, D.J., Sims, K., MacCollin, M., Louis, D.N., and Ramesh, V. (2001). Survey of somatic mutations in tuberous sclerosis complex (TSC) hamartomas suggests different genetic mechanisms for pathogenesis of TSC lesions. Am J Hum Genet 69, 493–503.

Norris, D.P., and Grimes, D.T. (2012). Mouse models of ciliopathies: the state of the art. Dis Model Mech 5, 299–312.

O'Driscoll, M., and Jeggo, P.A. (2008). The role of the DNA damage response pathways in brain development and microcephaly: insight from human disorders. DNA Repair (Amst.) 7, 1039–1050.

O'Driscoll, M., Ruiz-Perez, V.L., Woods, C.G., Jeggo, P.A., and Goodship, J.A. (2003). A splicing mutation affecting expression of ataxia-telangiectasia and Rad3-related protein (ATR) results in Seckel syndrome. Nat Genet 33, 497–501.

O'Roak, B.J., Vives, L., Fu, W., Egertson, J.D., Stanaway, I.B., Phelps, I.G., Carvill, G., Kumar, A., Lee, C., Ankenman, K., et al. (2012). Multiplex targeted sequencing identifies recurrently mutated genes in autism spectrum disorders. Science 338, 1619–1622.

Ogi, T., Walker, S., Stiff, T., Hobson, E., Limsirichaikul, S., Carpenter, G., Prescott, K., Suri, M., Byrd, P.J., Matsuse, M., et al. (2012). Identification of the first ATRIP-deficient patient and novel mutations in ATR define a clinical spectrum for ATR-ATRIP Seckel Syndrome. PLoS Genet 8, e1002945.

Peterson, R.L., and Pennington, B.F. (2012). Developmental dyslexia. Lancet 379, 1997–2007.

Piao, X., Hill, R.S., Bodell, A., Chang, B.S., Basel-Vanagaite, L., Straussberg, R., Dobyns, W.B., Qasrawi, B., Winter, R.M., Innes, A.M., et al. (2004). G protein-coupled receptor-dependent development of human frontal cortex. Science 303, 2033–2036.

Pilz, D.T., Kuc, J., Matsumoto, N., Bodurtha, J., Bernadi, B., Tassinari, C.A., Dobyns, W.B., and Ledbetter, D.H. (1999). Subcortical band heterotopia in rare affected males can be caused by missense mutations in DCX (XLIS) or LIS1. Hum Mol Genet 8, 1757–1760.

Poduri, A., Evrony, G.D., Cai, X., Elhosary, P.C., Beroukhim, R., Lehtinen, M.K., Hills, L.B., Heinzen, E.L., Hill, A., Hill, R.S., et al. (2012). Somatic activation of AKT3 causes hemispheric developmental brain malformations. Neuron 74, 41–48.

Poirier, K., Keays, D.A., Francis, F., Saillour, Y., Bahi, N., Manouvrier, S., Fallet-Bianco, C., Pasquier, L., Toutain, A., Tuy, F.P.D., et al. (2007). Large spectrum of lissencephaly and pachygyria phenotypes resulting from de novo missense mutations in tubulin alpha 1A (TUBA1A). Hum Mutat 28, 1055–1064.

Poirier, K., Lebrun, N., Broix, L., Tian, G., Saillour, Y., Boscheron, C., Parrini, E., Valence, S., Pierre,

B.S., Oger, M., et al. (2013). Mutations in TUBG1, DYNC1H1, KIF5C and KIF2A cause malformations of cortical development and microcephaly. Nat Genet 45, 639–647.

Poirier, K., Saillour, Y., Bahi-Buisson, N., Jaglin, X.H., Fallet-Bianco, C., Nabbout, R., Castelnau-Ptakhine, L., Roubertie, A., Attié-Bitach, T., Desguerre, I., et al. (2010). Mutations in the neuronal ß-tubulin subunit TUBB3 result in malformation of cortical development and neuronal migration defects. Hum Mol Genet 19, 4462–4473.

Poolos, N.P., Das, S., Clark, G.D., Lardizabal, D., Noebels, J.L., Wyllie, E., and Dobyns, W.B. (2002). Males with epilepsy, complete subcortical band heterotopia, and somatic mosaicism for DCX. Neurology 58, 1559–1562.

des Portes, V., Pinard, J.M., Billuart, P., Vinet, M.C., Koulakoff, A., Carrié, A., Gelot, A., Dupuis, E., Motte, J., Berwald-Netter, Y., et al. (1998). A novel CNS gene required for neuronal migration and involved in X-linked subcortical laminar heterotopia and lissencephaly syndrome. Cell 92, 51–61.

Pozniak, C.D., and Pleasure, S.J. (2006). A tale of two signals: Wnt and Hedgehog in dentate neurogenesis. Science's STKE 2006, pe5.

Qin, W., Kozlowski, P., Taillon, B.E., Bouffard, P., Holmes, A.J., Janne, P., Camposano, S., Thiele, E., Franz, D., and Kwiatkowski, D.J. (2010). Ultra deep sequencing detects a low rate of mosaic mutations in tuberous sclerosis complex. Hum Genet 127, 573–582.

Qvist, P., Huertas, P., Jimeno, S., Nyegaard, M., Hassan, M.J., Jackson, S.P., and Børglum, A.D. (2011). CtIP mutations cause Seckel and Jawad syndromes. PLoS Genet 7, e1002310.

Radmanesh, F., Cağlayan, A.O., Silhavy, J.L., Yilmaz, C., Cantagrel, V., Omar, T., Rosti, B., Kaymakçalan, H., Gabriel, S., Li, M., et al. (2013). Mutations in LAMB1 cause cobblestone brain malformation without muscular or ocular abnormalities. Am J Hum Genet 92, 468–474.

Reillo, I., de Juan Romero, C., García-Cabezas, M.Á., and Borrell, V. (2011). A role for intermediate radial glia in the tangential expansion of the mammalian cerebral cortex. Cereb Cortex 21, 1674–1694.

Reiner, O., Carrozzo, R., Shen, Y., Wehnert, M., Faustinella, F., Dobyns, W.B., Caskey, C.T., and Ledbetter, D.H. (1993). Isolation of a Miller-Dieker lissencephaly gene containing G

protein beta-subunit-like repeats. Nature 364, 717–721.

Reynolds, J.J., Walker, A.K., Gilmore, E.C., Walsh, C.A., and Caldecott, K.W. (2012). Impact of PNKP mutations associated with microcephaly, seizures and developmental delay on enzyme activity and DNA strand break repair. Nucleic Acids Res 40, 6608–6619.

Rivière, J.-B., Mirzaa, G.M., O'Roak, B.J., Beddaoui, M., Alcantara, D., Conway, R.L., St-Onge, J., Schwartzentruber, J.A., Gripp, K.W., Nikkel, S.M., et al. (2012a). De novo germline and postzygotic mutations in AKT3, PIK3R2 and PIK3CA cause a spectrum of related megalencephaly syndromes. Nat Genet 44, 934–940.

Rivière, J.-B., van Bon, B.W.M., Hoischen, A., Kholmanskikh, S.S., O'Roak, B.J., Gilissen, C., Gijsen, S., Sullivan, C.T., Christian, S.L., Abdul-Rahman, O.A., et al. (2012b). De novo mutations in the actin genes ACTB and ACTG1 cause Baraitser-Winter syndrome. Nat Genet 44, 440–444.

Robin, N.H., Taylor, C.J., Mcdonald-Mcginn, D.M., Zackai, E.H., Bingham, P., Collins, K.J., Earl, D., Gill, D., Granata, T., Guerrini, R., et al. (2006). Polymicrogyria and deletion 22q11.2 syndrome: window to the etiology of a common cortical malformation. Am J Med Genet A 140, 2416–2425.

Roscioli, T., Kamsteeg, E.-J., Buysse, K., Maystadt, I., Van Reeuwijk, J., Van Den Elzen, C., van Beusekom, E., Riemersma, M., Pfundt, R., Vissers, L.E.L.M., et al. (2012). Mutations in ISPD cause Walker-Warburg syndrome and defective glycosylation of [alpha]-dystroglycan. Nat Genet 44, 581–585.

Rosenberg, M.J., Agarwala, R., Bouffard, G., Davis, J., Fiermonte, G., Hilliard, M.S., Koch, T., Kalikin, L.M., Makalowska, I., Morton, D.H., et al. (2002). Mutant deoxynucleotide carrier is associated with congenital microcephaly. Nat Genet 32, 175–179.

Sattar, S., and Gleeson, J.G. (2011). The ciliopathies in neuronal development: a clinical approach to investigation of Joubert syndrome and Joubert syndrome-related disorders. Dev Med Child Neurol 53, 793–798.

Satz, J.S., Barresi, R., Durbeej, M., Willer, T., Turner, A., Moore, S.A., and Campbell, K.P. (2008). Brain and eye malformations resembling Walker-Warburg syndrome are recapitulated in mice by dystroglycan deletion in the epiblast. J Neurosci 28, 10567–10575.

Sepp, T., Yates, J.R., and Green, A.J. (1996). Loss of heterozygosity in tuberous sclerosis hamartomas. J Med Genet 33, 962–964.

Sheen, V.L., Ganesh, V.S., Topcu, M., Sebire, G., Bodell, A., Hill, R.S., Grant, P.E., Shugart, Y.Y., Imitola, J., Khoury, S.J., et al. (2004). Mutations in ARFGEF2 implicate vesicle trafficking in neural progenitor proliferation and migration in the human cerebral cortex. Nat Genet 36, 69–76.

Shen, J., Gilmore, E.C., Marshall, C.A., Haddadin, M., Reynolds, J.J., Eyaid, W., Bodell, A., Barry, B., Gleason, D., Allen, K., et al. (2010). Mutations in PNKP cause microcephaly, seizures and defects in DNA repair. Nat Genet 42, 245–249.

Sicca, F., Kelemen, A., Genton, P., Das, S., Mei, D., Moro, F., Dobyns, W.B., and Guerrini, R. (2003). Mosaic mutations of the LIS1 gene cause subcortical band heterotopia. Neurology 61, 1042–1046.

Sir, J.-H., Barr, A.R., Nicholas, A.K., Carvalho, O.P., Khurshid, M., Sossick, A., Reichelt, S., D'Santos, C., Woods, C.G., and Gergely, F. (2011). A primary microcephaly protein complex forms a ring around parental centrioles. Nat Genet 43, 1147–1153.

Smith, D.J., Stevens, M.E., Sudanagunta, S.P., Bronson, R.T., Makhinson, M., Watabe, A.M., O'Dell, T.J., Fung, J., Weier, H.U., Cheng, J.F., et al. (1997). Functional screening of 2 Mb of human chromosome 21q22.2 in transgenic mice implicates minibrain in learning defects associated with Down syndrome. Nat Genet 16, 28–36.

Sotelo, C. (2004). Cellular and genetic regulation of the development of the cerebellar system. Prog Neurobiol 72, 295–339.

Stevens, E., Carss, K.J., Cirak, S., Foley, A.R., Torelli, S., Willer, T., Tambunan, D.E., Yau, S., Brodd, L., Sewry, C.A., et al. (2013). Mutations in B3GALNT2 cause congenital muscular dystrophy and hypoglycosylation of α-dystroglycan. Am J Hum Genet 92, 354–365.

Sullivan, P.F., Daly, M.J., and O'Donovan, M. (2012). Genetic architectures of psychiatric disorders: the emerging picture and its implications. Nat Rev Genet 13, 537–551.

Sumigray, K.D., Chen, H., and Lechler, T. (2011). Lis1 is essential for cortical microtubule organization and desmosome stability in the epidermis. T J Cell Biol 194, 631–642.

Tarrant, A., Garel, C., Germanaud, D., de Villemeur, T.B., Mignot, C., Lenoir, M., and le Pointe, H.D.

(2009). Microcephaly: a radiological review. Pediatr Radiol 39, 772–80.

Tejedor, F., Zhu, X.R., Kaltenbach, E., Ackermann, A., Baumann, A., Canal, I., Heisenberg, M., Fischbach, K.F., and Pongs, O. (1995). minibrain: a new protein kinase family involved in postembryonic neurogenesis in Drosophila. Neuron 14, 287–301.

Thornton, G.K., and Woods, C.G. (2009). Primary microcephaly: do all roads lead to Rome? Trends Genet 25, 501–510.

Tischfield, M.A., Baris, H.N., Wu, C., Rudolph, G., Van Maldergem, L., He, W., Chan, W.-M., Andrews, C., Demer, J.L., Robertson, R.L., et al. (2010). Human TUBB3 mutations perturb microtubule dynamics, kinesin interactions, and axon guidance. Cell 140, 74–87.

Tischfield, M.A., Cederquist, G.Y., Gupta, M.L., and Engle, E.C. (2011). Phenotypic spectrum of the tubulin-related disorders and functional implications of disease-causing mutations. Curr Opin Genet Dev 21, 286–294.

Tory, K., Lacoste, T., Burglen, L., Morinière, V., Boddaert, N., Macher, M.-A., Llanas, B., Nivet, H., Bensman, A., Niaudet, P., et al. (2007). High NPHP1 and NPHP6 mutation rate in patients with Joubert syndrome and nephronophthisis: potential epistatic effect of NPHP6 and AHI1 mutations in patients with NPHP1 mutations. J Am Soc Nephrol 18, 1566–1575.

Tsukada, M., Prokscha, A., Ungewickell, E., and Eichele, G. (2005). Doublecortin association with actin filaments is regulated by neurabin II. J Biol Chem 280, 11361–11368.

Vallee, R.B., and Tsai, J.-W. (2006). The cellular roles of the lissencephaly gene LIS1, and what they tell us about brain development. Genes Dev 20, 1384–1393.

van Bon, B.W.M., Hoischen, A., Hehir-Kwa, J., de Brouwer, A.P.M., Ruivenkamp, C., Gijsbers, A.C.J., Marcelis, C.L., de Leeuw, N., Veltman, J.A., Brunner, H.G., et al. (2011). Intragenic deletion in DYRK1A leads to mental retardation and primary microcephaly. Clin Genet 79, 296–299.

Van Reeuwijk, J., Maugenre, S., Van Den Elzen, C., Verrips, A., Bertini, E., Muntoni, F., Merlini, L., Scheffer, H., Brunner, H.G., Guicheney, P., et al. (2006). The expanding phenotype of

POMT1 mutations: from Walker-Warburg syndrome to congenital muscular dystrophy, microcephaly, and mental retardation. Hum Mutat 27, 453–459.

Vulprecht, J., David, A., Tibelius, A., Castiel, A., Konotop, G., Liu, F., Bestvater, F., Raab, M.S., Zentgraf, H., Izraeli, S., et al. (2012). STIL is required for centriole duplication in human cells. J Cell Sci 125, 1353–1362.

Wang, X., Tsai, J.-W., Imai, J.H., Lian, W.-N., Vallee, R.B., and Shi, S.-H. (2009). Asymmetric centrosome inheritance maintains neural progenitors in the neocortex. Nature 461, 947–955.

Weiss, L.A., Shen, Y., Korn, J.M., Arking, D.E., Miller, D.T., Fossdal, R., Saemundsen, E., Stefansson, H., Ferreira, M.A.R., Green, T., et al. (2008). Association between microdeletion and microduplication at 16p11.2 and autism. N Engl J Med 358, 667–675.

te Welscher, P., Zuniga, A., Kuijper, S., Drenth, T., Goedemans, H.J., Meijlink, F., and Zeller, R. (2002). Progression of vertebrate limb development through SHH-mediated counteraction of GLI3. Science 298, 827–830.

Willemsen, M.H., Vissers, L.E.L., Willemsen, M.A.A.P., van Bon, B.W.M., Kroes, T., de Ligt, J., de Vries, B.B., Schoots, J., Lugtenberg, D., Hamel, B.C.J., et al. (2012). Mutations in DYNC1H1 cause severe intellectual disability with neuronal migration defects. J Med Genet 49, 179–183.

Willer, T., Lee, H., Lommel, M., Yoshida-Moriguchi, T., de Bernabe, D.B.V., Venzke, D., Cirak, S., Schachter, H., Vajsar, J., Voit, T., et al. (2012). ISPD loss-of-function mutations disrupt dystroglycan O-mannosylation and cause Walker-Warburg syndrome. Nat Genet 44, 575–580.

Yamada, K., Andrews, C., Chan, W.-M., McKeown, C.A., Magli, A., de Berardinis, T., Loewenstein, A., Lazar, M., O'Keefe, M., Letson, R., et al. (2003). Heterozygous mutations of the kinesin KIF21A in congenital fibrosis of the extraocular muscles type 1 (CFEOM1). Nat Genet 35, 318–321.

Yang, Y.J., Baltus, A.E., Mathew, R.S., Murphy, E.A., Evrony, G.D., Gonzalez, D.M., Wang, E.P., Marshall-Walker, C.A., Barry, B.J., Murn, J., et al. (2012). Microcephaly gene links trithorax and REST/NRSF to control neural stem cell proliferation and differentiation. Cell 151, 1097–1112.

Yoneda, Y., Haginoya, K., Kato, M., Osaka, H., Yokochi, K., Arai, H., Kakita, A., Yamamoto, T., Otsuki, Y., Shimizu, S.-I., et al. (2013). Phenotypic spectrum of COL4A1 mutations: porencephaly to schizencephaly. Ann Neurol 73, 48–57.

Yu, T.W., Chahrour, M.H., Coulter, M.E., Jiralerspong, S., Okamura-Ikeda, K., Ataman, B., Schmitz-Abe, K., Harmin, D.A., Adli, M., Malik, A.N., et al. (2013). Using whole-exome sequencing to identify inherited causes of autism. Neuron 77, 259–273.

Yu, T.W., Mochida, G.H., Tischfield, D.J., Sgaier, S.K., Flores-Sarnat, L., Sergi, C.M., Topçu, M., Mcdonald, M.T., Barry, B.J., Felie, J.M., et al. (2010). Mutations in WDR62, encoding a centrosome-associated protein, cause microcephaly with simplified gyri and abnormal cortical architecture. Nat Genet 42, 1015–1020.

8

DISORDERS OF AXON GUIDANCE

HEIKE BLOCKUS[1,2,3] AND ALAIN CHÉDOTAL[1,2,3]
[1]*Sorbonne Universités, UPMC Univ Paris, UMRS968 and CNRS, UMR 7210, Institut de la Vision, Paris, F-75012, France*
[2]*INSERM, Institut de la Vision, UMRS_968, Paris, F-75012, France*
[3]*CNRS, UMR_7210, Paris, F-75012, France*

8.1 INTRODUCTION

Growing axons are guided by molecular cues in their environment, along stereotyped pathways, often via a series of intermediate choice points, to finally reach their appropriate target region. Guidance cues are recognized by receptors expressed in specific combinations at the surface of the axonal growth cone. Axon guidance molecules also shape the topography of connections and their lamination. Additional cues subsequently specify cell-type-specific synaptic connectivity (see Chapter 9). The initial pattern of connectivity is subsequently refined by activity-dependent processes and experience-dependent plasticity. Mutations in genes encoding axon guidance molecules can impair initial connectivity and also alter activity-dependent maturation by changing the input patterns of activity, shifting the subsequent developmental trajectory. Specific mutations in axon guidance genes have been linked to a number of neurological disorders (Table 8.1), where gross disturbances in axonal tracts are often visible with magnetic resonance imaging (MRI). More recent findings suggest that such mutations may also be implicated in some psychiatric diseases (Table 8.2).

8.2 AXON GUIDANCE MOLECULES

During the past 20 years, many proteins that are able to guide growing axons were identified using biochemical and genetic methods. These axon guidance molecules are secreted or bound to the cell membrane and can either attract axons or repel them (Dickson, 2002; Kolodkin and Tessier-Lavigne, 2011; Kolodkin and Pasterkamp, 2013; Pasterkamp and Kolodkin,

The Genetics of Neurodevelopmental Disorders, First Edition. Edited by Kevin J. Mitchell.
© 2015 John Wiley & Sons, Inc. Published 2015 by John Wiley & Sons, Inc.

TABLE 8.1 Axon guidance genes mutated in discrete neurological disorders

Gene	Disease/Phenotype	Type of study	Experimental approach	References
Oculomotor system				
CHN1	Duane Syndrome	Zebrafish	LOF/GOF	Clark et al. (2013)
CHN1	Duane Syndrome	Human genetics	Not investigated	Rama et al. (2012)
Kif21a	CFEOM1	Human genetics	Not investigated	Yamada et al. (2003); Demer et al. (2005)
Kif21a	CFEOM1	Transgenics	Kif21a R954W knockin	Cheng et al. (2014)
Map1b	CFEOM1	KO mice	$Map1b^{-/-}$	Cheng et al. (2014)
TUBB3	CFEOM3	Human genetics	Not investigated	Tischfield et al. (2010)
TUBB3	CFEOM3	Transgenics	Tubb3 knockin	Tischfield et al. (2010)
Visual system				
Tyrosinase	Visual deficits	Human genetics	Not investigated	Kwon et al. (1987)
Tyrosinase	RGCs	Axon targeting	Reduction of ipsilateral RGCs	Lund, 1965; Guillery and Kaas, 1973; Neveu et al. (2003)
Corticospinal tract				
Shh, Wnt, PI, PCP	JSRD	Human genetics	Not investigated	Lee et al. (2011)
DCC	MM	Human genetics	Not investigated	Srour et al. (2010), Depienne et al. (2011), Djarmati-Westenberger et al. (2011)
DCC	MM	Hypomorph	DCC^{kanga}	Finger et al. (2002)
Rad51	MM	Human genetics	Not investigated	Méneret et al. (2014); Depienne et al. (2012)
Robo3	HGPPS	Human genetics	Not investigated	Jen et al. (2004); Chan et al. (1996); Abu-Amero et al. (2009)
Corpus callosum				
DISC1	Callosal agenesis	Human genetics	Not investigated	Osbun et al. (2011); Duff et al. (2013)
DISC1	Callosal agenesis	KO mice	$Disc1^{-/-}$	Shen et al. (2008)
NFIA	Callosal agenesis	Human genetics	Not investigated	Shu et al. (2003); Lu et al. (2007); Rao et al. (2014); Ji et al. (2014)
L1CAM	MASA/CRASH	Human genetics	Not investigated	Fransen et al. (1995)
DISC1	Callosal agenesis	Human genetics	Not investigated	Osbun et al. (2011), Duff et al. (2013)

TABLE 8.2 Axon guidance genes associated with common psychiatric disorders

Gene	Disease/Phenotype	Type of study	Experimental approach	References
Neuropsychiatric diseases				
Sema3A	Schizophrenia	Human genetics	Not investigated	Eastwood et al. (2003)
Sema3D	Schizophrenia	Human genetics	Not investigated	Fujii et al. (2011)
Sema4B	Synaptic development	*In vitro*	RNAi screen, hippocampus	Paradis et al. (2007)
Sema4D	Synaptic development	*In vitro*	RNAi screen, hippocampus	Paradis et al. (2007)
Sema5A	Autism	Human genetics	Not investigated	Melin et al. (2006); Weiss et al. (2009)
Sema5A	Autism	KO mice	$Sema5A^{-/-}$, no phenotype	Gunn et al. (2011)
Sema6A	Schizophrenia	KO mice	$Sema6A^{-/-}$, behavior	Rünker et al. (2011)
PlxnA2	Schizophrenia	Human genetics	Not investigated	Mah et al. (2006); Fujii et al. (2007); Allen et al. (2008)
PlxnB3	Schizophrenia	Human genetics	Not investigated	Rujescu et al. (2007)
CRMP1	Schizophrenia	KO mice	$CRMP1^{-/-}$	Su et al. (2007)
CRMP2	Schizophrenia	Human genetics	Not investigated	Edgar et al. (2000)
CRMP2	Alzheimer's Disease	Transgenics	APP/PS1	Williamson et al. (2011)
St8Sia2	Schizophrenia	Human genetics	Not investigated	Kamien et al. (2014); Anney et al. (2010); Lee et al. (2011)
St8Sia2	Fear behavior	KO mice	$St8Sia2^{-/-}$, hippocampus	Angata et al. (2004)
Slitrk1	GTS	Human genetics	Not investigated	Paschou (2013)
Slitrk1	Fear behavior	KO mice	$Slitrk1^{-/-}$	Katayama et al. (2009)
Slitrk5	OCD, Depression	KO mice	$Slitrk5^{-/-}$	Proenca et al. (2011)
Slitrk6	Auditory impairment	Human patients	Auditory assessment	Morlet et al. (2014)
Slitrk6	Auditory impairment	KO mice	$Slitrk6^{-/-}$	Matsumoto et al. (2011)
APP	Alzheimer's Disease	Human genetics	APP transgenics	Nelson et al. (2012)
APP	Commissure formation	Transgenics	APP transgenics	Rama et al. (2012)
APP	Growth cone adhesion	*In vitro*	Primary culture	Sosa et al. (2013)
APP	Down Syndrome	*In vitro*	Primary culture	Sosa et al. (2014)
Fe65	Alzheimer's Disease	KO mice	$Fe65^{-/-}\ Fe65L1^{-/-}$	Borquez et al. (2012)
Bace1	Axon guidance	KO mice	$BACE1^{-/-}$, axon targeting	Vassar et al. (2014)
Robo1, Robo2	Autism	Biomarker	Peripheral lymphocytes	Hu et al. (2006)
Robo3, Robo4	Autism	Human genetics	SNP analysis	Anitha et al. (2008)

2013). The trajectories of specific cell types are determined by the repertoire of receptors that they express, which can be dynamically regulated during development. Their molecular structure and mechanism of action appear highly conserved across animal species and they play additional roles outside the nervous system in the regulation of cell–cell interactions in developing, mature, and diseased organs (Mehlen et al., 2011; Ypsilanti et al., 2010).

We will first introduce the main families of axon guidance molecules and their receptors, focusing on those that have been linked to neurological disorders and thus will be the main subject of this chapter.

8.2.1 Netrin-1 and Its Receptors

Netrin-1 is the main chemoattractant for axons projecting across the midline of the central nervous system (CNS), the so-called commissural axons. It is an extracellular matrix protein related to laminins, which was first discovered in *C. elegans* and chick embryos (Hedgecock et al., 1990; Serafini et al., 1994). Netrin-1 displays versatile functions and can repel some classes of axons or control other developmental processes such as apoptosis (Lai Wing Sun et al., 2011). This variety of biological activities of Netrin-1 is associated with a diversity of receptors expressed on axonal growth cones.

Deleted in colorectal cancer (DCC), an immunoglobulin superfamily member appears to be the main receptor mediating Netrin-1 attractive activity (Chan et al., 1996; Keino-Masu et al., 1996; Kolodziej et al., 1996). However, other receptors or co-receptors could also be involved such as A2b, an adenosine receptor (Corset et al., 2000; Shewan et al., 2002) and DSCAM (Down syndrome cell adhesion molecule) (Ly et al., 2008), but in both cases, *in vivo* support is missing and their role in netrin-1 signaling is still debated (Palmesino et al., 2012; Stein et al., 2001). Recently, APP (amyloid precursor protein), a transmembrane receptor, which after proteolytic cleavage generates β-amyloid (Aβ) and is involved in Alzheimer's disease pathogenesis, was shown

to interact with DCC and to potentiate netrin-1 attraction in spinal cord commissural neurons (Rama et al., 2012).

Netrin-1 repulsion requires Unc-5 receptors (Unc5a–Unc5d), which also belong to the IgCAM family (Leonardo et al., 1997). Although Unc-5 receptors bind netrin-1, it is still unclear if the formation of Unc5/DCC complex is required to trigger repulsion as initially proposed (Hong et al., 1999). Some studies rather suggest that Unc5 receptors might induce a repulsive response in axons independently of DCC (Keleman and Dickson, 2001; Watanabe et al., 2006; Poon et al., 2008).

Of note, these receptors have other ligands than netrin-1, such as Draxin for DCC (Ahmed et al., 2011) and FLRT2/3 or Robo4 for UNC5 (Koch et al., 2011; Yamagishi et al., 2011) respectively. As most IgCAM molecules, they can bind to themselves or other IgCAMs to form homo- or heteromeric complexes (Stein and Tessier-Lavigne, 2001).

8.2.2 Slits and Robo Receptors

Slits are secreted proteins, which, like netrin-1, were discovered for their role in axon guidance at the CNS midline (Brose et al., 1999; Kidd et al., 1999). Mammalian Slits are ECM proteins containing four leucine-rich domains (D1–D4) followed by nine EGF (epidermal growth factor) repeats and a C terminal cysteine knot. Slits bind to the Roundabout receptors (Robo) triggering axon repulsion (Brose et al., 1999; Li et al., 1999). In mammals, three Slits (Slit1–3) and three Robo receptors (Robo1–3) were characterized and are broadly expressed in the developing nervous system (Brose et al., 1999; Marillat et al., 2002). A fourth divergent Robo, Robo4 is expressed in the vasculature and does not bind Slits (Huminiecki et al., 2002; Koch et al., 2011). So far, most studies have shown that Slits have a repulsive activity on growing axons. However, Slit/Robo signaling not only controls axon guidance but also neuronal migration and proliferation as well as dendritic extension/polarity, axonal branching and targeting (Blockus and Chédotal, 2014; Chédotal,

2007; Ypsilanti et al., 2010). Glycoproteins such as heparan sulfate proteoglycans (HSPGs) and alpha-Dystroglycan (α-DG) influence Slit/Robo signaling possibly by stabilizing the Slit/Robo complex at the cell surface and by limiting Slit diffusion (Chanana et al., 2009; Hu, 2001; Johnson et al., 2004; Kastenhuber et al., 2009; Piper et al., 2006; Ronca et al., 2001; Wright et al., 2012). Robo receptors are IgCAMs and interact with other IgCAM receptors, in particular DCC (Stein and Tessier-Lavigne, 2001). *In vitro* studies in Xenopus neurons, suggest that the binding of Slits to Robo not only activates axonal repulsion but also induces Robo cis-interaction with DCC, which in turn silences Netrin-1/DCC attraction (Stein and Tessier-Lavigne, 2001).

8.2.3 Semaphorins, Neuropilins, and Plexins

Semaphorins were discovered in insects for their role in axon guidance and were later found in most vertebrate species and in some viruses (Kolodkin et al., 1993; Messersmith et al., 1995; Pasterkamp, 2012). They all contain a signature "Sema domain" of about 500 amino acids, and, depending on the subclass, additional conserved motifs such as thrombospondin repeats (class 5) or an Ig domain (classes 3, 4 and 7). Most semaphorins are transmembrane proteins (classes 1, 4, 5, and 6), whereas others are either anchored to the membrane by a glycosylphosphatidylinositol link (GPI; class 7), or secreted (classes 2 and 3). In mammals, about twenty distinct semaphorin genes are known to date. In most cases, semaphorin ligands are repulsive for growing axons expressing their receptors, although a few studies supports an attractive activity of some secreted semaphorins on axons. Like Slits, semaphorins participate in a large range of neurodevelopmental processes, from neuronal migration, myelination, neurite extension, branching and pruning, to apoptosis, which are mediated by multiple receptor complexes (Pasterkamp, 2012; Tran et al., 2007). In mammals, six out of seven secreted class 3 semaphorins (Sema3A, B,

C, D, F and G), bind to neuropilin receptors (Npn1 or Npn2; Chen et al., 1997; Giger et al., 1998; He and Tessier-Lavigne, 1997; Kolodkin et al., 1997). Neuropilins do not transduce signals into axons themselves, but interact with two other transmembrane proteins, type A plexins (PlexinA1-A4) and an IgCAM (L1CAM or NrCAM), which together transduce the semaphorin signal (Castellani et al., 2000; Falk et al., 2005; Takahashi et al., 1999; Tamagnone et al., 1999). However, the last class 3 semaphorin, Sema3E, directly binds to PlexinD1 (Chauvet et al., 2007; Gu et al., 2005). Transmembrane semaphorins bind and signal through Plexins, but other receptors or co-receptors, such as HSPGs, integrins, and VEGFR2 (vascular endothelial growth factor receptor 2) are also involved (Bellon et al., 2010; Pasterkamp et al., 2003; Serini et al., 2003). Of note, in some cells, class 6 transmembrane semaphorins can act as receptors for type A Plexins (Renaud et al., 2008; Toyofuku et al., 2004a; 2004b).

8.2.4 Ephrins and Eph

Ephrins are ligands of the Eph receptor tyrosine kinase family. Ephrin-A*s* (A1–A5 in mammals) are GPI anchored and ephrin-B*s* (B1–B3) are transmembrane (Klein, 2012). They bind to EphA (A1–A8, A10) and EphB (B1–B4, B6) respectively although some cross-binding between A and B classes has been observed (Lisabeth et al., 2013). Unlike most other axon guidance molecules, ephrin–Eph signaling is bidirectional: ephrins can act as receptors (or co-receptors) for Ephs and vice versa (Holland et al., 1996; Marquardt et al., 2005). Moreover, there are extensive cis-interactions between ephrins and Eph receptors, which modulate signaling in trans. In most cases, ephrin/Eph interaction initiates a repulsive response in axon, leading to growth cone collapse. Ephrin/Eph signaling has been shown to play a major role in the development of topographic axonal projection maps, in particular in the visual system where gradients of ephrin ligands organize the targeting of RGC axons in visual centers such as the colliculus and thalamus (Cheng et al., 1995; Drescher et al., 1995; Nakamoto et al., 1996; Triplett and Feldheim, 2012).

8.3 AXON GUIDANCE DEFECTS OF OCULOMOTOR NERVES

Vision depends upon the stabilization of images close to the center of the fovea to prevent image drifting. This is a very complex task, requiring the coordination of many neuronal inputs (see subsequent sections). The complexity of the oculomotor circuit (more complex in animals with fovea and binocular vision) and the high precision of oculomotor projections, probably explain why the oculomotor system is prone to diseases (strabismus affect about 1–5% of the population; Leigh and Zee, 2006; Table 8.1). Moreover, oculomotor defects are easily diagnosed by clinicians and optometrists.

8.3.1 Organization of the Oculomotor System

In mammals, eye movements are controlled by three antagonistic pairs of extraocular muscles (EOM; 4 recti and 2 obliques), which move the eyeball in all directions: the lateral rectus muscle (LR) and medial rectus (MR) horizontally, the superior oblique (SO) and inferior oblique (IO) provide torsion, the inferior rectus (IR) and superior rectus (SR) move the eye vertically. EOM are connected to three pairs of oculomotor nuclei all located in the brainstem. Neurons in the abducens motor nuclei (VI) only innervate the LR, the trochlear (IV) motor neurons only innervate the SO muscle, whereas the oculomotor nucleus (III) projects to the four other muscles (IO, IR, SR, and MR) and to the upper eyelid muscle (*levator palpebrae superioris*, LPS), contralaterally in the mouse, and bilaterally in humans. Axons from abducens and most of the IIIrd nuclei project to the ipsilateral eyeball whereas the caudal part of the IIIrd and the trochlear nucleus innervate muscles on the contralateral eye (the SR and SO respectively; Buttner-Ennever, 2006).

Bilateral connections between internuclear neurons in the abducens and oculomotor nuclei coordinate movements of both eyes. Lastly, many other neurons, in particular in the cerebellar, vestibular and precerebellar systems also play a key role in fine-tuning eye movements and integrating various stimuli, such as vestibular inputs from the inner ear, which arise during head movements and acceleration (Leigh and Zee, 2006). Although congenital forms of strabismus and eye movement disorders such as Duane's syndrome have been known for a very long time (Duane, 1905), their etiology remained largely unexplained until recently. These disorders were initially classified as congenital fibrosis of extraocular muscles (CFEOM) based on the assumption that they were all directly affecting EOMs. However, more recent studies have shown that most of these diseases, now collectively referred to as congenital innervation disorders (CID; Assaf, 2011) or congenital cranial dysinnervation disorders (CCDDs ; Gutowski et al., 2003), are caused by either a lack or a mistargeting of oculomotor axons and that the muscle fibrosis is only secondary (Engle, 2006). Before discussing these syndromes and their cause further, we will briefly describe the normal development of the oculomotor system.

8.3.2 Development of Oculomotor Nerves

Fate-map studies and the analysis of mutant mice have shown that the three oculomotor nuclei are born in distinct segments of the posterior neural tube. In mice, rhombomere 1 generates trochlear neurons, rhombomere 5 the abducens, and the mesencephalon the third oculomotor nuclei (Gilland and Baker, 2005). In the mouse, oculomotor axons exit the hindbrain early, around embryonic day 9–9.5 (Mastick et al., 1996), reach the eye around E10.5–E11 and the innervation pattern has a mature configuration by E14.5 (Wahl et al., 1994). In human embryos, the oculomotor and trochlear axons leave the brain between 5 and 6 weeks of gestation, Cargenie stage 14 (Cooper, 1946; Muller and O'Rahilly, 1988).

Not much is known about the molecular mechanisms that govern axon pathfinding in the oculomotor system. However, a few molecules that can influence the growth of oculomotor axons, at least in explant cultures, were identified. In the chick embryo, the chemokine CXCL12 or SDF1 (stromal derived factor 1) and the hepatocyte growth factor (HGF; Naeem et al., 2002) are expressed near oculomotor exit point and in mesenchyme surrounding the EOM (Lerner et al., 2010). Their respective receptors, CXCR4 and Met are expressed in IIIrd and IV nuclei (Caton et al., 2000; Lerner et al., 2010). HGF and SDF1 attract and stimulate oculomotor axon growth and branching *in vitro*. *In vitro* experiments also suggest that the trochlear axons are repelled from the ventral midline by repellents secreted by floor plate cells such as netrin-1 (Colamarino and Tessier-Lavigne, 1995), and by semaphorin 3A (Sema3A), which is enriched in the ventral part of the hindbrain. However, no guidance defect of the trochlear nerve was detected in mice deficient for Netrin-1, Sema3A, or their receptors (Serafini et al., 1996). Trochlear axons express neuropilin-2 receptors and are prevented from entering the mesencephalon by Semaphorin 3F (Sema3F; Chen et al., 2000; Giger et al., 2000; Watanabe et al., 2004). In parallel, the morphogen fibroblast growth factor 8 (Fgf8) might attract trochlear axons (Irving et al., 2002). In chick embryo, Sema3A/3C is expressed in and around EOMs and the knockdown of PlexinA2/A1 receptors leads to oculomotor axon defasciculation, abnormal projection to LR, and overgrowth (Ferrario et al., 2012). Furthermore, PlexinA4 is expressed in many cranial nerves, including the oculomotor nerve (Gutekunst and Gross, 2014).

How oculomotor axons recognize their specific EOM is also an open question.

Many genetic studies in Drosophila have shown that motor axons are guided to their correct body wall muscles by combination of secreted and membrane-bound molecules expressed by subsets of muscles and also by factors which control the fasciculation and defasciculation of motor axons at specific choice points (Kohsaka et al., 2012). Transplantation experiments in the chick spinal cord also support the existence of specific guidance cues for subtypes of motor axons (Tosney and Landmesser, 1984). In mammals, repellents and attractants also control the innervation of limb muscles by motor axons (Bonanomi et al., 2012; Huber et al., 2005; Kao and Kania, 2011). However, how the different types of oculomotor axons are guided to their correct muscles is still largely unknown. The surgical ablation of the abducens neurons in chick embryos does not lead to the abnormal innervation of the LR by the remaining oculomotor axons (Chilton and Guthrie, 2004), which would support the existence of muscle specific cues. By contrast, there is evidence in *Wnt-1* null mutant embryos, where the III and IV motor nuclei fail to develop, that the abducens axons (Fritzsch et al., 1995; Porter and Baker, 1997) not only project to the LR, but also to EOM normally innervated by III and IV. In addition, in *Xenopus* larvae, the IIIrd motor axons can abnormally innervate the SO muscle if the trochlear nerve is cut (Fritzsch and Sonntag, 1990). Last, in chick embryos, abducens neurons transplanted to the midbrain innervate other muscles than the LR (Lance-Jones et al., 2012). This would argue against the existence of muscle specific cues in the oculomotor system.

8.3.3 Congenital Cranial Dysinnervation Disorders

Although most CCDDs/CIDs, have a neurogenic origin, axon guidance *per se* is perturbed in only some of these disorders whereas in others motor neuron differentiation is affected (7 CCDD have been reported: *KIF21A*, *TUBB3*, *PHOX2A*, *SALL4*, *HOXA1*, *ROBO3*, *CHN1*). *HOXA1* mutations lead to EOM dysinnervation, possibly due to a lack of differentiation of abducens neurons (Tischfield et al., 2005). Likewise, in CFEOM2, autosomal recessive mutations in the *PHOXA2* transcription factor prevent the formation of trochlear and oculomotor axons (Nakano et al., 2001; Bosley et al., 2006). Last, homozygous mutations in the homeobox gene

HOXA1 prevent the generation of rhombomere 5 and therefore of abducens neurons (Lufkin et al., 1991; Tischfield et al., 2005).

Herein, we will only discuss Duane syndrome, CFEOM1, CFEOM3, and HGPPS, for which abnormal axon guidance appears to be the primary cause of the disease.

In Duane Retraction syndrome (Duane, DRS; 0.1% incidence in population, about 2–4% of strabismic cases), postmortem studies revealed an absence or strong reduction of the abducens nerve. An abnormal innervation of the LR by oculomotor III axons triggers the co-contraction of the LR and MR and eye globe retraction (Parsa et al., 1998). MRI studies confirmed the lack or atrophic abducens but also showed that in some patients, the oculomotor nerves are also hypoplastic. (Demer et al., 2007; Xia et al., 2014). Vertical gaze abnormalities can also occur, penetrance is incomplete and three clinically distinguishable variants of DRS exist (DRS1-3; (Alexandrakis and Saunders, 2001; Ye et al., 2014)).

Duane Syndrome   Recent studies have shown that some patients with DRS harbor heterozygous missense mutations in alpha2-chimaerin (*CHN1*), a cytosolic Rac guanosine triphosphatase (GTPase) activating protein, which is active when bound to GTP and inactivates Rac. All mutations are thought to act mechanistically similarly (including Y148F, P141L, P252S; Chan et al., 2011; Miyake et al., 2011) are thought to hyperactivate alpha2-chimaerin, thereby reducing Rac-GTP level. Alpha2-chimaerin is broadly expressed throughout the developing brain, including oculomotor nuclei, and in zebrafish, expression of hyperactive alpha2-chimaerin as well as its inactivation result in defects of axon guidance and branching of oculomotor axons (Clark et al., 2013). These findings raise the question of up- and downstream integration in signaling pathways of alpha2-chimaerin.

It was shown that alpha2-chimaerin acts downstream of the receptor tyrosine kinase EphA4 (Beg et al., 2007; Iwasato et al., 2007; Wegmeyer et al., 2007) to control the development of locomotor circuits in the spinal cord. However, a role for ephrin/eph signaling in the development of the oculomotor system has not been demonstrated. There is also evidence linking alpha2-chimaerin and semaphorin signaling, as alpha2-chimaerin loss-of-function in oculomotor axons blocks Sema3A/Plexina repulsion and perturbs axon guidance (Ferrario et al., 2012). However, the guidance pathway affected in alpha2-chimaerin patients is still unknown.

Interestingly, alpha2 chimaerin is a candidate gene for other disorders such as epilepsy, autism, and schizophrenia (Bacchelli et al., 2003; Davidsson et al., 2008; Lencz et al., 2007). As mentioned before, alpha2-chimaerin is broadly expressed in the CNS and was involved in the control of neuronal migration in the neocortex (Ip et al., 2012). In the hippocampus, alpha2-chimaerin and beta2-chimaerin control dendritic pruning (Buttery et al., 2006).

CFEOM1   CFEOM1 patients exhibit bilateral restriction of gaze in several directions and restricted vertical gaze, variably restricted horizontal gaze, and droopy eyelids (ptosis). They seem to lack two subnuclei of the III which projects to SR and LPS (Yamagishi et al., 2011) and the abducens nerve might also be affected. Patients were shown to carry autosomal dominant heterozygous missense mutations in the kinesin KIF21A (Demer et al., 2005; Yamada et al., 2003). Kinesins are motor proteins, which in axons and dendrites transport molecular complexes and vesicles along microtubules (Hirokawa et al., 2010; van der Vaart et al., 2013). KIF21A is expressed in all oculomotor nuclei and in EOMs (Desai et al., 2012) and why the oculomotor system is selectively affected is unknown. Very recently, a knockin mouse model for the most common human *Kif21a* mutation found in CFEOM1 patients has been described (*Kif21a* R954W; Cheng et al., 2014). This mutation attenuates KIF21A autoregulation keeping it in an intermediately active state, and thus acts in a gain-of-function manner that manifests in a thinner oculomotor nerve with a hypoplastic superior division and aberrant branches in the inferior divison. On a cellular level, in *Kif21a* R954W knockins a subset of oculomotor axons terminate prematurely in the proximal nerve and these misdirected axons are hyper-rich in filopodia and have enlarged growth cones. Building on that finding molecularly, the study furthermore reveals that interaction of Kif21a with the microtubule-associated protein 1b (Map1b) is important for microtubule growth cone dynamics crucial for axon elongation and targeting. The study finishes by confirming that *Map1b* knockout mice develop CFEOM1, thus highlighting the importance of the KIF21a-microtubule interaction *in vivo*.

CFEOM3 It was recently demonstrated that patients suffering from CFEOM3, a rare form of oculomotor disorders (Doherty et al., 1999), carry autosomal dominant missense mutations in *TUBB3*, a gene encoding the neuron specific β-tubulin isotype III (βIII-tubulin; Chew et al., 2013; Tischfield et al., 2010). MRI showed that oculomotor nerves, SR and LPS are hypoplastic in CFEOM3 patients.

The spectrum of axon guidance disorders linked to mutations in *TUBB3* is not restricted to cranial nerves and the corpus callosum and internal capsule can be also abnormal (Tischfield et al., 2010). Moreover, in several families, brain development is more severely affected and in addition to strabismus, cortical and cerebellar dysgenesis and mental retardation were described (Poirier et al., 2010). The mutations might alter the ability of βIII tubulin to heterodimerize with alpha-tubulin or its interaction with microtubule associated proteins such as kinesins. This would perturb microtubule dynamics, which is essential for axonal growth and cell motility. The main axon guidance defects are recapitulated in *Tubb3* knockin mouse mutants (Tischfield et al., 2010).

Interestingly, mutations in further tubulin-coding genes, *TUBB2B*, *TUBA8*, *TUBA1A*, and *TUBB5* (Breuss et al., 2012; Fallet-Bianco et al., 2008; Jaglin et al., 2009; Keays et al., 2007), have been identified and these lead to severe neuronal migration and axon guidance defects including oculomotor nerves (Cederquist et al., 2012). This suggests that so-called "tubulinopathies" might define a large group of neurological diseases affecting neuronal migration in most cases, and axon guidance in some. (Cushion et al., 2013; Jaglin and Chelly, 2009; Romaniello et al., 2015). Of note, DCC

was shown to interact with Tubb3 (Qu et al., 2013).

8.3.4 Midline Crossing Disorders

Most animal species have a symmetrical nervous system, divided longitudinally in left and right halves. During development, commissural neurons project their axon across the longitudinal axis or midline to contact targets on the opposite side. Commissural neurons play a very important role in the control of locomotion and in sensory systems (Goulding, 2009; Peng and Charron, 2013). Mounting evidence links neurological diseases to developmental defects of commissural axon guidance.

Visual System A classic example is albinism (Table 8.1). In Albino patients (oculocutaneous albinism type 1, OCA1) retinal pigmented epithelium (RPE) and melanocytes do not synthetize normal levels of the pigment melanin due to anomalies affecting the melanin synthetic pathways, such as mutations of the enzyme tyrosinase (Kwon et al., 1987). In addition to a loss of melanin, they often suffer from nystagmus and strabismus, with altered depth perception (Ray et al., 2007).

In the visual system of primates, retinal ganglion cells (RGCs) in the nasal retina project to the contralateral geniculate nucleus (LGN) whereas RGCs of the temporal retina project to the ipsilateral LGN. Therefore, in both eyes, the RGCs that process information from the same half of the visual field converge onto the same side of the brain. This anatomical feature is at the basis of binocular vision. By contrast, in the mouse, less than 3% of the temporal RGCs project ipsilaterally (compared to about 45% in primates) and binocular vision is limited (Fukuda et al., 1989; Guillery et al., 1995). The choice made by growing RGC axons to cross or not to cross occurs at the optic chiasm, around E13 in the mouse (Godement et al., 1990). Many studies have shown that in albino mammals, including humans, there is an important reduction of the size of the ipsilateral contingent or RGC axons, which underlies the visual deficits (Guillery and Kaas, 1973; Lund, 1965; Neveu et al., 2003). How tyrosinase, which is expressed in the developing retina, controls axon guidance is still unknown (Ray et al., 2007). In albino mice, less ipsilaterally projecting RGCs are generated in the retina, suggesting that temporal RGCs do not differentiate properly and fail to express molecules that are required to prevent their axon from crossing upon reaching the chiasm (Rebsam et al., 2012). The identity of these molecules is still unknown but in rodents, recent progress has been made on the characterization of the genetic determinants that specify ipsilaterally and contralaterally projecting RGCs. Transcription factors such as Zic2 and islet2 are involved as well as the axon guidance molecules NrCAM, Semaphorins, EphB1 and even VEGF (Erskine et al., 2011; Herrera et al., 2003; Kuwajima et al., 2012; Pak et al., 2004; Petros et al., 2008; Williams et al., 2006).

Other extreme cases of visual projection defects have been described in congenital achiasmatic patients (Nondecussating retinal-fugal syndrome; Apkarian et al., 1994) whose optic nerves only project ipsilaterally. Interestingly, these patients not only lack binocular vision, but also show a profound rearrangement of their retinotopic map in the visual striate cortex; such as a significant overlap of the temporal and nasal retina representations (Hoffmann et al., 2012). In humans, there is to date no clear genetic basis for congenital achiasma, but one strain of achiasmatic Belgian sheepdogs has been identified (Williams et al., 1994).

Corticospinal Tract In mammals, the corticospinal tract (CST) connects layer 5 pyramidal neurons in the motor cortex to the spinal cord. In rodents CST axons innervate mostly interneurons in the dorsal spinal cord, whereas in primates they make direct contacts with motor neurons (Canty and Murphy, 2008; ten Donkelaar et al., 2004). In the mouse, CST axons reach the spinal cord around birth but the CST still develops for 2–3 more weeks postnatally (Canty and Murphy, 2008). Initially, many neurons outside the motor cortex also project to the spinal cord but they are eliminated later (Stanfield et al., 1982). Likewise, during development, CST axons send collateral

branches to various brain areas, most of which are being pruned later except in the basilar pons (Luo and O'Leary, 2005). Upon reaching the spinal cord, about 85% of the CST axons leave the ventral part of the medulla (the pyramids) to grow dorsally and cross the midline to continue contralaterally in the dorsal funiculus (Canty and Murphy, 2008; ten Donkelaar et al., 2004). The CST crossover point is also known as the pyramidal decussation.

In several human neurological diseases, the crossing of CST axons is perturbed (Table 8.1), which can lead to to motor deficits, such as mirror movements (MM). MM patients involuntary perform a bilateral and symmetric movement when intending a unilateral one (Gallea et al., 2011). MM have been described in Joubert syndrome and related disorders (JSRD), Klippel-feil and Kalmann syndrome (Engle, 2010). In all these cases, the molecular and cellular mechanisms underlying the abnormal pyramidal decussation are still unknown and neurological deficits are quite extensive. For instance, at least seven genes are mutated in JSRD patients and they affect primary cilia or ciliogenesis without any obvious link to CST axon guidance (Lee and Gleeson, 2011a). However, recent studies have shed light onto the etiology of other MM disorders.

Autosomal dominant mutations in the DCC receptor were identified in several MM families, without other obvious neurological defects (Depienne et al., 2011; Djarmati-Westenberger et al., 2011; Srour et al., 2010). In these patients, truncated DCC receptors (interrupted after Ig domain 2 or 3) are produced, which most likely alters DCC/netrin1 signaling. CST axons express the receptors DCC and UNC5c and their ligand netrin-1 is highly expressed by floor plate cells (Finger et al., 2002). However, the mis-positioning of the CST could rather be linked to the abnormal and lateral location of the inferior olive seen in DCC and Netrin-1 KO (Marcos et al., 2009), as this brainstem nucleus was proposed to guide CST axons (Runker et al., 2008). In the Unc5h3 mutant, there is a defasciculation and abnormal decussation of CST axons, and DCC[kanga] mutants (which is a hypomorphic DCC allele) exhibit synchronous movements of their hindlimbs (kangaroo-gait) and bilateral projection of the CST in the spinal cord. This suggests that in the patients abnormal CST crossing is at the origin of MM. However, reduced commissural projections of spinal cord interneurons across the midline has also been described in DCC and Netrin-1 knockout mice and might contribute to the locomotor deficits (Rabe Bernhardt et al., 2012; Rabe et al., 2009).

More recently, autosomal dominant mutations in the *RAD51* gene were found in other MM families (Depienne et al., 2012; Méneret et al., 2014). RAD51 plays a role in DNA repair (Suwaki et al., 2011), and although it is expressed in the mouse CST, how it influences CST axon guidance is still mysterious (Klar, 2014).

Other molecules, which control the development of mouse CST, have been identified but there is so far no genetic evidence supporting their involvement in MM. CST axons express EphA4 (Kuwajima et al., 2012) and EphA7 (Rogers et al., 1999) when its ligand ephrinB3 is expressed in the floor plate. In EphA4 and ephrinB3 knockout mice, which exhibit kangaroo gait, reduced repulsion results in an increase of midline crossing by CST and spinal cord commissural axons (Coonan et al., 2001; Rashid et al., 2005). Abnormal CST crossing and defasciculation have also been observed in L1CAM knockout mice (Castellani et al., 2000; Cohen et al., 1998), which could be due to abnormal Sema3A signaling. Although patients with mutations in L1-CAM were first thought to have CST axon guidance defect, this was not confirmed by more recent analyses (Dobson et al., 2001; Fransen et al., 1998; Graf et al., 2000). Last, in mice deficient for Sema6A or its receptor PlexinA4, a significant subset of CTS axons extends ventrally in the ipsilateral spinal cord (Faulkner et al., 2008; Runker et al., 2008).

HGPPS Horizontal gaze palsy with progressive scoliosis (HGPPS) is a rare autosomal recessive disorder, which is associated with oculomotor disorders and a severe scoliosis (Dretakis and Kondoyannis, 1974).

Physiological and brain imaging studies have shown that in most HGPPS patients the CST does not decussate and projects in the ipsilateral spinal cord (Amoiridis et al., 2006; Bosley et al., 2005; Jen et al., 2004). In addition, ascending sensory projections from the spinal cord are also ipsilateral and major hindbrain commissures seem to lack (Haller et al., 2008). However, the corpus callosum and anterior commissure are still present. All HGPPS patients carry mutations in the *ROBO3* gene (Abu-Amero et al., 2009; Chan et al., 2006; Jen et al., 2004), which encodes a transmembrane receptor of the Ig superfamily (Yuan et al., 1999). In *Robo3* knockout mice, all hindbrain and spinal cord commissures fail to form and axons contact their targets but on the ipsilateral side of the brain (Badura et al., 2013; Marillat et al., 2004; Michalski et al., 2013; Renier et al., 2010; Sabatier et al., 2004). Although *Robo3* knockout mice die at birth of respiratory failure (Bouvier et al., 2010), before the CST enters the spinal cord, the absence of Robo3 expression in layer V pyramidal neurons (Barber et al., 2009) suggests that CST defects might be secondary to the existence of a midline cleft along the brainstem, which could physically prevent CST axons from crossing. Conditional deletion of the *Robo3* gene in a mouse model showed that the migration of the abducens neurons is perturbed, but that the abducens nerve still connects to the LR. By contrast, the abducens interneurons project to the ipsilateral III nucleus instead of the contralateral one. These mice also exhibit horizontal gaze palsy. This phenotype is also observed in Robo3 mutant mice, which lack the inferior olivary commissure. Together, these data suggest that in HGPPS patients the abnormal eye movements are caused by a miswiring of commissural connections in the hindbrain and not by hypoplasia of oculomotor nuclei or a defect of EOM innervation.

Corpus Callosum It is estimated that about half of the commissural axons belong to the corpus callosum, which primarily connects homotopic areas of the two cerebral hemispheres (Paul et al., 2007). Complete or partial cortical agenesis (about 0.1–0.6% individuals) is observed in a variety of human diseases (most often together with other defects). DTI studies suggest that human cortical agenesis results in noticeable rearrangements of interhemispheric and subcortical projections (Owen et al., 2013). Likewise, in some acallosal mouse mutants, a large fraction of cortical neurons are rerouted to the anterior commissure (Britanova et al., 2008). Callosal agenesis is a heterogeneous and multifactorial condition but in a few cases, mutations in axon guidance molecules have been found (Paul et al., 2007; Table 1). Mutations in Disrupted-in-Schizoprenia-1 (DISC1), a gene previously involved schizophrenia, have been discovered in individuals with agenesis of the corpus callosum (Duff et al., 2013; Osbun et al., 2011). Callosal dysgenesis has also been described in DISC1 mutant mice (Shen et al., 2008). DISC1 is a cytosolic protein that interacts with multiple partners, many of which, such as GSK3β, Kinesin-1, LIS1 (lissencephaly-1), and NDEL1 (nuclear distribution element-like 1), play a role in the regulation of cytoskeleton dynamics during axon guidance and neuronal migration (Porteous et al., 2011). Interestingly, a subset of *TUBB3* mutations can also lead to corpus callosum defects (Poirier et al., 2010; Tischfield et al., 2010).

Corpus callosum agenesis was observed in human and mouse with mutations in the transcription factor Nf1a (Nuclear factor Ia; Ji et al., 2014; Rao et al., 2014; Shu et al., 2003). This is most likely due to the abnormal development of cortical midline glia structures, which normally guide callosal axons (Kang et al., 2012). In addition, Nf1a also regulates the expression of N-cadherin and ephrinB1 (Wang et al., 2007).

Last, in MASA syndrome (Mental retardation, Aphasia, Shuffling gait and Adducted thumbs) also known as CRASH syndrome (Corpus callosum hypoplasia, Retardation, Adducted thumbs, Spastic paraplegia, and Hydrocephalus), patients suffer from multiple neurological deficits and exhibit callosal hypoplasia (Fransen et al., 1998). They carry mutations in the L1CAM gene, which is on the X chromosome. As mentioned before, L1 plays multiple roles in axon guidance both as a homophilic cell-adhesion molecule and as a component of the semaphorin 3A receptor complex (Castellani et al., 2000).

8.4 CONTRIBUTION OF AXON GUIDANCE GENES TO NEUROPSYCHIATRIC DISORDERS

Recently, genetic, functional, and experimental evidence has linked axon guidance genes to a wide array of neurodevelopmental disorders with neuropsychiatric manifestations (Table 2). Given the incomplete knowledge of molecular hallmarks of many of these diseases, the exact nature of underlying aberrancies remains debatable at this point. Interestingly, although obvious wiring deficits are not always readily observable in these diseases, a growing body of evidence suggests new mechanisms of well-known axon guidance molecules in different cellular functions such as synaptogenesis, possibly contributing to the appearance of diverse clinical conditions characteristic for many neurological disorders.

8.4.1 Axon Guidance Molecules in Neuropsychiatric Diseases – Emerging Concepts

The Neurodevelopmental Hypothesis of Schizophrenia Schizophrenia is a multifactorial psychiatric illness affecting about 1% of the human population worldwide. Its wide range of symptoms is commonly subdivided into three categories, including positive symptoms (hallucinations, delusions, thought and movement disorders), negative symptoms (avolition, anhedonia, flattened affect) and cognitive deficits, majorly related to working memory impairment as well as attentive and executive dysfunctions (Napal et al., 2012). On top of fMRI studies shedding light on global and regional dysconnectivity occurrences in schizophrenia, today's molecular understanding of the disease ranks primarily around two neurotransmitter-based hypotheses, where the classical dopamine-centered approach recently finds itself more and more subverted by emerging evidence for a glutamatergic hypofunction as the firsthand underlying cause of the schizophrenic phenotype (Gordon, 2010). In this paragraph, we will summarize findings supporting the involvement of genes that regulate axon guidance in schizophrenia.

Disconnectivity Hypothesis of the Schizophrenic Brain – A Developmental Origin? In addition to cellular and genetic underpinnings of schizophrenia discussed subsequently, neuroimaging connectomic studies using functional or structural MRI and diffusion tensor imaging (DTI) have greatly contributed to fuel our understanding of the disease in a translational way. The "disconnectivity hypothesis" of schizophrenia has already gained a lot of attention early on in the history of schizophrenia research. Fundamental improvements in imaging techniques have allowed for unprecedented insight into brain connectivity in patients. Given the heterogeneous causes of schizophrenia, inconsistency in findings across studies is not surprising; however, certain structural hallmarks of gray and white matter abnormalities in schizophrenia have emerged (Canu et al., 2014; van den Heuvel and Fornito, 2014; Wheeler and Voineskos, 2014). While the long-reaching white matter tracts are greatly important for interregional connectivity, gray matter connections play a role in both, inter- and intraregional neuronal communication. Thus, both components are likely to be altered in a disconnected schizophrenic brain. Risk factors for schizophrenia have been identified already in pre- and perinatal life periods and are thought to affect neuronal migration and wiring of early neural circuitry (Karlsgodt et al., 2008), hence supporting a strong developmental component long before occurrence of the symptomatic clinical condition. Building on this conceptual framework, microarray data from primate cortex shows differential expression of a wide variety of axon guidance molecules including Semaphorins, Plexins, Eph and ephrins, Cxcr4,

Robos, and Slits between 3 and 6 months of age (Sasaki et al., 2014), which corresponds to a cycle of axon target refinement and pruning, known to be a susceptibility period for autism and schizophrenia. Further evidence for this hypothesis stems from the observation of a correlation of dynamic changes in structural and functional connectivity during normal development, which seems to be uncoupled in schizophrenia (Griffa et al., 2013).

8.4.2 Semaphorins and Plexins in Schizophrenia

Genetic Studies Identifying Semaphorin and Plexin Risk Loci in Schizophrenia Genome-wide association studies on single nucleotide polymorphisms (SNPs) have lead to the investigation of PlexinA2 (PLXNA2) on chromosome 1q32 as a susceptibility locus for schizophrenia. However, following the first identification of an intronic SNP in the PLXNA2 gene as a candidate locus in a European-American population (Mah et al., 2006), a Japanese study failed to confirm the finding (Fujii et al., 2007). In 2008, a meta-analysis combining the data from both studies supported a positive link to schizophrenia (Allen et al., 2008). In the latest and largest GWAS, PLXNA2 did not emerge as a candidate gene for schizophrenia (Ripke et al., 2013), but interestingly, Sema3G was identified as a possible risk locus. The discrepancy of these large genetic studies, does not rule out the possibility that rare mutations in PLXNA2 could contribute to the disease in some individuals. Interestingly, a common variant in the *SEMA3D* gene, leading to an amino acid change (Lys701Gln), seems to be prevalent among control subjects as compared to schizophrenic patients and may thus confer a protective effect (Fujii et al., 2011). Investigating the biological consequence of this mutation on Sema3D structure and signaling may help reveal novel molecular mechanisms in schizophrenia. Intriguingly, the same study identifies a distinct haplotype in the *SEMA3D* gene that does not include the Lys701Gln mutation, but yet is associated with schizophrenia, providing additional proof that Semaphorins are promising candidates in the hunt for susceptibility genes in schizophrenia.

Schizophrenia and Autism – Genetic Implication of Axon Guidance Networks Considering several converging symptoms and neurobiological correlates in schizophrenia and autism (de Lacy and King, 2013), it is worth briefly mentioning genetic findings implicating axon guidance molecules in autism.

A few studies show a possible involvement of Robo genes in autism (Anitha et al., 2008), identifying SNPs in Robo3 and Robo4 gene in autistic patients alongside mRNA-changes in Robo1 and Robo2 in peripheral lymphocytes, making Robo genes a putative candidate for a peripheral biomarker in this disease. Interestingly, in Drosophila, the Serotonin-transporter SerT is under positive transcriptional control of Robo2 and Robo3 (Couch et al., 2004). The serotonergic system is critical for higher cognitive functions and networks underlying social interactions disrupted in ASD (Ciranna and Catania, 2014).

Even though decreased Sema5A expression has been found in genetic studies on autistic patients (Melin et al., 2006; Weiss et al., 2009), an exhaustive behavioral analysis of Sema5A knockout mice did not show gross abnormalities and thus questions the importance of this gene or at least suitability of this model in autism pathogenesis (Gunn et al., 2011).

A study analyzing the correlation between several haplotypes of the PlexinB2 (*PLXNB2*) gene with white matter volume and cognitive performance in healthy versus schizophrenic individuals failed to show any direct association with the disease (Rujescu et al., 2007).

A thorough and exhaustive behavioral analysis of the *Sema6A* knockout mice has elegantly proven its suitability as a model for schizophrenia and autism spectrum disorders. Behavioral phenotypes reminiscent of schizophrenic symptoms could be reversed by treatment of the animals with antipsychotics, further supporting the credibility and pathophysiological relevance of the described model (Rünker et al., 2011).

A recent computational approach to clustering schizophrenia susceptibility genes and assigning the identified clusters to biological functions shows that most of the implied networks rank around axon guidance, neuronal migration, synaptic processes, and chromatin remodeling. Further specific analysis of individual genes in these clusters may provide additional insight into the implementations of axon guidance molecules in the manifestation of schizophrenia (Gilman et al., 2012).

Semaphorins and Plexins in Schizophrenia – Axonal Guidance versus Synaptic Functions Considering the widespread and multifaceted functions of Semaphorins and Plexins, it is not surprising that their genetic dysregulation may contribute to a variety of diseases. Increased expression of Sema3A in the cerebellum has been proposed to cause a decrease of synaptic markers at the granule cell – Purkinje synapse in the molecular layer in postmortem studies of schizophrenic patients (Eastwood et al., 2003). Coincidently, increased hippocampal levels of the Sema3A effector collapsin response mediator 2 (CRMP2) have been reported (Edgar et al., 2000) in schizophrenia, suggesting that the chemorepulsive activity of Semaphorins contributes to the synaptic pathology seen in schizophrenic patients. Interestingly, CRMP1 knockout mice show deficits in hippocampal long-term potentiation and perform poorly in spatial learning and memory tasks (Su et al., 2007), which may correlate with some of the cognitive symptoms seen in schizophrenic patients.

Several lines of evidence specifically address the contribution of Semaphorins to synaptogenesis and synaptic plasticity, from which putative hypotheses about the molecular mechanism of the schizophrenic phenotype may be derived: a high-throughput RNAi-based screen in cultured hippocampal neurons reveals the involvement of Sema4B in glutamatergic and GABAergic synaptic development, whereas Sema4D appears to only regulate the formation of GABAergic synapses (Paradis et al., 2007). Intriguingly, these two transmitter systems are central to the neurochemical paradigm of schizophrenia pathogenesis (see Introduction). Knockdown of Sema5B in primary hippocampal neurons leads to an increase in synapse number and size of pre- and postsynaptical compartments (O'Connor et al., 2009). Additionally, the phenotypes of *Sema3F*, *Neuropilin-2*, and *PlexinA3* knockout mice include increased spine densities in defined hippocampal and cortical neuronal populations (Reviewed in Tran et al., 2007).

Taken together, these mechanistic studies on Semaphorin function at the synapse and the phenotypic consequences that can be drawn thereof, suggest the schizophrenic phenotype may more likely depend on post-axonal guidance functions of these developmentally important molecules.

Schizophrenia – Axon Guidance or Synaptic Disease? In summary, not only these and other genetic studies (Gilman et al., 2012; Meda et al., 2014), but also proteomic profiling of susceptible brain regions, such as the amygdala (Fernandez-Irigoyen et al., 2014), make schizophrenia appear as a mixed, synaptic, and axonal disease, which comprehensively reflects multifaceted symptoms seen in patients.

The findings reviewed in this paragraph propose a role for molecules originally described for their function in axon guidance during neural circuit formation in the developing CNS in schizophrenia. However, the cellular mechanisms underlying the observed phenotypes often remain elusive, and one can only speculate about a possible link to axon guidance, especially considering the growing body of evidence supporting a role for these molecules in synaptogenesis and plasticity (reviewed in Shen and Cowan, 2010).

To integrate these findings in a broader picture, one should consider the nature of molecular imprints related to schizophrenia seamlessly, taking into account several concerted steps of neuronal circuit formation such as axon navigation and synaptogenesis – two intricately coupled and overlapping processes. An example of molecular support for the hypothesis that schizophrenia is a manifestation of errors in multiple steps of establishing neuronal networks

during development, stems from studies on SynCAMs (synaptic cell adhesion molecules), which have been shown to function in both, synaptogenesis and axon guidance (Frei and Stoeckli, 2014) and mutations have been identified in patients suffering from neurodevelopmental disorders (Melom and Littleton, 2011; Zoghbi and Bear, 2012).

Atypical Mechanisms of Axon Guidance Molecules in Schizophrenia Further unconventional – and to date speculative – molecular hypotheses about the neurobiology of schizophrenia involving axon guidance events have been proposed. For example, knockout mice for the NCAM (neural cell adhesion molecule) to PSA-NCAM (polysialylated-neural cell adhesion molecule) glycosylation enzyme ST8SIA2 show hippocampal axon guidance defects and ectopic synapses (Angata et al., 2004) altering fear behavior. An importance for this finding in human patients furthermore stems from genetic studies of the *St8Sia2* locus (Anney et al., 2010; Kamien et al., 2014; Lee and Gleeson, 2011b).

Evidence for a crucial role of glycosylation events in axon guidance during development is widespread (Avram et al., 2014), and analyses of functional consequences are constantly emerging. One study shows that sensory deficits related to olfaction seen in schizophrenic patients might be partly due to aberrant CSPG (chondroitin sulfate proteoglycan) expression on olfactory receptor neurons disrupting axon targeting in the olfactory epithelium (Pantazopoulos et al., 2013).

An increased risk of schizophrenia and autism linked to maternal infection during gestation has been shown by various studies (Meyer et al., 2011) and a recent study (Lucchese et al., 2014) takes on an original explanatory approach to this issue by showing that axon guidance proteins such as Semaphorins, Robo receptors, and others share unique pentapeptide sequences with known Influenza hemagglutinin epitopes, speculating about possible immune-cross-reactivity mechanisms between these molecules leading to autoimmune attacks in the fetus.

8.4.3 Slitrks in Tourette Syndrome and Other Neuronal Diseases

Gilles de la Tourette Syndrome (GTS) Gilles de la Tourette syndrome (GTS) is a neurodevelopmental disease characterized by behavioral abnormalities such as motor tics and phonic tics, which usually follow a few years later. GTS is a worldwide disease of biological origin with a prevalence between 0.4% and 3.8% in children between 5 and 17 years, depending on country and study (Deng et al., 2012). The average childhood onset of GTS is 7 years, with a significant decrease in symptom severity in early adulthood (18–21 years (Paschou, 2013). Motor tics are involuntary, recurrent, and arythmic rapid or slow movements such as eye blinking, throat clearing, or coughing and verbal tics include echolalia, palilalia, and coprolalia. The consistent observation that the condition is eased during adolescence points to a developmental origin of the disease, which may be partially suppressed or compensated for during brain maturation through remodeling and plasticity mechanisms (Jackson et al., 2011; see the subsequent sections). The etiology of GTS is thought to be primarily rooted in genetic abnormalities; however, its heterogeneous phenotype and an up to 90% comorbidity rate of neuropsychological complications such as ADHD (attention deficit hyperactivity disorder) and OCD (obsessive compulsive disorder), as well as certain genetic similarities to ASD (autism spectrum disorders) suggest a combination of genetic and environmental causes in the pathogenesis of the disease (Robertson, 2012). There is no cure for GTS and its waxing and waning nature makes pharmacological approaches quite challenging (McNaught and Mink, 2011).

The Family of Slitrks Initial name giving suggested structural similarities of the six Slitrks with two other members of the LRR family of proteins, the Slits (reflected by the presence of two LRR domains in their extracellular domain) and the Trk neurotrophin receptors (Ntrks) (for their intracellular domain; Aruga and

Mikoshiba, 2003). However, a comprehensive *in silico* analysis of the LRR superfamily proteome across species reveals evolutionary divergence among Slits, Ntrks, and Slitrks (Dolan et al., 2007). Within the Slitrk family, Slitrk1 with its short cytoplasmic tail structurally stands out, since it lacks the common Trk-like tyrosine residues found in other Slitrks. In humans and rodents, genes encoding the Slitrk proteins are clustered within three chromosomal locations (Aruga et al., 2003).

The unique and only partially overlapping expression patterns of the six Slitrks in the developing CNS suggest different roles in the regulation and maintenance of neuronal circuits. Slitrk mRNAs can be detected as early as embryonic stage E9 in the mouse and continuous expression of Slitrk isoforms is observed throughout embryogenesis and up to postnatal day 10 (for more detailed regional expression data, the reader is referred to (Beaubien and Cloutier, 2009)). Remarkably, Slitrk1 has been found in projection neurons of the CSTC (cortico-striatal-thalamocortical) system, a neuronal network implicated in the pathophysiology of GTS. Furthermore, Slitrk expression was reported in somatodendritic compartments and intracellular vesicles in cortical pyramidal neurons in an evolutionarily conserved manner (Stillman et al., 2009). Slitrk6 expression differs the most from other family members in that it is restricted to only a few brain regions (thalamus, putamen, lateral geniculate nucleus, and auditory system).

Genetic Evidence for Slitrk1 in GTS Since the first case study of a de novo chromosomal inversion on 13q31.1 in a child with Tourette syndrome led to a candidate-driven identification of Slitrk1 350 bp from the breakpoint (Abelson et al., 2005), the implications of Slitrk1 in GTS have been a matter of intense debate. Motivated by the single-case study, the Slitrk1 gene was resequenced in larger cohorts of patients with GTS ($n = 174$), revealing two additional mutations with functional consequences referred to as varCDf, producing a truncated protein and the missense variant 321 (var321) respectively (O'Roak et al., 2010). The frameshift mutation leading to the truncated gene product (varCDf) was shown to be less efficient in promoting dendritic outgrowth in cortical pyramidal neurons. var321 shows altered binding to hsa-miR-189, a micro RNA whose expression overlaps significantly with Slitrk1 mRNA during development in neuronal circuits implicated in GTS and presence of var321 decreased Slitrk1 wildtype mRNA. The contradictory results of a huge variety of genetic GTS studies aiming at elucidating the role of abnormalities in the Slitrk1 gene are most likely attributable to population stratifications; however, a recent review (Paschou, 2013) summarizing the genetic data concludes with an overall importance of the Slitrk1 gene as a susceptibility locus for the development of GTS.

Network Imbalances and Cellular Mechanisms in GTS Related to Slitrk1 The clinical condition of GTS is accompanied by a wide variety of neuroanatomical changes that have led to the identification of certain neuronal networks as the most promising target regions for treatment options. However, it remains unclear, whether these neurological differences are the actual underlying causes of the disease or rather manifestations of adaptations that have occurred to compensate for behavioral deficits such as involuntary tic movements (Felling and Singer, 2011). The cellular paradigm that has received broad attention centers the CSTC network as responsible for neuronal activity imbalances in GTS. As also described for other hyperkinetic movement disorders, the motor tics are thought to stem from cortical over-excitability and basal ganglia circuit dysfunction. Stillman et al. (2009) have taken a direct approach to probing the possible involvement of Slitrk1 in CSTC function, by studying its expression and subcellular localization in mice, monkeys, and humans. Interestingly, during development, Slitrk1 was detected in apical dendrites of pyramidal neurons found in cortical layers 3, 5, and 6. Correlated with a role for basal ganglia circuits in GTS, Slitrk1 expression was confined to medium-size spiny neurons,

which are indicative of the direct excitatory output pathway from the striatum to the medial globus pallidus and substantia nigra, providing evidence for the importance of this signaling axis in the pathophysiology of the disease. Slitrk1 did not colocalize with markers for the indirect pathway. In the adult, Slitrk expression in the striatum was only found in cholinergic interneurons.

Overall, these findings support the genetic observations for a possible implication of Slitrk in GTS and further cellular and molecular studies of Slitrk function may additionally shed light on the pathogenesis of the disease. Two knockout mouse models for Slitrk1 and Slitrk5 (see the subsequent section) also aided in clarifying the genomical studies regarding the importance of Slitrk gene loci in the neuropsychological phenotype of GTS. Behavioral studies on *Slitrk1*$^{-/-}$ mice reported increased anxiety and depressive traits in this model, which could be eased by treatment with α-adrenergic agonists, also commonly used for treatment of tics and comorbidities in GTS patients (Katayama et al., 2010). Furthermore, increases in norepinephrine in various brain regions of Slitrk1 null mice mirror a hallmark of GTS in human patients (Leckman et al., 2010).

Another interesting neuroanatomical feature in GTS patients is a reduced area and decreased number of inter-hemispheric axonal connections in the corpus callosum (Paul, 2011; Plessen et al., 2006). Given the number of axon guidance diseases that are accompanied with a dysgenesis of the corpus callosum, it will be of great interest to study a possible axon guidance defect in GTS models, which may reveal further insight into pathophysiological mechanisms underlying this disease during early brain development.

Are Slitrks More Broadly Implicated in Neuropsychological Disorders? Considering the heterogenous phenotype and the strikingly high comorbidity rate of GTS with other neuropsychological disorders, it is not far-fetched to investigate a possible role of Slitrk molecules in a broader context of comorbid phenotypes of GTS. Slitrk5$^{-/-}$ mice have recently been described (Shmelkov et al., 2010) with increased anxiety and self-grooming behavior, a phenotype, which could be partially rescued by treatment with SSRIs (selective serotonin reuptake inhibitors), commonly used to treat OCD and depression. This mouse model further resembles functional disruptions seen in human patients with OCD that show a basal-ganglia dependent overactivation of orbitofrontal–subcortical circuits. Substantially, the striatum of Slitrk5$^{-/-}$ mice shows cell morphological aberrancies, another important aspect that relates Slitrk5 function to the underlying neuroanatomical changes responsible for the clinical manifestation of OCD.

Trichotillomania (TTM), the incessant need to pull out one's own hair, is considered an OCD spectrum disorder that has attracted the attention of geneticists in a follow-up study (Zuchner et al., 2006) to the first finding of Slitrk1 mutations in GTS, since the mother of an affected child had been diagnosed with TTM. Two amino acid substitutions, distinct from what had been described for Slitrk1 in GTS, were thus found in a population screening of European descent further underlining the implications of the Slitrk protein family in neuropsychological disorders (Chattopadhyay and Chatterjee, 2012).

Slitrk6-Related Defects in Cochlear Development Apart from neuropsychological diseases, Slitrk6 has been shown to be crucially important for the development of the vestibular and auditory system in mice (Katayama et al., 2009) and very recently the auditory phenotype of human subjects with Slitrk6 nonsense mutations has been described in great detail (Morlet et al., 2014). Slitrk6 is prominently expressed in thalamic nuclei and sensory epithelia of the inner ear. Slitrk6$^{-/-}$ mice have reduced innervation in the cochlea and misguided innervation in the vestibular system alongside with increased apoptosis of spiral and vestibular ganglion cells. Slitrk6 knockout animals have decreased mRNA levels of NT-3 and BDNF as well decreased protein levels of TrkB, TrkC, and phospho-Trk suggesting that

this global reduction in neurotrophic signaling causes auditory and vestibular phenotypes in Slitrk6$^{-/-}$ mice. However, it does not explain the axon guidance defects also observed in this model. Interestingly, Slitrk6 knockout animals show almost no behavioral phenotype, besides an altered response to a novel environment hinting at a subtle function possibly in cognitive processing (Matsumoto et al., 2011).

8.4.4 Neurodegenerative Lessons From Neurodevelopmental Concepts?

The inclusion of a neurodegenerative disease such as AD in a comprehensive review of neurodevelopmental disorders may appear counterintuitive at first; however, as discussed subsequently, certain lines of evidence reveal surprising coadjutant mechanisms regulating neurodevelopment and particular aspects of neurodegeneration.

The intriguing possibility of a mechanistic connection between generation and degeneration of the nervous system has been extensively fueled by the establishment of transgenic mouse models allowing for an investigation of brain phenotypes that initially attracted attention in neurodegenerative research for the field of neurodevelopment. As the following paragraph will summarize, this can be exemplified by taking an unconventional perspective on the biology of the Alzheimer-related amyloid precursor protein (APP), especially by investigating its physiological role in development, which may give hints to cellular pathogenic mechanisms in disease.

Alzheimer's Disease Alzheimer's Disease (AD) is the most common form of dementia in the elderly and given the demographic change of western societies, its burden not only for the individual, but also for the health care system is detrimental. The estimate for prevalence of AD by 2050 calculates the number of affected individuals at about 106 million, which reflects an at least four times increase as compared to reported cases in 2006 (Brookmeyer et al., 2007; D'Onofrio et al., 2012).

The pathological hallmarks of AD are extracellular deposits of fibrillogenic amyloid beta peptide aggregates (senile plaques), chronologically followed by the intracellular appearance of neurofibrillary tangles (NFTs) with paired helical filaments (PHFs), containing hyperphosphorylated tau and other specific phosphoproteins (Rudrabhatla et al., 2011; Serrano-Pozo et al., 2011). These pathological lesions coincide with reactive astrogliosis and activation of microglial cells, which altogether ultimately lead to synaptic loss and neuronal cell death thought to be the molecular correlate for the clinically manifestant cognitive decline seen in AD patients (Walsh and Selkoe, 2004).

The amyloid hypothesis states that the over-accumulation of oligomeric Aβ species triggers the pathological cascade and is supported by genomic evidence of familial Alzheimer's Disease (FAD), in which mutations in three genes have shown to be causative for AD symptoms: Amyloid Precursor Protein (APP), and Presenilin-1 (PS1) and -2 (PS2; Bettens et al., 2013) alongside with a recent finding of a point mutation in APP that confers a protective effect against AD (Jonsson et al., 2012). Functional disruption in these genes shares a common outcome, namely the overproduction of fibrillogenic Aβ species by favoring the amyloidogenic APP processing pathway mediated by initial β-secretase cleavage (β-Site Amyloid Precursor Protein (APP)-cleaving Enzyme 1, BACE1) followed by the intramembraneous gamma-secretase complex cleavage (including presenilin as the catalytic core), ultimately releasing the 40–42 amino acid peptide Aβ (Wang et al., 2012). A decreased ratio of Aβ42/40 in the cerebrospinal fluid serves as an early indicator for at risk individuals (Hansson et al., 2007). Interestingly, the protective mutation found in an Icelandic population (Jonsson et al., 2012) is situated near the BACE cleavage site and may thus hint at over-activity of β-secretase being pathologically inclined in the disease. However, further studies are warranted to confirm this.

Nevertheless, certain obstacles about the pathogenesis of AD and current molecular hypothesis remain, especially given the fact that to date no transgenic mouse model exists that faithfully and completely resembles the human condition (Ashe and Zahs, 2010; Aydin et al., 2012). Furthermore, post mortem studies show that Aβ load and plaque deposition by itself is a poor predictability factor for cognitive decline; however, the chronological occurrence of NFTs (and PHF) correlates strongly with clinically apparent memory impairment and is furthermore the sole underlying cause of other types of dementia in the class of neurodegenerative tauopathies (Arriagada et al., 1992).

APP Dependent Axon Pruning During Development – A Role in Neurodegeneration?

During the establishment of neuronal networks in the developing brain, a delicate balance between formation of proper connections and removal of improperly targeted interactions is crucial to the construction of final functional synaptic connectivity. It has been met with the appropriate excitement when death receptor 6 (DR6) was described as a cognate receptor for an N-terminal APP fragment, mediating axonal pruning during development (Nikolaev et al., 2009). The striking finding that DR6 was also found in the adult brain in regions implicated in AD (primarily cortical and hippocampal localizations) and the fact that both, APP and DR6 have shown to be enriched in damaged axons (Medana, 2003), make assumptions about a putative role in neurodegeneration not far-fetched. This possibility is especially intriguing given that the exact function of DR6 has already been described in a developmental context, suggesting that a similar "self-destruction" – mechanism may be exploited patho-physiologically in the degeneration of neurons during later-on diseases.

It is noteworthy that the APP-triggered DR6-dependent axonal degeneration described (Nikolaev et al., 2009) is initiated by trophic factor deprivation, in turn, leading to BACE dependent APP-cleavage. This finding may be complementary to the so called axonal transport (Stokin et al., 2005) and "neurotrophic hypothesis" of AD, which suggests that axonal injury leads to impaired axonal transport of neurotrophic factors and their receptors consequently imbalancing the localization of these molecules (Schindowski et al., 2008).

FE65- an APP Binding Protein with Axonal Guidance Properties during Development The family of Fe65 proteins (Fe65, Fe65L1, Fe65L2) interacts with the APP intracellular domain created (AICD) by γ-secretase cleavage of APP and APP like proteins (APLP1, APLP2) and is involved in transcriptional activation after translocation to the nucleus either together or separately from APP (for review see (Bórquez and González-Billault, 2012; King and Scott Turner, 2004; McLoughlin and Miller, 2008; Schettini et al., 2010)). Even though somewhat controversial in the consistency of their finding, transcriptional target genes of Fe65 may include BACE1, GSK3β, Neprilysin, and APP itself- all of which are implicated in the pathogenesis of AD. BACE1$^{-/-}$ mice, exhibit olfactory sensory neuron and hippocampal axon guidance defects, most likely due to aberrant processing of the BACE1 substrate CHL1 (close homolog of L1; Cao et al., 2012; Hitt et al., 2012; Rajapaksha et al., 2011; Vassar et al., 2014). Although Fe65 is the only isoform exclusively found in the brain (Kesavapany et al., 2002), Fe65 knockout mice have no phenotypic abnormalities. However, *Fe65/Fe65L1* double knockouts exhibit neuronal heterotopia and severe axon mistargeting defects (Guénette et al., 2006) such as an agenesis of the corpus callosum and a lack of hippocampal infrapyramidal mossy fibers. This phenotype is reminiscent of *APP:APLP1:APLP2* triple knockout animals as well as *Mena*$^{-/-}$ transgenic mice (Herms et al., 2004; Lanier et al., 1999) and furthermore lissencephalopathic conditions in humans (Ross and Walsh, 2001). Fe65 and Mena interact through the Fe65WW domain, suggesting a role for this protein complex in actin cytoskeleton remodeling of growth cone architecture during development (Minopoli et al., 2012). Further mechanistic analysis comes from a recent study showing that Fe65 regulates neurite outgrowth via activation of Arf6 (Cheung et al., 2014).

The Physiological Role of APP in Axon Guidance and Cortical Migration Although the pathological role of APP processing in AD is rather well established, the physiological function of APP *in vivo* has long remained elusive. Strikingly, recent findings pinpoint a critical role during development, especially related to cortical migration and chemoattractive axonal signaling in commissure formation at the ventral midline of the CNS.

It has been shown that acute knockdown of APP by RNA interference lead to a decrease of neuronal precursors entering the cortical plate, whereas overexpression of APP accelerated migration, thus suggesting APP may be normally required for correct formation of cortical layering in the rodent brain. This also involves disrupted-in-schizophrenia-1 (DISC1), which acts downstream of APP to regulate cortical migration (Young-Pearse et al., 2010). A recent study provides evidence for a role of APP in commissure formation in the developing CNS. Netrin1 binds to APP and increases the recruitment of downstream adaptor proteins such as Fe65 (see the previous section) and DAB-1 to AICD in turn increasing nuclear transactivation of APP-dependent gene transcription (Lourenço et al., 2009). Remarkably, Netrin1 hemizygotes have increased cerebral Aβ concentrations. Moreover, APP acts as a coreceptor for DCC at axonal growth cones to mediate commissure formation at the ventral midline of the developing mammalian spinal cord (Rama et al., 2012).

Further axonal guidance properties have been attributed to APP by its identification as a growth cone adhesion molecule mediating contact guidance and possibly axonal pathfinding *in vivo* in Down syndrome neurons (Sosa, 2013, 2014). Other studies also support a role for APP in neuritogenesis and neuronal differentiation from neural cell precursors (Chen and Tang, 2006; Khandekar et al., 2012). Given that DCC as well as APP are both targets of Presenilin1 (PS1)-encoded gamma-secretase activity during development, it is noteworthy in this context that the PS1 catalytic activity is required in axon guidance of motor neurons in the spinal cord. The cleavage of DCC by PS1 in motor axons prevents them from being attracted by the netrin-1 secreted by floor plate. Whether or how this mechanism plays a role in AD pathogenesis remains to be investigated (Bai et al., 2011).

The Sema3A Downstream Component CRMP2 in Neurofibrillary Tangles

Since there is to date no cure for AD, the early diagnosis by disease-related biomarkers is crucially relevant to the efficiency of palliative treatments. In order to successfully identify biomarkers, it is of outmost importance to precisely analyze the components of the senile plaques and neurofibrillary tangles. A screen for monoclonal antibodies that would specifically react with NFTs (Yoshida et al., 1998) resulted in the identification of the 3F4 antibody, whose epitope was later shown to map to a highly phosphorylated C-terminal portion of CRMP2 (Collapsin-response mediator protein 2), mostly associated with NFTs and occasionally with senile plaques (Gu et al., 2000). The importance of hyperphosphorylated CRMP2 as an early-stage biomarker specific to ADs and not other neurodegenerative diseases was further substantiated by the detailed biochemical analysis of CRMP2-phosphorylation status in APP and PS1 transgenic mice (Williamson et al., 2011).

The whole story ranking around CRMP2 phosphorylation in the brains of AD patients becomes interesting in a neurodevelopmental context when taking signaling studies into account showing that stimulation of dorsal root ganglion neurons with the axon guidance cue Sema3A leads to subsequent phosphorylation of CRMP2 by Cdk5 followed by GSK3β, hence increasing epitope reactivity with the 3F4 antibody (Uchida et al., 2005). CRMP2 may function as a hub for distinct phosphorylation events mediated by Cdk5 and GSK3β, which also act on tau- concomitantly providing possible new targets for Alzheimer's Disease

and insights into axon guidance signaling mechanisms.

Axon Guidance Molecules Contribute to the Synaptic Phenotype Seen in AD

A recent microarray study on sporadic early onset AD (sEOAD) or familial AD (FAD) patients with PSEN-1 mutations comparing posterior cingulate area gene expression profiles with healthy control subjects reveals a large list of axon guidance molecules differentially regulated in AD patients (Antonell et al., 2013). This study provides intriguing conceptual support that axon guidance and synaptogenesis mechanisms may be dysregulated in neurodegenerative diseases.

There are numerous exciting studies addressing the role of Aβ in the regulation of the axon-guidance relevant EphB2-ephrinB2 bidirectional signaling in the pathogenesis of Alzheimer's Disease. However, thorough cellular and molecular investigations have concluded on this phenomenon most likely being a synaptic phenotype, which predominantly involves impaired NMDA receptor trafficking. Thus, this highlights the role of Ephs and Ephrin in plasticity and memory formation, unrelated to their role in axon guidance (Sheffler-Collins and Dalva, 2012), a functional context that shall therefore not be discussed herein.

Genomic Pathway Approaches for a More Complete Picture of Complex Diseases

A pressing requirement in the field of Genetics – in addition to studying rare gene mutations seen in individual patients – is the identification of common gene variants that may underlie the development of complex diseases, such as Parkinson (PD) or Alzheimer's Disease. A few years ago, the notion has come up that it may be advantageous to study whole pathways or sets of genes involved in specific physiological functions instead of single loci, as complex interactions between various players acting in concert are usually essential to achieve a certain physiological function (Lesnick et al., 2007). Thus, it may be speculated that when facing the pathogenesis of a complex disease, it is unlikely that a single molecule is fully responsible for the phenotype. However, it is a reasonable assumption that molecules tightly involved in the same functional context contribute concertedly to disease manifestations. Lesnick et al. (2007) approached this hypothesis by analyzing whether polymorphism in axon guidance genes may predispose to Parkinson's Disease. Their results were encouraging in their identification of certain SNPs in axon guidance genes that conferred predictability to PD. This pioneering study thus seems like a promising model for extrapolation to further complex diseases, such as AD and others, and may help to complete our genetic understanding of multifaceted pathological conditions.

8.5 CONCLUSION/PERSPECTIVES

One should keep in mind that mutations in genes not encoding axon guidance molecules or their receptors could still perturb axon guidance in an indirect manner. Growing axons follow precise pathways and make guidance decision at specific choice points where they often need to make contact with so-called guidepost cells to continue their journey. If these guidepost cells do not differentiate or migrate properly to their normal position, axons can make guidance errors or fail to grow beyond the choice point. One good example is the "corridor cells" (Lopez-Bendito et al., 2006), which, through neuregulin-1/ErbB4 signaling, act as a permissive bridge allowing thalamocortical and corticothalamic axons to extend and grow. Interestingly, Slit2 orchestrates corridor cell migration and in *Slit2* knockout, the distortion/displacement or the corridor makes thalamic axons deviate from their normal trajectory (Bielle et al., 2011). Such cells were also recently discovered in the corpus callosum and shown to play a role in the development of callosal projections (Niquille et al., 2009). Axon guidance disorders can also have some unexpected consequences. Hypothalamic neuroendocrine cells secreting the Gonadotropin-releasing hormone (GnRH) originate in the nasal placode and migrate

into the CNS along olfactory/vomeronasal axons, a process known as axophilic migration (Schwanzel-Fukuda and Pfaff, 1989). In Kallmann syndrome, an absence of GnRH neurons results in hypogonadism. Many Kallmann patients are also anosmic. Ten causative genes have been identified so far accounting for about one third of Kalmann cases: *KAL1*, which is X-linked and encodes Anosmin-1 (Legouis et al., 1991), Prokineticin-2 (*PROK2*, and its receptor *PROKR2* (Dode et al., 2006; Pitteloud et al., 2007), Fibroblast growth factor 8 (*FGF8*) and its receptor *FGFR1* (Falardeau et al., 2008), *HS6ST1* (Tornberg et al., 2011), *WDR11* (Kim et al., 2010), CHD7 (Jongmans et al., 2009), and *SEMA3A* (Hanchate et al., 2012). The analysis of the corresponding animal models has shown that in at least four cases (*PROK2, PROKR2, KAL1* and *SEMA3A*), the inability of GnRH to enter the brain is, probably secondary to a failure of olfactory axons to penetrate into the olfactory bulb.

8.5.1 Axonal Pruning

In many neuronal circuits, the initial projections are exuberant, with axons forming extra branches that are later eliminated or pruned (Vanderhaeghen and Cheng, 2010). Like other skeletal muscles, EOM are initially multi-innervated by several motor axons before synaptic remodeling and elimination results in a one axon/ muscle fiber ratio (Fox et al., 2011). However, in the case of EOMS, multiple innervation persists at so-called "en-grappe synapses" longer than in other muscles (specially for the LPS). Therefore, abnormal axonal remodeling could also result in miswiring and abnormal circuit function.

The findings discussed in this chapter exemplify the nonlinear relationship between genotype and phenotype by showing that the genetically determined expression of single proteins is highly context-specific in its function, leading to an extraordinarily vast spectrum of outcomes, ranging from the control of axon guidance during development to neuropsychiatric diseases and even neurodegeneration.

REFERENCES

Abelson, J.F., Kwan, K.Y., O'Roak, B.J., Baek, D.Y., Stillman, A.a., Morgan, T.M., Mathews, C.a., Pauls, D.L., Rasin, M.-R., Gunel, M., et al. (2005). Sequence variants in SLITRK1 are associated with Tourette's syndrome. Science 310, 317–320.

Abu-Amero, K.K., al Dhalaan, H., al Zayed, Z., Hellani, A., and Bosley, T.M. (2009). Five new consanguineous families with horizontal gaze palsy and progressive scoliosis and novel ROBO3 mutations. J Neurol Sci 276, 22–26.

Ahmed, G., Shinmyo, Y., Ohta, K., Islam, S.M., Hossain, M., Naser, I.B., Riyadh, M.A., Su, Y., Zhang, S., Tessier-Lavigne, M., et al. (2011). Draxin inhibits axonal outgrowth through the netrin receptor DCC. J Neurosci 31, 14018–14023.

Alexandrakis, G., and Saunders, R.A. (2001). Duane retraction syndrome. Ophthalmol Clin North Am 14, 407–417.

Allen, N.C., Bagade, S., McQueen, M.B., Ioannidis, J.P., Kavvoura, F.K., Khoury, M.J., Tanzi, R.E., and Bertram, L. (2008). Systematic meta-analyses and field synopsis of genetic association studies in schizophrenia: the SzGene database. Nat Genet 40, 827–834.

Amoiridis, G., Tzagournissakis, M., Christodoulou, P., Karampekios, S., Latsoudis, H., Panou, T., Simos, P., and Plaitakis, A. (2006). Patients with horizontal gaze palsy and progressive scoliosis due to ROBO3 E319K mutation have both uncrossed and crossed central nervous system pathways and perform normally on neuropsychological testing. J Neurol Neurosurg Psychiatry 77, 1047–1053.

Angata, K., Long, J.M., Bukalo, O., Lee, W., Dityatev, A., Wynshaw-Boris, A., Schachner, M., Fukuda, M., and Marth, J.D. (2004). Sialyltransferase ST8Sia-II assembles a subset of polysialic acid that directs hippocampal axonal targeting and promotes fear behavior. J Biol Chem 279, 32603–32613.

Anitha, A., Nakamura, K., Yamada, K., Suda, S., Thanseem, I., Tsujii, M., Iwayama, Y., Hattori, E., Toyota, T., Miyachi, T., et al. (2008). Genetic analyses of Roundabout (ROBO) axon guidance receptors in autism. Am J Med Genet Part B.

Anney, R., Klei, L., Pinto, D., Regan, R., Conroy, J., Magalhaes, T.R., Correia, C., Abrahams, B.S., Sykes, N., Pagnamenta, A.T., et al. (2010). A genome-wide scan for common alleles affecting risk for autism. Hum Mol Genet 19, 4072–4082.

Antonell, A., Llado, A., Altirriba, J., Botta-Orfila, T., Balasa, M., Fernandez, M., Ferrer, I., Sanchez-Valle, R., and Molinuevo, J.L. (2013). A preliminary study of the whole-genome expression profile of sporadic and monogenic early-onset Alzheimer's disease. Neurobiol Aging 34, 1772–1778.

Apkarian, P., Bour, L., and Barth, P.G. (1994). A unique achiasmatic anomaly detected in non-albinos with misrouted retinal-fugal projections. Eur J Neurosci 6, 501–507.

Arriagada, P.V., Growdon, J.H., Hedley-Whyte, E.T., and Hyman, B.T. (1992). Neurofibrillary tangles but not senile plaques parallel duration and severity of Alzheimer's disease. Neurology 42, 631–639.

Aruga, J., and Mikoshiba, K. (2003). Identification and characterization of Slitrk, a novel neuronal transmembrane protein family controlling neurite outgrowth. Mol Cell Neurosci 24, 117–129.

Aruga, J., Yokota, N., and Mikoshiba, K. (2003). Human SLITRK family genes: genomic organization and expression profiling in normal brain and brain tumor tissue. Gene 315, 87–94.

Ashe, K.H., and Zahs, K.R. (2010). Probing the biology of Alzheimer's disease in mice. Neuron 66, 631–645.

Assaf, A.A. (2011). Congenital innervation dysgenesis syndrome (CID)/congenital cranial dysinnervation disorders (CCDDs). Eye (Lond) 25, 1251–1261.

Avram, S., Shaposhnikov, S., Buiu, C., and Mernea, M. (2014). Chondroitin sulfate proteoglycans: structure-function relationship with implication in neural development and brain disorders. BioMed Res Int 2014, 642798.

Aydin, D., Weyer, S.W., and Müller, U.C. (2012). Functions of the APP gene family in the nervous system: insights from mouse models. Exp Brain Res 217, 423–434.

Bacchelli, E., Blasi, F., Biondolillo, M., Lamb, J.A., Bonora, E., Barnby, G., Parr, J., Beyer, K.S., Klauck, S.M., Poustka, A., et al. (2003). Screening of nine candidate genes for autism on chromosome 2q reveals rare nonsynonymous variants in the cAMP-GEFII gene. Mol Psychiatry 8, 916–924.

Badura, A., Schonewille, M., Voges, K., Galliano, E., Renier, N., Gao, Z., Witter, L., Hoebeek, F.E.,

Chédotal, A., and De Zeeuw, C.I. (2013). Climbing fiber input shapes reciprocity of Purkinje cell firing. Neuron 78, 700–713.

Bai, G., Chivatakarn, O., Bonanomi, D., Lettieri, K., Franco, L., Xia, C., Stein, E., Ma, L., Lewcock, J.W., and Pfaff, S.L. (2011). Presenilin-dependent receptor processing is required for axon guidance. Cell 144, 106–118.

Barber, M., Di Meglio, T., Andrews, W.D., Hernandez-Miranda, L.R., Murakami, F., Chédotal, A., and Parnavelas, J.G. (2009). The Role of Robo3 in the Development of Cortical Interneurons. Cereb Cortex 19, i22–i31.

Beaubien, F., and Cloutier, J.-F. (2009). Differential expression of Slitrk family members in the mouse nervous system. Dev Dyn 238, 3285–3296.

Beg, A.A., Sommer, J.E., Martin, J.H., and Scheiffele, P. (2007). alpha2-Chimaerin is an essential EphA4 effector in the assembly of neuronal locomotor circuits. Neuron 55, 768–778.

Bellon, A., Luchino, J., Haigh, K., Rougon, G., Haigh, J., Chauvet, S., and Mann, F. (2010). VEGFR2 (KDR/Flk1) signaling mediates axon growth in response to semaphorin 3E in the developing brain. Neuron 66, 205–219.

Bettens, K., Sleegers, K., and Van Broeckhoven, C. (2013). Genetic insights in Alzheimer's disease. Lancet Neurol 12, 92–104.

Bielle, F., Marcos-Mondejar, P., Keita, M., Mailhes, C., Verney, C., Nguyen Ba-Charvet, K., Tessier-Lavigne, M., Lopez-Bendito, G., and Garel, S. (2011). Slit2 activity in the migration of guidepost neurons shapes thalamic projections during development and evolution. Neuron 69, 1085–1098.

Blockus, H., and Chédotal, A. (2014). The multifaceted roles of Slits and Robos in cortical circuits: from proliferation to axon guidance and neurological diseases. Curr Opin Neurobiol 27, 82–88.

Bonanomi, D., Chivatakarn, O., Bai, G., Abdesselem, H., Lettieri, K., Marquardt, T., Pierchala, B.A., and Pfaff, S.L. (2012). Ret is a multifunctional coreceptor that integrates diffusible- and contact-axon guidance signals. Cell 148, 568–582.

Bórquez, D.a., and González-Billault, C. (2012). The amyloid precursor protein intracellular domain-fe65 multiprotein complexes: a challenge to the amyloid hypothesis for Alzheimer's disease? Int J Alzheimer's Dis 2012, 353145.

Bosley, T.M., Oystreck, D.T., Robertson, R.L., al Awad, A., Abu-Amero, K., and Engle, E.C. (2006). Neurological features of congenital fibrosis of the extraocular muscles type 2 with mutations in PHOX2A. Brain 129, 2363–2374.

Bosley, T.M., Salih, M.A., Jen, J.C., Lin, D.D., Oystreck, D., Abu-Amero, K.K., MacDonald, D.B., al Zayed, Z., al Dhalaan, H., Kansu, T., et al. (2005). Neurologic features of horizontal gaze palsy and progressive scoliosis with mutations in ROBO3. Neurology 64, 1196–1203.

Bouvier, J., Thoby-Brisson, M., Renier, N., Dubreuil, V., Ericson, J., Champagnat, J., Pierani, A., Chédotal, A., and Fortin, G. (2010). Hindbrain interneurons and axon guidance signaling critical for breathing. Nat Neurosci 13, 1066–1074.

Breuss, M., Heng, J.I., Poirier, K., Tian, G., Jaglin, X.H., Qu, Z., Braun, A., Gstrein, T., Ngo, L., Haas, M., et al. (2012). Mutations in the beta-tubulin gene TUBB5 cause microcephaly with structural brain abnormalities. Cell Rep 2, 1554–1562.

Britanova, O., de Juan Romero, C., Cheung, A., Kwan, K.Y., Schwark, M., Gyorgy, A., Vogel, T., Akopov, S., Mitkovski, M., Agoston, D., et al. (2008). Satb2 is a postmitotic determinant for upper-layer neuron specification in the neocortex. Neuron 57, 378–392.

Brookmeyer, R., Johnson, E., Ziegler-Graham, K., and Arrighi, H.M. (2007). Forecasting the global burden of Alzheimer's disease. Alzheimers Dement 3, 186–191.

Brose, K., Bland, K.S., Wang, K.H., Arnott, D., Henzel, W., Goodman, C.S., Tessier-Lavigne, M., and Kidd, T. (1999). Slit proteins bind Robo receptors and have an evolutionarily conserved role in repulsive axon guidance. Cell 96, 795–806.

Buttery, P., Beg, A.A., Chih, B., Broder, A., Mason, C.A., and Scheiffele, P. (2006). The diacylglycerol-binding protein alpha1-chimaerin regulates dendritic morphology. Proc Natl Acad Sci U S A 103, 1924–1929.

Buttner-Ennever, J.A. (2006). The extraocular motor nuclei: organization and functional neuroanatomy. Prog Brain Res 151, 95–125.

Canty, A.J., and Murphy, M. (2008). Molecular mechanisms of axon guidance in the developing corticospinal tract. Prog Neurobiol 85, 214–235.

Canu, E., Agosta, F., and Filippi, M. (2014). A selective review of structural connectivity abnormalities of schizophrenic patients at different stages of the disease. Schizophr Res.

Cao, L., Rickenbacher, G.T., Rodriguez, S., Moulia, T.W., and Albers, M.W. (2012). The precision of axon targeting of mouse olfactory sensory neurons requires the BACE1 protease. Sci Rep 2, 231.

Castellani, V., Chédotal, A., Schachner, M., Faivre-Sarrailh, C., and Rougon, G. (2000). Analysis of the L1-deficient mouse phenotype reveals cross-talk between Sema3A and L1 signaling pathways in axonal guidance. Neuron 27, 237–249.

Caton, A., Hacker, A., Naeem, A., Livet, J., Maina, F., Bladt, F., Klein, R., Birchmeier, C., and Guthrie, S. (2000). The branchial arches and HGF are growth-promoting and chemoattractant for cranial motor axons. Development 127, 1751–1766.

Cederquist, G.Y., Luchniak, A., Tischfield, M.A., Peeva, M., Song, Y., Menezes, M.P., Chan, W.M., Andrews, C., Chew, S., Jamieson, R.V., et al. (2012). An inherited TUBB2B mutation alters a kinesin-binding site and causes polymicrogyria, CFEOM and axon dysinnervation. Hum Mol Genet 21, 5484–5499.

Chan, S.S., Zheng, H., Su, M.W., Wilk, R., Killeen, M.T., Hedgecock, E.M., and Culotti, J.G. (1996). UNC-40, a C. elegans homolog of DCC (Deleted in Colorectal Cancer), is required in motile cells responding to UNC-6 netrin cues. Cell 87, 187–195.

Chan, W.M., Miyake, N., Zhu-Tam, L., Andrews, C., and Engle, E.C. (2011). Two novel CHN1 mutations in 2 families with Duane retraction syndrome. Arch Ophthalmol 129, 649–652.

Chan, W.M., Traboulsi, E.I., Arthur, B., Friedman, N., Andrews, C., and Engle, E.C. (2006). Horizontal gaze palsy with progressive scoliosis can result from compound heterozygous mutations in ROBO3. J Med Genet 43, e11.

Chanana, B., Steigemann, P., Jackle, H., and Vorbruggen, G. (2009). Reception of Slit requires only the chondroitin-sulphate-modified extracellular domain of Syndecan at the target cell surface. Proc Natl Acad Sci U S A 106, 11984–11988.

Chattopadhyay, K., and Chatterjee, K. (2012). The genetic factors influencing the development of trichotillomania. J Genet 91, 259–262.

Chauvet, S., Cohen, S., Yoshida, Y., Fekrane, L., Livet, J., Gayet, O., Segu, L., Buhot, M.C., Jessell, T.M., Henderson, C.E., et al. (2007). Gating of Sema3E/PlexinD1 signaling by neuropilin-1 switches axonal repulsion to attraction during brain development. Neuron 56, 807–822.

Chédotal, A. (2007). Slits and their receptors. Adv Exp Med Biol 621, 65–80.

Chen, H., Bagri, A., Zupicich, J.A., Zou, Y., Stoeckli, E., Pleasure, S.J., Lowenstein, D.H., Skarnes, W.C., Chédotal, A., and Tessier-Lavigne, M. (2000). Neuropilin-2 regulates the development of selective cranial and sensory nerves and hippocampal mossy fiber projections. Neuron 25, 43–56.

Chen, H., Chédotal, A., He, Z., Goodman, C.S., and Tessier-Lavigne, M. (1997). Neuropilin-2, a novel member of the neuropilin family, is a high affinity receptor for the semaphorins Sema E and Sema IV but not Sema III. Neuron 19, 547–559.

Chen, Y., and Tang, B.L. (2006). The amyloid precursor protein and postnatal neurogenesis/neuroregeneration. Biochem Biophys Res Commun 341, 1–5.

Cheng, H.J., Nakamoto, M., Bergemann, A.D., and Flanagan, J.G. (1995). Complementary gradients in expression and binding of ELF-1 and Mek4 in development of the topographic retinotectal projection map. Cell 82, 371–381.

Cheng, L., Desai, J., Miranda, C.J., Duncan, J.S., Qiu, W., Nugent, A.A., Kolpak, A.L., Wu, C.C., Drokhlyansky, E., Delisle, M.M., et al. (2014). Human CFEOM1 mutations attenuate KIF21A autoinhibition and cause oculomotor axon stalling. Neuron 82, 334–349.

Cheung, H.N., Dunbar, C., Morotz, G.M., Cheng, W.H., Chan, H.Y., Miller, C.C., and Lau, K.F. (2014). FE65 interacts with ADP-ribosylation factor 6 to promote neurite outgrowth. FASEB J 28, 337–349.

Chew, S., Balasubramanian, R., Chan, W.M., Kang, P.B., Andrews, C., Webb, B.D., MacKinnon, S.E., Oystreck, D.T., Rankin, J., Crawford, T.O., et al. (2013). A novel syndrome caused by the E410K amino acid substitution in the neuronal beta-tubulin isotype 3. Brain 136, 522–535.

Chilton, J.K., and Guthrie, S. (2004). Development of oculomotor axon projections in the chick embryo. J Comp Neurol 472, 308–317.

Ciranna, L., and Catania, M.V. (2014). 5-HT7 receptors as modulators of neuronal excitability, synaptic transmission and plasticity: physiological role and possible implications in autism spectrum disorders. Front Cell Neurosci 8, 250.

Clark, C., Austen, O., Poparic, I., and Guthrie, S. (2013). alpha2-Chimaerin regulates a key axon guidance transition during development of the oculomotor projection. J Neurosci 33, 16540–16551.

Cohen, N.R., Taylor, J.S., Scott, L.B., Guillery, R.W., Soriano, P., and Furley, A.J. (1998). Errors in corticospinal axon guidance in mice lacking the neural cell adhesion molecule L1. Curr Biol 8, 26–33.

Colamarino, S.A., and Tessier-Lavigne, M. (1995). The axonal chemoattractant netrin-1 is also a chemorepellent for trochlear motor axons. Cell 81, 621–629.

Coonan, J.R., Greferath, U., Messenger, J., Hartley, L., Murphy, M., Boyd, A.W., Dottori, M., Galea, M.P., and Bartlett, P.F. (2001). Development and reorganization of corticospinal projections in EphA4 deficient mice. J Comp Neurol 436, 248–262.

Cooper, E.R.A. (1946). The development of the nuclei of the oculomotor and trochlear nerves (somatic efferent column). Brain 4, 50–57.

Corset, V., Nguyen-Ba-Charvet, K.T., Forcet, C., Moyse, E., Chédotal, A., and Mehlen, P. (2000). Netrin-1-mediated axon outgrowth and cAMP production requires interaction with adenosine A2b receptor. Nature 407, 747–750.

Couch, J.A., Chen, J., Rieff, H.I., Uri, E.M., and Condron, B.G. (2004). robo2 and robo3 interact with eagle to regulate serotonergic neuron differentiation. Development 131, 997–1006.

Cushion, T.D., Dobyns, W.B., Mullins, J.G., Stoodley, N., Chung, S.K., Fry, A.E., Hehr, U., Gunny, R., Aylsworth, A.S., Prabhakar, P., et al. (2013). Overlapping cortical malformations and mutations in TUBB2B and TUBA1A. Brain 136, 536–548.

D'Onofrio, G., Panza, F., Frisardi, V., Solfrizzi, V., Imbimbo, B.P., Paroni, G., Cascavilla, L., Seripa, D., and Pilotto, A. (2012). Advances in the identification of γ-secretase inhibitors for the treatment of Alzheimer's disease. Expert Opin Drug Discovery 7, 19–37.

Davidsson, J., Collin, A., Olsson, M.E., Lundgren, J., and Soller, M. (2008). Deletion of the SCN gene cluster on 2q24.4 is associated with severe epilepsy: an array-based genotype-phenotype correlation and a comprehensive review of previously published cases. Epilepsy Res 81, 69–79.

Demer, J.L., Clark, R.A., and Engle, E.C. (2005). Magnetic resonance imaging evidence for widespread orbital dysinnervation in congenital fibrosis of extraocular muscles due to mutations in KIF21A. Invest Ophthalmol Vis Sci 46, 530–539.

Demer, J.L., Clark, R.A., Lim, K.H., and Engle, E.C. (2007). Magnetic resonance imaging of innervational and extraocular muscle abnormalities in Duane-radial ray syndrome. Invest Ophthalmol Vis Sci 48, 5505–5511.

Deng, H., Gao, K., and Jankovic, J. (2012). The genetics of Tourette syndrome. Nat Rev Neurol 8, 203–213.

Depienne, C., Bouteiller, D., Meneret, A., Billot, S., Groppa, S., Klebe, S., Charbonnier-Beaupel, F., Corvol, J.C., Saraiva, J.P., Brueggemann, N., et al. (2012). RAD51 haploinsufficiency causes congenital mirror movements in humans. Am J Hum Genet 90, 301–307.

Depienne, C., Cincotta, M., Billot, S., Bouteiller, D., Groppa, S., Brochard, V., Flamand, C., Hubsch, C., Meunier, S., Giovannelli, F., et al. (2011). A novel DCC mutation and genetic heterogeneity in congenital mirror movements. Neurology 76, 260–264.

Desai, J., Velo, M.P., Yamada, K., Overman, L.M., and Engle, E.C. (2012). Spatiotemporal expression pattern of KIF21A during normal embryonic development and in congenital fibrosis of the extraocular muscles type 1 (CFEOM1). Gene Expr Patterns 12, 180–188.

Dickson, B.J. (2002). Molecular mechanisms of axon guidance. Science 298, 1959–1964.

Djarmati-Westenberger, A., Bruggemann, N., Espay, A.J., Bhatia, K.P., and Klein, C. (2011). A novel DCC mutation and genetic heterogeneity in congenital mirror movements. Neurology 77, 1580.

Dobson, C.B., Villagra, F., Clowry, G.J., Smith, M., Kenwrick, S., Donnai, D., Miller, S., and Eyre, J.A. (2001). Abnormal corticospinal function but normal axonal guidance in human L1CAM mutations. Brain: A Journal of Neurology 124, 2393–2406.

Dode, C., Teixeira, L., Levilliers, J., Fouveaut, C., Bouchard, P., Kottler, M.L., Lespinasse, J., Lienhardt-Roussie, A., Mathieu, M., Moerman, A., et al. (2006). Kallmann syndrome: mutations in the genes encoding prokineticin-2 and prokineticin receptor-2. PLoS Genet 2, e175.

Doherty, E.J., Macy, M.E., Wang, S.M., Dykeman, C.P., Melanson, M.T., and Engle, E.C. (1999). CFEOM3: a new extraocular congenital fibrosis syndrome that maps to 16q24.2-q24.3. Invest Ophthalmol Vis Sci 40, 1687–1694.

Dolan, J., Walshe, K., Alsbury, S., Hokamp, K., O'Keeffe, S., Okafuji, T., Miller, S.F.C., Tear, G., and Mitchell, K.J. (2007). The extracellular leucine-rich repeat superfamily; a comparative survey and analysis of evolutionary relationships and expression patterns. BMC Genomics 8, 320.

Drescher, U., Kremoser, C., Handwerker, C., Loschinger, J., Noda, M., and Bonhoeffer, F. (1995). In vitro guidance of retinal ganglion cell axons by RAGS, a 25 kDa tectal protein related to ligands for Eph receptor tyrosine kinases. Cell 82, 359–370.

Dretakis, E.K., and Kondoyannis, P.N. (1974). Congenital scoliosis associated with encephalopathy in five children of two families. J Bone Joint Surg Am 56, 1747–1750.

Duane, A. (1905). Congenital deficiency of abduction associated with impairment of adduction, retraction movements, contraction of palpebral fissure and oblique movements of the eye. Arch Ophtalmol 34, 133–159.

Duff, B.J., Macritchie, K.A., Moorhead, T.W., Lawrie, S.M., and Blackwood, D.H. (2013). Human brain imaging studies of DISC1 in schizophrenia, bipolar disorder and depression: a systematic review. Schizophr Res 147, 1–13.

Eastwood, S.L., Law, a.J., Everall, I.P., and Harrison, P.J. (2003). The axonal chemorepellant semaphorin 3A is increased in the cerebellum in schizophrenia and may contribute to its synaptic pathology. Mol Psychiatry 8, 148–155.

Edgar, P.F., Douglas, J.E., Cooper, G.J., Dean, B., Kydd, R., and Faull, R.L. (2000). Comparative proteome analysis of the hippocampus implicates chromosome 6q in schizophrenia. Mol Psychiatry 5, 85–90.

Engle, E.C. (2006). The genetic basis of complex strabismus. Pediatr Res 59, 343–348.

Engle, E.C. (2010). Human genetic disorders of axon guidance. Cold Spring Harb Perspect Biol 2, a001784.

Erskine, L., Reijntjes, S., Pratt, T., Denti, L., Schwarz, Q., Vieira, J.M., Alakakone, B., Shewan, D., and Ruhrberg, C. (2011). VEGF signaling through neuropilin 1 guides commissural axon crossing at the optic chiasm. Neuron 70, 951–965.

Falardeau, J., Chung, W.C., Beenken, A., Raivio, T., Plummer, L., Sidis, Y., Jacobson-Dickman, E.E., Eliseenkova, A.V., Ma, J., Dwyer, A., et al. (2008). Decreased FGF8 signaling causes deficiency of gonadotropin-releasing hormone in humans and mice. J Clin Invest 118, 2822–2831.

Falk, J., Bechara, A., Fiore, R., Nawabi, H., Zhou, H., Hoyo-Becerra, C., Bozon, M., Rougon, G., Grumet, M., Puschel, A.W., et al. (2005). Dual functional activity of semaphorin 3B is required for positioning the anterior commissure. Neuron 48, 63–75.

Fallet-Bianco, C., Loeuillet, L., Poirier, K., Loget, P., Chapon, F., Pasquier, L., Saillour, Y., Beldjord, C., Chelly, J., and Francis, F. (2008). Neuropathological phenotype of a distinct form of lissencephaly associated with mutations in TUBA1A. Brain 131, 2304–2320.

Faulkner, R.L., Low, L.K., Liu, X.B., Coble, J., Jones, E.G., and Cheng, H.J. (2008). Dorsal turning of motor corticospinal axons at the pyramidal decussation requires plexin signaling. Neural Dev 3, 21.

Felling, R.J., and Singer, H.S. (2011). Neurobiology of tourette syndrome: current status and need for further investigation. J Neurosci 31, 12387–12395.

Fernandez-Irigoyen, J., Zelaya, M.V., and Santamaria, E. (2014). Applying mass spectrometry-based qualitative proteomics to human amygdaloid complex. Front Cell Neurosci 8, 80.

Ferrario, J.E., Baskaran, P., Clark, C., Hendry, A., Lerner, O., Hintze, M., Allen, J., Chilton, J.K., and Guthrie, S. (2012). Axon guidance in the developing ocular motor system and Duane retraction syndrome depends on Semaphorin signaling via alpha2-chimaerin. Proc Natl Acad Sci U S A 109, 14669–14674.

Finger, J.H., Bronson, R.T., Harris, B., Johnson, K., Przyborski, S.A., and Ackerman, S.L. (2002). The netrin 1 receptors Unc5h3 and Dcc are necessary at multiple choice points for the guidance of corticospinal tract axons. J Neurosci 22, 10346–10356.

Fox, M.A., Tapia, J.C., Kasthuri, N., and Lichtman, J.W. (2011). Delayed synapse elimination in mouse levator palpebrae superioris muscle. J Comp Neurol 519, 2907–2921.

Fransen, E., Lemmon, V., Van Camp, G., Vits, L., Coucke, P., Willems, P.J. (1995). CRASH syndrome: clinical spectrum of corpus callosum hypoplasia, retardation, adducted thumbs, spastic paraparesis and hydrocephalus due to mutations in one single gene, L1. Eur J Hum Genet 3, 273–84.

Fransen, E., Van Camp, G., D'Hooge, R., Vits, L., and Willems, P.J. (1998). Genotype-phenotype correlation in L1 associated diseases. J Med Genet 35, 399–404.

Frei, J.A., and Stoeckli, E.T. (2014). SynCAMs extend their functions beyond the synapse. Eur J Neurosci 39, 1752–1760.

Fritzsch, B., Nichols, D.H., Echelard, Y., and McMahon, A.P. (1995). Development of midbrain and anterior hindbrain ocular motoneurons in normal and Wnt-1 knockout mice. J Neurobiol 27, 457–469.

Fritzsch, B., and Sonntag, R. (1990). Oculomotor (N III) motoneurons can innervate the superior oblique muscle of Xenopus after larval trochlear (N IV) nerve surgery. Neurosci Lett 114, 129–134.

Fujii, T., Iijima, Y., Kondo, H., Shizuno, T., Hori, H., Nakabayashi, T., Arima, K., Saitoh, O., and Kunugi, H. (2007). Failure to confirm an association between the PLXNA2 gene and schizophrenia in a Japanese population. Prog Neuropsychopharmacol Biol Psychiatry 31, 873–877.

Fujii, T., Uchiyama, H., Yamamoto, N., Hori, H., Tatsumi, M., Ishikawa, M., Arima, K., Higuchi, T., and Kunugi, H. (2011). Possible association of the semaphorin 3D gene (SEMA3D) with schizophrenia. J Psychiatr Res 45, 47–53.

Fukuda, Y., Sawai, H., Watanabe, M., Wakakuwa, K., and Morigiwa, K. (1989). Nasotemporal overlap of crossed and uncrossed retinal ganglion cell projections in the Japanese monkey (Macaca fuscata). J Neurosci 9, 2353–2373.

Gallea, C., Popa, T., Billot, S., Meneret, A., Depienne, C., and Roze, E. (2011). Congenital mirror movements: a clue to understanding bimanual motor control. J Neurol 258, 1911–1919.

Giger, R.J., Cloutier, J.F., Sahay, A., Prinjha, R.K., Levengood, D.V., Moore, S.E., Pickering, S., Simmons, D., Rastan, S., Walsh, F.S., et al. (2000). Neuropilin-2 is required in vivo for selective axon guidance responses to secreted semaphorins. Neuron 25, 29–41.

Giger, R.J., Urquhart, E.R., Gillespie, S.K., Levengood, D.V., Ginty, D.D., and Kolodkin, A.L. (1998). Neuropilin-2 is a receptor for semaphorin IV: insight into the structural basis of receptor function and specificity. Neuron 21, 1079–1092.

Gilland, E., and Baker, R. (2005). Evolutionary patterns of cranial nerve efferent nuclei in vertebrates. Brain Behav Evol 66, 234–254.

Gilman, S.R., Chang, J., Xu, B., Bawa, T.S., Gogos, J.a., Karayiorgou, M., and Vitkup, D. (2012). Diverse types of genetic variation converge on functional gene networks involved in schizophrenia. Nat Neurosci 15, 1723–1728.

Godement, P., Salaun, J., and Mason, C.A. (1990). Retinal axon pathfinding in the optic chiasm: divergence of crossed and uncrossed fibers. Neuron 5, 173–186.

Gordon, J.A. (2010). Testing the glutamate hypothesis of schizophrenia. Nat Neurosci 13, 2–4.

Goulding, M. (2009). Circuits controlling vertebrate locomotion: moving in a new direction. Nat Rev Neurosci 10, 507–518.

Graf, W.D., Born, D.E., Shaw, D.W., Thomas, J.R., Holloway, L.W., and Michaelis, R.C. (2000). Brainstem diffusion-weighted MRI in boys with L1CAM mutations. Ann Neurol 47, 113–117.

Griffa, A., Baumann, P.S., Thiran, J.-P., and Hagmann, P. (2013). Structural connectomics in brain diseases. Neuroimage 80, 515–526.

Gu, C., Yoshida, Y., Livet, J., Reimert, D.V., Mann, F., Merte, J., Henderson, C.E., Jessell, T.M., Kolodkin, A.L., and Ginty, D.D. (2005). Semaphorin 3E and plexin-D1 control vascular pattern independently of neuropilins. Science 307, 265–268.

Gu, Y., Hamajima, N., and Ihara, Y. (2000). Neurofibrillary tangle-associated collapsin response mediator protein-2 (CRMP-2) is highly phosphorylated on Thr-509, Ser-518, and Ser-522. Biochemistry 39, 4267–4275.

Guénette, S., Chang, Y., Hiesberger, T., Richardson, J.a., Eckman, C.B., Eckman, E.a., Hammer, R.E., and Herz, J. (2006). Essential roles for the FE65 amyloid precursor protein-interacting proteins in brain development. EMBO J 25, 420–431.

Guillery, R.W., and Kaas, J.H. (1973). Genetic abnormality of the visual pathways in a "white" tiger. Science 180, 1287–1289.

Guillery, R.W., Mason, C.A., and Taylor, J.S. (1995). Developmental determinants at the mammalian optic chiasm. J Neurosci 15, 4727–4737.

Gunn, R.K., Huentelman, M.J., and Brown, R.E. (2011). Are Sema5a mutant mice a good model of autism? A behavioral analysis of sensory systems, emotionality and cognition. Behav Brain Res 225, 142–150.

Gutekunst, C.A., and Gross, R.E. (2014) Plexina4 expression in adult rat cranial nerves. J Chem Neuroanat 61, 13–19.

Gutowski, N.J., Bosley, T.M., and Engle, E.C. (2003). 110th ENMC International Workshop: the congenital cranial dysinnervation disorders (CCDDs). Naarden, The Netherlands, 25–27 October, 2002. Neuromuscul Disord 13, 573–578.

Haller, S., Wetzel, S.G., and Lutschg, J. (2008). Functional MRI, DTI and neurophysiology in horizontal gaze palsy with progressive scoliosis. Neuroradiology.

Hanchate, N.K., Giacobini, P., Lhuillier, P., Parkash, J., Espy, C., Fouveaut, C., Leroy, C., Baron, S., Campagne, C., Vanacker, C., et al. (2012). SEMA3A, a gene involved in axonal pathfinding, is mutated in patients with Kallmann syndrome. PLoS Genet 8, e1002896.

Hansson, O., Zetterberg, H., Buchhave, P., Andreasson, U., Londos, E., Minthon, L., and Blennow, K. (2007). Prediction of Alzheimer's disease using the CSF Abeta42/Abeta40 ratio in patients with mild cognitive impairment. Dement Geriatr Cogn Disord 23, 316–320.

He, Z., and Tessier-Lavigne, M. (1997). Neuropilin is a receptor for the axonal chemorepellent Semaphorin III. Cell 90, 739–751.

Hedgecock, E.M., Culotti, J.G., and Hall, D.H. (1990). The unc-5, unc-6, and unc-40 genes guide circumferential migrations of pioneer axons and mesodermal cells on the epidermis in C. elegans. Neuron 4, 61–85.

Herms, J., Anliker, B., Heber, S., Ring, S., Fuhrmann, M., Kretzschmar, H., Sisodia, S., and Müller, U. (2004). Cortical dysplasia resembling human type 2 lissencephaly in mice lacking all three APP family members. EMBO J 23, 4106–4115.

Herrera, E., Brown, L., Aruga, J., Rachel, R.A., Dolen, G., Mikoshiba, K., Brown, S., and Mason, C.A. (2003). Zic2 patterns binocular vision by specifying the uncrossed retinal projection. Cell 114, 545–557.

Hirokawa, N., Niwa, S., and Tanaka, Y. (2010). Molecular motors in neurons: transport mechanisms and roles in brain function, development, and disease. Neuron 68, 610–638.

Hitt, B., Riordan, S.M., Kukreja, L., Eimer, W.a., Rajapaksha, T.W., and Vassar, R. (2012). β-Site amyloid precursor protein (APP)-cleaving enzyme 1 (BACE1)-deficient mice exhibit a close homolog of L1 (CHL1) loss-of-function phenotype involving axon guidance defects. J Biol Chem 287, 38408–38425.

Hoffmann, M.B., Kaule, F.R., Levin, N., Masuda, Y., Kumar, A., Gottlob, I., Horiguchi, H., Dougherty, R.F., Stadler, J., Wolynski, B., et al. (2012). Plasticity and stability of the visual system in human achiasma. Neuron 75, 393–401.

Holland, S.J., Gale, N.W., Mbamalu, G., Yancopoulos, G.D., Henkemeyer, M., and Pawson, T. (1996). Bidirectional signalling through the EPH-family receptor Nuk and its transmembrane ligands. Nature 383, 722–725.

Hong, K., Hinck, L., Nishiyama, M., Poo, M.M., Tessier-Lavigne, M., and Stein, E. (1999). A ligand-gated association between cytoplasmic domains of UNC5 and DCC family receptors converts netrin-induced growth cone attraction to repulsion. Cell 97, 927–941.

Hu, H. (2001). Cell-surface heparan sulfate is involved in the repulsive guidance activities of Slit2 protein. Nat Neurosci 4, 695–701.

Hu, V.W., Frank, B.C., Heine, S., Lee, N.H., Quackenbush, J. (2006). Gene expression profiling of lymphoblastoid cell lines from monozygotic twins discordant in severity of autism reveals differential regulation of neurologically relevant genes. BMC Genomics 7, 118.

Huber, A.B., Kania, A., Tran, T.S., Gu, C., De Marco Garcia, N., Lieberam, I., Johnson, D., Jessell, T.M., Ginty, D.D., and Kolodkin, A.L. (2005). Distinct roles for secreted semaphorin signaling in spinal motor axon guidance. Neuron 48, 949–964.

Huminiecki, L., Gorn, M., Suchting, S., Poulsom, R., and Bicknell, R. (2002). Magic roundabout is a new member of the roundabout receptor family that is endothelial specific and expressed at sites of active angiogenesis. Genomics 79, 547–552.

Ip, J.P., Shi, L., Chen, Y., Itoh, Y., Fu, W.Y., Betz, A., Yung, W.H., Gotoh, Y., Fu, A.K., and Ip, N.Y. (2012). alpha2-chimaerin controls neuronal migration and functioning of the cerebral cortex through CRMP-2. Nat Neurosci 15, 39–47.

Irving, C., Malhas, A., Guthrie, S., and Mason, I. (2002). Establishing the trochlear motor axon trajectory: role of the isthmic organiser and Fgf8. Development 129, 5389–5398.

Iwasato, T., Katoh, H., Nishimaru, H., Ishikawa, Y., Inoue, H., Saito, Y.M., Ando, R., Iwama, M., Takahashi, R., Negishi, M., et al. (2007). Rac-GAP alpha-chimerin regulates motor-circuit formation as a key mediator of EphrinB3/EphA4 forward signaling. Cell 130, 742–753.

Jackson, S.R., Parkinson, A., Jung, J., Ryan, S.E., Morgan, P.S., Hollis, C., and Jackson, G.M. (2011). Compensatory neural reorganization in Tourette syndrome. Curr Biol 21, 580–585.

Jaglin, X.H., and Chelly, J. (2009). Tubulin-related cortical dysgeneses: microtubule dysfunction underlying neuronal migration defects. Trends Genet 25, 555–566.

Jaglin, X.H., Poirier, K., Saillour, Y., Buhler, E., Tian, G., Bahi-Buisson, N., Fallet-Bianco, C., Phan-Dinh-Tuy, F., Kong, X.P., Bomont, P., et al. (2009). Mutations in the beta-tubulin gene TUBB2B result in asymmetrical polymicrogyria. Nat Genet 41, 746–752.

Jen, J.C., Chan, W.M., Bosley, T.M., Wan, J., Carr, J.R., Rub, U., Shattuck, D., Salamon, G., Kudo, L.C., Ou, J., et al. (2004). Mutations in a human ROBO gene disrupt hindbrain axon pathway crossing and morphogenesis. Science 304, 1509–1513.

Ji, J., Salamon, N., and Quintero-Rivera, F. (2014). Microdeletion of 1p32-p31 involving NFIA in a patient with hypoplastic corpus callosum, ventriculomegaly, seizures and urinary tract defects. Eur J Med Genet 57, 267–268.

Johnson, K.G., Ghose, A., Epstein, E., Lincecum, J., O'Connor, M.B., and Van Vactor, D. (2004). Axonal heparan sulfate proteoglycans regulate the distribution and efficiency of the repellent slit during midline axon guidance. Curr Biol 14, 499–504.

Jongmans, M.C., van Ravenswaaij-Arts, C.M., Pitteloud, N., Ogata, T., Sato, N., Claahsen-van der Grinten, H.L., van der Donk, K., Seminara, S., Bergman, J.E., Brunner, H.G., et al. (2009). CHD7 mutations in patients initially diagnosed with Kallmann syndrome--the clinical overlap with CHARGE syndrome. Clin Genet 75, 65–71.

Jonsson, T., Atwal, J.K., Steinberg, S., Snaedal, J., Jonsson, P.V., Bjornsson, S., Stefansson, H., Sulem, P., Gudbjartsson, D., Maloney, J., et al. (2012). A mutation in APP protects against Alzheimer's disease and age-related cognitive decline. Nature 488, 96–99.

Kamien, B., Harraway, J., Lundie, B., Smallhorne, L., Gibbs, V., Heath, A., and Fullerton, J.M. (2014). Characterization of a 520 kb deletion on chromosome 15q26.1 including ST8SIA2 in a patient with behavioral disturbance, autism spectrum disorder, and epilepsy. Am J Med Genet A 164A, 782–788.

Kang, P., Lee, H.K., Glasgow, S.M., Finley, M., Donti, T., Gaber, Z.B., Graham, B.H., Foster, A.E., Novitch, B.G., Gronostajski, R.M., et al. (2012). Sox9 and NFIA coordinate a transcriptional regulatory cascade during the initiation of gliogenesis. Neuron 74, 79–94.

Kao, T.J., and Kania, A. (2011). Ephrin-mediated cis-attenuation of Eph receptor signaling is essential for spinal motor axon guidance. Neuron 71, 76–91.

Karlsgodt, K.H., Sun, D., Jimenez, A.M., Lutkenhoff, E.S., Willhite, R., van Erp, T.G.M., and Cannon, T.D. (2008). Developmental disruptions in neural connectivity in the pathophysiology of schizophrenia. Dev Psychopathol 20, 1297–1327.

Kastenhuber, E., Kern, U., Bonkowsky, J.L., Chien, C.B., Driever, W., and Schweitzer, J. (2009). Netrin-DCC, Robo-Slit, and heparan sulfate proteoglycans coordinate lateral positioning of longitudinal dopaminergic diencephalospinal axons. J Neurosci 29, 8914–8926.

Katayama, K., Yamada, K., Ornthanalai, V.G., Inoue, T., Ota, M., Murphy, N.P., and Aruga, J. (2010). Slitrk1-deficient mice display elevated anxiety-like behavior and noradrenergic abnormalities. Mol Psychiatry 15, 177–184.

Katayama, K.-i., Zine, A., Ota, M., Matsumoto, Y., Inoue, T., Fritzsch, B., and Aruga, J. (2009). Disorganized innervation and neuronal loss in the inner ear of Slitrk6-deficient mice. PLoS One 4, e7786.

Keays, D.A., Tian, G., Poirier, K., Huang, G.J., Siebold, C., Cleak, J., Oliver, P.L., Fray, M., Harvey, R.J., Molnar, Z., et al. (2007). Mutations in alpha-tubulin cause abnormal neuronal migration in mice and lissencephaly in humans. Cell 128, 45–57.

Keino-Masu, K., Masu, M., Hinck, L., Leonardo, E.D., Chan, S.S., Culotti, J.G., and Tessier-Lavigne, M. (1996). Deleted in Colorectal Cancer (DCC) encodes a netrin receptor. Cell 87, 175–185.

Keleman, K., and Dickson, B.J. (2001). Short- and long-range repulsion by the Drosophila Unc5 netrin receptor. Neuron 32, 605–617.

Kesavapany, S., Banner, S.J., Lau, K.-F., Shaw, C.E., Miller, C.C.J., Cooper, J.D., and McLoughlin, D.M. (2002). Expression of the Fe65 adapter protein in adult and developing mouse brain. Neuroscience 115, 951–960.

Khandekar, N., Lie, K.H., Sachdev, P.S., and Sidhu, K.S. (2012). Amyloid precursor proteins, neural differentiation of pluripotent stem cells and its relevance to Alzheimer's disease. Stem Cells Dev 21, 997–1006.

Kidd, T., Bland, K.S., and Goodman, C.S. (1999). Slit is the midline repellent for the robo receptor in Drosophila. Cell 96, 785–794.

Kim, H.G., Ahn, J.W., Kurth, I., Ullmann, R., Kim, H.T., Kulharya, A., Ha, K.S., Itokawa, Y., Meliciani, I., Wenzel, W., et al. (2010). WDR11, a WD protein that interacts with transcription factor EMX1, is mutated in idiopathic hypogonadotropic hypogonadism and Kallmann syndrome. Am J Hum Genet 87, 465–479.

King, G.D., and Scott Turner, R. (2004). Adaptor protein interactions: modulators of amyloid precursor protein metabolism and Alzheimer's disease risk? Exp Neurol 185, 208–219.

Klar, A.J. (2014). Selective Chromatid Segregation Mechanism Invoked For the Human Congenital Mirror Hand Movement Disorder Development by Mutations: A Hypothesis. Int J Biol Sci 10, 1018–1023.

Klein, R. (2012). Eph/ephrin signalling during development. Development 139, 4105–4109.

Koch, A.W., Mathivet, T., Larrivee, B., Tong, R.K., Kowalski, J., Pibouin-Fragner, L., Bouvree, K., Stawicki, S., Nicholes, K., Rathore, N., et al. (2011). Robo4 maintains vessel integrity and inhibits angiogenesis by interacting with UNC5B. Dev Cell 20, 33–46.

Kohsaka, H., Okusawa, S., Itakura, Y., Fushiki, A., and Nose, A. (2012). Development of larval motor circuits in Drosophila. Dev Growth Differ 54, 408–419.

Kolodkin, A.L., Levengood, D.V., Rowe, E.G., Tai, Y.T., Giger, R.J., and Ginty, D.D. (1997). Neuropilin is a semaphorin III receptor. Cell 90, 753–762.

Kolodkin, A.L., Matthes, D.J., and Goodman, C.S. (1993). The semaphorin genes encode a family of transmembrane and secreted growth cone guidance molecules. Cell 75, 1389–1399.

Kolodkin, A.L., and Pasterkamp, R.J. (2013). SnapShot: Axon guidance II. Cell 153, 722 e721.

Kolodkin, A.L., and Tessier-Lavigne, M. (2011). Mechanisms and molecules of neuronal wiring: a primer. Cold Spring Harb Perspect Biol 3.

Kolodziej, P.A., Timpe, L.C., Mitchell, K.J., Fried, S.R., Goodman, C.S., Jan, L.Y., and Jan, Y.N. (1996). frazzled encodes a Drosophila member of the DCC immunoglobulin subfamily and is required for CNS and motor axon guidance. Cell 87, 197–204.

Kuwajima, T., Yoshida, Y., Takegahara, N., Petros, T.J., Kumanogoh, A., Jessell, T.M., Sakurai, T., and Mason, C. (2012). Optic chiasm presentation

of Semaphorin6D in the context of Plexin-A1 and Nr-CAM promotes retinal axon midline crossing. Neuron 74, 676–690.

Kwon, B.S., Haq, A.K., Pomerantz, S.H., and Halaban, R. (1987). Isolation and sequence of a cDNA clone for human tyrosinase that maps at the mouse c-albino locus. Proc Natl Acad Sci U S A 84, 7473–7477.

De Lacy, N., and King, B.H. (2013) Revisiting the relationship between autism and schizophrenia: toward and integrated neurobiology. Annu Rev Clin Psychol 9, 555–587.

Lai Wing Sun, K., Correia, J.P., and Kennedy, T.E. (2011). Netrins: versatile extracellular cues with diverse functions. Development 138, 2153–2169.

Lance-Jones, C., Shah, V., Noden, D.M., and Sours, E. (2012). Intrinsic properties guide proximal abducens and oculomotor nerve outgrowth in avian embryos. Dev Neurobiol 72, 167–185.

Lanier, L.M., Gates, M.a., Witke, W., Menzies, a.S., Wehman, a.M., Macklis, J.D., Kwiatkowski, D., Soriano, P., and Gertler, F.B. (1999). Mena is required for neurulation and commissure formation. Neuron 22, 313–325.

Leckman, J.F., Bloch, M.H., Smith, M.E., Larabi, D., and Hampson, M. (2010). Neurobiological substrates of Tourette's disorder. J Child Adolesc Psychopharmacol 20, 237–247.

Lee, J.E., and Gleeson, J.G. (2011a). Cilia in the nervous system: linking cilia function and neurodevelopmental disorders. Curr Opin Neurol 24, 98–105.

Lee, J.E., and Gleeson, J.G. (2011b). A systems-biology approach to understanding the ciliopathy disorders. Genome Med 3, 59.

Lee, M.T., Chen, C.H., Lee, C.S., Chen, C.C., Chong, M.Y., Ouyang, W.C., Chiu, N.Y., Chuo, L.J., Chen, C.Y., Tan, H.K., Lane, H.Y., Chang, T.J., Lin, C.H., Jou, S.H., Hou, Y.M., Feng, J., Lai, T.J., Tung, C.L., Chen, T.J., Chang, C.J., Lung, F.W., Chen, C.K., Shiah, I.S., Liu, C.Y., Teng, P.R., Chen, K.H., Shen, L.J., Cheng, C.S., Chang, T.P., Li, C.F., Chou, C.H., Chen, C.Y., Wang, K.H., Fann, C.S., Wu, J.Y., Chen, Y.T., Cheng, A.T. (2011). Genome-wide association study of bipolar I disorder in the Han Chinese population. Mol Psychiatry 16, 548–56.

Legouis, R., Hardelin, J.P., Levilliers, J., Claverie, J.M., Compain, S., Wunderle, V., Millasseau, P., Le Paslier, D., Cohen, D., Caterina, D., et al. (1991). The candidate gene for the X-linked Kallmann syndrome encodes a protein related to adhesion molecules. Cell 67, 423–435.

Leigh, J.R., and Zee, D.S. (2006). The neurology of eye movements, 4th edn Oxford: Oxford university press.

Lencz, T., Lambert, C., DeRosse, P., Burdick, K.E., Morgan, T.V., Kane, J.M., Kucherlapati, R., and Malhotra, A.K. (2007). Runs of homozygosity reveal highly penetrant recessive loci in schizophrenia. Proc Natl Acad Sci U S A 104, 19942–19947.

Leonardo, E.D., Hinck, L., Masu, M., Keino-Masu, K., Ackerman, S.L., and Tessier-Lavigne, M. (1997). Vertebrate homologues of C. elegans UNC-5 are candidate netrin receptors. Nature 386, 833–838.

Lerner, O., Davenport, D., Patel, P., Psatha, M., Lieberam, I., and Guthrie, S. (2010). Stromal cell-derived factor-1 and hepatocyte growth factor guide axon projections to the extraocular muscles. Dev Neurobiol 70, 549–564.

Lesnick, T.G., Papapetropoulos, S., Mash, D.C., Ffrench-Mullen, J., Shehadeh, L., de Andrade, M., Henley, J.R., Rocca, W.a., Ahlskog, J.E., and Maraganore, D.M. (2007). A genomic pathway approach to a complex disease: axon guidance and Parkinson disease. PLoS Genet 3, e98.

Li, H.S., Chen, J.H., Wu, W., Fagaly, T., Zhou, L., Yuan, W., Dupuis, S., Jiang, Z.H., Nash, W., Gick, C., et al. (1999). Vertebrate slit, a secreted ligand for the transmembrane protein roundabout, is a repellent for olfactory bulb axons. Cell 96, 807–818.

Lisabeth, E.M., Falivelli, G., and Pasquale, E.B. (2013). Eph receptor signaling and ephrins. Cold Spring Harb Perspect Biol 5.

Lopez-Bendito, G., Cautinat, A., Sanchez, J.A., Bielle, F., Flames, N., Garratt, A.N., Talmage, D.A., Role, L.W., Charnay, P., Marin, O., et al. (2006). Tangential neuronal migration controls axon guidance: A role for neuregulin-1 in thalamocortical axon navigation. Cell 125, 127–142.

Lourenço, F.C., Galvan, V., Fombonne, J., Corset, V., Llambi, F., Müller, U., Bredesen, D.E., and Mehlen, P. (2009). Netrin-1 interacts with amyloid precursor protein and regulates amyloid-beta production. Cell Death Differ 16, 655–663.

Lu, W., Quintero-Rivera, F., Fan, Y., Alkuraya, F.S., Donovan, D.J., Xi, Q., Turbe-Doan, A., Li, Q.G., Campbell, C.G., Shanske, A.L., Sherr, E.H.,

Ahmad, A., Peters, R., Rilliet, B., Parvex, P., Bassuk, A.G., Harris, D.J., Ferguson, H., Kelly, C., Walsh, C.A., Gronostajski, R.M., Devriendt, K., Higgins, A., Ligon, A.H., Quade, B.J., Morton, C.C., Gusella, J.F., Maas, R.L. (2007). NFIA haploinsufficiency is associated with a CNS malformation syndrome and urinary tract defects. PLoS Genet 3, e80.

Lucchese, G., Capone, G., and Kanduc, D. (2014). Peptide sharing between influenza A H1N1 hemagglutinin and human axon guidance proteins. Schizophr Bull 40, 362–375.

Lufkin, T., Dierich, A., LeMeur, M., Mark, M., and Chambon, P. (1991). Disruption of the Hox-1.6 homeobox gene results in defects in a region corresponding to its rostral domain of expression. Cell 66, 1105–1119.

Lund, R.D. (1965). Uncrossed Visual Pathways of Hooded and Albino Rats. Science 149, 1506–1507.

Luo, L., and O'Leary, D.D. (2005). Axon retraction and degeneration in development and disease. Annu Rev Neurosci 28, 127–156.

Ly, A., Nikolaev, A., Suresh, G., Zheng, Y., Tessier-Lavigne, M., and Stein, E. (2008). DSCAM is a netrin receptor that collaborates with DCC in mediating turning responses to netrin-1. Cell 133, 1241–1254.

Mah, S., Nelson, M.R., Delisi, L.E., Reneland, R.H., Markward, N., James, M.R., Nyholt, D.R., Hayward, N., Handoko, H., Mowry, B., et al. (2006). Identification of the semaphorin receptor PLXNA2 as a candidate for susceptibility to schizophrenia. Mol Psychiatry 11, 471–478.

Marcos, S., Backer, S., Causeret, F., Tessier-Lavigne, M., and Bloch-Gallego, E. (2009). Differential roles of Netrin-1 and its receptor DCC in inferior olivary neuron migration. Mol Cell Neurosci 41, 429–439.

Marillat, V., Cases, O., Nguyen-Ba-Charvet, K.T., Tessier-Lavigne, M., Sotelo, C., and Chédotal, A. (2002). Spatiotemporal expression patterns of slit and robo genes in the rat brain. J Comp Neurol 442, 130–155.

Marillat, V., Sabatier, C., Failli, V., Matsunaga, E., Sotelo, C., Tessier-Lavigne, M., and Chédotal, A. (2004). The slit receptor Rig-1/Robo3 controls midline crossing by hindbrain precerebellar neurons and axons. Neuron 43, 69–79.

Marquardt, T., Shirasaki, R., Ghosh, S., Andrews, S.E., Carter, N., Hunter, T., and Pfaff, S.L. (2005). Coexpressed EphA receptors and ephrin-A ligands mediate opposing actions on growth cone navigation from distinct membrane domains. Cell 121, 127–139.

Mastick, G.S., Fan, C.M., Tessier-Lavigne, M., Serbedzija, G.N., McMahon, A.P., and Easter, S.S., Jr. (1996). Early deletion of neuromeres in Wnt-1$^{-/-}$ mutant mice: evaluation by morphological and molecular markers. J Comp Neurol 374, 246–258.

Matsumoto, Y., Katayama, K., Okamoto, T., Yamada, K., Takashima, N., Nagao, S., and Aruga, J. (2011). Impaired auditory-vestibular functions and behavioral abnormalities of Slitrk6-deficient mice. PLoS One 6, e16497.

McLoughlin, D.M., and Miller, C.C.J. (2008). The FE65 proteins and Alzheimer's disease. J Neurosci Res 86, 744–754.

McNaught, K.S.P., and Mink, J.W. (2011). Advances in understanding and treatment of Tourette syndrome. Nat Rev Neurol 7, 667–676.

Meda, S.A., Ruano, G., Windemuth, A., O'Neil, K., Berwise, C., Dunn, S.M., Boccaccio, L.E., Narayanan, B., Kocherla, M., Sprooten, E., et al. (2014). Multivariate analysis reveals genetic associations of the resting default mode network in psychotic bipolar disorder and schizophrenia. Proc Natl Acad Sci U S A 111, E2066–E2075.

Medana, I.M. (2003). Axonal damage: a key predictor of outcome in human CNS diseases. Brain 126, 515–530.

Mehlen, P., Delloye-Bourgeois, C., and Chédotal, A. (2011). Novel roles for Slits and netrins: axon guidance cues as anticancer targets? Nat Rev Cancer 11, 188–197.

Melin, M., Carlsson, B., Anckarsater, H., Rastam, M., Betancur, C., Isaksson, A., Gillberg, C., and Dahl, N. (2006). Constitutional downregulation of SEMA5A expression in autism. Neuropsychobiology 54, 64–69.

Melom, J.E., and Littleton, J.T. (2011). Synapse development in health and disease. Curr Opin Genet Dev 21, 256–261.

Méneret, A., Depienne, C., Riant, F., Trouillard, O., Bouteiller, D., Cincotta, M., Bitoun, P., Wickert, J., Lagroua, I., Westenberger, A., et al. (2014). Congenital mirror movements: mutational analysis of RAD51 and DCC in 26 cases. Neurology 82, 1999–2002.

Messersmith, E.K., Leonardo, E.D., Shatz, C.J., Tessier-Lavigne, M., Goodman, C.S., and Kolodkin, A.L. (1995). Semaphorin III can function as a selective chemorepellent to pattern sensory projections in the spinal cord. Neuron 14, 949–959.

Meyer, U., Feldon, J., and Dammann, O. (2011). Schizophrenia and autism: both shared and disorder-specific pathogenesis via perinatal inflammation? Pediatr Res 69, 26R–33R.

Michalski, N., Babai, N., Renier, N., Perkel, D.J., Chédotal, A., and Schneggenburger, R. (2013). Robo3-driven axon midline crossing conditions functional maturation of a large commissural synapse. Neuron 78, 855–868.

Minopoli, G., Gargiulo, A., Parisi, S., and Russo, T. (2012). Fe65 matters: new light on an old molecule. IUBMB Life 64, 936–942.

Miyake, N., Demer, J.L., Shaaban, S., Andrews, C., Chan, W.M., Christiansen, S.P., Hunter, D.G., and Engle, E.C. (2011). Expansion of the CHN1 strabismus phenotype. Invest Ophthalmol Vis Sci 52, 6321–6328.

Morlet, T., Rabinowitz, M.R., Looney, L.R., Riegner, T., Greenwood, L.A., Sherman, E.A., Achilly, N., Zhu, A., Yoo, E., O'Reilly, R.C., et al. (2014). A homozygous SLITRK6 nonsense mutation is associated with progressive auditory neuropathy in humans. Laryngoscope 124, E95–E103.

Muller, F., and O'Rahilly, R. (1988). The first appearance of the future cerebral hemispheres in the human embryo at stage 14. Anat Embryol 177, 495–511.

Naeem, A., Abbas, L., and Guthrie, S. (2002). Comparison of the effects of HGF, BDNF, CT-1, CNTF, and the branchial arches on the growth of embryonic cranial motor neurons. J Neurobiol 51, 101–114.

Nakamoto, M., Cheng, H.J., Friedman, G.C., McLaughlin, T., Hansen, M.J., Yoon, C.H., O'Leary, D.D., and Flanagan, J.G. (1996). Topographically specific effects of ELF-1 on retinal axon guidance in vitro and retinal axon mapping in vivo. Cell 86, 755–766.

Nakano, M., Yamada, K., Fain, J., Sener, E.C., Selleck, C.J., Awad, A.H., Zwaan, J., Mullaney, P.B., Bosley, T.M., and Engle, E.C. (2001). Homozygous mutations in ARIX(PHOX2A) result in congenital fibrosis of the extraocular muscles type 2. Nat Genet 29, 315–320.

Napal, O., Ojeda, N., Elizagárate, E., Peña, J., Ezcurra, J., and Gutiérrez, M. (2012). The course of the schizophrenia and its impact on cognition: a review of literature. Actas Esp Psiquiatr 40, 198–220.

Nelson, P.T., Alafuzoff, I., Bigio, E.H., Bouras, C., Braak, H., Cairns, N.J., Castellani, R.J., Crain, B.J., Davies, P., Del Tredici, K., Duyckaerts, C., Frosch, M.P., Haroutunian, V., Hof, P.R., Hulette, C.M., Hyman, B.T., Iwatsubo, T., Jellinger, K.A., Jicha, G.A., Kövari, E., Kukull, W.A., Leverenz, J.B., Love, S., Mackenzie, I.R., Mann, D.M., Masliah, E., McKee, A.C., Montine, T.J., Morris, J.C., Schneider, J.A., Sonnen, J.A., Thal, D.R., Trojanowski, J.Q., Troncoso, J.C., Wisniewski, T., Woltjer, R.L., Beach, T.G. (2012). Correlation of Alzheimer disease neuropathologic changes with cognitive status: a review of the literature. J Neuropathol Exp Neurol 71, 362–81.

Neveu, M.M., Jeffery, G., Burton, L.C., Sloper, J.J., and Holder, G.E. (2003). Age-related changes in the dynamics of human albino visual pathways. Eur J Neurosci 18, 1939–1949.

Nikolaev, A., McLaughlin, T., O'Leary, D.D., and Tessier-Lavigne, M. (2009). APP binds DR6 to trigger axon pruning and neuron death via distinct caspases. Nature 457, 981–989.

Niquille, M., Garel, S., Mann, F., Hornung, J.P., Otsmane, B., Chevalley, S., Parras, C., Guillemot, F., Gaspar, P., Yanagawa, Y., et al. (2009). Transient neuronal populations are required to guide callosal axons: a role for semaphorin 3C. PLoS Biol 7, e1000230.

O'Connor, T.P., Cockburn, K., Wang, W., Tapia, L., Currie, E., and Bamji, S.X. (2009). Semaphorin 5B mediates synapse elimination in hippocampal neurons. Neural Dev 4, 18.

O'Roak, B.J., Morgan, T.M., Fishman, D.O., Saus, E., Alonso, P., Gratacòs, M., Estivill, X., Teltsh, O., Kohn, Y., Kidd, K.K., et al. (2010). Additional support for the association of SLITRK1 var321 and Tourette syndrome. Mol Psychiatry 15, 447–450.

Osbun, N., Li, J., O'Driscoll, M.C., Strominger, Z., Wakahiro, M., Rider, E., Bukshpun, P., Boland, E., Spurrell, C.H., Schackwitz, W., et al. (2011). Genetic and functional analyses identify DISC1 as a novel callosal agenesis candidate gene. Am J Med Genet A 155A, 1865–1876.

Owen, J.P., Li, Y.O., Ziv, E., Strominger, Z., Gold, J., Bukhpun, P., Wakahiro, M., Friedman, E.J., Sherr, E.H., and Mukherjee, P. (2013). The structural connectome of the human brain in agenesis of the corpus callosum. Neuroimage 70, 340–355.

Pak, W., Hindges, R., Lim, Y.S., Pfaff, S.L., and O'Leary, D.D. (2004). Magnitude of binocular vision controlled by islet-2 repression of a genetic program that specifies laterality of retinal axon pathfinding. Cell 119, 567–578.

Palmesino, E., Haddick, P.C., Tessier-Lavigne, M., and Kania, A. (2012). Genetic analysis of DSCAM's role as a Netrin-1 receptor in vertebrates. J Neurosci 32, 411–416.

Pantazopoulos, H., Boyer-Boiteau, A., Holbrook, E.H., Jang, W., Hahn, C.G., Arnold, S.E., and Berretta, S. (2013). Proteoglycan abnormalities in olfactory epithelium tissue from subjects diagnosed with schizophrenia. Schizophr Res 150, 366–372.

Paradis, S., Harrar, D.B., Lin, Y., Koon, A.C., Hauser, J.L., Griffith, E.C., Zhu, L., Brass, L.F., Chen, C., and Greenberg, M.E. (2007). An RNAi-based approach identifies molecules required for glutamatergic and GABAergic synapse development. Neuron 53, 217–232.

Parsa, C.F., Grant, P.E., Dillon, W.P., Jr., du Lac, S., and Hoyt, W.F. (1998). Absence of the abducens nerve in Duane syndrome verified by magnetic resonance imaging. Am J Ophthalmol 125, 399–401.

Paschou, P. (2013). The genetic basis of Gilles de la Tourette Syndrome. Neurosci Biobehav Rev, 1–14.

Pasterkamp, R.J. (2012). Getting neural circuits into shape with semaphorins. Nat Rev Neurosci 13, 605–618.

Pasterkamp, R.J., and Kolodkin, A.L. (2013). SnapShot: Axon Guidance. Cell 153, 494, e491–e492.

Pasterkamp, R.J., Peschon, J.J., Spriggs, M.K., and Kolodkin, A.L. (2003). Semaphorin 7A promotes axon outgrowth through integrins and MAPKs. Nature 424, 398–405.

Paul, L.K. (2011). Developmental malformation of the corpus callosum: a review of typical callosal development and examples of developmental disorders with callosal involvement. J Neurodev Disord 3, 3–27.

Paul, L.K., Brown, W.S., Adolphs, R., Tyszka, J.M., Richards, L.J., Mukherjee, P., and Sherr, E.H. (2007). Agenesis of the corpus callosum: genetic, developmental and functional aspects of connectivity. Nat Rev Neurosci 8, 287–299.

Peng, J., and Charron, F. (2013). Lateralization of motor control in the human nervous system: genetics of mirror movements. Curr Opin Neurobiol 23, 109–118.

Petros, T.J., Rebsam, A., and Mason, C.A. (2008). Retinal axon growth at the optic chiasm: to cross or not to cross. Annu Rev Neurosci 31, 295–315.

Piper, M., Anderson, R., Dwivedy, A., Weinl, C., van Horck, F., Leung, K.M., Cogill, E., and Holt, C. (2006). Signaling mechanisms underlying Slit2-induced collapse of Xenopus retinal growth cones. Neuron 49, 215–228.

Pitteloud, N., Zhang, C., Pignatelli, D., Li, J.D., Raivio, T., Cole, L.W., Plummer, L., Jacobson-Dickman, E.E., Mellon, P.L., Zhou, Q.Y., et al. (2007). Loss-of-function mutation in the prokineticin 2 gene causes Kallmann syndrome and normosmic idiopathic hypogonadotropic hypogonadism. Proc Natl Acad Sci U S A 104, 17447–17452.

Plessen, K.J., Grüner, R., Lundervold, A., Hirsch, J.G., Xu, D., Bansal, R., Hammar, A., Lundervold, A.J., Wentzel-Larsen, T., Lie, S.A., et al. (2006). Reduced white matter connectivity in the corpus callosum of children with Tourette syndrome. J Child Psychol Psychiatry 47, 1013–1022.

Poirier, K., Saillour, Y., Bahi-Buisson, N., Jaglin, X.H., Fallet-Bianco, C., Nabbout, R., Castelnau-Ptakhine, L., Roubertie, A., Attie-Bitach, T., Desguerre, I., et al. (2010). Mutations in the neuronal ss-tubulin subunit TUBB3 result in malformation of cortical development and neuronal migration defects. Hum Mol Genet 19, 4462–4473.

Poon, V.Y., Klassen, M.P., and Shen, K. (2008). UNC-6/netrin and its receptor UNC-5 locally exclude presynaptic components from dendrites. Nature 455, 669–673.

Porteous, D.J., Millar, J.K., Brandon, N.J., and Sawa, A. (2011). DISC1 at 10: connecting psychiatric genetics and neuroscience. Trends Mol Med 17, 699–706.

Porter, J.D., and Baker, R.S. (1997). Absence of oculomotor and trochlear motoneurons leads to altered extraocular muscle development in the Wnt-1 null mutant mouse. Dev Brain Res 100, 121–126.

Proenca, C.C., Gao, K.P., Shmelkov, S.V., Rafii, S., Lee, F.S. (2011). Slitrks as emerging candidate genes involved in neuropsychiatric disorders. Trends Neurosci 34, 143–53.

Qu, C., Dwyer, T., Shao, Q., Yang, T., Huang, H., and Liu, G. (2013). Direct binding of TUBB3 with DCC couples netrin-1 signaling to intracellular microtubule dynamics in axon outgrowth and guidance. J Cell Sci 126, 3070–3081.

Rabe Bernhardt, N., Memic, F., Gezelius, H., Thiebes, A.L., Vallstedt, A., and Kullander, K. (2012). DCC mediated axon guidance of spinal interneurons is essential for normal locomotor central pattern generator function. Dev Biol 366, 279–289.

Rabe, N., Gezelius, H., Vallstedt, A., Memic, F., and Kullander, K. (2009). Netrin-1-dependent spinal interneuron subtypes are required for the formation of left-right alternating locomotor circuitry. J Neurosci 29, 15642–15649.

Rajapaksha, T.W., Eimer, W.A., Bozza, T.C., and Vassar, R. (2011). The Alzheimer's beta-secretase enzyme BACE1 is required for accurate axon guidance of olfactory sensory neurons and normal glomerulus formation in the olfactory bulb. Mol Neurodegener 6, 88.

Rama, N., Goldschneider, D., Corset, V., Lambert, J., Pays, L., and Mehlen, P. (2012). Amyloid precursor protein regulates netrin-1-mediated commissural axon outgrowth. J Biol Chem 287, 30014–30023.

Rao, A., O'Donnell, S., Bain, N., Meldrum, C., Shorter, D., and Goel, H. (2014). An intragenic deletion of the NFIA gene in a patient with a hypoplastic corpus callosum, craniofacial abnormalities and urinary tract defects. Eur J Med Genet 57, 65–70.

Rashid, T., Upton, A.L., Blentic, A., Ciossek, T., Knoll, B., Thompson, I.D., and Drescher, U. (2005). Opposing gradients of ephrin-As and EphA7 in the superior colliculus are essential for topographic mapping in the mammalian visual system. Neuron 47, 57–69.

Ray, K., Chaki, M., and Sengupta, M. (2007). Tyrosinase and ocular diseases: some novel thoughts on the molecular basis of oculocutaneous albinism type 1. Prog Retinal Eye Res 26, 323–358.

Rebsam, A., Bhansali, P., and Mason, C.A. (2012). Eye-specific projections of retinogeniculate axons are altered in albino mice. J Neurosci 32, 4821–4826.

Renaud, J., Kerjan, G., Sumita, I., Zagar, Y., Georget, V., Kim, D., Fouquet, C., Suda, K., Sanbo,

M., Suto, F., et al. (2008). Plexin-A2 and its ligand, Sema6A, control nucleus-centrosome coupling in migrating granule cells. Nat Neurosci 11, 440–449.

Renier, N., Schonewille, M., Giraudet, F., Badura, A., Tessier-Lavigne, M., Avan, P., De Zeeuw, C.I., and Chédotal, A. (2010). Genetic dissection of the function of hindbrain axonal commissures. PLoS Biol 8, e1000325.

Ripke, S., O'Dushlaine, C., Chambert, K., Moran, J.L., Kahler, A.K., Akterin, S., Bergen, S.E., Collins, A.L., Crowley, J.J., Fromer, M., et al. (2013). Genome-wide association analysis identifies 13 new risk loci for schizophrenia. Nat Genet 45, 1150–1159.

Robertson, M.M. (2012). The Gilles de la Tourette syndrome: the current status. Arch Dis Child Educ Pract Ed 97, 166–175.

Rogers, J.H., Ciossek, T., Ullrich, A., West, E., Hoare, M., and Muir, E.M. (1999). Distribution of the receptor EphA7 and its ligands in development of the mouse nervous system. Brain Res Mol Brain Res 74, 225–230.

Romaniello, F., Arrigoni, F., Bassi, M.T., and Borgatti, R. (2015) Mutations in α- and β-tubulin encoding genes: Implications in brain malformations. Brain Dev 37(3), 273–280.

Ronca, F., Andersen, J.S., Paech, V., and Margolis, R.U. (2001). Characterization of Slit protein interactions with glypican-1. J Biol Chem 276, 29141–29147.

Ross, M.E., and Walsh, C.A. (2001). Human brain malformations and their cortical malformation: Disorders of Neuronal Position. Annu Rev Neurosci 24, 1041–1070.

Rudrabhatla, P., Jaffe, H., and Pant, H.C. (2011). Direct evidence of phosphorylated neuronal intermediate filament proteins in neurofibrillary tangles (NFTs): phosphoproteomics of Alzheimer's NFTs. FASEB J 25, 3896–3905.

Rujescu, D., Meisenzahl, E.M., Krejcova, S., Giegling, I., Zetzsche, T., Reiser, M., Born, C.M., Moller, H.J., Veske, A., Gal, A., et al. (2007). Plexin B3 is genetically associated with verbal performance and white matter volume in human brain. Mol Psychiatry 12(190–194), 115.

Runker, A.E., Little, G.E., Suto, F., Fujisawa, H., and Mitchell, K.J. (2008). Semaphorin-6A controls guidance of corticospinal tract axons at multiple choice points. Neural Dev 3, 34.

Rünker, A.E., O'Tuathaigh, C., Dunleavy, M., Morris, D.W., Little, G.E., Corvin, A.P., Gill, M., Henshall, D.C., Waddington, J.L., and Mitchell, K.J. (2011). Mutation of Semaphorin-6A disrupts limbic and cortical connectivity and models neurodevelopmental psychopathology. PLoS One 6, e26488.

Sabatier, C., Plump, A.S., Le, M., Brose, K., Tamada, A., Murakami, F., Lee, E.Y., and Tessier-Lavigne, M. (2004). The divergent Robo family protein rig-1/Robo3 is a negative regulator of slit responsiveness required for midline crossing by commissural axons. Cell 117, 157–169.

Sasaki, T., Oga, T., Nakagaki, K., Sakai, K., Sumida, K., Hoshino, K., Miyawaki, I., Saito, K., Suto, F., and Ichinohe, N. (2014). Developmental expression profiles of axon guidance signaling and the immune system in the marmoset cortex: potential molecular mechanisms of pruning of dendritic spines during primate synapse formation in late infancy and prepuberty (I). Biochem Biophys Res Commun 444, 302–306.

Schettini, G., Govoni, S., Racchi, M., and Rodriguez, G. (2010). Phosphorylation of APP-CTF-AICD domains and interaction with adaptor proteins: signal transduction and/or transcriptional role--relevance for Alzheimer pathology. J Neurochem 115, 1299–1308.

Schindowski, K., Belarbi, K., and Buée, L. (2008). Neurotrophic factors in Alzheimer's disease: role of axonal transport. Genes, Brain Behav 7(Suppl 1), 43–56.

Schwanzel-Fukuda, M., and Pfaff, D.W. (1989). Origin of luteinizing hormone-releasing hormone neurons. Nature 338, 161–164.

Serafini, T., Colamarino, S.A., Leonardo, E.D., Wang, H., Beddington, R., Skarnes, W.C., and Tessier-Lavigne, M. (1996). Netrin-1 is required for commissural axon guidance in the developing vertebrate nervous system. Cell 87, 1001–1014.

Serafini, T., Kennedy, T.E., Galko, M.J., Mirzayan, C., Jessell, T.M., and Tessier-Lavigne, M. (1994). The netrins define a family of axon outgrowth-promoting proteins homologous to C. elegans UNC-6. Cell 78, 409–424.

Serini, G., Valdembri, D., Zanivan, S., Morterra, G., Burkhardt, C., Caccavari, F., Zammataro, L., Primo, L., Tamagnone, L., Logan, M., et al. (2003). Class 3 semaphorins control vascular morphogenesis by inhibiting integrin function. Nature 424, 391–397.

Serrano-Pozo, A., Frosch, M.P., Masliah, E., and Hyman, B.T. (2011). Neuropathological alterations in Alzheimer disease. Cold Spring Harbor Perspect Med 1, a006189.

Sheffler-Collins, S.I., and Dalva, M.B. (2012). EphBs: an integral link between synaptic function and synaptopathies. Trends Neurosci 35, 293–304.

Shen, K., and Cowan, C.W. (2010). Guidance molecules in synapse formation and plasticity. Cold Spring Harb Perspect Biol 2, a001842.

Shen, S., Lang, B., Nakamoto, C., Zhang, F., Pu, J., Kuan, S.L., Chatzi, C., He, S., Mackie, I., Brandon, N.J., et al. (2008). Schizophrenia-related neural and behavioral phenotypes in transgenic mice expressing truncated Disc1. J Neurosci 28, 10893–10904.

Shewan, D., Dwivedy, A., Anderson, R., and Holt, C.E. (2002). Age-related changes underlie switch in netrin-1 responsiveness as growth cones advance along visual pathway. Nat Neurosci 5, 955–962.

Shmelkov, S.V., Hormigo, A., Jing, D., Proenca, C.C., Bath, K.G., Milde, T., Shmelkov, E., Kushner, J.S., Baljevic, M., Dincheva, I., et al. (2010). Slitrk5 deficiency impairs corticostriatal circuitry and leads to obsessive-compulsive-like behaviors in mice. Nat Med 16, 598–602.

Shu, T., Butz, K.G., Plachez, C., Gronostajski, R.M., and Richards, L.J. (2003). Abnormal development of forebrain midline glia and commissural projections in Nfia knock-out mice. J Neurosci 23, 203–212.

Sosa L.J., Bergman J., Estrada-Bernal A., Glorioso T.J., Kittelson J.M., and Pfenninger K.H. (2013). Amyloid precursor protein is an autonomous growth cone adhesion molecule engaged in contact guidance. PLoS One, 8:e64521.

Sosa L.J., Postma N.L., Estrada-Bernal A., Hanna M., Guo R., Busciglio J., and Pfenninger K.H. (2014) Dosage of amyloid precursor protein affects axonal contact guidance in Down syndrome. FASEB J 1,195–205.

Srour, M., Riviere, J.B., Pham, J.M., Dube, M.P., Girard, S., Morin, S., Dion, P.A., Asselin, G., Rochefort, D., Hince, P., et al. (2010). Mutations in DCC cause congenital mirror movements. Science 328, 592.

Stanfield, B.B., O'Leary, D.D., and Fricks, C. (1982). Selective collateral elimination in early postnatal development restricts cortical distribution of rat pyramidal tract neurones. Nature 298, 371–373.

Stein, E., and Tessier-Lavigne, M. (2001). Hierarchical organization of guidance receptors: silencing of netrin attraction by slit through a Robo/DCC receptor complex. Science 291, 1928–1938.

Stein, E., Zou, Y., Poo, M., and Tessier-Lavigne, M. (2001). Binding of DCC by netrin-1 to mediate axon guidance independent of adenosine A2B receptor activation. Science 291, 1976–1982.

Stillman, A.a., Krsnik, Z., Sun, J., Rasin, M.-R., State, M.W., Sestan, N., and Louvi, A. (2009). Developmentally regulated and evolutionarily conserved expression of SLITRK1 in brain circuits implicated in Tourette syndrome. J Comp Neurol 513, 21–37.

Stokin, G.B., Lillo, C., Falzone, T.L., Brusch, R.G., Rockenstein, E., Mount, S.L., Raman, R., Davies, P., Masliah, E., Williams, D.S., et al. (2005). Axonopathy and transport deficits early in the pathogenesis of Alzheimer's disease. Science 307, 1282–1288.

Su, K.Y., Chien, W.L., Fu, W.M., Yu, I.S., Huang, H.P., Huang, P.H., Lin, S.R., Shih, J.Y., Lin, Y.L., Hsueh, Y.P., et al. (2007). Mice deficient in collapsin response mediator protein-1 exhibit impaired long-term potentiation and impaired spatial learning and memory. J Neurosci 27, 2513–2524.

Suwaki, N., Klare, K., and Tarsounas, M. (2011). RAD51 paralogs: roles in DNA damage signalling, recombinational repair and tumorigenesis. Semin Cell Dev Biol 22, 898–905.

Takahashi, T., Fournier, A., Nakamura, F., Wang, L.H., Murakami, Y., Kalb, R.G., Fujisawa, H., and Strittmatter, S.M. (1999). Plexin-neuropilin-1 complexes form functional semaphorin-3A receptors. Cell 99, 59–69.

Tamagnone, L., Artigiani, S., Chen, H., He, Z., Ming, G.I., Song, H., Chédotal, A., Winberg, M.L., Goodman, C.S., Poo, M., et al. (1999). Plexins are a large family of receptors for transmembrane, secreted, and GPI-anchored semaphorins in vertebrates. Cell 99, 71–80.

ten Donkelaar, H.J., Lammens, M., Wesseling, P., Hori, A., Keyser, A., and Rotteveel, J. (2004). Development and malformations of the human pyramidal tract. J Neurol 251, 1429–1442.

Tischfield, M.A., Baris, H.N., Wu, C., Rudolph, G., Van Maldergem, L., He, W., Chan, W.M., Andrews, C., Demer, J.L., Robertson, R.L., et al.

(2010). Human TUBB3 mutations perturb microtubule dynamics, kinesin interactions, and axon guidance. Cell 140, 74–87.

Tischfield, M.A., Bosley, T.M., Salih, M.A., Alorainy, I.A., Sener, E.C., Nester, M.J., Oystreck, D.T., Chan, W.M., Andrews, C., Erickson, R.P., et al. (2005). Homozygous HOXA1 mutations disrupt human brainstem, inner ear, cardiovascular and cognitive development. Nat Genet 37, 1035–1037.

Tornberg, J., Sykiotis, G.P., Keefe, K., Plummer, L., Hoang, X., Hall, J.E., Quinton, R., Seminara, S.B., Hughes, V., Van Vliet, G., et al. (2011). Heparan sulfate 6-O-sulfotransferase 1, a gene involved in extracellular sugar modifications, is mutated in patients with idiopathic hypogonadotrophic hypogonadism. Proc Natl Acad Sci U S A 108, 11524–11529.

Tosney, K.W., and Landmesser, L.T. (1984). Pattern and specificity of axonal outgrowth following varying degrees of chick limb bud ablation. J Neurosci 4, 2518–2527.

Toyofuku, T., Zhang, H., Kumanogoh, A., Takegahara, N., Suto, F., Kamei, J., Aoki, K., Yabuki, M., Hori, M., Fujisawa, H., et al. (2004a). Dual roles of Sema6D in cardiac morphogenesis through region-specific association of its receptor, Plexin-A1, with off-track and vascular endothelial growth factor receptor type 2. Genes Dev 18, 435–447.

Toyofuku, T., Zhang, H., Kumanogoh, A., Takegahara, N., Yabuki, M., Harada, K., Hori, M., and Kikutani, H. (2004b). Guidance of myocardial patterning in cardiac development by Sema6D reverse signalling. Nat Cell Biol 6, 1204–1211.

Tran, T.S., Kolodkin, A.L., and Bharadwaj, R. (2007). Semaphorin regulation of cellular morphology. Annu Rev Cell Dev Biol 23, 263–292.

Triplett, J.W., and Feldheim, D.A. (2012). Eph and ephrin signaling in the formation of topographic maps. Semin Cell Dev Biol 23, 7–15.

Uchida, Y., Ohshima, T., Sasaki, Y., Suzuki, H., Yanai, S., Yamashita, N., Nakamura, F., Takei, K., Ihara, Y., Mikoshiba, K., et al. (2005). Semaphorin3A signalling is mediated via sequential Cdk5 and GSK3beta phosphorylation of CRMP2: implication of common phosphorylating mechanism underlying axon guidance and Alzheimer's disease. Genes Cells 10, 165–179.

van den Heuvel, M.P., and Fornito, A. (2014). Brain networks in schizophrenia. Neuropsychol Rev 24, 32–48.

van der Vaart, B., van Riel, W.E., Doodhi, H., Kevenaar, J.T., Katrukha, E.A., Gumy, L., Bouchet, B.P., Grigoriev, I., Spangler, S.A., Yu, K.L., et al. (2013). CFEOM1-associated kinesin KIF21A is a cortical microtubule growth inhibitor. Dev Cell 27, 145–160.

Vanderhaeghen, P., and Cheng, H.J. (2010). Guidance molecules in axon pruning and cell death. Cold Spring Harb Perspect Biol 2, a001859.

Vassar, R., Kuhn, P.H., Haass, C., Kennedy, M.E., Rajendran, L., Wong, P.C., and Lichtenthaler, S.F. (2014). Function, therapeutic potential and cell biology of BACE proteases: current status and future prospects. J Neurochem 130, 4–28.

Wahl, C.M., Noden, D.M., and Baker, R. (1994). Developmental relations between sixth nerve motor neurons and their targets in the chick embryo. Dev Dyn 201, 191–202.

Walsh, D.M., and Selkoe, D.J. (2004). Deciphering the molecular basis of memory failure in Alzheimer's disease. Neuron 44, 181–193.

Wang, H., Megill, A., He, K., Kirkwood, A., and Lee, H.-K. (2012). Consequences of inhibiting amyloid precursor protein processing enzymes on synaptic function and plasticity. Neural Plast 2012, 272374.

Wang, W., Mullikin-Kilpatrick, D., Crandall, J.E., Gronostajski, R.M., Litwack, E.D., and Kilpatrick, D.L. (2007). Nuclear factor I coordinates multiple phases of cerebellar granule cell development via regulation of cell adhesion molecules. J Neurosci 27, 6115–6127.

Watanabe, K., Tamamaki, N., Furuta, T., Ackerman, S.L., Ikenaka, K., and Ono, K. (2006). Dorsally derived netrin 1 provides an inhibitory cue and elaborates the 'waiting period' for primary sensory axons in the developing spinal cord. Development 133, 1379–1387.

Watanabe, Y., Toyoda, R., and Nakamura, H. (2004). Navigation of trochlear motor axons along the midbrain-hindbrain boundary by neuropilin 2. Development 131, 681–692.

Wegmeyer, H., Egea, J., Rabe, N., Gezelius, H., Filosa, A., Enjin, A., Varoqueaux, F., Deininger, K., Schnutgen, F., Brose, N., et al. (2007). EphA4-dependent axon guidance is mediated by the RacGAP alpha2-chimaerin. Neuron 55, 756–767.

Weiss, L.A., Arking, D.E., Daly, M.J., and Chakravarti, A. (2009). A genome-wide linkage and association scan reveals novel loci for autism. Nature 461, 802–808.

Wheeler, A.L., and Voineskos, A.N. (2014). A review of structural neuroimaging in schizophrenia: from connectivity to connectomics. Front Hum Neurosci 8, 653.

Williams, R.W., Hogan, D., and Garraghty, P.E. (1994). Target recognition and visual maps in the thalamus of achiasmatic dogs. Nature 367, 637–639.

Williams, S.E., Grumet, M., Colman, D.R., Henkemeyer, M., Mason, C.A., and Sakurai, T. (2006). A role for Nr-CAM in the patterning of binocular visual pathways. Neuron 50, 535–547.

Williamson, R., van Aalten, L., Mann, D.M.a., Platt, B., Plattner, F., Bedford, L., Mayer, J., Howlett, D., Usardi, A., Sutherland, C., et al. (2011). CRMP2 hyperphosphorylation is characteristic of Alzheimer's disease and not a feature common to other neurodegenerative diseases. J Alzheimers Dis 27, 615–625.

Wright, K.M., Lyon, K.A., Leung, H., Leahy, D.J., Ma, L., and Ginty, D.D. (2012). Dystroglycan organizes axon guidance cue localization and axonal pathfinding. Neuron 76, 931–944.

Xia, S., Li, R.L., Li, Y.P., Qian, X.H., Chong, V., and Qi, J. (2014). MRI findings in Duane's ocular retraction syndrome. Clin Radiol 69, e191–198.

Yamada, K., Andrews, C., Chan, W.M., McKeown, C.A., Magli, A., de Berardinis, T., Loewenstein, A., Lazar, M., O'Keefe, M., Letson, R., et al. (2003). Heterozygous mutations of the kinesin KIF21A in congenital fibrosis of the extraocular muscles type 1 (CFEOM1). Nat Genet 35, 318–321.

Yamagishi, S., Hampel, F., Hata, K., Del Toro, D., Schwark, M., Kvachnina, E., Bastmeyer, M., Yamashita, T., Tarabykin, V., Klein, R., et al. (2011). FLRT2 and FLRT3 act as repulsive guidance cues for Unc5-positive neurons. EMBO J 30, 2920–2933.

Ye, X.C., Pegado, V., Patel, M.S. and Wasserman, W.W. (2014) Strabismus genetic across a spectrum of eye misalignment disorders. Clin Genet 86, 103–111.

Yoshida, H., Watanabe, A., and Ihara, Y. (1998). Collapsin response mediator protein-2 is associated with neurofibrillary tangles in Alzheimer's disease. J Biol Chem 273, 9761–9768.

Young-Pearse, T.L., Suth, S., Luth, E.S., Sawa, A., and Selkoe, D.J. (2010). Biochemical and functional interaction of disrupted-in-schizophrenia 1 and amyloid precursor protein regulates neuronal migration during mammalian cortical development. J Neurosci 30, 10431–10440.

Ypsilanti, A.R., Zagar, Y., and Chédotal, A. (2010). Moving away from the midline: new developments for Slit and Robo. Development 137, 1939–1952.

Yuan, S.S., Cox, L.A., Dasika, G.K., and Lee, E.Y. (1999). Cloning and functional studies of a novel gene aberrantly expressed in RB-deficient embryos. Dev Biol 207, 62–75.

Zoghbi, H.Y., and Bear, M.F. (2012). Synaptic dysfunction in neurodevelopmental disorders associated with autism and intellectual disabilities. Cold Spring Harb Perspect Biol 4.

Zuchner, S., Cuccaro, M.L., Tran-Viet, K.N., Cope, H., Krishnan, R.R., Pericak-Vance, M.a., Wright, H.H., and Ashley-Koch, a. (2006). SLITRK1 mutations in trichotillomania. Mol Psychiatry 11, 887–889.

9

SYNAPTIC DISORDERS

CATALINA BETANCUR[1,2,3] AND KEVIN J. MITCHELL[4]

[1]*INSERM U1130, 75005 Paris, France*
[2]*CNRS UMR 8246, 75005 Paris, France*
[3]*Sorbonne Universités, UPMC Univ Paris 6, Neuroscience Paris Seine, 75005 Paris, France*
[4]*Smurfit Institute of Genetics and Institute of Neuroscience, Trinity College Dublin, Dublin 2, Ireland*

9.1 INTRODUCTION

The last few years have brought substantial advancement in our knowledge on the genetic architecture of neurodevelopmental disorders. Genome-wide studies of copy number variants (CNVs), and more recently exome sequencing studies, have identified hundreds of causative genetic variants in disorders such as autism spectrum disorders (ASD), intellectual disability (ID), schizophrenia, and epilepsy, revealing a far more extensive genetic heterogeneity than previously recognized. These studies have shown an important contribution of rare variants in neurodevelopmental conditions for which the underlying genetic causes had remained elusive, and have contributed to a profound paradigm shift in psychiatric genetics. The

significant enrichment of *de novo* structural variants and sequence mutations together with low population frequencies implies purifying selection and large effects on disease risk. Many of these genetic variants confer risk for a broad range of neurologic and psychiatric phenotypes, revealing common pathogenic mechanisms in conditions conceptualized as distinct.

A large number of genetic variants associated with neurodevelopmental disorders have been shown to affect genes related to synaptic development and function, highlighting this as a core neural substrate dysregulated in these conditions. Synaptic genes have thus become a focus of research on neurodevelopmental disorders, contributing to our understanding of disease pathogenesis and providing promising therapeutic targets. Here, we briefly consider the

The Genetics of Neurodevelopmental Disorders, First Edition. Edited by Kevin J. Mitchell.
© 2015 John Wiley & Sons, Inc. Published 2015 by John Wiley & Sons, Inc.

molecular processes of synapse formation and plasticity and review the evidence that genes with roles in these processes constitute a major mutational target for both rare and common neurodevelopmental disorders.

9.2 PROCESSES OF SYNAPSE FORMATION AND PLASTICITY

The mammalian nervous system is characterized by an astounding diversity of cell types, which are interconnected with exquisite specificity. The synaptic interconnections show an equal level of diversity in electrophysiological characteristics, biochemical profiles, and patterns of synaptic plasticity (O'Rourke et al., 2012). The specification of these connections is achieved through diverse molecular mechanisms that direct highly stereotyped initial wiring, followed by extensive refinement of connectivity through activity-dependent and maturational processes.

Growing axons select appropriate target regions for innervation using similar cues and receptors as those that direct axonal pathfinding (netrins, semaphorins, Wnts, ephrins, cadherins, etc; see Chapter 8 (Shen and Cowan, 2010)). Within large regions, axons may select specific nuclei, cellular layers, or even sublayers of neuropil. Following invasion of the appropriate subregion, synapses must be formed in a cell-type-specific manner, which requires recognition between appropriate pre- and postsynaptic partners, mediated by matching homophilic cell adhesion molecules or heterophilic partners (Sanes and Yamagata, 2009). Finding the right cell is just the start of this process. Many synapses are localized to subcellular regions, such as the soma, axon initial segment, or proximal or distal dendrites, in response to the localization of synaptogenic cues to these compartments.

A growing number of molecules have been discovered to direct the formation of synapses between specific cell types, and there is reason to expect an even greater diversity of cellular labels to specify the vast number of pairwise connectivity relationships in the mammalian brain. In addition to guidance molecules listed earlier, these include proteins such as neuroligins and neurexins, along with many members of the immunoglobulin (e.g., contactins, CNT-NAPs, neuregulin-1, L1-CAMs) or leucine-rich repeat (LRR) superfamilies (e.g., LRRTMs, Slitrks, NGLs, Lrfns), as well as protocadherins, BMPs, FGFs and other molecules (reviewed in Sanes and Yamagata, 2009; Yang et al., 2014).

Forming a synapse requires both cellular recognition/physical adhesion between pre- and postsynaptic partners and the induction of biochemical and cellular processes involved in building the highly specialized pre- and postsynaptic structures. There is, moreover, an enormous level of diversity and complexity in the *types of synapses* that are made. This extends far beyond the obvious distinctions in major neurotransmitters and neuromodulators used (glutamate, GABA, acetylcholine, dopamine, serotonin, oxytocin, etc.) to include selective expression of a huge variety of neurotransmitter receptor subunits – which can be combined in multiple ways – as well as a vast array of ion channels, G-protein-coupled receptors, transporters, and many other proteins affecting neural communication and plasticity (O'Rourke et al., 2012).

These proteins are recruited to the synapse and organized by an equally diverse set of scaffolding proteins, including members of the membrane-associated guanylate kinase (MAGUK) family (e.g., discs large [DLG]/postsynaptic density [PSD] proteins), SHANKs, GKAPs, AKAPs, gephyrin, homers, and others postsynaptically (Sheng and Kim, 2011), and bassoon, piccolo, CASK, RIMs, and others presynaptically (Schoch and Gundelfinger, 2006). Members of each of these protein families interact combinatorially and are differentially expressed in overlapping patterns in different cells (Emes and Grant, 2012). They are also deployed differentially to individual synapses within cells, generating even greater diversity in synapse types. Scaffolding proteins of this sort mediate not just the formation of particular synaptic structures but are also involved in the constant and highly dynamic trafficking of proteins in and out of synapses (Choquet and Triller, 2013).

The formation of synapses during early neural development is followed by an extended period of activity-dependent refinement and by ongoing synaptic plasticity in the adult. In both cases, regressive events of synaptic weakening and pruning are as important as the strengthening or formation of new synapses. While the outcomes of these processes are not driven by information encoded in the genome, the processes themselves still rely on biochemical mechanisms that can be disrupted by mutations and can thus be a focus for genetic disease.

Synaptic plasticity is best known as a cellular mechanism for various forms of learning and memory, for example, through long-term potentiation or depression (LTP or LTD) in the hippocampus or cortex. But many other forms of plasticity exist, which in some way alter the functional parameters of a synapse in response to patterns of activity (Citri and Malenka, 2008). For example, various forms of short-term plasticity (STP) may last only tens of seconds but play important roles in information transfer and neural dynamics. The particular type of STP at any synapse depends in part on the profile of metabotropic glutamate receptors and kainate receptors on the presynaptic side (Cosgrove et al., 2011; Sihra et al., 2014). This profile may in turn be determined in a target-specific way by proteins expressed by the postsynaptic cell (such as Elfn1) (Blackman et al., 2013; Sylwestrak and Ghosh, 2012).

Additional forms of plasticity include biochemical changes that do not alter the strength of synaptic connectivity between cells but the types of plasticity at those synapses (metaplasticity) (Hulme et al., 2013). The input−output relationship between two cells can also be altered indirectly by changes at synapses from a third cell (such as an inhibitory interneuron), mediating network-level plasticity (Ramaswami, 2014; Xue et al., 2014). Homeostatic mechanisms at the level of individual synapses and across networks also play a crucial role in maintaining neural network set points within an appropriate range (Davis, 2013).

A number of pathways have been defined that detect or measure activity levels or patterns at individual synapses and induce biochemical changes in response to them. In the postsynaptic compartment, many of these begin with NMDA receptors and calcium channels, which mediate ionic flux in response to neurotransmitter release. Among other effects, these fluxes initiate signaling cascades that regulate the translation of mRNAs that are held in an inaccessible complex in dendrites, allowing the rapid production of new proteins to mediate synaptic plasticity. Plasticity also often involves communication from synapses to the nucleus of the cell and resultant changes in gene expression, which feed back to the relevant synapses. These are mediated by a variety of activity-dependent transcription factors and chromatin regulatory proteins (Greer and Greenberg, 2008).

Subsequently, we consider how mutations in many genes encoding members of each of these classes can result in developmental brain dysfunction, with a variety of clinical effects. Many of these are associated with rare, recognized clinical syndromes but mutations in this class of genes also explain a growing number of cases of more common clinical categories.

9.3 RARE SYNDROMES

Multiple rare genetic disorders characterized by ID and other neuropsychiatric phenotypes are associated with synaptic dysfunction, including aberrant synaptic formation, function, and plasticity. Classic examples include fragile X syndrome, Rett syndrome, tuberous sclerosis, Angelman syndrome, and *PTEN*-related syndromes; their mechanistic roles have been the subject of several recent reviews (Mabb et al., 2011; Na et al., 2013; Sidorov et al., 2013; Tsai and Sahin, 2011). Other genetic disorders associated with abnormal synaptic function are listed in Table 9.1. Although many of these syndromes and the causative genes have been known for a long time, others have been identified more recently, for example, Kleefstra syndrome (*EHMT1*), cortical

TABLE 9.1 Synaptic genes involved in neurodevelopmental disorders through rare mutations (*See insert for color representation of this table.*)

Gene	Gene name	Cytoband	Function	Disorder	Evidence	Selected references
Cell–cell interactions/synaptic adhesion						
CNTNAP2	Contactin associated protein-like 2	7q35-q36.1	Neurexin family member	Cortical dysplasia-focal epilepsy syndrome, associated with ID and ASD (recessive); Pitt–Hopkins-like syndrome-1 (recessive). Deletions or chromosomal rearrangements disrupting a *single* copy of *CNTNAP2* have been reported in patients with ASD, ID, epilepsy, schizophrenia, and bipolar disorder as well as in healthy subjects; their clinical significance is unknown	Recessive point mutations, deletions	(Strauss et al., 2006; Zweier et al., 2009)
IL1RAPL1	Interleukin 1 receptor accessory protein-like 1	Xp21.2-p21.3	Cell adhesion, synapse formation	X-linked ID and ASD, with or without dysmorphic features	Point mutations, deletions, intragenic duplications	(Franek et al., 2011; Pinto et al., 2010; Piton et al., 2008; Valnegri et al., 2011)
L1CAM	L1 cell adhesion molecule	Xq28	Cell adhesion, synapse formation and development	Syndromic X-linked ID with hydrocephalus, adducted thumbs, spastic paraplegia, and hypoplasia of the corpus callosum	Deletions, point mutations	(Saghatelyan et al., 2004; Schafer and Altevogt, 2010; Schrander-Stumpel and Vos, 2010)

Gene	Name	Location	Function	Disorder	Mutation type	References
LGI1	Leucine-rich glioma inactivated-1	10q24	Secreted LRR protein, synapse formation	Autosomal dominant lateral temporal lobe epilepsy and sporadic epilepsy	Point mutations, deletions	(Kegel et al., 2013)
NLGN3	Neuroligin 3	Xq13.1	Cell adhesion, inhibitory synapse formation	Nonsyndromic X-linked ASD and ID	Point mutation, deletion	(Jamain et al., 2003; Sanders et al., 2011)
NLGN4X	Neuroligin 4, X-linked	Xp22.32-p22.31	Cell adhesion, synapse formation	Nonsyndromic X-linked ASD and/or ID	Point mutations, deletions	(Jamain et al., 2003; Laumonnier et al., 2004)
NRXN1	Neurexin 1	2p16.3	Cell adhesion, synapse formation	Disrupted in ASD, ID, schizophrenia, ADHD, Tourette syndrome and other neurodevelopmental and psychiatric disorders (dominant); deletions also reported in unaffected parents and controls. Pitt–Hopkins-like syndrome-2 (recessive)	Deletions, point mutations, translocations	(Ching et al., 2010; Pinto et al., 2010; Rujescu et al., 2009; Szatmari et al., 2007; Zweier et al., 2009)
PCDH19	Protocadherin 19	Xq22.1	Cell adhesion, synapse formation	X-linked female-limited epilepsy, with or without cognitive impairment and ASD; early infantile epileptic encephalopathy	Point mutations, deletions	(Camacho et al., 2012; Depienne and LeGuern, 2012)
SLITRK1	SLIT and NTRK-like family, member 1	13q31.1	Cell adhesion, neurite outgrowth	Tourette syndrome, trichotillomania, obsessive-compulsive disorder	Point mutations	(Abelson et al., 2005; Ozomaro et al., 2013; Zuchner et al., 2006)

(continued)

TABLE 9.1 *(Continued)*

Gene	Gene name	Cytoband	Function	Disorder	Evidence	Selected references
Scaffolding proteins						
CASK	Calcium/calmodulin-dependent serine protein kinase	Xp11.4	Adaptor/scaffold protein, synapse plasticity	X-linked ID and micro-cephaly with pontine and cerebellar hypoplasia (loss-of-function mutations, mainly in females); hypomorphic mutations cause non-syndromic ID with or without nystagmus and ASD in males	Point mutations, deletions	(Hackett et al., 2010; Lin et al., 2013; Najm et al., 2008; Tarpey et al., 2009)
DISC1	disrupted in schizophrenia 1	1q42.2	Scaffold protein, synapse development	Balanced translocation t(1;11) cosegregates with schizophrenia, bipolar disorder and depression in a single large Scottish family	Translocation	(Brandon and Sawa, 2011)
DLG3	Discs, large homolog 3	Xq13.1	Synaptic scaffolding (MAGUK)	Nonsyndromic X-linked ID	Point mutations	(Tarpey et al., 2004; Zanni et al., 2010)
SHANK2	SH3 and multiple ankyrin repeat domains 2	11q13.3	Synaptic scaffolding	ID, ASD	Deletions, point mutations	(Berkel et al., 2010; Leblond et al., 2012; Pinto et al., 2010)
SHANK3	SH3 and multiple ankyrin repeat domains 3	22q13.33	Synaptic scaffolding	Phelan-McDermid syndrome, associated with ID, absent or severely delayed speech, ASD, hypotonia; mutations reported in 2 families with schizophrenia and ID	Deletions, point mutations	(Durand et al., 2007; Gauthier et al., 2010; Gong et al., 2012; Hamdan et al., 2011b; Leblond et al., 2014; Moessner et al., 2007)

Receptors and channels

CACNA1C	Calcium channel, voltage-dependent, L type, alpha 1C subunit	12p13.33	Voltage-gated calcium channel	Timothy syndrome (arrhythmias with syndactyly, congenital heart disease, immune deficiency, ID, and ASD)	Gain-of-function mutations	(Splawski et al., 2004)
CHRNA7	Cholinergic receptor, nicotinic, alpha 7	15q13.3	Ligand gated ion channel, nicotinic acetylcholine receptor	15q13.3 microdeletion syndrome characterized by variable phenotype and incomplete penetrance, including ID, seizures, ASD, schizophrenia, and other neuropsychiatric disorders. The common deletion is approximately 1.3 Mb; smaller deletions affecting only CHRNA7 suggest that this is the causative gene for the majority of the phenotypes	Deletions	(Hoppman-Chaney et al., 2013; Levinson et al., 2011; Sharp et al., 2008; Shinawi et al., 2009)
GRIA3	Glutamate receptor, ionotrophic, AMPA 3	Xq25	Ligand gated ion channel, ionotropic glutamate receptor, AMPA	X-linked ASD and ID	Deletions, duplications, point mutations, translocations	(Chiyonobu et al., 2007; Wu et al., 2007)
GRIN2A	Glutamate receptor, ionotropic, N-methyl D-aspartate 2A	16p13.2	Ligand gated ion channel, ionotropic glutamate receptor, NMDA	Focal epilepsy with speech disorder, with or without ID	Point mutations, deletions, translocations	(Carvill et al., 2013; Endele et al., 2010; Lesca et al., 2013)

(continued)

201

TABLE 9.1 *(Continued)*

Gene	Gene name	Cytoband	Function	Disorder	Evidence	Selected references
GRIN2B	Glutamate receptor, ionotropic, N-methyl D-aspartate 2B	12p13.1	Ligand gated ion channel, ionotropic glutamate receptor, NMDA	ID, ASD, seizures	Point mutations, translocations	(Endele et al., 2010; O'Roak et al., 2012a)
SCN1A	Sodium channel, voltage-gated, type I, alpha subunit	2q24.3	Voltage-gated sodium channel	Severe myoclonic epilepsy of infancy (Dravet syndrome), ID, ASD	Deletions, point mutations	(Carvill et al., 2013; Marini et al., 2009; O'Roak et al., 2011)
SCN2A	Sodium channel, voltage-gated, type II, alpha subunit	2q24.3	Voltage-gated sodium channel	Early infantile epileptic encephalopathy; benign familial infantile seizures, ID, ASD	Deletions, point mutations	(Carvill et al., 2013; Neale et al., 2012; Sanders et al., 2012)
Signal transduction, translation						
CDKL5	Cyclin-dependent kinase-like 5 (kinase)	Xp22.13	Synapse development and plasticity	Early infantile epileptic encephalopathy, ID, ASD	Point mutations, deletions	(Archer et al., 2006a; Fehr et al., 2013; Russo et al., 2009; Su and Tsai, 2011)
CUL4B	Cullin 4B	Xq24	Ubiquitin E3 ligase subunit, synapse formation	Syndromic X-linked ID, Cabezas type (short stature, hypogonadism, and abnormal gait)	Point mutations, deletions	(Chen et al., 2012; Tarpey et al., 2007)
FMR1	Fragile X mental retardation 1	Xq27.3	Translation repressor of numerous synaptic proteins	Fragile X syndrome, associated with ID, ASD, ADHD, and epilepsy	(CGG)n expansion, point mutations	(Sidorov et al., 2013)
IQSEC2	IQ motif and Sec7 domain 2	Xp11.22	Arf6-GEF, synaptic plasticity (also known as BRAG1)	Nonsyndromic X-linked ID, autistic traits, epilepsy	Point mutations, intragenic duplications	(Gandomi et al., 2014; Shoubridge et al., 2010)

Gene	Protein/Name	Locus	Function	Disorder	Mutation type	References
NF1	Neurofibromin 1	17q11.2	MAPK signaling pathway (RAS-GTPase activator protein)	Neurofibromatosis type 1, associated with ID and ASD	Deletions, point mutations	(Garg et al., 2013)
PTEN	Phosphatase and tensin homolog	10q23.31	AKT-mTOR signaling pathway (tyrosine phosphatase), synaptic development, activity-dependent synaptic plasticity	PTEN hamartoma-tumor syndrome (including Bannayan–Riley–Ruvalcaba syndrome and Cowden syndrome); macrocephaly/autism syndrome	Deletions, point mutations	(Butler et al., 2005; Buxbaum et al., 2007; McBride et al., 2010)
RAB39B	RAB39B, member RAS oncogene family	Xq28	Synapse formation and maintenance	X-linked ID associated with ASD, epilepsy, and macrocephaly	Point mutations	(Giannandrea et al., 2010)
STXBP1	Syntaxin binding protein 1	9q34.11	Synaptic vesicle fusion (SNARE protein)	Early infantile epileptic encephalopathy, nonsyndromic ID without epilepsy, ASD, corpus callosum abnormalities, and frontal cortical hypoplasia	Point mutations, deletions	(Barcia et al., 2014; Hamdan et al., 2011c; Milh et al., 2011; Neale et al., 2012)
SYN1	Synapsin I	Xp11.23	Synaptic vesicle phosphoprotein, modulates neurotransmitter release, synaptic vesicle trafficking, and synaptogenesis	X-linked epilepsy with variable learning disabilities and behavior disorders	Point mutations, deletions	(Boido et al., 2010; Cesca et al., 2010; Fassio et al., 2011; Garcia et al., 2004)
SYNGAP1	Synaptic Ras GTPase activating protein 1	6p21.32	RAS signaling pathway, regulation of glutamate receptor trafficking and synaptic efficacy, maturation of excitatory synapses	Nonsyndromic ID, ASD, and epilepsy; epileptic encephalopathy	Deletions, point mutations	(Berryer et al., 2013; Carvill et al., 2013; Clement et al., 2012; Hamdan et al., 2011a; Pinto et al., 2010)

(continued)

TABLE 9.1 (*Continued*)

Gene	Gene name	Cytoband	Function	Disorder	Evidence	Selected references
TSC1 *TSC2*	Tuberous sclerosis 1/2	9q34.13, 16p13.3	mTOR pathway inhibitor (tumor suppressor protein)	Tuberous sclerosis complex, associated with ID, ASD and epilepsy	Deletions, point mutations	(Numis et al., 2011)
UBE3A	Ubiquitin protein ligase E3A	15q11.2	Ubiquitin ligase, marks proteins for degradation; synapse formation	Angelman syndrome, associated with ID, ASD, lack of speech, and seizures (haploin-sufficiency); 15q11-q13 duplication syndrome, maternally derived, associated with ID, ASD, schizophrenia, language impairment, and seizures	Deletions, point mutations, duplications	(Hogart et al., 2010; Ingason et al., 2011; Mabb et al., 2011)
Transcription/chromatin regulation						
ARID1A	AT rich interactive domain 1A (SWI-like)	1p36.11	Chromatin remodeling	Coffin–Siris syndrome (ID with marked language impairment, hypoplasia/aplasia of the fifth finger/toenail, and facial coarseness)	Point mutations	(Tsurusaki et al., 2012)
ARID1B	AT rich interactive domain 1B (SWI1-like)	6q25.3	Neuron-specific chromatin remodeling, synaptic plasticity	ID, speech impairment, ASD, corpus callosum abnor-malities, Coffin-Siris syndrome	Point mutations, deletions	(Halgren et al., 2012; Santen et al., 2012; Wieczorek et al., 2013)
CREBBP *EP300*	CREB binding protein, E1A binding protein p300	16p13.3, 22q13.2	Transcription modulator (histone acetyl-transferase)	Rubinstein-Taybi syndrome (ID, characteristic facial features, broad thumbs and great toes)	Point mutations, deletions	(Schorry et al., 2008)

Gene	Gene name	Location	Function	Syndrome/phenotype	Type of mutation	References
EHMT1	euchromatic histone-lysine *N*-methyltransferase 1	9q34.3	Transcription regulation (histone methyltransferase), synapse development	Kleefstra syndrome/9q subtelomeric deletion syndrome (ID, distinctive facial features, microcephaly, and hypotonia), ASD, schizophrenia	Deletions, point mutations	(Balemans et al., 2013; Kirov et al., 2012; Willemsen et al., 2012)
HDAC4	Histone deacetylase 4	2q37.3	Transcription regulation (histone deacetylase), synapse plasticity	Brachydactyly mental retardation syndrome (2q37 deletion syndrome), associated with ID and ASD	Deletions, point mutations	(Kim et al., 2012; Sando et al., 2012; Williams et al., 2010b)
MECP2	Methyl-CpG-binding protein 2	Xq28	Transcription factor (methyl DNA binding)	Haploinsufficiency: Rett syndrome in females; congenital encephalopathy or nonsyndromic ID in males, 1 case with schizophrenia; *MECP2* duplication syndrome, mostly in males, ASD	Deletions, point mutations, duplications	(Carney et al., 2003; Cohen et al., 2002; Na et al., 2013; Ramocki et al., 2010)
MEF2C	Myocyte enhancer factor 2C	5q14.3	Regulation of synapse formation and function	5q14.3 microdeletion syndrome, ID, stereotypic movements, epilepsy, cerebral malformations, and ASD	Deletions, point mutations	(Barbosa et al., 2008b; Novara et al., 2010; Zweier et al., 2010)
SMARCA2	SWI/SNF-related matrix-associated, actin dependent regulator of chromatin, subfamily a, member 2	9p24.3	Neuron-specific chromatin remodeling (ATPase/helicase), synaptic plasticity	Nicolaides-Baraitser syndrome (severe ID with marked language impairment, seizures, short stature, microcephaly, facial coarseness, and sparse hair), Coffin-Siris syndrome, ID, ASD	Point mutations, deletions	(Sousa et al., 2009; Van Houdt et al., 2012)

(continued)

TABLE 9.1 *(Continued)*

Gene	Gene name	Cytoband	Function	Disorder	Evidence	Selected references
SMARCA4 *SMARCB1* *SMARCE1*	SWI/SNF-related matrix-associated, actin dependent regulator of chromatin, subfamily a, member 4 subfamily b, member 1 subfamily e, member 1	19p13.2 22q11.23 17q21.2	Chromatin remodeling	Coffin–Siris syndrome	Point mutations	(Tsurusaki et al., 2012)
SRCAP	Snf2-related CREBBP activator protein	16p11.2	Neuron-specific chromatin remodeling (ATPase), synaptic plasticity	Floating-Harbor syndrome (short stature, language delay, and distinctive facial appearance), variable ID, ADHD, ASD	Point mutations	(Hood et al., 2012; White et al., 2010)
TBR1	T-box, brain-1	2q24.2	Transcription factor, neuronal specification, and synaptic plasticity	ID, ASD	Deletions, point mutations	(Neale et al., 2012; O'Roak et al., 2012a; O'Roak et al., 2012b)

Abbreviations: ADHD, attention-deficit hyperactivity disorder; ASD, autism spectrum disorder; ID, intellectual disability; MAGUK, membrane-associated guanylate kinase; mTOR, mammalian target of rapamycin; SNARE, soluble *N*-ethylmaleimide-sensitive-factor attachment protein receptor.

dysplasia-focal epilepsy syndrome (*CNTNAP2*), X-linked female-limited epilepsy (*PCDH19*), and Coffin–Siris syndrome, a genetically heterogeneous ID syndrome caused by mutations in several chromatin remodeling genes.

Many of these syndromes are multisystemic disorders and can be recognized by their characteristic dysmorphic features or other physical abnormalities. However, numerous genes can have syndromic or nonsyndromic presentations; in the latter cases, the diagnosis is based on the identification of the molecular defect. For instance, mutations in *MECP2* mostly affect females with Rett syndrome and are usually lethal in males. However, they have also been reported in females with a diagnosis of autism (without Rett syndrome) (Carney et al., 2003; Zappella et al., 2003) as well as in males with nonsyndromic ID (Couvert et al., 2001) and in rare patients with schizophrenia (Cohen et al., 2002; McCarthy et al., 2014).

9.4 ENRICHMENT FOR SYNAPTIC GENES IN PATHOGENIC COPY NUMBER VARIANTS

Structural genomic variants are an important source of genetic variation among healthy individuals and are now recognized as major determinants of neurodevelopmental disorders (Chapter 3). Numerous studies have documented an increased burden of large rare copy number variants (CNVs; <1% population frequency) in patients with neuropsychiatric and neurological conditions compared to controls, including schizophrenia (International Schizophrenia Consortium, 2008; Kirov et al., 2009; Walsh et al., 2008), ASD (Pinto et al., 2014; Pinto et al., 2010; Sanders et al., 2011), epilepsy (Heinzen et al., 2010), ADHD (Williams et al., 2012), and Tourette syndrome (Nag et al., 2013). By contrast, no increased CNV burden was observed in bipolar disorder (Grozeva et al., 2013). Large *de novo* CNVs are significantly enriched among probands with ASD or schizophrenia when compared to unaffected siblings or controls (Sanders et al., 2011; Xu et al., 2008).

Together with whole-genome and whole-exome sequencing approaches (reviewed subsequently), CNV studies have shown that *de novo* mutations play a prominent role in the etiology of neurodevelopmental disorders. In ASD and schizophrenia, for instance, *de novo* CNVs are observed in 5–10% of cases, compared to 1–2% in unaffected subjects (Kirov et al., 2012; Malhotra et al., 2011; Pinto et al., 2014; Pinto et al., 2010; Sanders et al., 2011; Xu et al., 2008). Interestingly, no significant difference was observed in the rate of *de novo* CNVs among sporadic and familial cases, either in autism or schizophrenia (Kirov et al., 2012; Malhotra et al., 2011; Pinto et al., 2014).

Rare recurrent CNVs at genomic hotspots rich in segmental duplications, either inherited or *de novo*, have been shown to substantially increase the susceptibility to various neurodevelopmental phenotypes, including 1q21.1, 15q13.3, 16p13.11, 16p11.2, 17q12, and 22q11.2 (Malhotra and Sebat, 2012). However, the majority of the increased CNV burden is driven by CNVs that are individually very rare or unique. None of the recurrent CNVs has been found to account for a significant proportion of the risk for any neuropsychiatric disorder and the most frequently occurring variants are found in ~1% of cases. Collectively, however, CNVs in ID and ASD provide an etiological diagnosis in 10% to 15% of cases, and chromosome microarray analysis is now recommended as a first-line test in the genetic workup of these patients (Miller et al., 2010).

Pinpointing the specific genes in the CNV involved in the abnormal phenotypes is challenging, since most recurrent CNVs are large and contain numerous genes. In some cases, the phenotypic effects of the genomic imbalances arise from the deletion of multiple genes; these are referred to as contiguous gene syndromes. Examples include Williams syndrome (7q11.23 deletion) and DiGeorge syndrome (22q11.2 deletion syndrome). In other cases, a single gene in the deleted region is responsible for the core phenotypic features of the deletion syndrome, so that large chromosome rearrangements as well as point mutations in this gene, small gene-specific deletions, or translocation breakpoints interrupting the gene lead to the same disorder. For instance, Phelan-McDermid syndrome, a neurodevelopmental disorder characterized by ID and severe speech impairment, frequently associated with ASD, is caused in the majority of cases by deletions in chromosome 22q13.33 of varying sizes encompassing the *SHANK3* gene, but can also arise through point mutations in *SHANK3* (Bonaglia et al., 2011; Durand et al., 2007). Other examples include Kleefstra syndrome, associated with 9q34.3 subtelomeric deletions and *EHMT1* mutations, and Sotos syndrome, resulting from 5q35 deletions and mutations involving *NSD1*.

Smaller rearrangements affecting single genes have also been associated with neurodevelopmental conditions, such as microdeletions of the gene *NRXN1*, encoding the cell adhesion molecule neurexin 1, and microduplications of *VIPR2* (vasoactive intestinal peptide receptor 2). As expected, because these rearrangements are not mediated by segmental duplications, their sizes are variable and the breakpoints are not recurrent. Heterozygous exonic deletions of *NRXN1* were first reported in two sisters with autism (Szatmari et al., 2007) and have since then been repeatedly identified in individuals with a wide phenotypic spectrum, including ASD, schizophrenia, ID, language impairment, Tourette syndrome, and epilepsy (Levinson et al., 2011; Moller et al., 2013; Nag et al., 2013; Pinto et al., 2014; Rujescu et al., 2009). The presence of *NRXN1* deletions in apparently unaffected parents and siblings suggests reduced penetrance and/or variable expressivity, similar to other well-documented CNVs conferring risk for neuropsychiatric disorders. Duplications at chromosome 7q36.3 overlapping the *VIPR2* gene or located within 89 kb upstream of the gene have been reported to be enriched in schizophrenia (Levinson et al., 2011; Vacic et al., 2011; Yuan et al., 2014). VIPR2 transcription and cyclic-AMP signaling were increased in lymphocytes from patients carrying 7q36.3 microduplications, but the exact genetic mechanism remains unclear (Vacic et al., 2011). The neuropeptide vasoactive intestinal peptide (VIP) is expressed in the brain, where it regulates synaptic transmission, neural excitability, and neurogenesis, both during embryonic development and in the adult (Zaben and Gray, 2013).

CNV studies in schizophrenia, ASD, ID, and ADHD have all shown an enrichment in synaptic genes. In schizophrenia, analysis of *de novo* CNVs in 662 parent-proband trios showed an enrichment in cases (5.1%) compared to controls (2.2%) (Kirov et al., 2012). Genes within the *de novo* CNVs were significantly enriched for components of the PSD, particularly for members of the *N*-Methyl-D-Aspartate receptor (NMDA-R) and neuronal activity-regulated cytoskeleton-associated protein complexes (ARC). NMDA-R and ARC complexes regulate synaptic plasticity at glutamatergic synapses and have been implicated in several forms of learning. Analysis of an independent sample of 7907 cases and 10,585 controls confirmed an enrichment for members of the NMDAR complex but not ARC. Multiple *de novo* CNVs implicated members of the DLG family of MAGUKs and *EHMT1*, a histone methyl transferase known to directly regulate DLG family members and involved in Kleefstra syndrome. These findings indicate that rare mutations of specific synaptic complexes implicated in cognitive function and neuronal plasticity contribute to the pathogenesis of schizophrenia.

Although the majority of the CNVs identified in ASD are rare and nonrecurrent, several studies in large ASD samples have identified gene networks with strong interconnectedness, pointing to pathways through which the effects of mutations in distinct genes may converge. Enrichment for synaptic functioning has been reported among *de novo* CNVs in subjects with sporadic or familial ASD (Gilman et al., 2011; Pinto et al., 2014), and among inherited CNVs (Gai et al., 2012). Analysis of functional gene sets affected by rare CNVs in ASD compared to controls identified an enrichment of rare deletions disrupting genes involved in neuronal development and function, and GTPase/Ras signaling (Pinto et al., 2010). The identified networks were strongly related to genes previously implicated in ID and ASD. Indeed, several Rho GTPases have been shown to regulate dendrite and spine plasticity and have been implicated in ID (Linseman and Loucks, 2008). Similarly, a number of monogenic ID syndromes associated with ASD are related to abnormal RAS signaling, including cardio-facio-cutaneous syndrome, Noonan syndrome, neurofibromatosis 1, and *SYNGAP1* haploinsufficiency (Table 9.1) (van Bokhoven, 2011). In an independent sample, Gilman et al. (2011) observed an enrichment of rare *de novo* CNVs within gene clusters related to actin network dynamics and reorganization, synaptogenesis, axonogenesis, cell–cell adhesion, small GTPase signaling, and neurite development. In addition, the functional network was significantly connected to PSD proteins identified by proteomic profiling of the human neocortex (Bayes et al., 2011). More recently, network analysis of *de novo* CNVs in 2,446 ASD families implicated chromatin/transcription regulation genes in ASD (Pinto et al., 2014). An increasing number of genes involved in monogenic forms of ASD, ID, and epilepsy are involved in chromatin regulation and transcription regulation, as discussed in the following sections (Table 9.1) (van Bokhoven, 2011).

In ADHD, rare inherited CNVs were significantly enriched for genes involved in learning, cell adhesion, and neurodevelopment, including several genes involved in synaptic transmission (Elia et al., 2010). In a follow-up study, rare recurrent CNVs affecting glutamatergic genes were overrepresented in multiple ADHD cohorts totaling 3506 cases and 13,327 controls (Elia et al., 2012). Specifically, metabotropic glutamate receptor genes were enriched across all cohorts, including *GRM5, GRM7,* and *GRM8* deletions, and *GRM1* duplications. Except for three *de novo GRM5* deletions, all the other CNVs for which parents were available were inherited. These CNVs account for 3.7% of the cases with ADHD, and this number increases to ~10% when genes interacting with the genes in the GRM family are included. However, the significance of some of these findings is unclear,

since several of the CNVs overlapping these genes are intronic.

Taken together, these pathway–based analyses add to an accumulating body of evidence from human and animal studies implicating synaptic dysfunction in the pathogenesis of neuropsychiatric disorders. However, further genetic and functional analyses are necessary before we can assign pathogenicity to the majority of the reported rare CNVs and identify the genes within the CNVs that contribute to the cognitive and behavioral deficits.

9.5 WHOLE-EXOME SEQUENCING AND PATHWAY ANALYSES IN ASD, SCHIZOPHRENIA, AND ID

Whole-exome sequencing (WES) provides an unbiased way to identify genes involved in neurodevelopmental disorders, and this approach is being widely pursued. WES can readily identify single nucleotide variants (SNVs), small insertions and deletions (indels), and small and large CNV. Since the SNVs, indels and small CNVs almost always impact just a single gene, pathway analysis making use of genes identified from these approaches is more straightforward.

The first four large concurrent WES studies in ASD focused on *de novo* loss-of-function mutations (nonsense, splice site, and frameshift) and generally agreed on several key points (Iossifov et al., 2012; Neale et al., 2012; O'Roak et al., 2012a; Sanders et al., 2012). First, *de novo* loss-of-function is about twice as common in ASD as compared to controls, making them a particularly enriched source of novel ASD genes. Second, there was agreement that the number of ASD genes that could be impacted by loss-of-function mutations was in the order of 1000 genes. Since *de novo* loss-of-function mutations are so rare, seeing a gene with two or more such mutations was considered enough to identify it as a bona fide ASD gene (with the total sample size of about 1000 nuclear families). Five genes emerged with two hits, including *CHD8, DYRK1A, KATNAL2, POGZ,* and *SCN2A.* Third, there is convergence on genes previously implicated in ID, as previously documented for CNVs. Fourth, the frequency of *de novo* mutation is dependent on paternal age, consistent with epidemiological studies showing increased incidence of certain genetic disorders in the progeny of older fathers, including ASD and schizophrenia.

Since, amongst the over 100 genes across the four studies that showed a *de novo* mutation, approximately half are going to be bona fide ASD genes (based on the rate of *de novo* loss-of-function mutations in unaffected siblings or controls) (Neale et al., 2012; Sanders et al., 2012), the results from these studies provide an opportunity for interesting pathway analyses. *De novo* loss-of-function sequence variants in ASD were enriched for genes found to interact with the fragile X mental retardation protein (FMRP) (Iossifov et al., 2012). This is consistent with evidence that FMRP targets belong to multiple signaling and interconnected pathways such as PTEN/PI3K/AKT/TSC/mTOR and RAS/MAPK, which have been linked to ID and ASD through deletions and mutations in numerous genes (Betancur, 2011).

A combined look at all of the genes with *de novo* mutations has been carried out in the context of coexpression networks (Willsey et al., 2013). The authors used microarray data from the Brainspan dataset, including gene expression from multiple brain regions across human development, to first ask where the mutant genes mapped to, spatially and temporally. They used both a high confidence gene set (arising from the WES noted earlier and follow-up studies and including *ANK2, CHD8, CUL3, DYRK1A, GRIN2B, KATNAL2, POGZ, SCN2A,* and *TBR1*) and 144 probable ASD genes with *de novo* loss-of-function mutations. These genes clearly mapped to (a) more frontal brain regions and (b) to midfetal development. Moreover, using additional datasets, the authors suggest that these genes mapped to cells in the midfetal inner cortical plate. A parallel study used RNAseq data from Brainspan (with about half the samples compared to Willsey et al., (2013)), and a larger set of potential ASD genes – using curated lists of genes as well as gene expression

data from ASD samples (Parikshak et al., 2013). This study mapped ASD genes to early fetal development. In addition, the ASD genes mapped to superficial layers of the cortex.

An important enhancement for ASD gene discovery was the developmental of methods for combining *de novo* and inherited findings in genes to leverage all available data for gene discovery. One such method, called TADA (transmitted and *de novo* association) was applied to all of the WES studies noted earlier, as well as case-control data (He et al., 2013). TADA nominated additional WES-derived genes (for a total of 15) as true ASD genes, based on the combined evidence from *de novo* mutations and inherited deleterious mutations. By the incorporation of inherited variation, TADA is able to provide evidence for or against all genes in the genome (unlike a strict focus on the very rare *de novo* mutations). This makes it an extremely powerful tool to merge with unbiased network analysis. For example, one can use gene expression data to create coexpression networks, use prior knowledge to identify ASD subnetworks, and layer in all genetic data of each gene in each subnetwork. Requiring that a potential ASD gene both resides in an ASD subnetwork and has some genetic evidence becomes a powerful tool for gene discovery. In fact, this approach (termed DAWN, for "detecting association within networks") is the only network-based approach that has been tested predictively and shown to significantly enrich for true ASD genes (Liu et al., 2014).

The potential ASD genes identified in a first run of DAWN (using coexpression networks derived from the prenatal developmental window identified in Willsey et al. (2013)) clustered into interesting functional groups, including synaptic development and function. While a large proportion of genes were involved in transcriptional regulation (including chromatin remodeling, see subsequently, RNA pol II categories, and regulation of translation), additional genes mapped onto neuronal migration and function, cell adhesion and cell migration, focal adhesion, ligase activity (including ubiquitin-protein ligase activity), and protein scaffolding and receptor signaling. Many of these clusters are synaptic, and as DAWN and similar models evolve, we will get a finer and finer unbiased view of the role of specific synaptic pathways implicated in ASD, as well as other neurodevelopmental disorders.

WES studies also can be analyzed for large and small CNVs. As noted earlier, the smaller CNVs can often encompass just one gene. When such approaches were applied to ASD, one study identified autophagy as a novel pathway in ASD risk (Poultney et al., 2013). While this needs to be replicated in independent samples, the role of autophagy in synaptic pruning during development makes this a potentially interesting pathway in ASD and possibly other neurodevelopmental conditions. In a similar study using an independent ASD dataset, genes disrupted by CNVs included several synaptic genes, including *ORC3*, a protein in the origin recognition complex, which regulates dendritic spines and dendrite arborization in postmitotic neurons (Krumm et al., 2013).

Two large WES studies have recently been reported for schizophrenia (Fromer et al., 2014; Purcell et al., 2014). In the first study with 623 trios, the authors focused on *de novo* mutations (Fromer et al., 2014). There were 637 *de novo* coding or splice site mutations, showing strong enrichment for ARC and NMDA complexes. FMRP targets were also enriched for *de novo* mutations, consistent with what has been observed in autism. Interestingly, there was enrichment of these variants in genes affected by *de novo* loss-of-function mutations in ASD and ID, highlighting overlapping risk for these neurodevelopmental disorders.

Purcell et al. (2014) examined over 2,500 cases and 2,500 controls and observed variants across a large number of genes, for what they term a polygenic burden of rare disruptive mutations. (Note that "polygenic" here simply means that many genes are involved across the population, not necessarily in individuals). Enrichment was again observed in ARC complex genes and FMRP targets. In addition, there was enrichment of rare disruptive variants

in voltage-gated calcium ion channels, critical modulators of synaptic transmission and plasticity.

Emerging WES studies in ID are showing similar kinds of findings, although sample sizes are still relatively modest (de Ligt et al., 2012; Rauch et al., 2012; Schuurs-Hoeijmakers et al., 2013). Diverse genes were identified with some having important roles in the synapse. For example *STXBP1*, *SYNGAP1*, and *SCN2A* were identified as recurrently mutated in one of these studies (Rauch et al., 2012).

Since WES is focused on rare variation, very large sample sizes will be required to interpret the clinical significance of the variants already identified and to identify additional genes. The emergence of large-scale, collaborative WES studies in multiple neurodevelopmental disorders (Allen et al., 2013; Buxbaum et al., 2012) will hasten the identification of genes contributing to these disorders (Hoischen et al., 2014; Zhu et al., 2014).

9.6 FUNCTIONAL CLASSES OF GENES IMPLICATED IN SYNAPTIC DISORDERS

Many of the genes implicated interact at the level of molecular pathways, suggesting common pathogenic mechanisms in the etiology of neurodevelopmental disorders and raising hope that common treatments could be developed. The following sections give examples of specific classes with strong evidence of involvement in neurodevelopmental disorders. It is not an exhaustive list at the level of individual genes but is intended to present the diversity of molecular mechanisms that, when impaired by mutations, can result in synaptic disorders.

9.6.1 Cell Adhesion Molecules

Synaptic cell adhesion proteins are involved in the formation and stabilization of synapses (Missler et al., 2012). The term "cell adhesion molecule" is actually far too limited for this group of proteins – while some do provide a physical adhesive force, most initiate some form of internal biochemical signaling pathways on binding of their trans-synaptic partners, often in both directions. They are thus probably better thought of as cell–cell interaction proteins.

Neuroligins and neurexins: Neuroligins and neurexins, encoding post- and presynaptic cell adhesion molecules, are canonical examples of synaptic genes and pathways that contribute to risk for multiple neurodevelopmental disorders (Betancur et al., 2009; Sudhof, 2008). Rare mutations in the genes encoding neuroligins *NLGN3* and *NLGN4X* have been associated with ASD and ID (Jamain et al., 2003; Laumonnier et al., 2004) whereas deletions of *NRXN1*, as mentioned previously, have been identified in various neurodevelopmental disorders, including ASD, schizophrenia, ID, and epilepsy (Levinson et al., 2011; Moller et al., 2013; Nag et al., 2013; Pinto et al., 2010; Rujescu et al., 2009). An inherited partial duplication of *NLGN1* and a *de novo* missense variant have also been reported in patients with ASD (Girirajan et al., 2013b; O'Roak et al., 2012b) as has a truncating mutation in *NRXN2* (Gauthier et al., 2011), though the evidence for pathogenicity is weaker in these cases.

CNTNAPs and contactins: Mutations in other members of the neurexin family called contactin-associated proteins (CNTNAPs) have also been observed in patients with neuropsychiatric conditions. The evidence for pathogenicity is strongest for mutations in *CNTNAP2*, which is involved in two recessive disorders, cortical dysplasia-focal epilepsy syndrome (Strauss et al., 2006) and Pitt-Hopkins-like syndrome (Zweier et al., 2009). In addition, deletions or chromosomal rearrangements disrupting one copy of the gene were first discovered in multiple members of a family with Tourette syndrome (Verkerk et al., 2003), and have been subsequently observed in patients with ASD (Alarcon et al., 2008; Bakkaloglu et al., 2008; O'Roak et al., 2011), schizophrenia (Friedman et al., 2008; International Schizophrenia Consortium, 2008), epilepsy (Friedman et al., 2008; Mefford et al., 2010), and ADHD (Elia et al., 2010). The clinical significance of these heterozygous

defects of *CNTNAP2* is unclear, since the parents of the children with recessive disorders are heterozygous carriers and are healthy (Strauss et al., 2006; Zweier et al., 2009). Disruptive mutations in the related genes *CNTNAP3* and *CNTNAP5* have also been reported in patients with ASD (An et al., 2014; Pagnamenta et al., 2010). Knockdown of *Cntnap2* in mice results in defects in dendritic arborization and spine development in pyramidal neurons, with concomitant effects on synaptic transmission (Anderson et al., 2012), while complete knockout is also associated with neuronal migration abnormalities, seizures, and autism-related behavioral phenotypes (Penagarikano et al., 2011). CNTNAP4 is also required for normal synapse function, playing distinct, presynaptic roles in fast-spiking interneurons and midbrain dopaminergic neurons (Karayannis et al., 2014).

CNTNAP proteins interact with contactins, members of the immunoglobulin domain-containing superfamily of proteins, which play important roles in many neurodevelopmental processes involving cell–cell interactions (Shimoda and Watanabe, 2009; Zuko et al., 2013). In particular, CNTN6 has been shown to be required for formation of glutamatergic synapses in both cerebellum and hippocampus (Sakurai et al., 2010; Sakurai et al., 2009). Rare CNVs in *CNTN4* have been reported in neuropsychiatric disorders, including ASD (Glessner et al., 2009; Nava et al., 2014; Williams et al., 2010a; Zuko et al., 2013) as well as in controls. No clear enrichment has been observed in cases, so the clinical significance of these CNVS is unknown. CNVs in the neighboring gene, encoding the highly related protein *CNTN6*, have also been observed in patients with similar conditions, as have larger chromosomal variants affecting both genes simultaneously (Guo et al., 2012; Zuko et al., 2013). Common variants in *CNTN4* also give genome-wide significant signals in a large genome-wide association study of schizophrenia (Schizophrenia Working Group of the Psychiatric Genomics Consortium, 2014).

Cadherins and protocadherins: Multiple members of these two families of cell adhesion molecules have been implicated in psychiatric disorders. However, the genetic evidence for pathogenicity is compelling only in the case of protocadherin 19 (*PCDH19*). Mutations in this X-linked gene have been found to cause some cases of Dravet syndrome (a condition characterized by severe epilepsy with onset in infancy and by associated developmental delays, including features of autism) (Camacho et al., 2012; Depienne and LeGuern, 2012; Dibbens et al., 2008). The clinical severity of *PCDH19* mutations is paradoxically dramatically higher in heterozygous females than in hemizygous males, who may show autistic-like traits but who typically do not have any clinical diagnosis (van Harssel et al., 2013). This suggests that the effect is due to cellular interference – it is not the absence of PCDH19 protein that is pathogenic, but an imbalance in levels between neighboring cells, which arises due to random X-inactivation in females.

The precise function of PCDH19 remains unknown but protocadherins generally play multiple important roles in nervous system development. Protocadherins in the *α*, *β*, and *γ* clusters undergo extensive alternative splicing and stochastic expression to generate specific combinations of protocadherin isoforms on their surface, which enable neurons to distinguish their own neurites (which are not an appropriate target for innervation) from those of other neurons (which may be) (Thu et al., 2014). The nonclustered protocadherins are selectively expressed in various regions of the developing brain (Kim et al., 2007) and PCDH17 and PCDH20 have both been shown to play active roles in synapse formation (Hoshina et al., 2013; Ke et al., 2013).

Homozygous mutations in *PCDH10* have been observed in families with apparently recessive inheritance of autism (Morrow et al., 2008) but this finding has not yet been replicated in other patients. Interestingly, the PCDH10 protein is involved in and required for a pathway by which the activity-dependent transcription factor MEF2 and the fragile X mental retardation protein FMRP downregulate levels of the postsynaptic scaffolding protein PSD95 and mediate synaptic elimination (Tsai et al., 2012).

The genetic evidence implicating members of the classic cadherin family is less solid. Rare familial microdeletions disrupting *CDH8* have been found in patients with autism and ID (Pagnamenta et al., 2011) and mutations in *CDH2* have been reported in individuals with obsessive-compulsive disorder (OCD) and Tourette syndrome (Moya et al., 2013) and also implicated in OCD in dogs (Tang et al., 2014). Finally, mutations in the cadherin family gene *FAT1* have been observed in multiple exome sequencing studies of patients with autism or schizophrenia (Cukier et al., 2014; Kenny et al., 2014; Neale et al., 2012), though pathogenicity remains unproven.

Netrin-G1 and CDKL5: De novo disruption of the *NTNG1* gene has been identified in a girl with Rett syndrome (Archer et al., 2006b; Borg et al., 2005) and in two sporadic autism cases (O'Roak et al., 2012b). *NTNG1* encodes a glycosyl phosphatidylinositol-linked protein that interacts with proteins of the Netrin-G-Ligand (NGL) family. NGLs are transmembrane proteins and members of the LRR superfamily, which in turn interact with postsynaptic density proteins and NMDA receptors (Woo et al., 2009). Interactions between these proteins, along with the receptor protein tyrosine phosphatase LAR regulate the formation of excitatory synapses (Kim et al., 2006; Song et al., 2013) and determine their localization on specific dendritic segments (Nishimura-Akiyoshi et al., 2007). Interestingly, mutations in cyclin-dependent kinase-like 5 (*CDKL5*), a rare cause of atypical Rett syndrome (Weaving et al., 2004), have been shown to affect the interaction between NGL-1 and PSD95, reducing synapse formation and stability and producing aberrant dendritic spines, in both mouse and human stem cell-derived neurons (Ricciardi et al., 2012).

L1CAM family: The L1 cell adhesion molecule family includes L1 itself, CHL1, NRCAM, and NFASC. These transmembrane proteins are members of the immunoglobulin superfamily that interact homophilically as well as with numerous heterophilic partners, including contactins. They play important roles in cell migration and axon guidance (Maness and Schachner, 2007), and also in the establishment of synaptic connectivity (Huang, 2006; Katidou et al., 2008; Sakurai, 2012), and synaptic plasticity (Dityatev et al., 2008). Mutations in the X-linked *L1CAM* gene result in a syndrome of ID with hydrocephalus, spastic paraplegia, and hypoplasia of the corpus callosum (Schrander-Stumpel and Vos, 2010).

More recently, mutations in the other members of the L1 family have also been reported in neurodevelopmental disorders, especially ASD. Deletions or disruptive microduplications of *CHL1* at 3p26.3 have been reported in subjects with ID, and are usually inherited from unaffected parents (Cuoco et al., 2011; Pohjola et al., 2010; Shoukier et al., 2013). CNVs disrupting *CHL1* have also been observed in ASD patients (Salyakina et al., 2011) and schizophrenia (Tam et al., 2010); their clinical significance is unknown. *CHL1* is adjacent to the contactin genes *CNTN4* and *CNTN6* and CNVs disrupting pairs of these genes or all three have also been observed in patients with ID and ASD (Zuko et al., 2013). Analysis of genes in ASD patients with *de novo* mutations or mutations inherited from a parent with a broad autism phenotype showed an enrichment of the L1CAM signaling pathway, including mutations in *NRCAM* and *NFASC* (An et al., 2014).

IL1RAPL1: Mutations in the *IL1RAPL1* gene, encoding the interleukin-1 receptor-associated protein-like 1 protein, are responsible for X-linked ID and ASD, with or without dysmorphic features (Franek et al., 2011; Pinto et al., 2010; Piton et al., 2008). In the immune system, this protein acts with the IL-1 receptor to mediate actions of this cytokine. In the nervous system, it carries out very different functions, interacting trans-synaptically with receptor protein tyrosine phosphatase delta to induce formation of excitatory presynaptic structures (Valnegri et al., 2011; Yoshida et al., 2011). Activation of this pathway also differentially affects the turnover and insertion of various subunits into AMPA receptors at the membrane,

via interactions with modulators of Rho GTPase (Hayashi et al., 2013; Valnegri et al., 2011).

SLITRKs: Although hundreds of genes have been identified as causes of ID, ASD, and epilepsy when mutated, discovery of clearly pathogenic genes in other neuropsychiatric disorders has so far had more limited success. One notable exception is the implication of *SLITRK1* (SLIT and NTRK-like family, member 1) in OCD and related conditions. Rare mutations in *SLITRK1* have been reported in patients with Tourette syndrome (Abelson et al., 2005), trichotillomania (Zuchner et al., 2006), and OCD (Ozomaro et al., 2013).

SLITRK1 encodes a transmembrane protein containing an extracellular LRR domain, which is mainly expressed in neural tissues (Aruga and Mikoshiba, 2003). Like several other subfamilies of the LRR superfamily (de Wit and Ghosh, 2014), SLITRK proteins can direct the formation of either excitatory or inhibitory synapses in neuronal cultures, in this case through interactions with distinct presynaptic receptor protein tyrosine phosphatases (Takahashi and Craig, 2013; Yim et al., 2013). *Slitrk1* knockout mice exhibit anxiety-like behaviors and increased levels of norepinephrine (Katayama et al., 2010). Interestingly, administration of clonidine, an alpha2-adrenergic agonist used in Tourette syndrome, attenuated the behavioral abnormalities of *Slitrk1* deficient mice. Mutation of *Slitrk5* in mice impairs corticostriatal synaptic connectivity and also results in obsessive-compulsive-like behaviors, including excessive grooming and anxiety (Shmelkov et al., 2010).

These findings suggest an unusual level of phenotypic specificity of mutations in these *SLITRK* family genes with respect to OCD and related conditions; it remains to be seen whether mutations in these genes also contribute to other common neurodevelopmental disorders. *SLITRK6* may play distinct roles, as mutations in this gene are associated with myopia and progressive auditory neuropathy resulting in deafness (Morlet et al., 2014; Tekin et al., 2013).

LGI1: Mutations in the leucine-rich, glioma-inactivated 1 (LGI1) gene are associated with autosomal dominant partial epilepsy with auditory features (also known as autosomal dominant lateral temporal lobe epilepsy) (Kalachikov et al., 2002; reviewed in Kegel et al., 2013), and also observed in about 2% of sporadic cases of temporal lobe epilepsy (Nobile et al., 2009). This gene encodes a secreted protein with an LRR domain and epitempin repeats. The LGI1 protein interacts with the transmembrane proteins ADAM22 and ADAM23 to organize a trans-synaptic complex, also including presynaptic potassium channels and postsynaptic AMPA receptor scaffolds containing PSD95 and stargazing (Fukata et al., 2010). This interaction enhances AMPA receptor-mediated synaptic transmission in hippocampal slices. Autoantibodies to LGI1 are implicated in autoimmune limbic encephalitis and have been found to block the interaction with ADAM22 and reduce synaptic AMPA receptors (Ohkawa et al., 2013). Mutation of *Adam22* or *Adam23* in mice also results in epilepsy (Mitchell et al., 2001; Sagane et al., 2005). Mutations in *LGI2* have been found to cause epilepsy in Belgian sheepdogs (Seppala et al., 2012). However, mutations in *LGI2*, *-3* or *-4* or in *ADAM22* or *-23* have not yet been reported in human epilepsy patients.

9.6.2 Synaptic Scaffolding Proteins

A diverse set of proteins contribute to the dynamic molecular organization of synaptic structures, both pre- and postsynaptically. Many of these scaffolding proteins fall into subfamilies, with individual members being differentially expressed across different synapse types. Combinatorial interactions between scaffolding proteins generate a diversity of heteromeric scaffolding complexes at different synapses (Emes and Grant, 2012). A recent proteomic analysis identified 1,461 proteins in the PSD from human neocortex (Bayes et al., 2011). Mutations in PSD genes cause 133 neurological and psychiatric diseases (including 40 genes involved in ID) and were enriched in cognitive and motor phenotypes (Bayes et al., 2011). Genes involved in X-linked ID are highly enriched for PSD genes (Laumonnier

et al., 2007), particularly the NMDA receptor complex/MAGUK–associated signaling complex, which play an essential role in the induction of neuronal plasticity and cognitive processes.

MAGUK proteins: The membrane-associated guanylate kinase (MAGUK) superfamily includes DLG proteins, CASK and MAGI proteins, all of which act as synaptic scaffolding proteins involved in synapse formation and plasticity (Zheng et al., 2011). There are four DLG homolog genes (the proteins are also variously known as Synaptic-Associated Proteins [SAP90, -97, -102], or Postsynaptic Density proteins [PSD93, -95]). These genes are differentially expressed across the brain and in an overlapping fashion in different synapse types (Emes and Grant, 2012; O'Rourke et al., 2012). DLG proteins help recruit and organize the postsynaptic components of the synapse, such as specific neurotransmitter receptor subunits, and also contribute to their dynamic trafficking in and out of the synapse in response to activity or stimulation (Sheng and Kim, 2011).

Mutations in *DLG3* are associated with nonsyndromic, X-linked ID (Tarpey et al., 2004; Zanni et al., 2010). A single-gene deletion of *DLG2* has also been reported in a patient with ID, ASD, and epilepsy, though pathogenicity has not been confirmed (Vulto-van Silfhout et al., 2013). *DLG1*, *DLG2*, and the genes encoding the DLG-associated proteins DLGAP1 and DLGAP2 (also known as GKAP1 and 2) are also contained within larger, recurrent CNVs with demonstrated pathogenicity for neuropsychiatric disorders (e.g., *DLG1* at 3q29) or with multiple observations of *de novo* occurrences in affected individuals (Kirov et al., 2012; Pinto et al., 2010). Members of the MAGUK family generally, including *MAGI1* and *-2* are also enriched among genes affected by CNVs in patients with schizophrenia (Raychaudhuri et al., 2009). Null mutations in *CASK* are associated with an X-linked ID syndrome characterized by hindbrain malformations in females, while hypomorphic mutations are observed in cases of nonsyndromic ID and ASD in males (Hackett et al., 2010; Lin et al., 2013;

Najm et al., 2008; Sanders et al., 2012; Tarpey et al., 2009).

Gephyrin: Gephyrin plays a similar scaffolding role to MAGUK proteins, but specifically at inhibitory synapses, where it helps cluster GABA(A) and glycine receptor subunits, regulating both synapse formation and plasticity (Tyagarajan and Fritschy, 2014). Heterozygous deletions in the gene *GPHN* have been associated with ASD, schizophrenia, and epilepsy (Dejanovic et al., 2014; Lionel et al., 2013) as well as in numerous controls, and their pathogenicity is uncertain. Homozygous mutations in *GPHN* cause molybdenum cofactor deficiency C, an autosomal recessive disorder characterized by a severe neurological phenotype and early death (Reiss et al., 2001).

SHANK genes: SHANK (or ProSAP) proteins are multidomain adaptors expressed in excitatory glutamatergic synapses that functionally cross-link membrane-proximal components of the postsynaptic density such as neurotransmitter receptors and neuroligins with the actin cytoskeleton in dendritic spines (Grabrucker et al., 2011). Deletions of the 22q13.33 region involving the *SHANK3* gene cause Phelan-McDermid syndrome, characterized by ID, severely delayed or absent speech, hypotonia, and ASD in the majority of patients (Soorya et al., 2013). Rare *de novo* mutations in *SHANK3* have been identified in individuals with idiopathic ASD (Durand et al., 2007; Gauthier et al., 2009; Moessner et al., 2007) and ID (Gong et al., 2012; Hamdan et al., 2011b), as well as in two families with schizophrenia (Gauthier et al., 2010). More recently, *de novo* deletions and mutations in *SHANK2* have been repeatedly identified in subjects with ASD and ID (Berkel et al., 2010; Leblond et al., 2012; Pinto et al., 2010; Sanders et al., 2011). Mutations in *SHANK1* have also been observed at a low rate in patients with ASD (Leblond et al., 2014; Sato et al., 2012); the clinical relevance of these findings remains to be determined.

9.6.3 Neurotransmitter Receptors and Ion Channels

Mutations in many different genes encoding neurotransmitter receptors and voltage-gated ion channels have been linked with various neurodevelopmental disorders, especially particular syndromes such as Timothy syndrome, Dravet syndrome, and many others (reviewed in Kullmann and Waxman, 2010; Russell et al., 2013). In particular, mutations in genes encoding GABA receptor subunits and channels for sodium, potassium, or calcium are well known in syndromic forms of epilepsy (Lerche et al., 2013). But mutations in many of the same genes or gene families are now also being observed in previously idiopathic cases of ID, ASD, and schizophrenia and in nonsyndromic epilepsy or epileptic encephalopathy (Allen et al., 2013; Schmunk and Gargus, 2013; Zhu et al., 2014).

Genes that are coming to prominence as harbouring likely pathogenic mutations in cases of "common disorders" include those encoding NMDA receptor subunits (*GRIN2A* and *-2B*), AMPA receptor subunits (*GRIA3*), cholinergic receptor subunit (*CHRNA7*), synaptic voltage-gated calcium channels (*CACNA1A* and *-1C* and possibly others), and sodium channels (*SCN1A*, *-2A* and others). Many of these proteins are not just involved in acute neurotransmission but also play prominent roles in synaptic plasticity. This is particularly well described for NMDA receptors and voltage-gated calcium channels, which mediate calcium fluxes in response to patterns of electrical activity, initiating biochemical pathways within dendrites that control local protein phosphorylation and mRNA translation, as well as signaling to the nucleus to direct activity-dependent gene expression (Greer and Greenberg, 2008). As noted earlier, CNVs in several metabotropic glutamate receptor genes have also been observed in ADHD patients (Elia et al., 2010; Elia et al., 2012) and several have been reported in individuals with schizophrenia (Ayoub et al., 2012) or ASD (Prasad et al., 2012), though pathogenicity remains unproven.

It is interesting that, among the long and growing list of neurotransmission-related genes implicated by mutations in patients with neurodevelopmental disorders, those encoding components of neuromodulatory systems, such as dopamine or serotonin, are conspicuously absent. These were natural candidate genes based on the known pharmacology of many psychiatric medications, but the search for pathogenic mutations in these genes has proven largely fruitless. These pathways also show no enrichment among genes disrupted by *de novo* or inherited mutations in ASD or schizophrenia (Fromer et al., 2014; Liu et al., 2014). If these genes are not haploinsufficient, then current methods of detecting pathogenic mutations may be biased against them; however, current evidence does not support a major role for mutations in these genes in the etiology of common neuropsychiatric disorders.

9.6.4 Signal Transduction, Translation

The genes implicated in several major neurodevelopmental syndromes converge on a biochemical pathway which mediates activity-dependent local translation of mRNAs at synapses. Many such mRNAs are ferried to synapses and maintained in a primed but quiescent state through sequestration in ribonucleoprotein (RNP) particles. Translation of these mRNAs is an essential mechanism underlying persistent changes in synaptic strength, such as long-term potentiation and depression (Buffington et al., 2014).

The fragile X protein, FMRP, is a major component of RNP particles and is required for normal responsiveness to activity. A pathway initiated through NMDA-R signaling and modulated by other surface receptors, including metabotropic glutamate receptors, induces PI3K activity and ultimately impinges on FMRP. This pathway notably involves the actions of several other genes also implicated in neurodevelopmental disorders, such as *PTEN* and the tuberous sclerosis genes, *TSC1* and *TSC2*.

A number of other synaptic signaling proteins in diverse but intersecting pathways are implicated in neurodevelopmental disorders.

These include, for example, the neurofibromatosis protein NF-1 (Diggs-Andrews and Gutmann, 2013), the ubiquitination enzyme Ube3A (Mabb et al., 2011), and the kinase CDKL5. As mentioned earlier, CDKL5 phosphorylates targets both at the synapse (such as NGL-1; Ricciardi et al., 2012) and in the nucleus (such as MeCP2; Mari et al., 2005). Mutations in *CDKL5* are a rare cause of Rett syndrome (Weaving et al., 2005), but are also found in nonsyndromic cases of ID and epileptic encephalopathy (Castren et al., 2011; Mirzaa et al., 2013).

Mutations in genes encoding several regulators of small GTPases can result in neurodevelopmental disorders. SYNGAP1 is a calcium-regulated Ras GTPase activating protein localized to the postsynaptic density. Mutations of this gene have been identified as a relatively common cause of ID, characterized by ASD and epilepsy (e.g., Berryer et al., 2013). Recent analyses have shown that mutation of one copy of the *Syngap1* gene in mice alters synaptic plasticity and maturation, resulting in cognitive deficits (Clement et al., 2013). Conditional mutagenesis in specific cell types has demonstrated that these defects result from reduced Syngap1 protein specifically in forebrain glutamatergic neurons, rather than other cell types, and specifically during development, rather than in postnatal life (Ozkan et al., 2014). This model also provides a nice illustration of how global defects in neural dynamics can emerge at later stages due to much earlier developmental deficits (Ozkan et al., 2014).

Mutations in *NF1*, which encodes neurofibromin, another protein with RasGAP activity, are the cause of neurofibromatosis, characterized by ID and high rates of ASD (Garg et al., 2013). This protein is the major negative regulator of Ras activity in dendrites and mutation of one copy in mice leads to altered synaptic plasticity, changes in expression of many synaptic genes, and behavioral and learning deficits (Costa et al., 2002; Oliveira and Yasuda, 2014; Park et al., 2009). Mutations in Ras pathway genes are responsible for numerous syndromes typically characterized by both cancer and neurological phenotypes and collectively termed

RASopathies. A recent analysis shows high rates of ASD among patients with several of these disorders (Adviento et al., 2014).

IQSEC2 (or BRAG1) is a guanine exchange factor for the Arf GTPase. Members of the IQSEC/BRAG family are differentially localized to distinct synapse types (Sakagami et al., 2013), with IQSEC2 localized at excitatory synapses where it interacts with NMDA-R subunits and PSD95 (Sakagami et al., 2008). In response to calcium-calmodulin and NMDA-R activation, IQSEC2 and Arf6 activity depresses AMPA-R-mediated neurotransmission by removal of GluA1 subunits (Myers et al., 2012). Mutations in *IQSEC2* have been found in patients with nonsyndromic ID (Shoubridge et al., 2010), severe syndromic ID (Tran Mau-Them et al., 2014), ID with seizures (Gandomi et al., 2014), and epileptic encephalopathy (Allen et al., 2013).

DISC1 was initially discovered as a gene disrupted by a translocation associated with schizophrenia, bipolar disorder, and other forms of mental illness in a large, single pedigree (Millar et al., 2000). Additional, very rare mutations in *DISC1* have been discovered in other families or individuals with neurodevelopmental disorders, especially schizophrenia (Sachs et al., 2005) and ASD (Girirajan et al., 2013a; Kenny et al., 2014; Williams et al., 2009). Deletions and mutations in *DISC1* have also been found in patients with agenesis of the corpus callosum (Osbun et al., 2011). *DISC1* encodes a multifunctional adaptor protein that interacts with many other proteins in many parts of the cell (Thomson et al., 2013). At the synapse, DISC1 also plays multiple roles and disruption of the gene affects synapse formation, synaptic transmission and plasticity (Randall et al., 2014). Recently, defects in synaptic transmission and plasticity have been demonstrated in neurons differentiated from induced pluripotent stem cells from patients carrying a DISC1 frameshift mutation (Sachs et al., 2005), which can be rescued by genetic correction of the DISC1 mutation (Wen et al., 2014). Collectively, the evidence is thus quite strong that rare mutations in DISC1 can affect synaptic biology and result in neurodevelopmental disorders.

9.6.5 Transcription Factors and Chromatin Regulators

Transcription factors: A growing number of neural transcription factors have been implicated in neurodevelopmental disorders, through specific syndromes or based on rare mutations in idiopathic cases of common disorders. Some of their effects may stem from dysregulation of genes controlling early neurodevelopmental processes such as cell migration, axon guidance, or synapse formation, but several also play roles in activity-dependent gene expression and synaptic plasticity.

For example, the TBR1 protein is involved in early development, where it regulates many genes (Bedogni et al., 2010), including *AUTS2*, itself a transcription factor implicated in ASD, ID, and schizophrenia (Oksenberg and Ahituv, 2013). However, TBR1 is also responsive to neural activity, acting in a complex with the MAGUK protein CASK, which has unusual functions in the nucleus in addition to acting as a synaptic scaffolding protein (Hsueh, 2006). The targets of this complex include the NMDA-R subunit GluN2B (encoded by *GRIN2B*) and *Reelin*, among many others. As mentioned earlier, mutations in *CASK* are associated with severe ID or nonsyndromic forms of ID and ASD, depending on the mutation. Haploinsufficiency of *TBR1* is thought to be a major contributor to neuropsychiatric phenotypes due to 2q24 microdeletions (Palumbo et al., 2014; Traylor et al., 2012) and point mutations in *TBR1* have also been observed in multiple cases of ASD (O'Roak et al., 2012a; O'Roak et al., 2012b). Removal of one copy of *Tbr1* in mice alters expression of many genes involved in synapse formation and plasticity, including *Netrin-G1*, *Cadherin-8*, and *Contactin-2*, and also blocks activity-dependent induction of *Grin2b* in the amygdala (Huang et al., 2014).

Another well-characterized example is the MEF2C protein, also an activity-responsive transcriptional regulator. Haploinsufficiency of the *MEF2C* gene is responsible for the manifestations of 5q14.3 microdeletion syndrome, characterized by ID, stereotypic movements, epilepsy, cerebral malformations, and ASD. *De novo* intragenic deletions or point mutations in *MEF2C* are found in sporadic cases of ID and ASD (Zweier and Rauch, 2012). Like TBR1, MEF2C is involved in early neurodevelopmental processes including neurogenesis and cell migration. However, it is also a key component of a pathway controlling gene expression in response to synaptic activity (West and Greenberg, 2011). Among other functions, MEF2C acts with FMRP to downregulate synapse number during development and in response to activity patterns that stimulate long-term depression (Barbosa et al., 2008a; Pfeiffer et al., 2010). At least part of this response depends on upregulation of the protocadherin PCDH10, along with ubiquitination of PSD95. An interaction between these two proteins leads to degradation of PSD95 and synapse elimination (Tsai et al., 2012).

Chromatin regulators: Recent exome sequencing studies in neurodevelopmental and neuropsychiatric disorders have identified causative mutations in many chromatin regulators, highlighting the role of chromatin regulatory mechanisms in neural development and cognitive function (McCarthy et al., 2014; Ronan et al., 2013). Chromatin regulator genes involved in ID, ASD, and epilepsy through dominant mutations include: (1) chromatin remodelers such as BAF (BRG1- and BRM-associated factor, also known as SWI/SNF-like) complexes (*ARID1A, ARID1B, SMARCA2, SMARCA4, SMARCB1, SMARCE1*, involved in Coffin–Siris syndrome, Nicolaides–Baraitser syndrome, ID and ASD), and *CHD2*, *CHD7*, and *CHD8* (chromodomain helicase DNA binding proteins involved in epileptic encephalopathy, CHARGE syndrome and ASD); and (2) chromatin modifiers such as *MECP2* (methyl-CpG-binding repressor, involved in Rett syndrome), *CREBBP* and *EP300* (histone acetyltransferases involved in Rubinstein–Taybi syndrome), and *HDAC4*

(histone deacetylase 4, involved in brachydactyly mental retardation syndrome). Of note, mutations in certain BAF complex components have roles in both neurodevelopmental disorders and cancer (Ronan et al., 2013).

Recently, whole-exome sequencing in ASD followed by targeted resequencing identified eight *de novo* truncating mutations in *CHD8* (O'Roak et al., 2012a; O'Roak et al., 2012b), a chromodomain protein that functions as an ATP-dependent chromatin remodeler involved in the regulation of the WNT/β-catenin signaling pathway (Thompson et al., 2008). Mutations in other CHD genes, including *CHD2* (Carvill et al., 2013; Chenier et al., 2014) and *CHD7* (Janssen et al., 2012) have also been implicated in neurodevelopmental disorders. While the targets of these genes have not been defined, the related protein CHD4 functions as part of the NuRD complex, the targets of which include genes that operate as critical regulators of presynaptic differentiation (Yamada et al., 2014).

2q37 deletion syndrome, also known as brachydactyly mental retardation syndrome, is characterized by developmental delay/ID, ASD, hypotonia, mild facial dysmorphism, short stature, obesity, and short digits. Recently, haploinsufficiency of *HDAC4* was shown to result in brachydactyly mental retardation syndrome (Williams et al., 2010b). *HDAC4* encodes a histone deacetylase that shuttles between the nucleus and cytoplasm in response to glutamatergic signaling (Sando et al., 2012). HDAC4 has been shown to regulate a transcriptional program essential for synaptic plasticity and memory; by repressing genes encoding synaptic proteins, it affects the strength and architecture of excitatory synapses (Sando et al., 2012). Conditional deletion of *Hdac4* in mouse forebrain neurons leads to impairments in spatial learning and memory and long-term synaptic plasticity (Kim et al., 2012).

Combined analysis of *de novo* loss-of-function SNVs identified in 965 ASD probands sequenced in four WES studies (121 genes) found significant enrichment for genes involved in chromatin regulation (Ben-David and Shifman, 2013), including the chromatin remodeling genes, *CHD8* and *ARID1B,* mentioned earlier, and *MBD5*, a DNA methylation binding protein such as *MECP2*. *MBD5* is the only gene contained in the critical region of the 2q23.1 microdeletion syndrome, associated with ID, epilepsy, and ASD (Talkowski et al., 2011). A particular enrichment was observed for genes involved in transcriptional regulation that are highly expressed during brain development, followed by a decrease in expression after birth. These findings, together with an ever-increasing list of chromatin regulator genes mutated in neurodevelopmental disorders (Ronan et al., 2013), highlight the key role of chromatin regulatory mechanisms in human brain development and function.

9.7 OVERVIEW OF CLINICAL GENETICS FINDINGS

Genetic disruption of the processes of synapse formation and plasticity clearly represents a major etiological mechanism for neurodevelopmental disorders. The numerous specific examples highlighted in earlier sections, along with the more general enrichment of mutations in synaptic genes in patients with common clinical diagnoses emphasize the importance of this class of genes, with new examples being discovered all the time.

While pathogenicity is well established for mutations in many of these genes (Table 9.1), the evidence for some others is currently inconclusive, at least based on human genetic data alone and considering each gene singly. However, the collective implication of this functional class of genes raises the prior probability of pathogenicity for any specific gene or subfamily member. Parallel functional analyses in cellular and animal models also provide strong biological plausibility for many. Nevertheless, caution is still warranted in inferring pathogenicity for any new variant.

As with mutations in other gene classes, the clinical outcomes can be highly variable, including ID, developmental delay, autism, psychosis, ADHD, OCD, seizures, and others. An emerging trend is that mutations in many genes initially associated with specific clinical syndromes may also contribute to idiopathic cases of more common diagnostic categories, such as ASD and schizophrenia. Phenotypic variability may be accounted for by allelic specificity in some cases or by additional variants in the genetic background. Indeed, many cases are likely to involve important contributions from more than one seriously disruptive mutation (Chapters 1 and 4). Phenotypic expression may also be affected by other modifying factors, including environmental variables or intrinsic developmental variation (as discussed in Chapter 1).

Perhaps the most striking impression from these findings is how many ways there are to disrupt synapses and how sensitive they are to removal of even one copy of so many different genes. There are clearly many biochemical processes involved in synapse function and plasticity, including cellular recognition, cell–cell adhesion and signaling, neurotransmission, multiple intersecting pathways of signal transduction, local translation, dynamic trafficking, and localization of hundreds of synaptic proteins, as well as activity-dependent gene expression mediated by sequence-specific transcription factors and an array of chromatin regulatory proteins. Perhaps the fragility of these structures is simply due to their biochemical complexity.

Another contributing factor may be that many of the proteins involved are members of protein families, which interact with each other or with members of other protein families in complexes with precise stoichiometry (Emes and Grant, 2012; Grant, 2003). This may explain why so many of these genes are dosage-sensitive (most obviously manifested as haploinsufficiency, but also apparent in pathogenic effects of gene duplications). This idea is reinforced by the evolutionary conservation of the relative number of paralogous genes in many of these gene families following whole-genome duplications (McLysaght et al., 2014), suggesting that changes in *relative* dosage are not well tolerated.

9.8 PATHOGENIC MECHANISMS

The diversity of genes and processes disrupted in synaptic disorders presents a challenge to understanding pathogenic mechanisms. How can mutations in so many different genes lead to the same spectrum of clinical defects? At what point do their effects converge to generate similar phenotypes?

Convergence may arise at multiple levels. On the one hand, many of the implicated genes can be linked functionally into pathways regulating synaptic plasticity, as described earlier. However, the temptation to place all these genes into one or a few pathways must be tempered by the realization that they are not all expressed at the same synapses or even in the same cells.

The question of how these diverse mutations produce the same spectrum of symptoms must thus, for many genes, involve convergence at the level of neural systems rather than molecular pathways. Mutations affecting synapses between different cell types within a circuit may all ultimately impinge on the neural dynamics within distributed systems and result in the emergence of pathophysiological states underlying specific psychiatric or neurological disturbances, such as psychosis or seizures.

9.9 CELLULAR AND ANIMAL MODELS AND THE DEVELOPMENT OF NEW THERAPIES

Understanding how any given mutation results in neuropsychiatric disease will require integration of analyses across many levels, from molecular and cellular levels to neural circuits and brain systems. Cellular models are obviously well suited to elucidation of molecular and cellular-level effects of pathogenic mutations (Chapter 10). The development of induced pluripotent stem cell technologies and protocols for differentiation into specific types of neurons has permitted the "virtual biopsy" of neurons from patients and analysis of their properties *in vitro*. For example, analyses of iPS cell-derived neurons from patients with mutations in *DISC1* revealed defects in synaptic transmission and plasticity and altered expression of many synaptic proteins (Wen et al., 2014). Neurons derived from patients with mutations in *CACNA1C* (the cause of Timothy syndrome), showed a pathological decrease in dendrite length in response to activity, rather than the normal increase (Krey et al., 2013). As a final example, neurons derived from patients with mutations in *SHANK3* showed major defects in excitatory, but not inhibitory, synaptic transmission, which could be corrected by restoration of *SHANK3* expression or treatment with insulin-like growth factor 1 (IGF1) (Shcheglovitov et al., 2013). The primary cellular defects associated with mutations leading to similar spectra of neurodevelopmental disorders may thus be quite diverse and may only be seen at specific synapses in specific cell types.

Animal models that recapitulate high-risk mutations are an essential, complementary tool to explore the propagation of cellular-level defects across higher levels of neural organization as circuits and systems develop in an activity-dependent manner (Chapter 11). They also provide the means to define pathophysiological states and link them with behavioral or neurological phenotypes that may underlie specific symptoms in humans.

Many mutations are pleiotropic, affecting multiple cell types in many regions of the brain (and often in other tissues, explaining particular spectra of comorbidities associated with specific mutations). It is thus essential to define the *cell types* and *synapse types* affected by any primary molecular pathology and to elucidate which cellular defects are responsible for the emergent brain-level dysfunction (e.g., Ozkan et al., 2014; Rothwell et al., 2014). Such efforts are greatly empowered by the continuing development of molecular tools to disrupt gene function in specific cell types, coupled with new methods such as optogenetics, which allow the activity of specific cell types to be linked to behavior on a moment-to-moment basis.

The definition of pathogenic mechanisms will hopefully yield a sufficient level of understanding of the nature of the defect that one can rationally design a new therapeutic to correct or compensate for the pathogenic dysfunction (Chapter 14). This may be achieved in two ways: first, for some disorders, it may be possible to target the primary molecular pathology, even in adults, and at least partially reverse the resultant effects at the level of electrophysiology and behavior. This approach may work for disorders characterized by an ongoing deficit in synaptic plasticity, such as fragile X syndrome or Rett syndrome (Ehninger et al., 2008).

On the other hand, disorders that result from a history of altered neurodevelopment and that lead to the indirect emergence of pathophysiological states may not be reversible by targeting the primary molecular pathology (the effects of which may have been important only during neurodevelopment; e.g., *SYNGAP1* (Ozkan et al., 2014); *DISC1* (Li et al., 2007)). Instead, it may be necessary to define the neural circuitry underlying the pathophysiological state in sufficient detail that a compensatory therapy can be developed to rebalance the neural system (Deisseroth, 2014). The traditional focus for such intervention has been through pharmacology, but direct brain stimulation methods are also showing promise in correcting pathological patterns of activity in specific circuits (Holtzheimer and Mayberg, 2011).

Recent findings have revealed a tremendous diversity of genetic causes of neurodevelopmental disorders and blurred the lines between rare syndromes and common psychiatric and neurological diagnostic categories. Within this diversity, there is a compelling convergence on the disruption of synapses as a major etiological mechanism. The ability to identify pathogenic mutations in individual patients coupled with an ever-increasing understanding of the associated pathogenic mechanisms promise a new personalized approach to treatment of these disorders in the coming years.

REFERENCES

Abelson, J.F., Kwan, K.Y., O'Roak, B.J., Baek, D.Y., Stillman, A.A., Morgan, T.M., Mathews, C.A., Pauls, D.L., Rasin, M.R., Gunel, M., et al. (2005). Sequence variants in SLITRK1 are associated with Tourette's syndrome. Science 310, 317–320.

Adviento, B., Corbin, I.L., Widjaja, F., Desachy, G., Enrique, N., Rosser, T., Risi, S., Marco, E.J., Hendren, R.L., Bearden, C.E., et al. (2014). Autism traits in the RASopathies. J Med Genet 51, 10–20.

Alarcon, M., Abrahams, B.S., Stone, J.L., Duvall, J.A., Perederiy, J.V., Bomar, J.M., Sebat, J., Wigler, M., Martin, C.L., Ledbetter, D.H., et al. (2008). Linkage, association, and gene-expression analyses identify CNTNAP2 as an autism-susceptibility gene. Am J Hum Genet 82, 150–159.

Allen, A.S., Berkovic, S.F., Cossette, P., Delanty, N., Dlugos, D., Eichler, E.E., Epstein, M.P., Glauser, T., Goldstein, D.B., Han, Y., et al. (2013). De novo mutations in epileptic encephalopathies. Nature 501, 217–221.

An, J.Y., Cristino, A.S., Zhao, Q., Edson, J., Williams, S.M., Ravine, D., Wray, J., Marshall, V.M., Hunt, A., Whitehouse, A.J., et al. (2014). Towards a molecular characterization of autism spectrum disorders: an exome sequencing and systems approach. Transl Psychiatry 4, e394.

Anderson, G.R., Galfin, T., Xu, W., Aoto, J., Malenka, R.C., and Sudhof, T.C. (2012). Candidate autism gene screen identifies critical role for cell-adhesion molecule CASPR2 in dendritic arborization and spine development. Proc Natl Acad Sci USA 109, 18120–18125.

Archer, H.L., Evans, J., Edwards, S., Colley, J., Newbury-Ecob, R., O'Callaghan, F., Huyton, M., O'Regan, M., Tolmie, J., Sampson, J., et al. (2006a). CDKL5 mutations cause infantile spasms, early onset seizures, and severe mental retardation in female patients. J Med Genet 43, 729–734.

Archer, H.L., Evans, J.C., Millar, D.S., Thompson, P.W., Kerr, A.M., Leonard, H., Christodoulou, J., Ravine, D., Lazarou, L., Grove, L., et al. (2006b). NTNG1 mutations are a rare cause of Rett syndrome. Am J Med Genet A 140, 691–694.

Aruga, J., and Mikoshiba, K. (2003). Identification and characterization of Slitrk, a novel neuronal transmembrane protein family controlling neurite outgrowth. Mol Cell Neurosci 24, 117–129.

Ayoub, M.A., Angelicheva, D., Vile, D., Chandler, D., Morar, B., Cavanaugh, J.A., Visscher, P.M., Jablensky, A., Pfleger, K.D., and Kalaydjieva, L. (2012). Deleterious GRM1 mutations in schizophrenia. PLoS One 7, e32849.

Bakkaloglu, B., O'Roak, B.J., Louvi, A., Gupta, A.R., Abelson, J.F., Morgan, T.M., Chawarska, K., Klin, A., Ercan-Sencicek, A.G., Stillman, A.A., et al. (2008). Molecular cytogenetic analysis and resequencing of contactin associated protein-like 2 in autism spectrum disorders. Am J Hum Genet 82, 165–173.

Balemans, M.C., Kasri, N.N., Kopanitsa, M.V., Afinowi, N.O., Ramakers, G., Peters, T.A., Beynon, A.J., Janssen, S.M., van Summeren, R.C., Eeftens, J.M., et al. (2013). Hippocampal dysfunction in the Euchromatin histone methyltransferase 1 heterozygous knockout mouse model for Kleefstra syndrome. Hum Mol Genet 22, 852–866.

Barbosa, A.C., Kim, M.S., Ertunc, M., Adachi, M., Nelson, E.D., McAnally, J., Richardson, J.A., Kavalali, E.T., Monteggia, L.M., Bassel-Duby, R., et al. (2008a). MEF2C, a transcription factor that facilitates learning and memory by negative regulation of synapse numbers and function. Proc Natl Acad Sci USA 105, 9391–9396.

Barbosa, A.C., Kim, M.S., Ertunc, M., Adachi, M., Nelson, E.D., McAnally, J., Richardson, J.A., Kavalali, E.T., Monteggia, L.M., Bassel-Duby, R., et al. (2008b). MEF2C, a transcription factor that facilitates learning and memory by negative regulation of synapse numbers and function. Proc Natl Acad Sci USA 105, 9391–9396.

Barcia, G., Chemaly, N., Gobin, S., Milh, M., Van Bogaert, P., Barnerias, C., Kaminska, A., Dulac, O., Desguerre, I., Cormier, V., et al. (2014). Early epileptic encephalopathies associated with STXBP1 mutations: Could we better delineate the phenotype? Eur J Med Genet 57, 15–20.

Bayes, A., van de Lagemaat, L.N., Collins, M.O., Croning, M.D., Whittle, I.R., Choudhary, J.S., and Grant, S.G. (2011). Characterization of the proteome, diseases and evolution of the human postsynaptic density. Nat Neurosci 14, 19–21.

Bedogni, F., Hodge, R.D., Elsen, G.E., Nelson, B.R., Daza, R.A., Beyer, R.P., Bammler, T.K., Rubenstein, J.L., and Hevner, R.F. (2010). Tbr1 regulates regional and laminar identity of postmitotic neurons in developing neocortex. Proc Natl Acad Sci USA 107, 13129–13134.

Ben-David, E., and Shifman, S. (2013). Combined analysis of exome sequencing points toward a major role for transcription regulation during brain development in autism. Mol Psychiatry 18, 1054–1056.

Berkel, S., Marshall, C.R., Weiss, B., Howe, J., Roeth, R., Moog, U., Endris, V., Roberts, W., Szatmari, P., Pinto, D., et al. (2010). Mutations in the SHANK2 synaptic scaffolding gene in autism spectrum disorder and mental retardation. Nat Genet 42, 489–491.

Berryer, M.H., Hamdan, F.F., Klitten, L.L., Moller, R.S., Carmant, L., Schwartzentruber, J., Patry, L., Dobrzeniecka, S., Rochefort, D., Neugnot-Cerioli, M., et al. (2013). Mutations in SYNGAP1 cause intellectual disability, autism, and a specific form of epilepsy by inducing haploinsufficiency. Hum Mutat 34, 385–394.

Betancur, C., Sakurai, T., and Buxbaum, J.D. (2009). The emerging role of synaptic cell-adhesion pathways in the pathogenesis of autism spectrum disorders. Trends Neurosci 32, 402–412.

Betancur, C. (2011). Etiological heterogeneity in autism spectrum disorders: more than 100 genetic and genomic disorders and still counting. Brain Res 1380, 42–77.

Blackman, A.V., Abrahamsson, T., Costa, R.P., Lalanne, T., and Sjostrom, P.J. (2013). Target-cell-specific short-term plasticity in local circuits. Front Synaptic Neurosci 5, 11.

Boido, D., Farisello, P., Cesca, F., Ferrea, E., Valtorta, F., Benfenati, F., and Baldelli, P. (2010). Cortico-hippocampal hyperexcitability in synapsin I/II/III knockout mice: age-dependency and response to the antiepileptic drug levetiracetam. Neuroscience 171, 268–283.

Bonaglia, M.C., Giorda, R., Beri, S., De Agostini, C., Novara, F., Fichera, M., Grillo, L., Galesi, O., Vetro, A., Ciccone, R., et al. (2011). Molecular mechanisms generating and stabilizing terminal 22q13 deletions in 44 subjects with Phelan/McDermid syndrome. PLoS Genet 7, e1002173.

Borg, I., Freude, K., Kubart, S., Hoffmann, K., Menzel, C., Laccone, F., Firth, H., Ferguson-Smith, M.A., Tommerup, N., Ropers, H.H., et al. (2005). Disruption of Netrin G1 by a balanced chromosome translocation in a girl with Rett syndrome. Eur J Hum Genet 13, 921–927.

Brandon, N.J., and Sawa, A. (2011). Linking neurodevelopmental and synaptic theories of mental illness through DISC1. Nat Rev Neurosci 12, 707–722.

Buffington, S.A., Huang, W., and Costa-Mattioli, M. (2014). Translational control in synaptic plasticity and cognitive dysfunction. Annu Rev Neurosci 37, 17–38.

Butler, M.G., Dasouki, M.J., Zhou, X.P., Talebizadeh, Z., Brown, M., Takahashi, T.N., Miles, J.H., Wang, C.H., Stratton, R., Pilarski, R., et al. (2005). Subset of individuals with autism spectrum disorders and extreme macrocephaly associated with germline PTEN tumour suppressor gene mutations. J Med Genet 42, 318–321.

Buxbaum, J.D., Cai, G., Chaste, P., Nygren, G., Goldsmith, J., Reichert, J., Anckarsater, H., Rastam, M., Smith, C.J., Silverman, J.M., et al. (2007). Mutation screening of the PTEN gene in patients with autism spectrum disorders and macrocephaly. Am J Med Genet B Neuropsychiatr Genet 144B, 484–491.

Buxbaum, J.D., Daly, M.J., Devlin, B., Lehner, T., Roeder, K., and State, M.W. (2012). The autism sequencing consortium: large-scale, high-throughput sequencing in autism spectrum disorders. Neuron 76, 1052–1056.

Camacho, A., Simon, R., Sanz, R., Vinuela, A., Martinez-Salio, A., and Mateos, F. (2012). Cognitive and behavioral profile in females with epilepsy with PDCH19 mutation: two novel mutations and review of the literature. Epilepsy Behav 24, 134–137.

Carney, R.M., Wolpert, C.M., Ravan, S.A., Shahbazian, M., Ashley-Koch, A., Cuccaro, M.L., Vance, J.M., and Pericak-Vance, M.A. (2003). Identification of MeCP2 mutations in a series of females with autistic disorder. Pediatr Neurol 28, 205–211.

Carvill, G.L., Heavin, S.B., Yendle, S.C., McMahon, J.M., O'Roak, B.J., Cook, J., Khan, A., Dorschner, M.O., Weaver, M., Calvert, S., et al. (2013). Targeted resequencing in epileptic encephalopathies identifies de novo mutations in CHD2 and SYNGAP1. Nat Genet 45, 825–830.

Castren, M., Gaily, E., Tengstrom, C., Lahdetie, J., Archer, H., and Ala-Mello, S. (2011). Epilepsy caused by CDKL5 mutations. Eur J Paediatr Neurol 15, 65–69.

Cesca, F., Baldelli, P., Valtorta, F., and Benfenati, F. (2010). The synapsins: key actors of synapse function and plasticity. Prog Neurobiol 91, 313–348.

Chen, C.Y., Tsai, M.S., Lin, C.Y., Yu, I.S., Chen, Y.T., Lin, S.R., Juan, L.W., Hsu, H.M., Lee, L.J., and Lin, S.W. (2012). Rescue of the genetically engineered Cul4b mutant mouse as a potential model for human X-linked mental retardation. Hum Mol Genet 21, 4270–4285.

Chenier, S., Yoon, G., Argiropoulos, B., Lauzon, J., Laframboise, R., Ahn, J.W., Ogilvie, C.M., Lionel, A.C., Marshall, C.R., Vaags, A.K., et al. (2014). CHD2 haploinsufficiency is associated with developmental delay, intellectual disability, epilepsy and neurobehavioural problems. J Neurodev Disord 6, 9.

Ching, M.S., Shen, Y., Tan, W.H., Jeste, S.S., Morrow, E.M., Chen, X., Mukaddes, N.M., Yoo, S.Y., Hanson, E., Hundley, R., et al. (2010). Deletions of NRXN1 (neurexin-1) predispose to a wide spectrum of developmental disorders. Am J Med Genet B Neuropsychiatr Genet 153B, 937–947.

Chiyonobu, T., Hayashi, S., Kobayashi, K., Morimoto, M., Miyanomae, Y., Nishimura, A., Nishimoto, A., Ito, C., Imoto, I., Sugimoto, T., et al. (2007). Partial tandem duplication of GRIA3 in a male with mental retardation. Am J Med Genet A 143A, 1448–1455.

Choquet, D., and Triller, A. (2013). The dynamic synapse. Neuron 80, 691–703.

Citri, A., and Malenka, R.C. (2008). Synaptic plasticity: multiple forms, functions, and mechanisms. Neuropsychopharmacology 33, 18–41.

Clement, J.P., Aceti, M., Creson, T.K., Ozkan, E.D., Shi, Y., Reish, N.J., Almonte, A.G., Miller, B.H., Wiltgen, B.J., Miller, C.A., et al. (2012). Pathogenic SYNGAP1 mutations impair cognitive development by disrupting maturation of dendritic spine synapses. Cell 151, 709–723.

Clement, J.P., Ozkan, E.D., Aceti, M., Miller, C.A., and Rumbaugh, G. (2013). SYNGAP1 links the maturation rate of excitatory synapses to the duration of critical-period synaptic plasticity. J Neurosci 33, 10447–10452.

Cohen, D., Lazar, G., Couvert, P., Desportes, V., Lippe, D., Mazet, P., and Heron, D. (2002). MECP2 mutation in a boy with language disorder and schizophrenia. Am J Psychiatry 159, 148–149.

Cosgrove, K.E., Galvan, E.J., Barrionuevo, G., and Meriney, S.D. (2011). mGluRs modulate strength and timing of excitatory transmission in hippocampal area CA3. Mol Neurobiol 44, 93–101.

Costa, R.M., Federov, N.B., Kogan, J.H., Murphy, G.G., Stern, J., Ohno, M., Kucherlapati, R., Jacks, T., and Silva, A.J. (2002). Mechanism for the learning deficits in a mouse model of neurofibromatosis type 1. Nature 415, 526–530.

Couvert, P., Bienvenu, T., Aquaviva, C., Poirier, K., Moraine, C., Gendrot, C., Verloes, A., Andres, C., Le Fevre, A.C., Souville, I., et al. (2001). MECP2 is highly mutated in X-linked mental retardation. Hum Mol Genet 10, 941–946.

Cukier, H.N., Dueker, N.D., Slifer, S.H., Lee, J.M., Whitehead, P.L., Lalanne, E., Leyva, N., Konidari, I., Gentry, R.C., Hulme, W.F., et al. (2014). Exome sequencing of extended families with autism reveals genes shared across neurodevelopmental and neuropsychiatric disorders. Mol Autism 5, 1.

Cuoco, C., Ronchetto, P., Gimelli, S., Bena, F., Divizia, M.T., Lerone, M., Mirabelli-Badenier, M., Mascaretti, M., and Gimelli, G. (2011). Microarray based analysis of an inherited terminal 3p26.3 deletion, containing only the CHL1 gene, from a normal father to his two affected children. Orphanet J Rare Dis 6, 12.

Davis, G.W. (2013). Homeostatic signaling and the stabilization of neural function. Neuron 80, 718–728.

de Ligt, J., Willemsen, M.H., van Bon, B.W., Kleefstra, T., Yntema, H.G., Kroes, T., Vulto-van Silfhout, A.T., Koolen, D.A., de Vries, P., Gilissen, C., et al. (2012). Diagnostic exome sequencing in persons with severe intellectual disability. N Engl J Med 367, 1921–1929.

de Wit, J., and Ghosh, A. (2014). Control of neural circuit formation by leucine-rich repeat proteins. Trends Neurosci 37, 539–550.

Deisseroth, K. (2014). Circuit dynamics of adaptive and maladaptive behaviour. Nature 505, 309–317.

Dejanovic, B., Lal, D., Catarino, C.B., Arjune, S., Belaidi, A.A., Trucks, H., Vollmar, C., Surges, R., Kunz, W.S., Motameny, S., et al. (2014). Exonic microdeletions of the gephyrin gene impair GABAergic synaptic inhibition in patients with idiopathic generalized epilepsy. Neurobiol Dis 67, 88–96.

Depienne, C., and LeGuern, E. (2012). PCDH19-related infantile epileptic encephalopathy: an unusual X-linked inheritance disorder. Hum Mutat 33, 627–634.

Dibbens, L.M., Tarpey, P.S., Hynes, K., Bayly, M.A., Scheffer, I.E., Smith, R., Bomar, J., Sutton, E., Vandeleur, L., Shoubridge, C., et al.

(2008). X-linked protocadherin 19 mutations cause female-limited epilepsy and cognitive impairment. Nat Genet 40, 776–781.

Diggs-Andrews, K.A., and Gutmann, D.H. (2013). Modeling cognitive dysfunction in neurofibromatosis-1. Trends Neurosci 36, 237–247.

Dityatev, A., Bukalo, O., and Schachner, M. (2008). Modulation of synaptic transmission and plasticity by cell adhesion and repulsion molecules. Neuron Glia Biol 4, 197–209.

Durand, C.M., Betancur, C., Boeckers, T.M., Bockmann, J., Chaste, P., Fauchereau, F., Nygren, G., Rastam, M., Gillberg, I.C., Anckarsater, H., et al. (2007). Mutations in the gene encoding the synaptic scaffolding protein SHANK3 are associated with autism spectrum disorders. Nat Genet 39, 25–27.

Ehninger, D., Li, W., Fox, K., Stryker, M.P., and Silva, A.J. (2008). Reversing neurodevelopmental disorders in adults. Neuron 60, 950–960.

Elia, J., Gai, X., Xie, H.M., Perin, J.C., Geiger, E., Glessner, J.T., D'Arcy, M., deBerardinis, R., Frackelton, E., Kim, C., et al. (2010). Rare structural variants found in attention-deficit hyperactivity disorder are preferentially associated with neurodevelopmental genes. Mol Psychiatry 15, 637–646.

Elia, J., Glessner, J.T., Wang, K., Takahashi, N., Shtir, C.J., Hadley, D., Sleiman, P.M., Zhang, H., Kim, C.E., Robison, R., et al. (2012). Genome-wide copy number variation study associates metabotropic glutamate receptor gene networks with attention deficit hyperactivity disorder. Nat Genet 44, 78–84.

Emes, R.D., and Grant, S.G. (2012). Evolution of synapse complexity and diversity. Annu Rev Neurosci 35, 111–131.

Endele, S., Rosenberger, G., Geider, K., Popp, B., Tamer, C., Stefanova, I., Milh, M., Kortum, F., Fritsch, A., Pientka, F.K., et al. (2010). Mutations in GRIN2A and GRIN2B encoding regulatory subunits of NMDA receptors cause variable neurodevelopmental phenotypes. Nat Genet 42, 1021–1026.

Fassio, A., Patry, L., Congia, S., Onofri, F., Piton, A., Gauthier, J., Pozzi, D., Messa, M., Defranchi, E., Fadda, M., et al. (2011). SYN1 loss-of-function mutations in autism and partial epilepsy cause impaired synaptic function. Hum Mol Genet 20, 2297–2307.

Fehr, S., Wilson, M., Downs, J., Williams, S., Murgia, A., Sartori, S., Vecchi, M., Ho, G., Polli, R., Psoni, S., et al. (2013). The CDKL5 disorder is an independent clinical entity associated with early-onset encephalopathy. Eur J Hum Genet 21, 266–273.

Franek, K.J., Butler, J., Johnson, J., Simensen, R., Friez, M.J., Bartel, F., Moss, T., DuPont, B., Berry, K., Bauman, M., et al. (2011). Deletion of the immunoglobulin domain of IL1RAPL1 results in nonsyndromic X-linked intellectual disability associated with behavioral problems and mild dysmorphism. Am J Med Genet A 155A, 1109–1114.

Friedman, J.I., Vrijenhoek, T., Markx, S., Janssen, I.M., van der Vliet, W.A., Faas, B.H., Knoers, N.V., Cahn, W., Kahn, R.S., Edelmann, L., et al. (2008). CNTNAP2 gene dosage variation is associated with schizophrenia and epilepsy. Mol Psychiatry 13, 261–266.

Fromer, M., Pocklington, A.J., Kavanagh, D.H., Williams, H.J., Dwyer, S., Gormley, P., Georgieva, L., Rees, E., Palta, P., Ruderfer, D.M., et al. (2014). De novo mutations in schizophrenia implicate synaptic networks. Nature 506, 179–184.

Fukata, Y., Lovero, K.L., Iwanaga, T., Watanabe, A., Yokoi, N., Tabuchi, K., Shigemoto, R., Nicoll, R.A., and Fukata, M. (2010). Disruption of LGI1-linked synaptic complex causes abnormal synaptic transmission and epilepsy. Proc Natl Acad Sci USA 107, 3799–3804.

Gai, X., Xie, H.M., Perin, J.C., Takahashi, N., Murphy, K., Wenocur, A.S., D'Arcy, M., O'Hara, R.J., Goldmuntz, E., Grice, D.E., et al. (2012). Rare structural variation of synapse and neurotransmission genes in autism. Mol Psychiatry 17, 402–411.

Gandomi, S.K., Farwell Gonzalez, K.D., Parra, M., Shahmirzadi, L., Mancuso, J., Pichurin, P., Temme, R., Dugan, S., Zeng, W., and Tang, S. (2014). Diagnostic exome sequencing identifies two novel IQSEC2 mutations associated with X-linked intellectual disability with seizures: implications for genetic counseling and clinical diagnosis. J Genet Couns 23, 289–298.

Garcia, C.C., Blair, H.J., Seager, M., Coulthard, A., Tennant, S., Buddles, M., Curtis, A., and Goodship, J.A. (2004). Identification of a mutation in synapsin I, a synaptic vesicle protein, in a family with epilepsy. J Med Genet 41, 183–186.

Garg, S., Lehtonen, A., Huson, S.M., Emsley, R., Trump, D., Evans, D.G., and Green, J. (2013). Autism and other psychiatric comorbidity in neurofibromatosis type 1: evidence from a population-based study. Dev Med Child Neurol 55, 139–145.

Gauthier, J., Spiegelman, D., Piton, A., Lafreniere, R.G., Laurent, S., St-Onge, J., Lapointe, L., Hamdan, F.F., Cossette, P., Mottron, L., et al. (2009). Novel de novo SHANK3 mutation in autistic patients. Am J Med Genet B Neuropsychiatr Genet 150B, 421–424.

Gauthier, J., Champagne, N., Lafreniere, R.G., Xiong, L., Spiegelman, D., Brustein, E., Lapointe, M., Peng, H., Cote, M., Noreau, A., et al. (2010). De novo mutations in the gene encoding the synaptic scaffolding protein SHANK3 in patients ascertained for schizophrenia. Proc Natl Acad Sci USA 107, 7863–7868.

Gauthier, J., Siddiqui, T.J., Huashan, P., Yokomaku, D., Hamdan, F.F., Champagne, N., Lapointe, M., Spiegelman, D., Noreau, A., Lafreniere, R.G., et al. (2011). Truncating mutations in NRXN2 and NRXN1 in autism spectrum disorders and schizophrenia. Hum Genet 130, 563–573.

Giannandrea, M., Bianchi, V., Mignogna, M.L., Sirri, A., Carrabino, S., D'Elia, E., Vecellio, M., Russo, S., Cogliati, F., Larizza, L., et al. (2010). Mutations in the small GTPase gene RAB39B are responsible for X-linked mental retardation associated with autism, epilepsy, and macrocephaly. Am J Hum Genet 86, 185–195.

Gilman, S.R., Iossifov, I., Levy, D., Ronemus, M., Wigler, M., and Vitkup, D. (2011). Rare de novo variants associated with autism implicate a large functional network of genes involved in formation and function of synapses. Neuron 70, 898–907.

Girirajan, S., Dennis, M.Y., Baker, C., Malig, M., Coe, B.P., Campbell, C.D., Mark, K., Vu, T.H., Alkan, C., Cheng, Z., et al. (2013a). Refinement and discovery of new hotspots of copy-number variation associated with autism spectrum disorder. Am J Hum Genet 92, 221–237.

Girirajan, S., Johnson, R.L., Tassone, F., Balciuniene, J., Katiyar, N., Fox, K., Baker, C., Srikanth, A., Yeoh, K.H., Khoo, S.J., et al. (2013b). Global increases in both common and rare copy number load associated with autism. Hum Mol Genet 22, 2870–2880.

Glessner, J.T., Wang, K., Cai, G., Korvatska, O., Kim, C.E., Wood, S., Zhang, H., Estes, A., Brune, C.W., Bradfield, J.P., et al. (2009). Autism genome-wide copy number variation reveals ubiquitin and neuronal genes. Nature 459, 569–573.

Gong, X., Jiang, Y.W., Zhang, X., An, Y., Zhang, J., Wu, Y., Wang, J., Sun, Y., Liu, Y., Gao, X., et al. (2012). High proportion of 22q13 deletions and SHANK3 mutations in Chinese patients with intellectual disability. PLoS One 7, e34739.

Grabrucker, A.M., Schmeisser, M.J., Schoen, M., and Boeckers, T.M. (2011). Postsynaptic ProSAP/Shank scaffolds in the cross-hair of synaptopathies. Trends Cell Biol 21, 594–603.

Grant, S.G. (2003). Synapse signalling complexes and networks: machines underlying cognition. Bioessays 25, 1229–1235.

Greer, P.L., and Greenberg, M.E. (2008). From synapse to nucleus: calcium-dependent gene transcription in the control of synapse development and function. Neuron 59, 846–860.

Grozeva, D., Kirov, G., Conrad, D.F., Barnes, C.P., Hurles, M., Owen, M.J., O'Donovan, M.C., and Craddock, N. (2013). Reduced burden of very large and rare CNVs in bipolar affective disorder. Bipolar Disord 15, 893–898.

Guo, H., Xun, G., Peng, Y., Xiang, X., Xiong, Z., Zhang, L., He, Y., Xu, X., Liu, Y., Lu, L., et al. (2012). Disruption of Contactin 4 in two subjects with autism in Chinese population. Gene 505, 201–205.

Hackett, A., Tarpey, P.S., Licata, A., Cox, J., Whibley, A., Boyle, J., Rogers, C., Grigg, J., Partington, M., Stevenson, R.E., et al. (2010). CASK mutations are frequent in males and cause X-linked nystagmus and variable XLMR phenotypes. Eur J Hum Genet 18, 544–552.

Halgren, C., Kjaergaard, S., Bak, M., Hansen, C., El-Schich, Z., Anderson, C., Henriksen, K., Hjalgrim, H., Kirchhoff, M., Bijlsma, E., et al. (2012). Corpus callosum abnormalities, intellectual disability, speech impairment, and autism in patients with haploinsufficiency of ARID1B. Clin Genet 2, 248–255.

Hamdan, F.F., Daoud, H., Piton, A., Gauthier, J., Dobrzeniecka, S., Krebs, M.O., Joober, R., Lacaille, J.C., Nadeau, A., Milunsky, J.M., et al. (2011a). De novo SYNGAP1 mutations in nonsyndromic intellectual disability and autism. Biol Psychiatry 69, 898–901.

Hamdan, F.F., Gauthier, J., Araki, Y., Lin, D.T., Yoshizawa, Y., Higashi, K., Park, A.R., Spiegelman, D., Dobrzeniecka, S., Piton, A., et al. (2011b). Excess of de novo deleterious mutations in genes associated with glutamatergic systems in nonsyndromic intellectual disability. Am J Hum Genet 88, 306–316.

Hamdan, F.F., Gauthier, J., Dobrzeniecka, S., Lortie, A., Mottron, L., Vanasse, M., D'Anjou, G., Lacaille, J.C., Rouleau, G.A., and Michaud, J.L. (2011c). Intellectual disability without epilepsy associated with STXBP1 disruption. Eur J Hum Genet 19, 607–609.

Hayashi, T., Yoshida, T., Ra, M., Taguchi, R., and Mishina, M. (2013). IL1RAPL1 associated with mental retardation and autism regulates the formation and stabilization of glutamatergic synapses of cortical neurons through RhoA signaling pathway. PLoS One 8, e66254.

He, X., Sanders, S.J., Liu, L., De Rubeis, S., Lim, E.T., Sutcliffe, J.S., Schellenberg, G.D., Gibbs, R.A., Daly, M.J., Buxbaum, J.D., et al. (2013). Integrated model of de novo and inherited genetic variants yields greater power to identify risk genes. PLoS Genet 9, e1003671.

Heinzen, E.L., Radtke, R.A., Urban, T.J., Cavalleri, G.L., Depondt, C., Need, A.C., Walley, N.M., Nicoletti, P., Ge, D., Catarino, C.B., et al. (2010). Rare deletions at 16p13.11 predispose to a diverse spectrum of sporadic epilepsy syndromes. Am J Hum Genet 86, 707–718.

Hogart, A., Wu, D., LaSalle, J.M., and Schanen, N.C. (2010). The comorbidity of autism with the genomic disorders of chromosome 15q11.2-q13. Neurobiol Dis 38, 181–191.

Hoischen, A., Krumm, N., and Eichler, E.E. (2014). Prioritization of neurodevelopmental disease genes by discovery of new mutations. Nat Neurosci 17, 764–772.

Holtzheimer, P.E., and Mayberg, H.S. (2011). Deep brain stimulation for psychiatric disorders. Annu Rev Neurosci 34, 289–307.

Hood, R.L., Lines, M.A., Nikkel, S.M., Schwartzentruber, J., Beaulieu, C., Nowaczyk, M.J., Allanson, J., Kim, C.A., Wieczorek, D., Moilanen, J.S., et al. (2012). Mutations in SRCAP, encoding SNF2-related CREBBP activator protein, cause Floating-Harbor syndrome. Am J Hum Genet 90, 308–313.

Hoppman-Chaney, N., Wain, K., Seger, P.R., Superneau, D.W., and Hodge, J.C. (2013). Identification of single gene deletions at 15q13.3: further evidence that CHRNA7 causes the 15q13.3 microdeletion syndrome phenotype. Clin Genet 83, 345–351.

Hoshina, N., Tanimura, A., Yamasaki, M., Inoue, T., Fukabori, R., Kuroda, T., Yokoyama, K., Tezuka, T., Sagara, H., Hirano, S., et al. (2013). Protocadherin 17 regulates presynaptic assembly in topographic corticobasal ganglia circuits. Neuron 78, 839–854.

Hsueh, Y.P. (2006). The role of the MAGUK protein CASK in neural development and synaptic function. Curr Med Chem 13, 1915–1927.

Huang, T.N., Chuang, H.C., Chou, W.H., Chen, C.Y., Wang, H.F., Chou, S.J., and Hsueh, Y.P. (2014). Tbr1 haploinsufficiency impairs amygdalar axonal projections and results in cognitive abnormality. Nat Neurosci 17, 240–247.

Huang, Z.J. (2006). Subcellular organization of GABAergic synapses: role of ankyrins and L1 cell adhesion molecules. Nat Neurosci 9, 163–166.

Hulme, S.R., Jones, O.D., and Abraham, W.C. (2013). Emerging roles of metaplasticity in behaviour and disease. Trends Neurosci 36, 353–362.

Ingason, A., Kirov, G., Giegling, I., Hansen, T., Isles, A.R., Jakobsen, K.D., Kristinsson, K.T., le Roux, L., Gustafsson, O., Craddock, N., et al. (2011). Maternally derived microduplications at 15q11-q13: implication of imprinted genes in psychotic illness. Am J Psychiatry 168, 408–417.

International Schizophrenia Consortium. (2008). Rare chromosomal deletions and duplications increase risk of schizophrenia. Nature 455, 237–241.

Iossifov, I., Ronemus, M., Levy, D., Wang, Z., Hakker, I., Rosenbaum, J., Yamrom, B., Lee, Y.H., Narzisi, G., Leotta, A., et al. (2012). De novo gene disruptions in children on the autistic spectrum. Neuron 74, 285–299.

Jamain, S., Quach, H., Betancur, C., Rastam, M., Colineaux, C., Gillberg, I.C., Soderstrom, H., Giros, B., Leboyer, M., Gillberg, C., et al. (2003). Mutations of the X-linked genes encoding neuroligins NLGN3 and NLGN4 are associated with autism. Nat Genet 34, 27–29.

Janssen, N., Bergman, J.E., Swertz, M.A., Tranebjaerg, L., Lodahl, M., Schoots, J., Hofstra, R.M., van Ravenswaaij-Arts, C.M., and Hoefsloot, L.H. (2012). Mutation update on the CHD7 gene involved in CHARGE syndrome. Hum Mutat 33, 1149–1160.

Kalachikov, S., Evgrafov, O., Ross, B., Winawer, M., Barker-Cummings, C., Martinelli Boneschi, F., Choi, C., Morozov, P., Das, K., Teplitskaya, E., et al. (2002). Mutations in LGI1 cause autosomal-dominant partial epilepsy with auditory features. Nat Genet 30, 335–341.

Karayannis, T., Au, E., Patel, J.C., Kruglikov, I., Markx, S., Delorme, R., Heron, D., Salomon, D., Glessner, J., Restituito, S., et al. (2014). Cntnap4 differentially contributes to GABAergic and dopaminergic synaptic transmission. Nature 511, 236–240.

Katayama, K., Yamada, K., Ornthanalai, V.G., Inoue, T., Ota, M., Murphy, N.P., and Aruga, J. (2010). Slitrk1-deficient mice display elevated anxiety-like behavior and noradrenergic abnormalities. Mol Psychiatry 15, 177–184.

Katidou, M., Vidaki, M., Strigini, M., and Karagogeos, D. (2008). The immunoglobulin superfamily of neuronal cell adhesion molecules: lessons from animal models and correlation with human disease. Biotechnol J 3, 1564–1580.

Ke, C., Li, C., Huang, X., Cao, F., Shi, D., He, W., Bu, H., Gao, F., Cai, T., Hinton, A.O., Jr., et al. (2013). Protocadherin20 promotes excitatory synaptogenesis in dorsal horn and contributes to bone cancer pain. Neuropharmacology 75, 181–190.

Kegel, L., Aunin, E., Meijer, D., and Bermingham, J.R. (2013). LGI proteins in the nervous system. ASN Neuro 5, 167–181.

Kenny, E.M., Cormican, P., Furlong, S., Heron, E., Kenny, G., Fahey, C., Kelleher, E., Ennis, S., Tropea, D., Anney, R., et al. (2014). Excess of rare novel loss-of-function variants in synaptic genes in schizophrenia and autism spectrum disorders. Mol Psychiatry 19, 872–879.

Kim, M.S., Akhtar, M.W., Adachi, M., Mahgoub, M., Bassel-Duby, R., Kavalali, E.T., Olson, E.N., and Monteggia, L.M. (2012). An essential role for histone deacetylase 4 in synaptic plasticity and memory formation. J Neurosci 32, 10879–10886.

Kim, S., Burette, A., Chung, H.S., Kwon, S.K., Woo, J., Lee, H.W., Kim, K., Kim, H., Weinberg, R.J., and Kim, E. (2006). NGL family PSD-95-interacting adhesion molecules regulate excitatory synapse formation. Nat Neurosci 9, 1294–1301.

Kim, S.Y., Chung, H.S., Sun, W., and Kim, H. (2007). Spatiotemporal expression pattern of non-clustered protocadherin family members in the developing rat brain. Neuroscience 147, 996–1021.

Kirov, G., Grozeva, D., Norton, N., Ivanov, D., Mantripragada, K.K., Holmans, P., Craddock, N.,

Owen, M.J., and O'Donovan, M.C. (2009). Support for the involvement of large copy number variants in the pathogenesis of schizophrenia. Hum Mol Genet 18, 1497–1503.

Kirov, G., Pocklington, A.J., Holmans, P., Ivanov, D., Ikeda, M., Ruderfer, D., Moran, J., Chambert, K., Toncheva, D., Georgieva, L., et al. (2012). De novo CNV analysis implicates specific abnormalities of postsynaptic signalling complexes in the pathogenesis of schizophrenia. Mol Psychiatry 17, 142–153.

Krey, J.F., Pasca, S.P., Shcheglovitov, A., Yazawa, M., Schwemberger, R., Rasmusson, R., and Dolmetsch, R.E. (2013). Timothy syndrome is associated with activity-dependent dendritic retraction in rodent and human neurons. Nat Neurosci 16, 201–209.

Krumm, N., O'Roak, B.J., Karakoc, E., Mohajeri, K., Nelson, B., Vives, L., Jacquemont, S., Munson, J., Bernier, R., and Eichler, E.E. (2013). Transmission disequilibrium of small CNVs in simplex autism. Am J Hum Genet 93, 595–606.

Kullmann, D.M., and Waxman, S.G. (2010). Neurological channelopathies: new insights into disease mechanisms and ion channel function. J Physiol 588, 1823–1827.

Laumonnier, F., Bonnet-Brilhault, F., Gomot, M., Blanc, R., David, A., Moizard, M.P., Raynaud, M., Ronce, N., Lemonnier, E., Calvas, P., et al. (2004). X-linked mental retardation and autism are associated with a mutation in the NLGN4 gene, a member of the neuroligin family. Am J Hum Genet 74, 552–557.

Laumonnier, F., Cuthbert, P.C., and Grant, S.G. (2007). The role of neuronal complexes in human X-linked brain diseases. Am J Hum Genet 80, 205–220.

Leblond, C.S., Heinrich, J., Delorme, R., Proepper, C., Betancur, C., Huguet, G., Konyukh, M., Chaste, P., Ey, E., Rastam, M., et al. (2012). Genetic and functional analyses of SHANK2 mutations suggest a multiple hit model of autism spectrum disorders. PLoS Genet 8, e1002521.

Leblond, C.S., Nava, C., Polge, A., Gauthier, J., Huguet, G., Lumbroso, S., Giuliano, F., Stordeur, C., Depienne, C., Mouzat, K., et al. (2014). Meta-analysis of SHANK mutations in autism spectrum disorders: a gradient of severity in cognitive impairments. PLoS Genet 10, e1004580.

Lerche, H., Shah, M., Beck, H., Noebels, J., Johnston, D., and Vincent, A. (2013). Ion channels in genetic and acquired forms of epilepsy. J Physiol 591, 753–764.

Lesca, G., Rudolf, G., Bruneau, N., Lozovaya, N., Labalme, A., Boutry-Kryza, N., Salmi, M., Tsintsadze, T., Addis, L., Motte, J., et al. (2013). GRIN2A mutations in acquired epileptic aphasia and related childhood focal epilepsies and encephalopathies with speech and language dysfunction. Nat Genet 45, 1061–1066.

Levinson, D.F., Duan, J., Oh, S., Wang, K., Sanders, A.R., Shi, J., Zhang, N., Mowry, B.J., Olincy, A., Amin, F., et al. (2011). Copy number variants in schizophrenia: confirmation of five previous findings and new evidence for 3q29 microdeletions and VIPR2 duplications. Am J Psychiatry 168, 302–316.

Li, W., Zhou, Y., Jentsch, J.D., Brown, R.A., Tian, X., Ehninger, D., Hennah, W., Peltonen, L., Lonnqvist, J., Huttunen, M.O., et al. (2007). Specific developmental disruption of disrupted-in-schizophrenia-1 function results in schizophrenia-related phenotypes in mice. Proc Natl Acad Sci USA 104, 18280–18285.

Lin, E.I., Jeyifous, O., and Green, W.N. (2013). CASK regulates SAP97 conformation and its interactions with AMPA and NMDA receptors. J Neurosci 33, 12067–12076.

Linseman, D.A., and Loucks, F.A. (2008). Diverse roles of Rho family GTPases in neuronal development, survival, and death. Front Biosci 13, 657–676.

Lionel, A.C., Vaags, A.K., Sato, D., Gazzellone, M.J., Mitchell, E.B., Chen, H.Y., Costain, G., Walker, S., Egger, G., Thiruvahindrapuram, B., et al. (2013). Rare exonic deletions implicate the synaptic organizer Gephyrin (GPHN) in risk for autism, schizophrenia and seizures. Hum Mol Genet 22, 2055–2066.

Liu, L., Lei, J., Sanders, S.J., Willsey, A.J., Kou, Y., Cicek, A.E., Klei, L., Lu, C., He, X., Li, M., et al. (2014). DAWN: a framework to identify autism genes and subnetworks using gene expression and genetics. Mol Autism 5, 22.

Mabb, A.M., Judson, M.C., Zylka, M.J., and Philpot, B.D. (2011). Angelman syndrome: insights into genomic imprinting and neurodevelopmental phenotypes. Trends Neurosci 34, 293–303.

Malhotra, D., McCarthy, S., Michaelson, J.J., Vacic, V., Burdick, K.E., Yoon, S., Cichon, S., Corvin,

A., Gary, S., Gershon, E.S., et al. (2011). High frequencies of de novo CNVs in bipolar disorder and schizophrenia. Neuron 72, 951–963.

Malhotra, D., and Sebat, J. (2012). CNVs: harbingers of a rare variant revolution in psychiatric genetics. Cell 148, 1223–1241.

Maness, P.F., and Schachner, M. (2007). Neural recognition molecules of the immunoglobulin superfamily: signaling transducers of axon guidance and neuronal migration. Nat Neurosci 10, 19–26.

Mari, F., Azimonti, S., Bertani, I., Bolognese, F., Colombo, E., Caselli, R., Scala, E., Longo, I., Grosso, S., Pescucci, C., et al. (2005). CDKL5 belongs to the same molecular pathway of MeCP2 and it is responsible for the early-onset seizure variant of Rett syndrome. Hum Mol Genet 14, 1935–1946.

Marini, C., Scheffer, I.E., Nabbout, R., Mei, D., Cox, K., Dibbens, L.M., McMahon, J.M., Iona, X., Carpintero, R.S., Elia, M., et al. (2009). SCN1A duplications and deletions detected in Dravet syndrome: implications for molecular diagnosis. Epilepsia 50, 1670–1678.

McBride, K.L., Varga, E.A., Pastore, M.T., Prior, T.W., Manickam, K., Atkin, J.F., and Herman, G.E. (2010). Confirmation study of PTEN mutations among individuals with autism or developmental delays/mental retardation and macrocephaly. Autism Res 3, 137–141.

McCarthy, S.E., Gillis, J., Kramer, M., Lihm, J., Yoon, S., Berstein, Y., Mistry, M., Pavlidis, P., Solomon, R., Ghiban, E., et al. (2014). De novo mutations in schizophrenia implicate chromatin remodeling and support a genetic overlap with autism and intellectual disability. Mol Psychiatry 19, 652–658.

McLysaght, A., Makino, T., Grayton, H.M., Tropeano, M., Mitchell, K.J., Vassos, E., and Collier, D.A. (2014). Ohnologs are overrepresented in pathogenic copy number mutations. Proc Natl Acad Sci USA 111, 361–366.

Mefford, H.C., Muhle, H., Ostertag, P., von Spiczak, S., Buysse, K., Baker, C., Franke, A., Malafosse, A., Genton, P., Thomas, P., et al. (2010). Genome-wide copy number variation in epilepsy: novel susceptibility loci in idiopathic generalized and focal epilepsies. PLoS Genet 6, e1000962.

Milh, M., Villeneuve, N., Chouchane, M., Kaminska, A., Laroche, C., Barthez, M.A., Gitiaux, C., Bartoli, C., Borges-Correia, A., Cacciagli, P., et al. (2011). Epileptic and nonepileptic features in patients with early onset epileptic encephalopathy and STXBP1 mutations. Epilepsia 52, 1828–1834.

Millar, J.K., Wilson-Annan, J.C., Anderson, S., Christie, S., Taylor, M.S., Semple, C.A., Devon, R.S., St Clair, D.M., Muir, W.J., Blackwood, D.H., et al. (2000). Disruption of two novel genes by a translocation co-segregating with schizophrenia. Hum Mol Genet 9, 1415–1423.

Miller, D.T., Adam, M.P., Aradhya, S., Biesecker, L.G., Brothman, A.R., Carter, N.P., Church, D.M., Crolla, J.A., Eichler, E.E., Epstein, C.J., et al. (2010). Consensus statement: chromosomal microarray is a first-tier clinical diagnostic test for individuals with developmental disabilities or congenital anomalies. Am J Hum Genet 86, 749–764.

Mirzaa, G.M., Paciorkowski, A.R., Marsh, E.D., Berry-Kravis, E.M., Medne, L., Alkhateeb, A., Grix, A., Wirrell, E.C., Powell, B.R., Nickels, K.C., et al. (2013). CDKL5 and ARX mutations in males with early-onset epilepsy. Pediatr Neurol 48, 367–377.

Missler, M., Sudhof, T.C., and Biederer, T. (2012). Synaptic cell adhesion. Cold Spring Harb Perspect Biol 4, a005694.

Mitchell, K.J., Pinson, K.I., Kelly, O.G., Brennan, J., Zupicich, J., Scherz, P., Leighton, P.A., Goodrich, L.V., Lu, X., Avery, B.J., et al. (2001). Functional analysis of secreted and transmembrane proteins critical to mouse development. Nat Genet 28, 241–249.

Moessner, R., Marshall, C.R., Sutcliffe, J.S., Skaug, J., Pinto, D., Vincent, J., Zwaigenbaum, L., Fernandez, B., Roberts, W., Szatmari, P., et al. (2007). Contribution of SHANK3 mutations to autism spectrum disorder. Am J Hum Genet 81, 1289–1297.

Moller, R.S., Weber, Y.G., Klitten, L.L., Trucks, H., Muhle, H., Kunz, W.S., Mefford, H.C., Franke, A., Kautza, M., Wolf, P., et al. (2013). Exon-disrupting deletions of NRXN1 in idiopathic generalized epilepsy. Epilepsia 54, 256–264.

Morlet, T., Rabinowitz, M.R., Looney, L.R., Riegner, T., Greenwood, L.A., Sherman, E.A., Achilly, N., Zhu, A., Yoo, E., O'Reilly, R.C., et al. (2014). A homozygous SLITRK6 nonsense mutation is associated with progressive auditory neuropathy in humans. Laryngoscope 124, E95–103.

Morrow, E.M., Yoo, S.Y., Flavell, S.W., Kim, T.K., Lin, Y., Hill, R.S., Mukaddes, N.M., Balkhy, S.,

Gascon, G., Hashmi, A., et al. (2008). Identifying autism loci and genes by tracing recent shared ancestry. Science 321, 218–223.

Moya, P.R., Dodman, N.H., Timpano, K.R., Rubenstein, L.M., Rana, Z., Fried, R.L., Reichardt, L.F., Heiman, G.A., Tischfield, J.A., King, R.A., et al. (2013). Rare missense neuronal cadherin gene (CDH2) variants in specific obsessive-compulsive disorder and Tourette disorder phenotypes. Eur J Hum Genet 21, 850–854.

Myers, K.R., Wang, G., Sheng, Y., Conger, K.K., Casanova, J.E., and Zhu, J.J. (2012). Arf6-GEF BRAG1 regulates JNK-mediated synaptic removal of GluA1-containing AMPA receptors: a new mechanism for nonsyndromic X-linked mental disorder. J Neurosci 32, 11716–11726.

Na, E.S., Nelson, E.D., Kavalali, E.T., and Monteggia, L.M. (2013). The impact of MeCP2 loss- or gain-of-function on synaptic plasticity. Neuropsychopharmacology 38, 212–219.

Nag, A., Bochukova, E.G., Kremeyer, B., Campbell, D.D., Muller, H., Valencia-Duarte, A.V., Cardona, J., Rivas, I.C., Mesa, S.C., Cuartas, M., et al. (2013). CNV analysis in Tourette syndrome implicates large genomic rearrangements in COL8A1 and NRXN1. PLoS One 8, e59061.

Najm, J., Horn, D., Wimplinger, I., Golden, J.A., Chizhikov, V.V., Sudi, J., Christian, S.L., Ullmann, R., Kuechler, A., Haas, C.A., et al. (2008). Mutations of CASK cause an X-linked brain malformation phenotype with microcephaly and hypoplasia of the brainstem and cerebellum. Nat Genet 40, 1065–1067.

Nava, C., Keren, B., Mignot, C., Rastetter, A., Chantot-Bastaraud, S., Faudet, A., Fonteneau, E., Amiet, C., Laurent, C., Jacquette, A., et al. (2014). Prospective diagnostic analysis of copy number variants using SNP microarrays in individuals with autism spectrum disorders. Eur J Hum Genet 22, 71–78.

Neale, B.M., Kou, Y., Liu, L., Ma'ayan, A., Samocha, K.E., Sabo, A., Lin, C.F., Stevens, C., Wang, L.S., Makarov, V., et al. (2012). Patterns and rates of exonic de novo mutations in autism spectrum disorders. Nature 485, 242–245.

Nishimura-Akiyoshi, S., Niimi, K., Nakashiba, T., and Itohara, S. (2007). Axonal netrin-Gs transneuronally determine lamina-specific subdendritic segments. Proc Natl Acad Sci USA 104, 14801–14806.

Nobile, C., Michelucci, R., Andreazza, S., Pasini, E., Tosatto, S.C., and Striano, P. (2009). LGI1 mutations in autosomal dominant and sporadic lateral temporal epilepsy. Hum Mutat 30, 530–536.

Novara, F., Beri, S., Giorda, R., Ortibus, E., Nageshappa, S., Darra, F., Bernardina, B.D., Zuffardi, O., and Van Esch, H. (2010). Refining the phenotype associated with MEF2C haploinsufficiency. Clin Genet 78, 471–477.

Numis, A.L., Major, P., Montenegro, M.A., Muzykewicz, D.A., Pulsifer, M.B., and Thiele, E.A. (2011). Identification of risk factors for autism spectrum disorders in tuberous sclerosis complex. Neurology 76, 981–987.

O'Roak, B.J., Deriziotis, P., Lee, C., Vives, L., Schwartz, J.J., Girirajan, S., Karakoc, E., Mackenzie, A.P., Ng, S.B., Baker, C., et al. (2011). Exome sequencing in sporadic autism spectrum disorders identifies severe de novo mutations. Nat Genet 43, 585–589.

O'Roak, B.J., Vives, L., Fu, W., Egertson, J.D., Stanaway, I.B., Phelps, I.G., Carvill, G., Kumar, A., Lee, C., Ankenman, K., et al. (2012a). Multiplex targeted sequencing identifies recurrently mutated genes in autism spectrum disorders. Science 338, 1619–1622.

O'Roak, B.J., Vives, L., Girirajan, S., Karakoc, E., Krumm, N., Coe, B.P., Levy, R., Ko, A., Lee, C., Smith, J.D., et al. (2012b). Sporadic autism exomes reveal a highly interconnected protein network of de novo mutations. Nature 485, 246–250.

O'Rourke, N.A., Weiler, N.C., Micheva, K.D., and Smith, S.J. (2012). Deep molecular diversity of mammalian synapses: why it matters and how to measure it. Nat Rev Neurosci 13, 365–379.

Ohkawa, T., Fukata, Y., Yamasaki, M., Miyazaki, T., Yokoi, N., Takashima, H., Watanabe, M., Watanabe, O., and Fukata, M. (2013). Autoantibodies to epilepsy-related LGI1 in limbic encephalitis neutralize LGI1-ADAM22 interaction and reduce synaptic AMPA receptors. J Neurosci 33, 18161–18174.

Oksenberg, N., and Ahituv, N. (2013). The role of AUTS2 in neurodevelopment and human evolution. Trends Genet 29, 600–608.

Oliveira, A.F., and Yasuda, R. (2014). Neurofibromin is the major ras inactivator in dendritic spines. J Neurosci 34, 776–783.

Osbun, N., Li, J., O'Driscoll, M.C., Strominger, Z., Wakahiro, M., Rider, E., Bukshpun, P., Boland,

E., Spurrell, C.H., Schackwitz, W., et al. (2011). Genetic and functional analyses identify DISC1 as a novel callosal agenesis candidate gene. Am J Med Genet A 155A, 1865–1876.

Ozkan, E.D., Creson, T.K., Kramar, E.A., Rojas, C., Seese, R.R., Babyan, A.H., Shi, Y., Lucero, R., Xu, X., Noebels, J.L., et al. (2014). Reduced cognition in Syngap1 mutants is caused by isolated damage within developing forebrain excitatory neurons. Neuron 82, 1317–1333.

Ozomaro, U., Cai, G., Kajiwara, Y., Yoon, S., Makarov, V., Delorme, R., Betancur, C., Ruhrmann, S., Falkai, P., Grabe, H.J., et al. (2013). Characterization of SLITRK1 variation in obsessive-compulsive disorder. PLoS One 8, e70376.

Pagnamenta, A.T., Bacchelli, E., de Jonge, M.V., Mirza, G., Scerri, T.S., Minopoli, F., Chiocchetti, A., Ludwig, K.U., Hoffmann, P., Paracchini, S., et al. (2010). Characterization of a family with rare deletions in CNTNAP5 and DOCK4 suggests novel risk loci for autism and dyslexia. Biol Psychiatry 68, 320–328.

Pagnamenta, A.T., Khan, H., Walker, S., Gerrelli, D., Wing, K., Bonaglia, M.C., Giorda, R., Berney, T., Mani, E., Molteni, M., et al. (2011). Rare familial 16q21 microdeletions under a linkage peak implicate cadherin 8 (CDH8) in susceptibility to autism and learning disability. J Med Genet 48, 48–54.

Palumbo, O., Fichera, M., Palumbo, P., Rizzo, R., Mazzolla, E., Cocuzza, D.M., Carella, M., and Mattina, T. (2014). TBR1 is the candidate gene for intellectual disability in patients with a 2q24.2 interstitial deletion. Am J Med Genet A 164A, 828–833.

Parikshak, N.N., Luo, R., Zhang, A., Won, H., Lowe, J.K., Chandran, V., Horvath, S., and Geschwind, D.H. (2013). Integrative functional genomic analyses implicate specific molecular pathways and circuits in autism. Cell 155, 1008–1021.

Park, C.S., Zhong, L., and Tang, S.J. (2009). Aberrant expression of synaptic plasticity-related genes in the NF1+/- mouse hippocampus. J Neurosci Res 87, 3107–3119.

Penagarikano, O., Abrahams, B.S., Herman, E.I., Winden, K.D., Gdalyahu, A., Dong, H., Sonnenblick, L.I., Gruver, R., Almajano, J., Bragin, A., et al. (2011). Absence of CNTNAP2 leads to epilepsy, neuronal migration abnormalities, and core autism-related deficits. Cell 147, 235–246.

Pfeiffer, B.E., Zang, T., Wilkerson, J.R., Taniguchi, M., Maksimova, M.A., Smith, L.N., Cowan, C.W., and Huber, K.M. (2010). Fragile X mental retardation protein is required for synapse elimination by the activity-dependent transcription factor MEF2. Neuron 66, 191–197.

Pinto, D., Pagnamenta, A.T., Klei, L., Anney, R., Merico, D., Regan, R., Conroy, J., Magalhaes, T.R., Correia, C., Abrahams, B.S., et al. (2010). Functional impact of global rare copy number variation in autism spectrum disorders. Nature 466, 368–372.

Pinto, D., Delaby, E., Merico, D., Barbosa, M., Merikangas, A., Klei, L., Thiruvahindrapuram, B., Xu, X., Ziman, R., Wang, Z., et al. (2014). Convergence of genes and cellular pathways dysregulated in autism spectrum disorders. Am J Hum Genet 94, 677–694.

Piton, A., Michaud, J.L., Peng, H., Aradhya, S., Gauthier, J., Mottron, L., Champagne, N., Lafreniere, R.G., Hamdan, F.F., Joober, R., et al. (2008). Mutations in the calcium-related gene IL1RAPL1 are associated with autism. Hum Mol Genet 17, 3965–3974.

Pohjola, P., de Leeuw, N., Penttinen, M., and Kaariainen, H. (2010). Terminal 3p deletions in two families--correlation between molecular karyotype and phenotype. Am J Med Genet A 152A, 441–446.

Poultney, C.S., Goldberg, A.P., Drapeau, E., Kou, Y., Harony-Nicolas, H., Kajiwara, Y., De Rubeis, S., Durand, S., Stevens, C., Rehnstrom, K., et al. (2013). Identification of small exonic CNV from whole-exome sequence data and application to autism spectrum disorder. Am J Hum Genet 93, 607–619.

Prasad, A., Merico, D., Thiruvahindrapuram, B., Wei, J., Lionel, A.C., Sato, D., Rickaby, J., Lu, C., Szatmari, P., Roberts, W., et al. (2012). A discovery resource of rare copy number variations in individuals with autism spectrum disorder. G3 (Bethesda) 2, 1665–1685.

Purcell, S.M., Moran, J.L., Fromer, M., Ruderfer, D., Solovieff, N., Roussos, P., O'Dushlaine, C., Chambert, K., Bergen, S.E., Kahler, A., et al. (2014). A polygenic burden of rare disruptive mutations in schizophrenia. Nature 506, 185–190.

Ramaswami, M. (2014). Network plasticity in adaptive filtering and behavioral habituation. Neuron 82, 1216–1229.

Ramocki, M.B., Tavyev, Y.J., and Peters, S.U. (2010). The MECP2 duplication syndrome. Am J Med Genet A 152A, 1079–1088.

Randall, A.D., Kurihara, M., Brandon, N.J., and Brown, J.T. (2014). Disrupted in schizophrenia 1 and synaptic function in the mammalian central nervous system. Eur J Neurosci 39, 1068–1073.

Rauch, A., Wieczorek, D., Graf, E., Wieland, T., Endele, S., Schwarzmayr, T., Albrecht, B., Bartholdi, D., Beygo, J., Di Donato, N., et al. (2012). Range of genetic mutations associated with severe non-syndromic sporadic intellectual disability: an exome sequencing study. Lancet 380, 1674–1682.

Raychaudhuri, S., Plenge, R.M., Rossin, E.J., Ng, A.C., Purcell, S.M., Sklar, P., Scolnick, E.M., Xavier, R.J., Altshuler, D., and Daly, M.J. (2009). Identifying relationships among genomic disease regions: predicting genes at pathogenic SNP associations and rare deletions. PLoS Genet 5, e1000534.

Reiss, J., Gross-Hardt, S., Christensen, E., Schmidt, P., Mendel, R.R., and Schwarz, G. (2001). A mutation in the gene for the neurotransmitter receptor-clustering protein gephyrin causes a novel form of molybdenum cofactor deficiency. Am J Hum Genet 68, 208–213.

Ricciardi, S., Ungaro, F., Hambrock, M., Rademacher, N., Stefanelli, G., Brambilla, D., Sessa, A., Magagnotti, C., Bachi, A., Giarda, E., et al. (2012). CDKL5 ensures excitatory synapse stability by reinforcing NGL-1-PSD95 interaction in the postsynaptic compartment and is impaired in patient iPSC-derived neurons. Nat Cell Biol 14, 911–923.

Ronan, J.L., Wu, W., and Crabtree, G.R. (2013). From neural development to cognition: unexpected roles for chromatin. Nat Rev Genet 14, 347–359.

Rothwell, P.E., Fuccillo, M.V., Maxeiner, S., Hayton, S.J., Gokce, O., Lim, B.K., Fowler, S.C., Malenka, R.C., and Sudhof, T.C. (2014). Autism-associated neuroligin-3 mutations commonly impair striatal circuits to boost repetitive behaviors. Cell 158, 198–212.

Rujescu, D., Ingason, A., Cichon, S., Pietilainen, O.P., Barnes, M.R., Toulopoulou, T., Picchioni, M., Vassos, E., Ettinger, U., Bramon, E., et al. (2009). Disruption of the neurexin 1 gene is associated with schizophrenia. Hum Mol Genet 18, 988–996.

Russell, J.F., Fu, Y.H., and Ptacek, L.J. (2013). Episodic neurologic disorders: syndromes, genes, and mechanisms. Annu Rev Neurosci 36, 25–50.

Russo, S., Marchi, M., Cogliati, F., Bonati, M.T., Pintaudi, M., Veneselli, E., Saletti, V., Balestrini, M., Ben-Zeev, B., and Larizza, L. (2009). Novel mutations in the CDKL5 gene, predicted effects and associated phenotypes. Neurogenetics 10, 241–250.

Sachs, N.A., Sawa, A., Holmes, S.E., Ross, C.A., DeLisi, L.E., and Margolis, R.L. (2005). A frameshift mutation in Disrupted in Schizophrenia 1 in an American family with schizophrenia and schizoaffective disorder. Mol Psychiatry 10, 758–764.

Sagane, K., Hayakawa, K., Kai, J., Hirohashi, T., Takahashi, E., Miyamoto, N., Ino, M., Oki, T., Yamazaki, K., and Nagasu, T. (2005). Ataxia and peripheral nerve hypomyelination in ADAM22-deficient mice. BMC Neurosci 6, 33.

Saghatelyan, A.K., Nikonenko, A.G., Sun, M., Rolf, B., Putthoff, P., Kutsche, M., Bartsch, U., Dityatev, A., and Schachner, M. (2004). Reduced GABAergic transmission and number of hippocampal perisomatic inhibitory synapses in juvenile mice deficient in the neural cell adhesion molecule L1. Mol Cell Neurosci 26, 191–203.

Sakagami, H., Sanda, M., Fukaya, M., Miyazaki, T., Sukegawa, J., Yanagisawa, T., Suzuki, T., Fukunaga, K., Watanabe, M., and Kondo, H. (2008). IQ-ArfGEF/BRAG1 is a guanine nucleotide exchange factor for Arf6 that interacts with PSD-95 at postsynaptic density of excitatory synapses. Neurosci Res 60, 199–212.

Sakagami, H., Katsumata, O., Hara, Y., Tamaki, H., Watanabe, M., Harvey, R.J., and Fukaya, M. (2013). Distinct synaptic localization patterns of brefeldin A-resistant guanine nucleotide exchange factors BRAG2 and BRAG3 in the mouse retina. J Comp Neurol 521, 860–876.

Sakurai, K., Toyoshima, M., Ueda, H., Matsubara, K., Takeda, Y., Karagogeos, D., Shimoda, Y., and Watanabe, K. (2009). Contribution of the neural cell recognition molecule NB-3 to synapse formation between parallel fibers and Purkinje cells in mouse. Dev Neurobiol 69, 811–824.

Sakurai, K., Toyoshima, M., Takeda, Y., Shimoda, Y., and Watanabe, K. (2010). Synaptic formation in subsets of glutamatergic terminals in the mouse hippocampal formation is affected by a deficiency in the neural cell recognition molecule NB-3. Neurosci Lett 473, 102–106.

Sakurai, T. (2012). The role of NrCAM in neural development and disorders–beyond a simple glue in the brain. Mol Cell Neurosci 49, 351–363.

Salyakina, D., Cukier, H.N., Lee, J.M., Sacharow, S., Nations, L.D., Ma, D., Jaworski, J.M., Konidari, I., Whitehead, P.L., Wright, H.H., et al. (2011). Copy number variants in extended autism spectrum disorder families reveal candidates potentially involved in autism risk. PLoS One 6, e26049.

Sanders, S.J., Ercan-Sencicek, A.G., Hus, V., Luo, R., Murtha, M.T., Moreno-De-Luca, D., Chu, S.H., Moreau, M.P., Gupta, A.R., Thomson, S.A., et al. (2011). Multiple recurrent de novo CNVs, including duplications of the 7q11.23 Williams syndrome region, are strongly associated with autism. Neuron 70, 863–885.

Sanders, S.J., Murtha, M.T., Gupta, A.R., Murdoch, J.D., Raubeson, M.J., Willsey, A.J., Ercan-Sencicek, A.G., Dilullo, N.M., Parikshak, N.N., Stein, J.L., et al. (2012). De novo mutations revealed by whole-exome sequencing are strongly associated with autism. Nature 485, 237–241.

Sando, R., 3rd, Gounko, N., Pieraut, S., Liao, L., Yates, J., 3rd, and Maximov, A. (2012). HDAC4 governs a transcriptional program essential for synaptic plasticity and memory. Cell 151, 821–834.

Sanes, J.R., and Yamagata, M. (2009). Many paths to synaptic specificity. Annu Rev Cell Dev Biol 25, 161–195.

Santen, G.W., Aten, E., Sun, Y., Almomani, R., Gilissen, C., Nielsen, M., Kant, S.G., Snoeck, I.N., Peeters, E.A., Hilhorst-Hofstee, Y., et al. (2012). Mutations in SWI/SNF chromatin remodeling complex gene ARID1B cause Coffin-Siris syndrome. Nat Genet 44, 379–380.

Sato, D., Lionel, A.C., Leblond, C.S., Prasad, A., Pinto, D., Walker, S., O'Connor, I., Russell, C., Drmic, I.E., Hamdan, F.F., et al. (2012). SHANK1 Deletions in Males with Autism Spectrum Disorder. Am J Hum Genet 90, 879–887.

Schafer, M.K., and Altevogt, P. (2010). L1CAM malfunction in the nervous system and human carcinomas. Cell Mol Life Sci 67, 2425–2437.

Schizophrenia Working Group of the Psychiatric Genomics Consortium. (2014). Biological insights from 108 schizophrenia-associated genetic loci. Nature 511, 421–427.

Schmunk, G., and Gargus, J.J. (2013). Channelopathy pathogenesis in autism spectrum disorders. Front Genet 4, 222.

Schoch, S., and Gundelfinger, E.D. (2006). Molecular organization of the presynaptic active zone. Cell Tissue Res 326, 379–391.

Schorry, E.K., Keddache, M., Lanphear, N., Rubinstein, J.H., Srodulski, S., Fletcher, D., Blough-Pfau, R.I., and Grabowski, G.A. (2008). Genotype-phenotype correlations in Rubinstein-Taybi syndrome. Am J Med Genet A 146A, 2512–2519.

Schrander-Stumpel, C., and Vos, Y.J. (2010). L1 syndrome. GeneReviews http://www.ncbi.nlm.nih.gov/books/NBK1484/ (18 December 2014).

Schuurs-Hoeijmakers, J.H., Vulto-van Silfhout, A.T., Vissers, L.E., van de Vondervoort, I.I., van Bon, B.W., de Ligt, J., Gilissen, C., Hehir-Kwa, J.Y., Neveling, K., del Rosario, M., et al. (2013). Identification of pathogenic gene variants in small families with intellectually disabled siblings by exome sequencing. J Med Genet 50, 802–811.

Seppala, E.H., Koskinen, L.L., Gullov, C.H., Jokinen, P., Karlskov-Mortensen, P., Bergamasco, L., Baranowska Korberg, I., Cizinauskas, S., Oberbauer, A.M., Berendt, M., et al. (2012). Identification of a novel idiopathic epilepsy locus in Belgian Shepherd dogs. PLoS One 7, e33549.

Sharp, A.J., Mefford, H.C., Li, K., Baker, C., Skinner, C., Stevenson, R.E., Schroer, R.J., Novara, F., De Gregori, M., Ciccone, R., et al. (2008). A recurrent 15q13.3 microdeletion syndrome associated with mental retardation and seizures. Nat Genet 40, 322–328.

Shcheglovitov, A., Shcheglovitova, O., Yazawa, M., Portmann, T., Shu, R., Sebastiano, V., Krawisz, A., Froehlich, W., Bernstein, J.A., Hallmayer, J.F., et al. (2013). SHANK3 and IGF1 restore synaptic deficits in neurons from 22q13 deletion syndrome patients. Nature 503, 267–271.

Shen, K., and Cowan, C.W. (2010). Guidance molecules in synapse formation and plasticity. Cold Spring Harb Perspect Biol 2, a001842.

Sheng, M., and Kim, E. (2011). The postsynaptic organization of synapses. Cold Spring Harb Perspect Biol 3, a005678.

Shimoda, Y., and Watanabe, K. (2009). Contactins: emerging key roles in the development and function of the nervous system. Cell Adh Migr 3, 64–70.

Shinawi, M., Schaaf, C.P., Bhatt, S.S., Xia, Z., Patel, A., Cheung, S.W., Lanpher, B., Nagl, S., Herding, H.S., Nevinny-Stickel, C., et al. (2009). A small recurrent deletion within 15q13.3 is associated with a range of neurodevelopmental phenotypes. Nat Genet 41, 1269–1271.

Shmelkov, S.V., Hormigo, A., Jing, D., Proenca, C.C., Bath, K.G., Milde, T., Shmelkov, E., Kushner, J.S., Baljevic, M., Dincheva, I., et al. (2010). Slitrk5 deficiency impairs corticostriatal circuitry and leads to obsessive-compulsive-like behaviors in mice. Nat Med 16, 598–602, 591p following 602.

Shoubridge, C., Tarpey, P.S., Abidi, F., Ramsden, S.L., Rujirabanjerd, S., Murphy, J.A., Boyle, J., Shaw, M., Gardner, A., Proos, A., et al. (2010). Mutations in the guanine nucleotide exchange factor gene IQSEC2 cause nonsyndromic intellectual disability. Nat Genet 42, 486–488.

Shoukier, M., Fuchs, S., Schwaibold, E., Lingen, M., Gartner, J., Brockmann, K., and Zirn, B. (2013). Microduplication of 3p26.3 in nonsyndromic intellectual disability indicates an important role of CHL1 for normal cognitive function. Neuropediatrics 44, 268–271.

Sidorov, M.S., Auerbach, B.D., and Bear, M.F. (2013). Fragile X mental retardation protein and synaptic plasticity. Mol Brain 6, 15.

Sihra, T.S., Flores, G., and Rodriguez-Moreno, A. (2014). Kainate receptors: multiple roles in neuronal plasticity. Neuroscientist 20, 29–43.

Song, Y.S., Lee, H.J., Prosselkov, P., Itohara, S., and Kim, E. (2013). Trans-induced cis interaction in the tripartite NGL-1, netrin-G1 and LAR adhesion complex promotes development of excitatory synapses. J Cell Sci 126, 4926–4938.

Soorya, L., Kolevzon, A., Zweifach, J., Lim, T., Dobry, Y., Schwartz, L., Frank, Y., Wang, A.T., Cai, G., Parkhomenko, E., et al. (2013). Prospective investigation of autism and genotype-phenotype correlations in 22q13 deletion syndrome and SHANK3 deficiency. Mol Autism 4, 18.

Sousa, S.B., Abdul-Rahman, O.A., Bottani, A., Cormier-Daire, V., Fryer, A., Gillessen-Kaesbach, G., Horn, D., Josifova, D., Kuechler, A., Lees, M., et al. (2009). Nicolaides-Baraitser syndrome: delineation of the phenotype. Am J Med Genet A 149A, 1628–1640.

Splawski, I., Timothy, K.W., Sharpe, L.M., Decher, N., Kumar, P., Bloise, R., Napolitano, C., Schwartz, P.J., Joseph, R.M., Condouris, K., et al. (2004). Ca(V)1.2 calcium channel dysfunction causes a multisystem disorder including arrhythmia and autism. Cell 119, 19–31.

Strauss, K.A., Puffenberger, E.G., Huentelman, M.J., Gottlieb, S., Dobrin, S.E., Parod, J.M., Stephan, D.A., and Morton, D.H. (2006). Recessive symptomatic focal epilepsy and mutant contactin-associated protein-like 2. N Engl J Med 354, 1370–1377.

Su, S.C., and Tsai, L.H. (2011). Cyclin-dependent kinases in brain development and disease. Annu Rev Cell Dev Biol 27, 465–491.

Sudhof, T.C. (2008). Neuroligins and neurexins link synaptic function to cognitive disease. Nature 455, 903–911.

Sylwestrak, E.L., and Ghosh, A. (2012). Elfn1 regulates target-specific release probability at CA1-interneuron synapses. Science 338, 536–540.

Szatmari, P., Paterson, A.D., Zwaigenbaum, L., Roberts, W., Brian, J., Liu, X.Q., Vincent, J.B., Skaug, J.L., Thompson, A.P., Senman, L., et al. (2007). Mapping autism risk loci using genetic linkage and chromosomal rearrangements. Nat Genet 39, 319–328.

Takahashi, H., and Craig, A.M. (2013). Protein tyrosine phosphatases PTPdelta, PTPsigma, and LAR: presynaptic hubs for synapse organization. Trends Neurosci 36, 522–534.

Talkowski, M.E., Mullegama, S.V., Rosenfeld, J.A., van Bon, B.W., Shen, Y., Repnikova, E.A., Gastier-Foster, J., Thrush, D.L., Kathiresan, S., Ruderfer, D.M., et al. (2011). Assessment of 2q23.1 microdeletion syndrome implicates MBD5 as a single causal locus of intellectual disability, epilepsy, and autism spectrum disorder. Am J Hum Genet 89, 551–563.

Tam, G.W., van de Lagemaat, L.N., Redon, R., Strathdee, K.E., Croning, M.D., Malloy, M.P., Muir, W.J., Pickard, B.S., Deary, I.J., Blackwood, D.H., et al. (2010). Confirmed rare copy number variants implicate novel genes in schizophrenia. Biochem Soc Trans 38, 445–451.

Tang, R., Noh, H.J., Wang, D., Sigurdsson, S., Swofford, R., Perloski, M., Duxbury, M., Patterson, E.E., Albright, J., Castelhano, M., et al. (2014). Candidate genes and functional noncoding variants identified in a canine model of obsessive-compulsive disorder. Genome Biol 15, R25.

Tarpey, P., Parnau, J., Blow, M., Woffendin, H., Bignell, G., Cox, C., Cox, J., Davies, H., Edkins, S., Holden, S., et al. (2004). Mutations in the DLG3 gene cause nonsyndromic X-linked mental retardation. Am J Hum Genet 75, 318–324.

Tarpey, P.S., Raymond, F.L., O'Meara, S., Edkins, S., Teague, J., Butler, A., Dicks, E., Stevens, C., Tofts, C., Avis, T., et al. (2007). Mutations in CUL4B, which encodes a ubiquitin E3 ligase subunit, cause an X-linked mental retardation syndrome associated with aggressive outbursts, seizures, relative macrocephaly, central obesity, hypogonadism, pes cavus, and tremor. Am J Hum Genet 80, 345–352.

Tarpey, P.S., Smith, R., Pleasance, E., Whibley, A., Edkins, S., Hardy, C., O'Meara, S., Latimer, C., Dicks, E., Menzies, A., et al. (2009). A systematic, large-scale resequencing screen of X-chromosome coding exons in mental retardation. Nat Genet 41, 535–543.

Tekin, M., Chioza, B.A., Matsumoto, Y., Diaz-Horta, O., Cross, H.E., Duman, D., Kokotas, H., Moore-Barton, H.L., Sakoori, K., Ota, M., et al. (2013). SLITRK6 mutations cause myopia and deafness in humans and mice. J Clin Invest 123, 2094–2102.

Thompson, B.A., Tremblay, V., Lin, G., and Bochar, D.A. (2008). CHD8 is an ATP-dependent chromatin remodeling factor that regulates beta-catenin target genes. Mol Cell Biol 28, 3894–3904.

Thomson, P.A., Malavasi, E.L., Grunewald, E., Soares, D.C., Borkowska, M., and Millar, J.K. (2013). DISC1 genetics, biology and psychiatric illness. Front Biol (Beijing) 8, 1–31.

Thu, C.A., Chen, W.V., Rubinstein, R., Chevee, M., Wolcott, H.N., Felsovalyi, K.O., Tapia, J.C., Shapiro, L., Honig, B., and Maniatis, T. (2014). Single-cell identity generated by combinatorial homophilic interactions between alpha, beta, and gamma protocadherins. Cell 158, 1045–1059.

Tran Mau-Them, F., Willems, M., Albrecht, B., Sanchez, E., Puechberty, J., Endele, S., Schneider, A., Ruiz Pallares, N., Missirian, C., Rivier, F., et al. (2014). Expanding the phenotype of IQSEC2 mutations: truncating mutations in severe intellectual disability. Eur J Hum Genet 22, 289–292.

Traylor, R.N., Dobyns, W.B., Rosenfeld, J.A., Wheeler, P., Spence, J.E., Bandholz, A.M., Bawle, E.V., Carmany, E.P., Powell, C.M., Hudson, B., et al. (2012). Investigation of TBR1 Hemizygosity: Four Individuals with 2q24 Microdeletions. Mol Syndromol 3, 102–112.

Tsai, N.P., Wilkerson, J.R., Guo, W., Maksimova, M.A., DeMartino, G.N., Cowan, C.W., and Huber, K.M. (2012). Multiple autism-linked genes mediate synapse elimination via proteasomal degradation of a synaptic scaffold PSD-95. Cell 151, 1581–1594.

Tsai, P., and Sahin, M. (2011). Mechanisms of neurocognitive dysfunction and therapeutic considerations in tuberous sclerosis complex. Curr Opin Neurol 24, 106–113.

Tsurusaki, Y., Okamoto, N., Ohashi, H., Kosho, T., Imai, Y., Hibi-Ko, Y., Kaname, T., Naritomi, K., Kawame, H., Wakui, K., et al. (2012). Mutations affecting components of the SWI/SNF complex cause Coffin-Siris syndrome. Nat Genet 44, 376–378.

Tyagarajan, S.K., and Fritschy, J.M. (2014). Gephyrin: a master regulator of neuronal function? Nat Rev Neurosci 15, 141–156.

Vacic, V., McCarthy, S., Malhotra, D., Murray, F., Chou, H.H., Peoples, A., Makarov, V., Yoon, S., Bhandari, A., Corominas, R., et al. (2011). Duplications of the neuropeptide receptor gene VIPR2 confer significant risk for schizophrenia. Nature 471, 499–503.

Valnegri, P., Montrasio, C., Brambilla, D., Ko, J., Passafaro, M., and Sala, C. (2011). The X-linked intellectual disability protein IL1RAPL1 regulates excitatory synapse formation by binding PTPdelta and RhoGAP2. Hum Mol Genet 20, 4797–4809.

van Bokhoven, H. (2011). Genetic and epigenetic networks in intellectual disabilities. Annu Rev Genet 45, 81–104.

van Harssel, J.J., Weckhuysen, S., van Kempen, M.J., Hardies, K., Verbeek, N.E., de Kovel, C.G., Gunning, W.B., van Daalen, E., de Jonge, M.V., Jansen, A.C., et al. (2013). Clinical and genetic aspects of PCDH19-related epilepsy syndromes and the possible role of PCDH19 mutations in males with autism spectrum disorders. Neurogenetics 14, 23–34.

Van Houdt, J.K., Nowakowska, B.A., Sousa, S.B., van Schaik, B.D., Seuntjens, E., Avonce, N., Sifrim, A., Abdul-Rahman, O.A., van den Boogaard, M.J., Bottani, A., et al. (2012). Heterozygous missense mutations in SMARCA2 cause Nicolaides-Baraitser syndrome. Nat Genet 44, 445–449.

Verkerk, A.J., Mathews, C.A., Joosse, M., Eussen, B.H., Heutink, P., and Oostra, B.A. (2003). CNTNAP2 is disrupted in a family with Gilles de la

Tourette syndrome and obsessive compulsive disorder. Genomics 82, 1–9.

Vulto-van Silfhout, A.T., Hehir-Kwa, J.Y., van Bon, B.W., Schuurs-Hoeijmakers, J.H., Meader, S., Hellebrekers, C.J., Thoonen, I.J., de Brouwer, A.P., Brunner, H.G., Webber, C., et al. (2013). Clinical significance of de novo and inherited copy-number variation. Hum Mutat 34, 1679–1687.

Walsh, T., McClellan, J.M., McCarthy, S.E., Addington, A.M., Pierce, S.B., Cooper, G.M., Nord, A.S., Kusenda, M., Malhotra, D., Bhandari, A., et al. (2008). Rare structural variants disrupt multiple genes in neurodevelopmental pathways in schizophrenia. Science 320, 539–543.

Weaving, L.S., Christodoulou, J., Williamson, S.L., Friend, K.L., McKenzie, O.L., Archer, H., Evans, J., Clarke, A., Pelka, G.J., Tam, P.P., et al. (2004). Mutations of CDKL5 cause a severe neurodevelopmental disorder with infantile spasms and mental retardation. Am J Hum Genet 75, 1079–1093.

Weaving, L.S., Ellaway, C.J., Gecz, J., and Christodoulou, J. (2005). Rett syndrome: clinical review and genetic update. J Med Genet 42, 1–7.

Wen, Z., Nguyen, H.N., Guo, Z., Lalli, M.A., Wang, X., Su, Y., Kim, N.S., Yoon, K.J., Shin, J., Zhang, C., et al. (2014). Synaptic dysregulation in a human iPS cell model of mental disorders. Nature 515, 414–418.

West, A.E., and Greenberg, M.E. (2011). Neuronal activity-regulated gene transcription in synapse development and cognitive function. Cold Spring Harb Perspect Biol 3, a005744.

White, S.M., Morgan, A., Da Costa, A., Lacombe, D., Knight, S.J., Houlston, R., Whiteford, M.L., Newbury-Ecob, R.A., and Hurst, J.A. (2010). The phenotype of Floating-Harbor syndrome in 10 patients. Am J Med Genet A 152A, 821–829.

Wieczorek, D., Bogershausen, N., Beleggia, F., Steiner-Haldenstatt, S., Pohl, E., Li, Y., Milz, E., Martin, M., Thiele, H., Altmuller, J., et al. (2013). A comprehensive molecular study on Coffin-Siris and Nicolaides-Baraitser syndromes identifies a broad molecular and clinical spectrum converging on altered chromatin remodeling. Hum Mol Genet 22, 5121–5135.

Willemsen, M.H., Vulto-van Silfhout, A.T., Nillesen, W.M., Wissink-Lindhout, W.M., van Bokhoven, H., Philip, N., Berry-Kravis, E.M., Kini, U., van Ravenswaaij-Arts, C.M., Delle Chiaie, B., et al.

(2012). Update on Kleefstra syndrome. Mol Syndromol 2, 202–212.

Williams, J.M., Beck, T.F., Pearson, D.M., Proud, M.B., Cheung, S.W., and Scott, D.A. (2009). A 1q42 deletion involving DISC1, DISC2, and TSNAX in an autism spectrum disorder. Am J Med Genet A 149A, 1758–1762.

Williams, N.M., Zaharieva, I., Martin, A., Langley, K., Mantripragada, K., Fossdal, R., Stefansson, H., Stefansson, K., Magnusson, P., Gudmundsson, O.O., et al. (2010a). Rare chromosomal deletions and duplications in attention-deficit hyperactivity disorder: a genome-wide analysis. Lancet 376, 1401–1408.

Williams, N.M., Franke, B., Mick, E., Anney, R.J., Freitag, C.M., Gill, M., Thapar, A., O'Donovan, M.C., Owen, M.J., Holmans, P., et al. (2012). Genome-wide analysis of copy number variants in attention deficit hyperactivity disorder: the role of rare variants and duplications at 15q13.3. Am J Psychiatry 169, 195–204.

Williams, S.R., Aldred, M.A., Der Kaloustian, V.M., Halal, F., Gowans, G., McLeod, D.R., Zondag, S., Toriello, H.V., Magenis, R.E., and Elsea, S.H. (2010b). Haploinsufficiency of HDAC4 causes brachydactyly mental retardation syndrome, with brachydactyly type E, developmental delays, and behavioral problems. Am J Hum Genet 87, 219–228.

Willsey, A.J., Sanders, S.J., Li, M., Dong, S., Tebbenkamp, A.T., Muhle, R.A., Reilly, S.K., Lin, L., Fertuzinhos, S., Miller, J.A., et al. (2013). Coexpression networks implicate human midfetal deep cortical projection neurons in the pathogenesis of autism. Cell 155, 997–1007.

Woo, J., Kwon, S.K., and Kim, E. (2009). The NGL family of leucine-rich repeat-containing synaptic adhesion molecules. Mol Cell Neurosci 42, 1–10.

Wu, Y., Arai, A.C., Rumbaugh, G., Srivastava, A.K., Turner, G., Hayashi, T., Suzuki, E., Jiang, Y., Zhang, L., Rodriguez, J., et al. (2007). Mutations in ionotropic AMPA receptor 3 alter channel properties and are associated with moderate cognitive impairment in humans. Proc Natl Acad Sci USA 104, 18163–18168.

Xu, B., Roos, J.L., Levy, S., van Rensburg, E.J., Gogos, J.A., and Karayiorgou, M. (2008). Strong association of de novo copy number mutations with sporadic schizophrenia. Nat Genet 40, 880–885.

Xue, M., Atallah, B.V., and Scanziani, M. (2014). Equalizing excitation-inhibition ratios across visual cortical neurons. Nature 511, 596–600.

Yamada, T., Yang, Y., Hemberg, M., Yoshida, T., Cho, H.Y., Murphy, J.P., Fioravante, D., Regehr, W.G., Gygi, S.P., Georgopoulos, K., et al. (2014). Promoter decommissioning by the NuRD chromatin remodeling complex triggers synaptic connectivity in the mammalian brain. Neuron 83, 122–134.

Yang, X., Hou, D., Jiang, W., and Zhang, C. (2014). Intercellular protein-protein interactions at synapses. Protein Cell 5, 420–444.

Yim, Y.S., Kwon, Y., Nam, J., Yoon, H.I., Lee, K., Kim, D.G., Kim, E., Kim, C.H., and Ko, J. (2013). Slitrks control excitatory and inhibitory synapse formation with LAR receptor protein tyrosine phosphatases. Proc Natl Acad Sci USA 110, 4057–4062.

Yoshida, T., Yasumura, M., Uemura, T., Lee, S.J., Ra, M., Taguchi, R., Iwakura, Y., and Mishina, M. (2011). IL-1 receptor accessory protein-like 1 associated with mental retardation and autism mediates synapse formation by trans-synaptic interaction with protein tyrosine phosphatase delta. J Neurosci 31, 13485–13499.

Yuan, J., Jin, C., Sha, W., Zhou, Z., Zhang, F., Wang, M., Wang, J., Li, J., Feng, X., and Yu, S. (2014). A competitive PCR assay confirms the association of a copy number variation in the VIPR2 gene with schizophrenia in Han Chinese. Schizophr Res 156, 66–70.

Zaben, M.J., and Gray, W.P. (2013). Neuropeptides and hippocampal neurogenesis. Neuropeptides 47, 431–438.

Zanni, G., van Esch, H., Bensalem, A., Saillour, Y., Poirier, K., Castelnau, L., Ropers, H.H., de Brouwer, A.P., Laumonnier, F., Fryns, J.P., et al. (2010). A novel mutation in the DLG3 gene encoding the synapse-associated protein 102 (SAP102) causes non-syndromic mental retardation. Neurogenetics 11, 251–255.

Zappella, M., Meloni, I., Longo, I., Canitano, R., Hayek, G., Rosaia, L., Mari, F., and Renieri, A. (2003). Study of MECP2 gene in Rett syndrome variants and autistic girls. Am J Med Genet B Neuropsychiatr Genet 119B, 102–107.

Zheng, C.Y., Seabold, G.K., Horak, M., and Petralia, R.S. (2011). MAGUKs, synaptic development, and synaptic plasticity. Neuroscientist 17, 493–512.

Zhu, X., Need, A.C., Petrovski, S., and Goldstein, D.B. (2014). One gene, many neuropsychiatric disorders: lessons from Mendelian diseases. Nat Neurosci 17, 773–781.

Zuchner, S., Cuccaro, M.L., Tran-Viet, K.N., Cope, H., Krishnan, R.R., Pericak-Vance, M.A., Wright, H.H., and Ashley-Koch, A. (2006). SLITRK1 mutations in trichotillomania. Mol Psychiatry 11, 887–889.

Zuko, A., Kleijer, K.T., Oguro-Ando, A., Kas, M.J., van Daalen, E., van der Zwaag, B., and Burbach, J.P. (2013). Contactins in the neurobiology of autism. Eur J Pharmacol 719, 63–74.

Zweier, C., de Jong, E.K., Zweier, M., Orrico, A., Ousager, L.B., Collins, A.L., Bijlsma, E.K., Oortveld, M.A., Ekici, A.B., Reis, A., et al. (2009). CNTNAP2 and NRXN1 are mutated in autosomal-recessive Pitt-Hopkins-like mental retardation and determine the level of a common synaptic protein in Drosophila. Am J Hum Genet 85, 655–666.

Zweier, M., Gregor, A., Zweier, C., Engels, H., Sticht, H., Wohlleber, E., Bijlsma, E.K., Holder, S.E., Zenker, M., Rossier, E., et al. (2010). Mutations in MEF2C from the 5q14.3q15 microdeletion syndrome region are a frequent cause of severe mental retardation and diminish MECP2 and CDKL5 expression. Hum Mutat 31, 722–733.

Zweier, M., and Rauch, A. (2012). The MEF2C-related and 5q14.3q15 microdeletion syndrome. Mol Syndromol 2, 164–170.

10

HUMAN STEM CELL MODELS OF NEURODEVELOPMENTAL DISORDERS

PETER KIRWAN AND FREDERICK J. LIVESEY
Gurdon Institute, Department of Biochemistry and Cambridge Stem Cell Institute, University of Cambridge, Tennis Court Road, Cambridge, CB2 1QN UK

10.1 INTRODUCTION

Mechanistic studies of the genetic basis of neurodevelopmental disorders have been underpinned for many years by the production of relevant mouse genetic models. Such models have been extensively used for behavioral and electrophysiological studies, particularly of monogenic forms of neurodevelopmental disorders. By contrast, cellular or in vitro models have commonly been used to study reductionist aspects of development such as cell growth, division, and differentiation. In neuroscience, they have been critical for understanding many of the specialized functions of the neuron such as axon guidance, neuronal firing properties, and synaptic function (see, for example, Kandel, 2012, for reviews and references).

Recent developments in stem cell and developmental biology have provided opportunities not only to produce human cell types affected by different diseases, but also to replay different aspects of development and tissue assembly

in vitro. These advances could enable future studies of the etiology and pathogenesis of neurodevelopmental disorders in human developing systems in vitro. Arguably, the ultimate usefulness of in vitro systems for studying neurodevelopmental disorders depends on the ability of those systems to accurately capture different aspects of human brain development, from neurogenesis to specific circuit formation and function. In this chapter, we will review the current status of the field in terms of progress in modeling human brain development in vitro and its application to the study of the etiology and pathogenesis of neurodevelopmental disorders.

10.2 MODELING HUMAN BRAIN DEVELOPMENT AND DISEASE IN RODENTS

Until recently, most attempts to study aspects of human cellular neurobiology have used postmortem tissue, including frozen tissue sections

(Harrison, 1999), primary neuronal cultures (Saud et al., 2006) and neural stem cell lines (Sun et al., 2008). While postmortem samples provide an opportunity to study neurobiology and disease in the humans, they are not by their nature ideal for functional analysis such as electrophysiology. Furthermore, they are often sourced at relatively late stages of development, rendering studies of early development and early disease pathologies difficult. Neural stem cell (NSC) lines have been derived from postmortem fetal brains, theoretically allowing for a long-term renewable source of neuronal cell types (Sun et al., 2008). However, neurons derived from NSC cultures are deficient at acquiring mature electrophysiological properties and over time NSCs in culture become gliogenic, losing their neurogenic capacity (Sun et al., 2008). Together with difficulties in obtaining materials, these factors have meant that rodents have been the favored models for studying nervous system development and disease.

While bearing notable similarities to rodents, the human nervous system is a great deal more complex. For example, the mouse cerebral cortex contains around eight million neurons (Schuz and Palm, 1989), while humans have in the region of 26 billion (Pakkenberg and Gundersen, 1997). As well as the absolute numbers of cells in the cerebral cortex, there is also increased cell type diversity in terms of progenitor subtypes and the neuronal population (DeFelipe et al., 2002; Hansen et al., 2010; Kriegstein et al., 2006). Together, this translates to a one thousand fold increase in brain surface area in humans (Rakic, 2009). An increase in complexity in the cortex is evidenced by the existence of 50 anatomically and functionally distinct cytoarchitectural regions in humans (Brodmann, 1908; Felleman and Van Essen, 1991) compared to a great deal fewer in mice (Rakic, 2009). Taken together, these enhancements in functional areas, cellular numbers, diversity and functionality are thought to result in an overall increase in the complexity of neural connectivity. These differences might allow for a much greater processing power in humans that

is clearly evident in the form of a vastly superior cognitive ability as well as complex behavioral characteristics.

There have been significant efforts toward modeling human neurodevelopmental disorders in rodents. These have exploited gene knock-in/knock-out technologies and have allowed aspects of several neurogenetic disorders to be studied in mice such as autism (Moy et al., 2006), Down syndrome (DS) (Reeves et al., 1995), fragile X syndrome (Bates and Gonitel, 2006), and schizophrenia (Chen et al., 2006). Such models have significantly advanced our understanding of the mechanisms behind these conditions. However, along with the previously mentioned differences between human and rodent brains, there are a number of other drawbacks to modeling human disorders in rodents (Bedell et al., 1997; Elsea and Lucas, 2002).

First of all, these are often very complex conditions that only affect humans and do not naturally occur in rodents. Therefore, it is often unclear if the full spectrum of symptoms and pathologies of human disorders can actually occur in mice. For example, in DS, primarily caused by a trisomy of human chromosome 21, efforts have been made to model this disorder in mice (O'Doherty et al., 2005; Reeves et al., 1995). However, it seems unlikely that all aspects of the condition could be replicated since mice do not have an equivalent chromosome 21. For example, it is striking that mouse models of DS do not fully develop tau pathologies typical of Alzheimer's disease, a common late feature of DS (Richardson and Burns, 2002; Vacano et al., 2012). In the case of fragile X syndrome, the molecular hallmark of the disorder is the inactivation of the *FMR1* gene due to a CGG triplet repeat expansion in the gene's 5'UTR region. However, *FMR1* is not silenced correctly in murine models of fragile X and aspects of the disease are only partially recapitulated (Berman et al., 2014).

A classic example of mouse models not recapitulating human pathologies is the case of the metabolic disorder Lesch–Nyhan disease. This is caused by a point mutation in the *HPRT* gene that codes for the hypoxanthine-guanine phosphoribosyltransferase, a key enzyme for purine metabolism. Loss of HPRT results in an accumulation of uric acid, which in turn causes neuronal dysfunction culminating in impaired motor function and intellectual disability (Jinnah et al., 2000). Several groups have made mouse models of this disorder (Hooper et al., 1987; Kuehn et al., 1987). However, despite displaying defects in purine metabolism, these mice do not exhibit any significant behavioral abnormalities.

It is noteworthy that many of the conditions that have been modeled to date in rodents are monogenic disorders. However, such disorders only represent a small fraction of the spectrum of neurodevelopmental conditions (Bishop, 2010). Additionally, most disorders have been modeled against an inbred genetic background. This can be problematic when trying to understand the impact of genetic diversity on such disorders as well as how they play out in different genetic backgrounds. The combined challenges of modeling neurodevelopmental disorders in animal models are perhaps most evident in clinical trials, where many therapeutics show that promise in animals have failed to translate to the clinic (van der Worp et al., 2010). Together, these significant drawbacks highlight a need for more representative systems when trying to model complex aspects of human biology as well as understanding and treating disease.

10.3 PLURIPOTENT STEM CELLS

Recently, advances stemming from our understanding of developmental biology and genetics are providing researchers with a better tool for modeling many aspects of human biology. The development of embryonic stem cell (ESC) (Thomson et al., 1998) and induced pluripotent stem cell (iPSC) technologies (Takahashi et al., 2007) (collectively referred to as human pluripotent stem cells; hPSCs) has allowed us to model many human cell types in vitro. In particular, techniques to differentiate hPSCs into populations of different neural subtypes are providing new potential to study human nervous system development, function, and the molecular and cellular defects that cause disease (Williams et al., 2012). Here, we will discuss the key milestones that have been achieved and current approaches that are used for generating pluripotent stem cells (Fig. 10.1).

10.3.1 Embryonic Stem Cells

During early mammalian embryogenesis, a fertilized zygote undergoes several rounds of division to form a structure called the blastocyst. The inner cell mass (ICM), a transient structure within the blastocyst, consists of a group of cells that divide and differentiate to eventually make up the entire organism (Cockburn and Rossant, 2010). In the blastocyst, ICM cells are pluripotent, having the potential to differentiate into all of the cell types that make the organism (Beddington and Robertson, 1999). In 1981, Evans and Kaufmann and Martin isolated the cells of the mouse ICM and showed that they could be maintained in a self-renewing, pluripotent state in culture (Fig. 10.1). Cultured ICM cells, referred to as ESCs, maintain the ability to differentiate into specialized cell types (Evans and Kaufman, 1981; Martin, 1981). The ability to manipulate ES cells provided the foundation for the study of pluripotency and differentiation, as well as allowing for the generation of transgenic mice through gene targeting (Evans, 2011; Thomas and Capecchi, 1987).

Crucially, the knowledge gained from mouse ES cell culture has led to the derivation and culture of human ES cells (hESCs) (Thomson et al., 1998). Thomson and colleagues also showed that hESCs can undergo multilineage differentiation (Odorico et al., 2001), offering much potential for the modeling of human cell types, tissue, and disease-causing defects in culture. hES cell lines have, however, only been derived from embryos for a small number of neurodevelopmental disorders including fragile X syndrome (Verlinsky et al., 2005) and Down Syndrome (Shi et al., 2012b). This limitation arises from the requirement for preimplantation genetic diagnosis of embryos

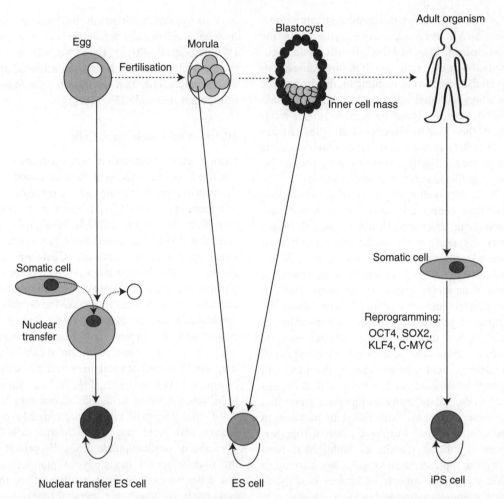

Fig. 10.1 Generation of pluripotent stem cells. (*See insert for color representation of this figure.*)

before derivation. This has also limited the ability to derive lines for complex disorders such as schizophrenia and autism where a large number of rare disease-associated mutations exist, which in addition may have different phenotypic consequences in different genetic backgrounds (Mitchell, 2011). Additionally, since the embryo is destroyed during the derivation, it is impossible to know whether disease pathologies would have developed *in vivo*. Finally, obtaining these lines is difficult due to the limited access to materials brought about by ethical concerns over the destruction of the embryo when deriving hESCs. Despite these

caveats, hESC technologies have significantly advanced our ability to study human biology as well as offering hope for the discovery of disease mechanisms and therapeutics.

10.3.2 Induced Pluripotent Stem Cells

Significant advances in developmental and stem cell biology over the last 50 years have paved the way for a new technology for investigating human biology. In 1962, John Gurdon demonstrated that the nuclei from somatic cells possess the potential to make a whole living organism (Gurdon, 1962). Taking nuclei from cells of the intestinal epithelium of tadpoles, Gurdon transferred them into enucleated unfertilized eggs. A small percentage of these eggs went on to develop into normal feeding tadpoles. These experiments demonstrated not only that differentiated cells are totipotent, containing all of the information required to make a fully functional organism, but also that their nuclei have the potential to be reprogrammed into an undifferentiated state. Over thirty years later, this principle was replicated in mammals by Ian Wilmut and colleagues, who successfully performed similar nuclear transfer experiments in sheep (Campbell et al., 1996). While nuclear transfer can in principle be used to generate pluripotent stem cells (Fig. 10.1), these techniques are not currently widely used for the generation of hPSCs due to the technical challenges involved. However, these nuclear transfer experiments established the biological principles that allow for conversion of somatic cells to pluripotent stem cells.

The nuclear transfer experiments pioneered by Gurdon implied that certain factors within an unfertilized egg can induce the reprogramming of an adult nucleus. A major consequence of this principle is that if supplied with the appropriate factors, a differentiated adult cell could potentially be reprogrammed into a pluripotent cell. In 2006, Takahashi and Yamanaka transformed mouse fibroblasts into an ESC-like state using four gene factors; *Oct4*, *Klf4*, *c-Myc*, and *Sox2*. These induced pluripotent stem cells (iPSCs or iPS cells) had similar properties to ES cells. They displayed ES cell-like morphology and gene expression, as well as an ability to self renew in culture and differentiate into cell types of all three germ layers. Furthermore, when injected into blastocysts, iPSCs contributed to the development of adult mice as well as making functional germ cells within the adult (Takahashi and Yamanaka, 2006). The next groundbreaking development came when Yamanaka and colleagues reprogrammed human fibroblasts into pluripotent stem cells (hiPSCs) using the same four gene factors (Takahashi

et al., 2007) (Fig. 10.1). Again these hiPSCs demonstrated a full capacity to be maintained in a self-renewing state *in vitro* as well as showing the developmental potential to be differentiated into different cell types.

The ability to reprogram human somatic cells into pluripotent stem cells had immediate implications for the study of human biology, as well as offering much promise for human translational medicine. iPS cells can be derived in theory from any kind of tissue, and to date have been derived from easily accessible human tissues such as keratinocytes, blood cells, and dermal fibroblasts (Aasen et al., 2008; Lowry et al., 2008; Ye et al., 2009). The ease of access to such materials means that a near unlimited amount of material from diverse genetic backgrounds and from patients with different disorders is now available. Encouragingly, it also means that the study of genetic conditions can be expanded to disorders such as schizophrenia and autism where many rare disease-associated mutations exist.

iPS cells have now been generated from patients of a host of different conditions including, Alzheimer's disease (Israel et al., 2012; Shi et al., 2012b), long-QT syndrome (Itzhaki et al., 2011), Huntington's disease (Camnasio et al., 2012), multiple sclerosis (Song et al., 2012), Turner syndrome (Li et al., 2012), and Lesch–Nyhan syndrome (Mekhoubad et al., 2012) to name but a few. Furthermore, many of these iPS lines are from individuals with neurodevelopmental disorders such as schizophrenia (Brennand et al., 2011), fragile X syndrome (Urbach et al., 2010), Angelman Syndrome, Prader-Willi syndrome(PWS) (Chamberlain et al., 2010), and Down Syndrome (Park et al., 2008; Shi et al., 2012b) and the autism spectrum disorders such as Rett syndrome (Marchetto et al., 2010) and Timothy syndrome (Pasca et al., 2011). The use of iPS cells means that these conditions can now be better defined at a molecular and cellular level as well as allowing investigation of how they develop over time.

10.4 DIRECTED DIFFERENTIATION OF HUMAN PLURIPOTENT STEM CELLS TO REPLAY NEURAL DEVELOPMENT

Early efforts to differentiate hESCs into neuronal subtypes utilized an embryoid body approach (Zhang et al., 2001). Here, hESCs were cultured as floating aggregates in the presence of FGF2. The resulting cultures produced cells reminiscent of an early neuroectodermal fate, comprising polarized neural tube-like structures that were enriched for neural progenitors. The neural progenitors then differentiated to produce neurons and glia. These experiments demonstrated the potential for directed differentiation of hESCs into neuronal tissue; however, this approach results in a mixture of undefined neuronal subtypes as well as an overproduction of glia (Zhang et al., 2001). Recently, however, through understanding how different parts of the human nervous system are generated during development, researchers have been able to manipulate hPSCs, generating an array of different defined cells types that make up a functional nervous system (Fig. 10.2).

A general principle is that, rather than making a particular cell type, fundamental developmental principles are followed to replay development of a particular region of the CNS. Dysfunction of the cerebral cortex occurs in a large number of neurodevelopmental and neurodegenerative disorders such as schizophrenia (Raedler et al., 1998), autism spectrum disorders (Geschwind and Levitt, 2007), epilepsy (Chang and Lowenstein, 2003), and Alzheimer's disease and DS. Therefore, we will discuss efforts to model neurodevelopmental disorders using cerebral cortex as our main example.

10.4.1 Replaying Human Cerebral Cortex Development In Vitro

Due to the importance of the cerebral cortex functionally, and in disease, significant efforts have been made to model this brain region using hPSCs. Early efforts demonstrated that mouse ES cells could be directed to a cortical fate, recapitulating all of the layers of the cortex (Eiraku

et al., 2008; Gaspard et al., 2008). Similar to their work in retina, Eiraku et al. demonstrated a self-organized layered structure formed when culturing mouse cortical neuroepithelium as embryoid bodies. Eiraku et al. also induced cortical-like neuroepithelium from hESCs in embryoid body cultures. However, these cultures failed to generate significant numbers of later born, upper layer cortical neurons subtypes. Additionally, it was not demonstrated whether the neurons became functional or developed synapses and networks.

Recently, we have shown a robust recapitulation of cortical development from hPSCs (Shi et al., 2012a; Shi et al., 2012c). By inducing a primitive neuroepithelium using dual SMAD inhibition (Chambers et al., 2009), together with exposure to retinoic acid and FGF2, cortical progenitors were induced from two ES lines and four iPS lines. The neuroepithelium formed polarized rosette structures containing a diverse population of human cortical progenitors including apical and basal progenitors, as well as a large population of outer radial glial (oRG) cells. The latter populations are proposed to underlie the considerable expansion in size of the human cerebral cortex, relative to that of nonhuman primates. Over the course of 100 days in vitro, the cortical progenitors divided to produce roughly equal proportions of all the major deep and upper layer excitatory cortical neuron subtypes as well as astrocytes. In keeping with a conserved program of cortical neurogenesis, the neurons and glia appeared in the same temporal order that is observed in vivo (Fig. 10.2).

Crucially, the cortical neurons matured to develop mature electrophysiological properties of excitatory neurons. Over weeks in culture, the cortical neurons also developed excitatory synapses. The excitatory synapses became functional, displaying both spontaneous and evoked excitatory activity. More complex network and circuit properties of human PSC-derived cortical neurons are areas of active research.

Excitatory, glutamatergic neurons make up 80% of the neurons in the cortex, with the other 20% comprising inhibitory GABAergic

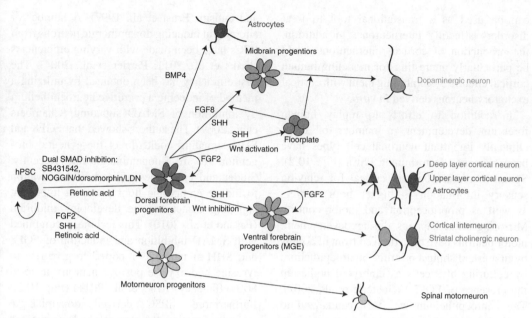

Fig. 10.2 Directed differentiation of human pluripotent stem cells (hPSCs) to different neural fates. (*See insert for color representation of this figure.*)

interneurons. The subcortical medial ganglionic eminence (MGE) acts as the primary source of GABAergic interneurons to the cerebral cortex and hippocampus, and cholinergic interneurons to the striatum (Anderson et al., 1997; Anderson et al., 2002; Lavdas et al., 1999). MGE-derived interneurons function as critical modulators of excitatory activity in the cortex (Markram et al., 2004) and contribute to a variety of neurodevelopmental disorders including schizophrenia (Lewis et al., 2012), autism (Casanova et al., 2006), Down syndrome (Bhattacharyya et al., 2009), and epilepsy (Powell et al., 2003). A number of signaling pathways including SHH have been shown to be important for the patterning of the MGE (Wilson and Rubenstein, 2000). The production of complete cortical networks that reflect in vivo biology will require the integration of excitatory and inhibitory neurons of the appropriate classes and in the correct proportions. A first step is the generation of interneurons from PSCs that reflect the complexity of this population in vivo.

A number of groups have now successfully manipulated hPSCs to derive MGE progenitor cells that differentiate into diverse subtypes of forebrain interneurons (Liu et al., 2013; Maroof et al., 2013; Nicholas et al., 2013) (Fig. 10.2). These groups induced a primitive neuroepithelium by inhibition of SMAD signaling. The neuroepithelium was subsequently induced to an MGE fate with over 90% efficiency by SHH signaling, and inhibition of Wnt. Over weeks in culture, MGE progenitors produced a diversity of GABAergic cortical interneurons as well as striatal cholinergic neurons. These neurons acquired mature functional properties and were cultured for up to 30 weeks *in vitro* (Maroof et al., 2013; Nicholas et al., 2013). Interestingly, when engrafted into mice, hPSC derived MGE progenitors produced GABA- and ChAT-positive interneurons that contributed to the development of the cortex and striatum and resulted in functional recovery in a Parkinson's disease model (Liu et al., 2013). This demonstration provides an encouraging proof of principle that *in vitro*-derived interneurons can be used as a translational tool to treat disorders affecting interneurons. In addition, the production of cortical interneurons could be particularly interesting for modeling human cortical circuits by combining them with cortical excitatory neurons derived *in vitro*.

In addition to efforts to replay human forebrain development, a number of other clinically important neuronal cell types have been generated from human PSCs (Fig. 10.2). Spinal motor neurons are critical for relaying sensory information to higher brain centers as well as proprioception and motor control. Mirroring what happens during development, motor neurons have been derived from hES cells by first establishing a primitive neuroepithelium by culturing hES cells as embryoid bodies in the presence of FGF2 (Wichterle et al., 2002). The neuroepithelium was then caudalized to a Hoxc5, Hoxc6 expressing motor neuron progenitor identity using retinoic acid. Using an agonist of SHH signaling at varying concentrations, the progenitors were induced to a ventral or motor neuron fate (Fig. 10.2). Thus the authors produced a diverse population of spinal motorneurons of dorsal, medial, and ventral identity, which integrated when engrafted into chick and mouse spinal cord (Wichterle et al., 2002). Crucially, hES-derived spinal motor neurons have been shown to be functional excitable cells that form synaptic connections (Li et al., 2005). Recently, efforts have utilized a similar embryoid body protocol to Wichterle et al. or an adherent culture protocol that also utilizes retinoid and SHH signaling to show that hiPSCs can be induced to a spinal motor neuron identity at an efficiency of ~60% (Karumbayaram et al., 2009).

The dopamine system in the brain is important for cognitive function, regulating movements and modulating reward pathways. While the dopaminergic system has been of keen interest due to its degeneration in Parkinson's disease (Dauer and Przedborski, 2003), a number of neurodevelopmental disorders also display defects in dopaminergic pathways including schizophrenia (Davis et al., 1991)

and autism (Ernst et al., 1997). A number of attempts at inducing dopaminergic neurons from PSCs have been made with varying efficiencies (Kriks et al., 2011; Perrier et al., 2004). The best efficiency has been obtained by utilizing a method of inducing a primitive neuroepithelium by inhibition of SMAD signaling (Chambers et al., 2009). The authors showed that FGF8 and SHH signaling could direct these neural progenitors toward a dopaminergic fate. Recently, Studer and colleagues utilized Wnt activation to induce embryonic floor plate, an important signaling center for the developing midbrain (Fasano et al., 2010). This technique combined with SMAD inhibition and induction of FGF8 and SHH signaling is reported to give rise to tyrosine hydroxylase positive neurons at up to 80% efficiency (Kriks et al., 2011) (Fig. 10.2). Furthermore, hPSC derived dopaminergic neurons functionally integrate when injected into rodent brains, offering hope for treating conditions where dopaminergic pathways are degraded (Kriks et al., 2011).

10.5 DIRECT DIFFERENTIATION AND TRANSDIFFERENTIATION

Alternative approaches to generating forebrain neurons and circuits are direct differentiation from PSCs and transdifferentiation from somatic cell types (Pang et al., 2011; Vierbuchen et al., 2010; Yoo et al., 2011). In both cases, technical efforts have focused on generating specific neuronal types, for example, dopaminergic or spinal motor neurons, rather than reconstitution of neural circuits. There has been a report of the production of neurons via a neural stem cell stage by transdifferentiation using a cocktail of small molecules together with proneural transcription factors (Ladewig, 2012). However, in general these approaches are designed for the rapid production of neurons, rather than for replaying developmental processes.

An advantage of this approach is the comparative speed of generation of neurons, compared with directed differentiation from PSCs. In addition, in principle, defined types of neurons can be produced. Current limitations to this approach are its relative inefficiency, plus the nonrenewable nature of the cells generated from primary fibroblasts, which puts a limit on the numbers of neurons that can be produced. Finally, in their current applications, these methods deliberately do not capture the complexity of the neuronal populations in any region of the brain. However, in principle, it should be possible to produce all of the elements of a given neuronal circuit using these approaches and to precisely engineer neuronal circuits using those elements to study circuit and network properties in health and disease.

10.6 GENERATION OF CEREBRAL CORTEX NEURAL CIRCUITRY

As neurodevelopmental disorders are conditions that ultimately affect neural circuit function, modeling neural circuits using iPS and ES cells should provide us with an optimal spatial, cellular, and temporal resolution that to date has not been possible for studying neural circuits in health and disease. In order to model human neurodevelopment, function, and disease, it is first necessary to replicate *in vitro* the diversity of neural subtypes that are present throughout the nervous system. It is crucial that the generation of cell types faithfully recapitulates neural development and that the correct neuronal classes affected by a given neurodevelopmental disorder are produced. For example, to model epilepsy, a condition in which seizures are caused by an imbalance of excitatory and inhibitory neuronal activity in the cerebral cortex, thalamus, and hippocampus (Chang and Lowenstein, 2003), it is critical that the appropriate subtypes of cortical, thalamic, and hippocampal neurons are generated so that the disorder can be modeled correctly, both functionally and developmentally.

However, it is an open question as to how best to reconstitute neural circuits in vitro in a manner that reflects in vivo circuits: whether to take advantage of the replay of developmental processes that occurs during differentiation from PSCs, which also typically includes the generation of complex neuronal populations, or to actively engineer circuits by assembling different neuronal types in a specific structure or order.

10.7 3D MODELS OF BRAIN DEVELOPMENT

While the majority of methods for generating human neural stem cells, neurons, and neural circuits are optimized for two-dimensional, monolayer culture, all regions of the brain, including the cerebral cortex, have pronounced spatial organization of cell types. In the cerebral cortex, this is manifested by the organization of excitatory neurons into discrete radial layers, with layer identity being a strong predictor of cell identity and connectivity. Therefore, precise circuit formation in vitro may require the reconstitution of the spatial relationships and orientation of the different cell types, ideally in three dimensions. Furthermore, some neurodevelopmental disorders may have their etiology in changes in neurogenesis, neuronal differentiation, and migration, aspects of which may be manifested more clearly in 3D systems. Considerable progress has been made in recent years in proof of concept studies of the feasibility of developing such systems.

In humans, the light-detecting retina comprises six major cell types spanning ten stratified layers (Cayouette et al., 2006; Cepko et al., 1996). A remarkable breakthrough toward modeling human retina *in vitro* has shown that self-organized multilayered retina can be derived from hESCs (Nakano et al., 2012). By culturing hESC aggregates in the presence of serum, Wnt inhibitor and SHH agonist, the retinal progenitors were derived at an efficiency of >70%. After weeks in culture, an invaginated, twin-walled optic cup structure formed. Over the course of ~130 days in culture, a pseudostratified retina-like structure formed containing multiple neuronal subtypes including interneurons, rod, cone, and ganglion cells. While the retinal layers lacked bipolar cells and the apical-most photoreceptors, the authors suggest that the recapitulation of retinal microenvironments, together with time in culture might result in the cultivation of a fully defined hPSC derived human retina *in vitro* (Nakano et al., 2012). While efforts to recapitulate retina *in vitro* are encouraging, it still remains to be demonstrated that the retina generated are functional. This will no doubt be crucial toward future transplantation therapies and treatment of retinal disorders.

In the case of the cerebral cortex, pioneering studies by Sasai and colleagues have found, as in the retina, that mouse embryoid body-derived neural tissue has the potential to self-organized and pattern into different regions of the forebrain, including the cerebral cortex (Eiraku et al., 2008). In those initial studies, similar results from human PSCs were reported, but with markedly reduced production of upper layer neurons and relatively poor lamination. More recently, the Knoblich and Sasai groups have reported the formation of complex mixtures of forebrain neural tissues from human PSCs (Kadoshima et al., 2013; Lancaster et al., 2013), which reached relatively large sizes. However, as for the previous studies, production of later born cells and lamination were both relatively low, compared with the previous mouse studies. However, it is clear that there will be marked progress in the near future in controlling this process to both increase the reproducibility of the process between experiments and also to extend the developmental process to include the production of all cortical neuron types and their spatial organization.

10.8 hPSC MODELS OF NEURODEVELOPMENTAL DISORDERS

The development of iPS cell technologies has provided new potential for the study of human neurodevelopmental disorders. A number of neurodevelopmental disorders have now been modeled from iPS cells, with many of them displaying disease-relevant phenotypes *in vitro* (Wang and Doering, 2012).

10.8.1 Autism Spectrum Disorders

Two autism spectrum disorders, Rett syndrome and Timothy syndrome have now been modeled from iPS cells. Rett syndrome is an X-linked, male-lethal autism spectrum disorder resulting from mutations in the *MeCP2* gene that encodes the transcriptional repressor Methyl CPG binding protein-2 (Armstrong, 2005). Neurons differentiated from iPS cells from Rett syndrome patients have smaller soma, fewer dendritic spines, reduced functional synaptic input and spontaneous calcium transients. The authors rescued the reduction in synapse numbers with two candidate drugs; however, they did not demonstrate a rescue of synaptic function (Marchetto et al., 2010).

Timothy syndrome is a rare autosomal dominant disorder that results in cardiac arrhythmias, heart disease, hypoglycemia, syndactyly, as well as autism. It arises from a missense mutation in the L-Type calcium channel $Ca_v1.2$ (Splawski et al., 2004). Functional analysis of Timothy syndrome iPS derived neurons revealed slower repolarization of action potentials compared to healthy control neurons . Furthermore, after depolarization of the neurons, the Timothy syndrome cells exhibited an increase in the sustained calcium rise (Pasca et al., 2011). These data are consistent with abnormal channel inactivation and calcium activity as a result of mutated $Ca_v1.2$ in Timothy syndrome (Splawski et al., 2004). Interestingly, some of the functional defects found in Timothy syndrome iPS-derived neurons could be rescued with the L-type calcium channel blocker nimodipine, demonstrating the promise for using these systems for testing candidate disease treating drugs (Pasca et al., 2011). In addition to defects in neuronal calcium activity caused by defective $Ca_v1.2$ channels in Timothy syndrome, iPS derived neurons from Timothy syndrome patients showed activity dependent retraction of dendrites, in contrast to healthy controls, which increased their dendrite arborization in response to activity (Krey et al., 2013). The dendritic retraction in Timothy syndrome neurons was shown not to be dependent of calcium activity, but driven through ectopic activation of RhoA signaling by $Ca_v1.2$, revealing a novel insight into the cellular and molecular defects in Timothy syndrome (Krey et al., 2013). This study highlights the usefulness of iPS cells for uncovering new mechanisms that contribute to neurodevelopmental disorders.

While Timothy and Rett syndrome represent classic, well defined forms of autism, they only represent a small percentage of autism spectrum disorders. Most cases of autism are sporadic and are likely caused by de novo mutations in the germline (Neale et al., 2012; O'Roak et al., 2012; Sanders et al., 2012). The underlying genetic variants that predispose individuals to autism are highly heterogeneous, suggesting that dysfunction in a large number molecular pathways can converge to produce an autistic phenotype. Additionally, the effects of many of the disease-related mutations in autism may vary depending on genetic background (Mitchell, 2011) (see Chapter 4). The existence of many rare disease-causing mutations combined with the effect of the genome on disease phenotypes highlights the advantage of using patient-derived cells for uncovering the molecular and cellular defects that lead to autism. Investigating iPS lines from large cohorts of patients and classifying them according to mutations that affect similar molecular and cellular pathways, as well as taking their genetic backgrounds into account, could therefore be the central to understanding the disease-causing mechanisms of autistic spectrum disorders.

10.8.2 Schizophrenia

Schizophrenia is a debilitating psychotic disorder affecting one percent of the population. Patients present with behavioral defects, suffering from auditory hallucinations, delusions, attention deficits, social withdrawal as well as cognitive impairments (Freedman, 2003). This complex neurodevelopmental disorder has a high heritability of 80–85% (Sullivan et al., 2003). Schizophrenia is a complex genetic disorder affecting many parts of the brain and as a result many neural pathways are dysfunctional (Freedman, 2003). As is the case with autism spectrum disorders, many different genetic variants have been identified that confer risk to schizophrenia, many of which affect pathways involved in neurodevelopment (Stone et al., 2008; Mitchell, 2011; Stefansson et al., 2008; Walsh et al., 2008)(see Chapter 4). Therefore, the use of patient-specific iPS cells lends itself well to study the molecular and cellular effects of the diversity of mutations that lead to schizophrenia.

Recently, hiPSCs have been derived from four schizophrenia patients and differentiated into neurons (Brennand et al., 2011). Schizophrenia patient-derived neurons showed abnormal gene expression, with 25% of genes that were abnormally expressed previously implicated in schizophrenia. These gene expression data also identified pathways that previously have not been implicated in the disorder such as NOTCH signaling, uncovering novel candidate disease-related molecular mechanisms. Schizophrenia neurons also displayed cellular defects, including reduced excitatory synapse numbers, and less neurite outgrowth. Coupled with this, the neurons also had reduced levels of neural connectivity, suggestive of defective neural networks in these patients. Interestingly, many of the defects in connectivity and gene expression could be partially rescued by the anti-psychotic drug loxapine (Brennand et al., 2011). This study, therefore, also provides a proof of principle for the testing of disease-modifying drugs. It is encouraging that when modeled from pluripotent stem cells, a complex neurodevelopmental disorder such as schizophrenia can converge on a number of easily studied phenotypes such as reduced synaptic connectivity.

While encouraging, this study does not clearly identify the underlying causes of schizophrenia in the patients from whom the iPS lines were derived. Given the complex genetic nature of the condition, a more complete understanding of schizophrenia will likely require investigation of larger patient cohorts and sub-grouping them according to shared molecular and cellular defects as well as genetics.

10.8.3   Imprinting Disorders

Imprinting disorders occur as a result of inheritance of epigenetic modifications from parents. Angelman syndrome occurs in 1 in 12,000–20,000 in the population and results from the loss of function of the maternal copy of the ubiquitin ligase E3A protein (UBE3A). Symptoms of Angelman syndrome include developmental delay, cognitive disability, speech impairment, ataxia, epilepsy, and hyperactivity (Williams et al., 2010). Despite the epigenetic changes that occur during reprogramming, iPS cells derived from Angelman syndrome patients showed retention of the disease-causing imprinting (Chamberlain et al., 2010). Despite this, neurons displayed no obvious cellular defects and had normal firing properties and functional synaptic inputs. This highlights a need to investigate more complex phenotypes such as dysfunction of neural networks in iPS models of neurodevelopmental disorders as it is unlikely that all neurodevelopmental disorders display relatively simple functional defects such as action potential firing and spontaneous synaptic function.

Prader-Willi syndrome (PWS), another imprinting disorder, occurs as a result of the lack of expression in a region of the paternally inherited chromosome 15q11-q13 that codes for a cluster of snoRNAs. Patients suffer from feeding problems likely due to hypothalamic dysfunction, as well as cognitive impairment and learning disabilities (Goldstone, 2004). iPS cells have been derived from PWS patients and it has been show that they retain the imprinting marks at the Prader-Willi imprinting center of their parental disease fibroblasts (Chamberlain et al., 2010). In a separate study, reduced expression of the disease-associated snoRNA cluster was found in Prader-Willi hiPSCs (Yang et al., 2010). To date, however, no study has investigated molecular, cellular, and functional phenotypes in neurons induced from iPS cells from PWS patients.

10.8.4   Fragile X Syndrome

Fragile X syndrome is an X-linked neurodevelopmental disorder that results from a CGG trinucleotide expansion in the 5'UTR of the *FMR1* gene. More than 200 CGG repeats results in silencing of the gene and loss of the FMRP protein (Crawford et al., 2001). FMRP is important for local protein synthesis in the dendrite and axon, playing a key role in circuit formation and synaptic plasticity (Bassell and Warren, 2008).

It has been shown in fragile X ES cells that the *FMR1* gene is actively transcribed. Indeed, upon differentiation of the ESCs to embryoid bodies or teratomas, the CGG expansion underwent significant methylation, histone modification, and gene silencing (Eiges et al., 2007). This suggests that the silencing of *FMR1* is a process that occurs during development.

By contrast, iPS cells generated from patients with fragile X failed to reactivate *FMR1*, and that methlyation and repressive histone modification marks present at the *FMR1* promoter (Urbach et al., 2010). These data suggested that these iPS lines are unsuitable for studying fragile X as a neurodevelopmental disorder due to the inability to replicate in culture the silencing that occurs during neuronal differentiation. In a separate study, however, iPSC lines were isolated containing an unmethylated and active FMR1 promoter (Sheridan et al., 2011). Neuronal differentiation of these fragile X iPS cells revealed that progenitors and neurons had abnormal processes. Additionally, the cultures displayed abnormal development, undergoing preferential gliogenesis. These observed defects coincided with promoter methylation and silencing of *FMR1* during the differentiation of iPS cells to neurons (Sheridan et al., 2011). While this study identified interesting cellular and developmental defects, further investigation of the underlying molecular defects as well as analysis of neuronal function and network development using fragile X iPS cells should provide further insight into the mechanisms of this condition.

While the progress at modeling neurodevelopmental disorders using pluripotent stem cells is encouraging, the aforementioned studies showed no clear and robust characterization of the neural subtypes that were induced for investigation. As these neurodevelopmental disorders are known to affect particular brain regions, cellular subtypes and neural circuits, inducing clearly defined cell types will be necessary to accurately study the molecular and cellular hallmarks of these disorders as well as understanding how cellular subtypes are differentially affected.

10.8.5 Microcephaly

Autosomal recessive primary microcephaly (MCPH) is a neurodevelopmental disorder characterized by a significantly reduced brain size, with the cerebral cortex exhibiting the greatest reduction in volume. Clinically MCPH patients suffer with intellectual disability. Most of the genes responsible for MCPH have been identified and characterized, all of which encode spindle associated proteins. Mutations in these proteins can cause defects in neurogenic mitosis. A consequence of deficient mitosis in MCPH is thought to result in premature neurogenesis during development and at the expense of neural progenitor self-renewal, ultimately leading to significantly fewer cells in the adult brain (Woods et al., 2005).

A recent study has used MCPH patient-derived iPS cells to generate three dimensional cortical "organoids" (Lancaster et al., 2013). These analyses revealed that MCPH organoids had smaller neuroepithelial volumes. There was an increase in the numbers of neurons present early in the development of MCPH cerebral organoids but with corresponding reductions in the numbers of neural progenitors, suggesting that premature neuronal differentiation was occurring. Examination of the spindle orientation in radial glia revealed that MCPH patient-derived cerebral organoids contained a large proportion of radial glia with oblique and vertically oriented spindles, compared to controls, which had horizontal oriented spindles. As a horizontal spindle orientation is important for symmetric divisions of neural progenitors (Chenn and McConnell, 1995; Konno et al., 2008; Yingling et al., 2008), the authors suggest that abnormally oriented spindles in microcephaly could result in reduced progenitor cell proliferation and drive them toward premature neurogenic divisions (Lancaster et al., 2013). This study demonstrated that key cellular mechanisms of neurodevelopmental disorders can be reproduced in culture using iPS cells.

10.8.6 Down Syndrome

DS is the most common inherited form of intellectual disability with a prevalence of 1 in 750 live births worldwide (Wiseman et al., 2009). DS mostly occurs as a result of a trisomy of chromosome 21 results, causing a gene dosage imbalance resulting in the neurodevelopmental disorder (Antonarakis et al., 2004). In a minority of cases, DS is caused by a Roberstsonian translocation where the long arm of chromosome 21 is joined to chromosome 14 or 15 (Petersen et al., 1991).

Individuals with DS suffer from heart abnormalities and are prone to certain forms of leukemia. Patients display a range of neurological defects including abnormal motor coordination and cognitive dysfunction as well as learning and memory deficits (Dierssen, 2012). Furthermore, they also suffer from early-onset Alzheimer's disease (Burger and Vogel, 1973), which is likely to be a result of having an extra copy of the amyloid precursor protein (APP) gene (Rumble et al., 1989). Pathologically, DS brains have been shown to have reduced cortical volumes, decreased numbers of upper layer neurons and abnormal dendritic spine morphologies (Ferrer and Gullotta, 1990; Ross et al., 1984; Schmidt-Sidor et al., 1990; Takashima et al., 1981).

Pluripotent stem cells provide an opportunity to gain new insights into the development and function of brains of individuals with DS. A number of iPS lines have now been derived from DS patients (Park et al., 2008; Weick et al., 2013). We have recently derived excitatory cortical neurons from two trisomy 21 (TS21) lines (DSES and DSiPS) (Shi et al., 2012b). TS21 lines differentiated to produce cortical neuroepithelium, replicating the diversity of progenitors observed *in vivo*, including apical and basal progenitors as well as oRG cells. Over weeks in culture, cortical progenitors produced the subtypes of upper and deep layer neurons observed *in vivo* in the same precise temporal order. TS21 neurons developed excitatory synapses and matured to acquire normal whole cell firing properties as well as functional synaptic inputs (Shi et al., 2012b). TS21 cortical neurons secreted higher levels of toxic amyloid Aβ40 and Aβ42 peptides. TS21 cortical cultures also showed a high accumulation of amyloid-β peptide deposits, highly reminiscent of Alzheimer's disease pathology. Furthermore, the levels of secreted amyloid peptides could be reduced using a drug that blocks the APP cleaving enzyme γ-secretase. As well as Aβ peptides, TS21 cortical neurons secreted higher levels of phosphorylated tau, in addition to abnormally localizing hyperphosphorylated Tau to cell bodies and dendrites (Shi et al., 2012b). Taken together, these data indicate that the pathologies of Alzheimer's disease develop in hiPSC derived TS21 cortical cultures. As well as providing a robust platform for studying early-onset dementia in individuals with DS, TS21 hPSCs should prove useful for performing drug screens for modifiers of the Alzheimer's disease phenotype.

A recent study has used TS21 lines with isogenic control lines that are genetically identical but are disomic for chromosome 21 (Weick et al., 2013). Neurons differentiated from these iPS cells displayed high levels of oxidative stress. Additionally, the authors reported a slight reduction in the presynaptic protein synapsin as well as mild defects in spontaneous synaptic activity. The use of disomic lines should prove ideal controls toward clearly identifying the defects in the brains of people with DS that are caused by a triplication of chromosome 21.

A recent breakthrough has allowed researchers to correct the dosage imbalance caused by trisomy 21 in culture (Jiang et al., 2013). Jiang et al. adapted the function of the *XIST* noncoding RNA toward silencing one chromosome 21 in trisomy 21 iPS cells. During mammalian development, *XIST* corrects dosage imbalance of X-linked genes in female XX embryos by inducing heterochromatic silencing of one X chromosome (Heard, 2005). In this study, the *XIST* gene under the control of a doxycycline inducible promoter was inserted into one of the copies of chorosome 21 in TS21 iPS lines. The induction of *XIST* transcription resulted in silencing of one copy of chromosome 21 in the iPS cells. The authors further showed that the *XIST*-induced correction of the chromosome 21 dosage imbalance resulted in an increase in neural progenitor cell proliferation in neuroepithelium induced for TS21 iPS cells. This suggests that this technology could be used to investigate developmental phenotypes in DS. *XIST* silencing of chromosome 21 should provide researchers with a powerful tool for studying molecular, cellular, and functional defects that occur during the nervous system development in individuals with DS.

While TS21 hPSC neurons are reported to display mild defects in spontaneous synaptic input at the level of the single cell, the development of cortical networks has not been investigated in TS21 hPSC neurons. Additionally, developmental phenotypes have not been investigated thoroughly in TS21 cortical neurons derived from hPSCs. In light of the observed developmental defects in the cortices of individuals with DS, hPSCs cortical cultures could be extremely useful toward identifying developmental abnormalities in the formation of the cortex as well as elucidating their mechanisms. As TS21 hPSCs can be differentiated into defined functional cortical cell types, aspects of neural circuitry in individuals with DS can also potentially be studied, as well as elucidating how networks develop. Taken together, hPSCs should prove extremely beneficial toward elucidating the molecular, cellular, and functional defects underlying this neurodevelopmental disorder.

10.9 FUTURE DIRECTIONS

Together, the aforementioned studies have demonstrated the potential for modeling human neurodevelopmental disorders using patient-derived iPS cells. Besides allowing for elucidating disease phenotypes, a number of the investigations have shown their use as drug screening platforms for modifiers of cellular and molecular defects that lead to disease pathology. Furthermore, the use of iPS cells circumvents the limitations of acquiring human material and provides an almost unlimited source of cells. As iPS cells can be derived from diverse genetic backgrounds, they also provide the opportunity to study the effects of genetic variation of disease phenotypes.

The usefulness of these and associated technologies, such as genome engineering, for studying neurodevelopmental disorders depends on question being addressed and the level of resolution required to answer that question. For example, analysis of neurogenesis, cell fate determination, cell migration, and synaptogenesis are relatively straightforward to study using current stem cell technologies. By contrast, more complex problems, such as neural network form and function, are areas of considerable research interest using these systems, but have not demonstrated their general utility.

REFERENCES

Aasen, T., Raya, A., Barrero, M.J., Garreta, E., Consiglio, A., Gonzalez, F., Vassena, R., Bilic, J., Pekarik, V., Tiscornia, G., et al. (2008). Efficient and rapid generation of induced pluripotent stem cells from human keratinocytes. Nat Biotechnol 26, 1276–1284.

Anderson, S.A., Eisenstat, D.D., Shi, L., and Rubenstein, J.L. (1997). Interneuron migration from basal forebrain to neocortex: dependence on Dlx genes. Science 278, 474–476.

Anderson, S.A., Kaznowski, C.E., Horn, C., Rubenstein, J.L., and McConnell, S.K. (2002). Distinct origins of neocortical projection neurons and interneurons in vivo. Cereb Cortex 12, 702–709.

Antonarakis, S.E., Lyle, R., Dermitzakis, E.T., Reymond, A., and Deutsch, S. (2004). Chromosome 21 and down syndrome: from genomics to pathophysiology. Nat Rev Genet 5, 725–738.

Armstrong, D.D. (2005). Neuropathology of Rett syndrome. J Child Neurol 20, 747–753.

Bassell, G.J., and Warren, S.T. (2008). Fragile X syndrome: loss of local mRNA regulation alters synaptic development and function. Neuron 60, 201–214.

Bates, G.P., and Gonitel, R. (2006). Mouse models of triplet repeat diseases. Mol Biotechnol 32, 147–158.

Beddington, R.S., and Robertson, E.J. (1999). Axis development and early asymmetry in mammals. Cell 96, 195–209.

Bedell, M.A., Largaespada, D.A., Jenkins, N.A., and Copeland, N.G. (1997). Mouse models of human disease. Part II: recent progress and future directions. Genes Dev 11, 11–43.

Berman, R.F., Buijsen, R.A., Usdin, K., Pintado, E., Kooy, F., Pretto, D., Pessah, I.N., Nelson, D.L., Zalewski, Z., Charlet-Bergeurand, N., et al. (2014). Mouse models of the fragile X premutation and fragile X-associated tremor/ataxia syndrome. Journal of neurodevelopmental disorders 6, 25.

Bhattacharyya, A., McMillan, E., Chen, S.I., Wallace, K., and Svendsen, C.N. (2009). A critical period in cortical interneuron neurogenesis in down syndrome revealed by human neural progenitor cells. Dev Neurosci 31, 497–510.

Bishop, D.V. (2010). Which neurodevelopmental disorders get researched and why? PLoS One 5, e15112.

Brennand, K.J., Simone, A., Jou, J., Gelboin-Burkhart, C., Tran, N., Sangar, S., Li, Y., Mu, Y., Chen, G., Yu, D., et al. (2011). Modelling schizophrenia using human induced pluripotent stem cells. Nature 473, 221–225.

Brodmann, K. (1908). Beitraege zur histologischen lokalisation der grosshirnrinde. VI Mitteilung: die cortexgliederung des menschen. J Psychol Neurol 10, 231–246.

Burger, P.C., and Vogel, F.S. (1973). The development of the pathologic changes of Alzheimer's disease and senile dementia in patients with Down's syndrome. Am J Pathol 73, 457–476.

Camnasio, S., Delli Carri, A., Lombardo, A., Grad, I., Mariotti, C., Castucci, A., Rozell, B., Lo Riso, P., Castiglioni, V., Zuccato, C., et al. (2012).

The first reported generation of several induced pluripotent stem cell lines from homozygous and heterozygous Huntington's disease patients demonstrates mutation related enhanced lysosomal activity. Neurobiol Dis 46, 41–51.

Campbell, K.H., McWhir, J., Ritchie, W.A., and Wilmut, I. (1996). Sheep cloned by nuclear transfer from a cultured cell line. Nature 380, 64–66.

Casanova, M.F., van Kooten, I.A., Switala, A.E., van Engeland, H., Heinsen, H., Steinbusch, H.W., Hof, P.R., Trippe, J., Stone, J., and Schmitz, C. (2006). Minicolumnar abnormalities in autism. Acta Neuropathol 112, 287–303.

Cayouette, M., Poggi, L., and Harris, W.A. (2006). Lineage in the vertebrate retina. Trends Neurosci 29, 563–570.

Cepko, C.L., Austin, C.P., Yang, X., Alexiades, M., and Ezzeddine, D. (1996). Cell fate determination in the vertebrate retina. Proc Natl Acad Sci U S A 93, 589–595.

Chamberlain, S.J., Chen, P.F., Ng, K.Y., Bourgois-Rocha, F., Lemtiri-Chlieh, F., Levine, E.S., and Lalande, M. (2010). Induced pluripotent stem cell models of the genomic imprinting disorders Angelman and Prader-Willi syndromes. Proc Natl Acad Sci U S A 107, 17668–17673.

Chambers, S.M., Fasano, C.A., Papapetrou, E.P., Tomishima, M., Sadelain, M., and Studer, L. (2009). Highly efficient neural conversion of human ES and iPS cells by dual inhibition of SMAD signaling. Nat Biotechnol 27, 275–280.

Chang, B.S., and Lowenstein, D.H. (2003). Epilepsy. N Engl J Med 349, 1257–1266.

Chen, J., Lipska, B.K., and Weinberger, D.R. (2006). Genetic mouse models of schizophrenia: from hypothesis-based to susceptibility gene-based models. Biol Psychiatry 59, 1180–1188.

Chenn, A., and McConnell, S.K. (1995). Cleavage orientation and the asymmetric inheritance of Notch1 immunoreactivity in mammalian neurogenesis. Cell 82, 631–641.

Cockburn, K., and Rossant, J. (2010). Making the blastocyst: lessons from the mouse. J Clin Invest 120, 995–1003.

Crawford, D.C., Acuna, J.M., and Sherman, S.L. (2001). FMR1 and the fragile X syndrome: human genome epidemiology review. Genet Med 3, 359–371.

Dauer, W., and Przedborski, S. (2003). Parkinson's disease: mechanisms and models. Neuron 39, 889–909.

Davis, K.L., Kahn, R.S., Ko, G., and Davidson, M. (1991). Dopamine in schizophrenia: a review and reconceptualization. Am J Psychiatry 148, 1474–1486.

DeFelipe, J., Alonso-Nanclares, L., and Arellano, J.I. (2002). Microstructure of the neocortex: comparative aspects. J Neurocytol 31, 299–316.

Dierssen, M. (2012). Down syndrome: the brain in trisomic mode. Nat Rev Neurosci 13, 844–858.

Eiges, R., Urbach, A., Malcov, M., Frumkin, T., Schwartz, T., Amit, A., Yaron, Y., Eden, A., Yanuka, O., Benvenisty, N., et al. (2007). Developmental study of fragile X syndrome using human embryonic stem cells derived from preimplantation genetically diagnosed embryos. Cell Stem Cell 1, 568–577.

Eiraku, M., Watanabe, K., Matsuo-Takasaki, M., Kawada, M., Yonemura, S., Matsumura, M., Wataya, T., Nishiyama, A., Muguruma, K., and Sasai, Y. (2008). Self-organized formation of polarized cortical tissues from ESCs and its active manipulation by extrinsic signals. Cell Stem Cell 3, 519–532.

Elsea, S.H., and Lucas, R.E. (2002). The mousetrap: what we can learn when the mouse model does not mimic the human disease. ILAR J 43, 66–79.

Ernst, M., Zametkin, A.J., Matochik, J.A., Pascualvaca, D., and Cohen, R.M. (1997). Low medial prefrontal dopaminergic activity in autistic children. Lancet 350, 638.

Evans, M. (2011). Discovering pluripotency: 30 years of mouse embryonic stem cells. Nat Rev Mol Cell Biol 12, 680–686.

Evans, M.J., and Kaufman, M.H. (1981). Establishment in culture of pluripotential cells from mouse embryos. Nature 292, 154–156.

Fasano, C.A., Chambers, S.M., Lee, G., Tomishima, M.J., and Studer, L. (2010). Efficient derivation of functional floor plate tissue from human embryonic stem cells. Cell Stem Cell 6, 336–347.

Felleman, D.J., and Van Essen, D.C. (1991). Distributed hierarchical processing in the primate cerebral cortex. Cereb Cortex 1, 1–47.

Ferrer, I., and Gullotta, F. (1990). Down's syndrome and Alzheimer's disease: dendritic spine counts in the hippocampus. Acta Neuropathol 79, 680–685.

Freedman, R. (2003). Schizophrenia. N Engl J Med 349, 1738–1749.

Gaspard, N., Bouschet, T., Hourez, R., Dimid-schstein, J., Naeije, G., van den Ameele, J., Espuny-Camacho, I., Herpoel, A., Passante, L., Schiffmann, S.N., et al. (2008). An intrinsic mechanism of corticogenesis from embryonic stem cells. Nature 455, 351–357.

Geschwind, D.H., and Levitt, P. (2007). Autism spectrum disorders: developmental disconnection syndromes. Curr Opin Neurobiol 17, 103–111.

Goldstone, A.P. (2004). Prader-Willi syndrome: advances in genetics, pathophysiology and treatment. Trends Endocrinol Metab 15, 12–20.

Gurdon, J.B. (1962). The developmental capacity of nuclei taken from intestinal epithelium cells of feeding tadpoles. J Embryol Exp Morphol 10, 622–640.

Hansen, D.V., Lui, J.H., Parker, P.R., and Kriegstein, A.R. (2010). Neurogenic radial glia in the outer subventricular zone of human neocortex. Nature 464, 554–561.

Harrison, P.J. (1999). The neuropathology of schizophrenia. A critical review of the data and their interpretation. Brain 122 (Pt 4), 593–624.

Heard, E. (2005). Delving into the diversity of facultative heterochromatin: the epigenetics of the inactive X chromosome. Curr Opin Genet Dev 15, 482–489.

Hooper, M., Hardy, K., Handyside, A., Hunter, S., and Monk, M. (1987). HPRT-deficient (Lesch-Nyhan) mouse embryos derived from germline colonization by cultured cells. Nature 326, 292–295.

Israel, M.A., Yuan, S.H., Bardy, C., Reyna, S.M., Mu, Y., Herrera, C., Hefferan, M.P., Van Gorp, S., Nazor, K.L., Boscolo, F.S., et al. (2012). Probing sporadic and familial Alzheimer's disease using induced pluripotent stem cells. Nature 482, 216–220.

Itzhaki, I., Maizels, L., Huber, I., Zwi-Dantsis, L., Caspi, O., Winterstern, A., Feldman, O., Gepstein, A., Arbel, G., Hammerman, H., et al. (2011). Modelling the long QT syndrome with induced pluripotent stem cells. Nature 471, 225–229.

Jiang, J., Jing, Y., Cost, G.J., Chiang, J.C., Kolpa, H.J., Cotton, A.M., Carone, D.M., Carone, B.R., Shivak, D.A., Guschin, D.Y., et al. (2013). Translating dosage compensation to trisomy 21. Nature 500, 296–300.

Jinnah, H.A., De Gregorio, L., Harris, J.C., Nyhan, W.L., and O'Neill, J.P. (2000). The spectrum of inherited mutations causing HPRT deficiency: 75 new cases and a review of 196 previously reported cases. Mutat Res 463, 309–326.

Kadoshima, T., Sakaguchi, H., Nakano, T., Soen, M., Ando, S., Eiraku, M., and Sasai, Y. (2013). Self-organization of axial polarity, inside-out layer pattern, and species-specific progenitor dynamics in human ES cell-derived neocortex. Proc Natl Acad Sci U S A 110, 20284–20289.

Kandel, E.R. (2012). Principles of Neural Science. New York: McGraw-Hill.

Karumbayaram, S., Novitch, B.G., Patterson, M., Umbach, J.A., Richter, L., Lindgren, A., Conway, A.E., Clark, A.T., Goldman, S.A., Plath, K., et al. (2009). Directed differentiation of human-induced pluripotent stem cells generates active motor neurons. Stem Cells 27, 806–811.

Konno, D., Shioi, G., Shitamukai, A., Mori, A., Kiyonari, H., Miyata, T., and Matsuzaki, F. (2008). Neuroepithelial progenitors undergo LGN-dependent planar divisions to maintain self-renewability during mammalian neurogenesis. Nat Cell Biol 10, 93–101.

Krey, J.F., Pasca, S.P., Shcheglovitov, A., Yazawa, M., Schwemberger, R., Rasmusson, R., and Dolmetsch, R.E. (2013). Timothy syndrome is associated with activity-dependent dendritic retraction in rodent and human neurons. Nat Neurosci 16, 201–209.

Kriegstein, A., Noctor, S., and Martinez-Cerdeno, V. (2006). Patterns of neural stem and progenitor cell division may underlie evolutionary cortical expansion. Nat Rev Neurosci 7, 883–890.

Kriks, S., Shim, J.W., Piao, J., Ganat, Y.M., Wakeman, D.R., Xie, Z., Carrillo-Reid, L., Auyeung, G., Antonacci, C., Buch, A., et al. (2011). Dopamine neurons derived from human ES cells efficiently engraft in animal models of Parkinson's disease. Nature 480, 547–551.

Kuehn, M.R., Bradley, A., Robertson, E.J., and Evans, M.J. (1987). A potential animal model for Lesch-Nyhan syndrome through introduction of HPRT mutations into mice. Nature 326, 295–298.

Ladewig, J., Mertens, J., Kesavan, J., Doerr, J., Poppe, D., Glaue, F., Herms, S., Wernet, P., Kogler, G., Muller, F.J., et al. (2012). Small molecules enable highly efficient neuronal conversion of human fibroblasts. Nature methods 9, 575–578.

Lancaster, M.A., Renner, M., Martin, C.A., Wenzel, D., Bicknell, L.S., Hurles, M.E., Homfray, T., Penninger, J.M., Jackson, A.P., and Knoblich,

J.A. (2013). Cerebral organoids model human brain development and microcephaly. Nature 501, 373–379.

Lavdas, A.A., Grigoriou, M., Pachnis, V., and Parnavelas, J.G. (1999). The medial ganglionic eminence gives rise to a population of early neurons in the developing cerebral cortex. J Neurosci 19, 7881–7888.

Lewis, D.A., Curley, A.A., Glausier, J.R., and Volk, D.W. (2012). Cortical parvalbumin interneurons and cognitive dysfunction in schizophrenia. Trends Neurosci 35, 57–67.

Li, W., Wang, X., Fan, W., Zhao, P., Chan, Y.C., Chen, S., Zhang, S., Guo, X., Zhang, Y., Li, Y., et al. (2012). Modeling abnormal early development with induced pluripotent stem cells from aneuploid syndromes. Hum Mol Genet 21, 32–45.

Li, X.J., Du, Z.W., Zarnowska, E.D., Pankratz, M., Hansen, L.O., Pearce, R.A., and Zhang, S.C. (2005). Specification of motoneurons from human embryonic stem cells. Nat Biotechnol 23, 215–221.

Liu, Y., Weick, J.P., Liu, H., Krencik, R., Zhang, X., Ma, L., Zhou, G.-m., Ayala, M., and Zhang, S.-C. (2013). Medial ganglionic eminence-like cells derived from human embryonic stem cells correct learning and memory deficits. Nat Biotech 31, 440–447.

Lowry, W.E., Richter, L., Yachechko, R., Pyle, A.D., Tchieu, J., Sridharan, R., Clark, A.T., and Plath, K. (2008). Generation of human induced pluripotent stem cells from dermal fibroblasts. Proc Natl Acad Sci U S A 105, 2883–2888.

Marchetto, M.C., Carromeu, C., Acab, A., Yu, D., Yeo, G.W., Mu, Y., Chen, G., Gage, F.H., and Muotri, A.R. (2010). A model for neural development and treatment of Rett syndrome using human induced pluripotent stem cells. Cell 143, 527–539.

Markram, H., Toledo-Rodriguez, M., Wang, Y., Gupta, A., Silberberg, G., and Wu, C. (2004). Interneurons of the neocortical inhibitory system. Nat Rev Neurosci 5, 793–807.

Maroof, A.M., Keros, S., Tyson, J.A., Ying, S.W., Ganat, Y.M., Merkle, F.T., Liu, B., Goulburn, A., Stanley, E.G., Elefanty, A.G., et al. (2013). Directed differentiation and functional maturation of cortical interneurons from human embryonic stem cells. Cell Stem Cell 12, 559–572.

Martin, G.R. (1981). Isolation of a pluripotent cell line from early mouse embryos cultured in medium

conditioned by teratocarcinoma stem cells. Proc Natl Acad Sci U S A 78, 7634–7638.

Mekhoubad, S., Bock, C., de Boer, A.S., Kiskinis, E., Meissner, A., and Eggan, K. (2012). Erosion of dosage compensation impacts human iPSC disease modeling. Cell Stem Cell 10, 595–609.

Mitchell, K.J. (2011). The genetics of neurodevelopmental disease. Curr Opin Neurobiol 21, 197–203.

Moy, S.S., Nadler, J.J., Magnuson, T.R., and Crawley, J.N. (2006). Mouse models of autism spectrum disorders: the challenge for behavioral genetics. Am J Med Genet C Semin Med Genet 142C, 40–51.

Nakano, T., Ando, S., Takata, N., Kawada, M., Muguruma, K., Sekiguchi, K., Saito, K., Yonemura, S., Eiraku, M., and Sasai, Y. (2012). Self-formation of optic cups and storable stratified neural retina from human ESCs. Cell Stem Cell 10, 771–785.

Neale, B.M., Kou, Y., Liu, L., Ma'ayan, A., Samocha, K.E., Sabo, A., Lin, C.F., Stevens, C., Wang, L.S., Makarov, V., et al. (2012). Patterns and rates of exonic de novo mutations in autism spectrum disorders. Nature 485, 242–245.

Nicholas, C.R., Chen, J., Tang, Y., Southwell, D.G., Chalmers, N., Vogt, D., Arnold, C.M., Chen, Y.J., Stanley, E.G., Elefanty, A.G., et al. (2013). Functional maturation of hPSC-derived forebrain interneurons requires an extended timeline and mimics human neural development. Cell Stem Cell 12, 573–586.

O'Doherty, A., Ruf, S., Mulligan, C., Hildreth, V., Errington, M.L., Cooke, S., Sesay, A., Modino, S., Vanes, L., Hernandez, D., et al. (2005). An aneuploid mouse strain carrying human chromosome 21 with Down syndrome phenotypes. Science 309, 2033–2037.

O'Roak, B.J., Vives, L., Girirajan, S., Karakoc, E., Krumm, N., Coe, B.P., Levy, R., Ko, A., Lee, C., Smith, J.D., et al. (2012). Sporadic autism exomes reveal a highly interconnected protein network of de novo mutations. Nature 485, 246–250.

Odorico, J.S., Kaufman, D.S., and Thomson, J.A. (2001). Multilineage differentiation from human embryonic stem cell lines. Stem Cells 19, 193–204.

Pakkenberg, B., and Gundersen, H.J. (1997). Neocortical neuron number in humans: effect of sex and age. J Comp Neurol 384, 312–320.

Pang, Z.P., Yang, N., Vierbuchen, T., Ostermeier, A., Fuentes, D.R., Yang, T.Q., Citri, A., Sebastiano, V., Marro, S., Sudhof, T.C., et al. (2011). Induction of human neuronal cells by defined transcription factors. Nature 476, 220–223.

Park, I.H., Arora, N., Huo, H., Maherali, N., Ahfeldt, T., Shimamura, A., Lensch, M.W., Cowan, C., Hochedlinger, K., and Daley, G.Q. (2008). Disease-specific induced pluripotent stem cells. Cell 134, 877–886.

Pasca, S.P., Portmann, T., Voineagu, I., Yazawa, M., Shcheglovitov, A., Pasca, A.M., Cord, B., Palmer, T.D., Chikahisa, S., Nishino, S., et al. (2011). Using iPSC-derived neurons to uncover cellular phenotypes associated with Timothy syndrome. Nat Med 17, 1657–1662.

Perrier, A.L., Tabar, V., Barberi, T., Rubio, M.E., Bruses, J., Topf, N., Harrison, N.L., and Studer, L. (2004). Derivation of midbrain dopamine neurons from human embryonic stem cells. Proc Natl Acad Sci U S A 101, 12543–12548.

Petersen, M.B., Adelsberger, P.A., Schinzel, A.A., Binkert, F., Hinkel, G.K., and Antonarakis, S.E. (1991). Down syndrome due to de novo Robertsonian translocation t(14q;21q): DNA polymorphism analysis suggests that the origin of the extra 21q is maternal. Am J Hum Genet 49, 529–536.

Powell, E.M., Campbell, D.B., Stanwood, G.D., Davis, C., Noebels, J.L., and Levitt, P. (2003). Genetic disruption of cortical interneuron development causes region- and GABA cell type-specific deficits, epilepsy, and behavioral dysfunction. J Neurosci 23, 622–631.

Raedler, T.J., Knable, M.B., and Weinberger, D.R. (1998). Schizophrenia as a developmental disorder of the cerebral cortex. Curr Opin Neurobiol 8, 157–161.

Rakic, P. (2009). Evolution of the neocortex: a perspective from developmental biology. Nat Rev Neurosci 10, 724–735.

Reeves, R.H., Irving, N.G., Moran, T.H., Wohn, A., Kitt, C., Sisodia, S.S., Schmidt, C., Bronson, R.T., and Davisson, M.T. (1995). A mouse model for Down syndrome exhibits learning and behaviour deficits. Nat Genet 11, 177–184.

Richardson, J.A., and Burns, D.K. (2002). Mouse models of Alzheimer's disease: a quest for plaques and tangles. ILAR J 43, 89–99.

Ross, M.H., Galaburda, A.M., and Kemper, T.L. (1984). Down's syndrome: is there a decreased population of neurons? Neurology 34, 909–916.

Rumble, B., Retallack, R., Hilbich, C., Simms, G., Multhaup, G., Martins, R., Hockey, A., Montgomery, P., Beyreuther, K., and Masters, C.L.

(1989). Amyloid A4 protein and its precursor in Down's syndrome and Alzheimer's disease. N Engl J Med 320, 1446–1452.

Sanders, S.J., Murtha, M.T., Gupta, A.R., Murdoch, J.D., Raubeson, M.J., Willsey, A.J., Ercan-Sencicek, A.G., DiLullo, N.M., Parikshak, N.N., Stein, J.L., et al. (2012). De novo mutations revealed by whole-exome sequencing are strongly associated with autism. Nature 485, 237–241.

Saud, K., Arriagada, C., Cardenas, A.M., Shimahara, T., Allen, D.D., Caviedes, R., and Caviedes, P. (2006). Neuronal dysfunction in Down syndrome: contribution of neuronal models in cell culture. J Physiol Paris 99, 201–210.

Schmidt-Sidor, B., Wisniewski, K.E., Shepard, T.H., and Sersen, E.A. (1990). Brain growth in Down syndrome subjects 15 to 22 weeks of gestational age and birth to 60 months. Clin Neuropathol 9, 181–190.

Schuz, A., and Palm, G. (1989). Density of neurons and synapses in the cerebral cortex of the mouse. J Comp Neurol 286, 442–455.

Sheridan, S.D., Theriault, K.M., Reis, S.A., Zhou, F., Madison, J.M., Daheron, L., Loring, J.F., and Haggarty, S.J. (2011). Epigenetic characterization of the FMR1 gene and aberrant neurodevelopment in human induced pluripotent stem cell models of fragile X syndrome. PLoS One 6, e26203.

Shi, Y., Kirwan, P., and Livesey, F.J. (2012a). Directed differentiation of human pluripotent stem cells to cerebral cortex neurons and neural networks. Nat Protoc 7, 1836–1846.

Shi, Y., Kirwan, P., Smith, J., MacLean, G., Orkin, S.H., and Livesey, F.J. (2012b). A human stem cell model of early Alzheimer's disease pathology in Down syndrome. Sci Transl Med 4, 124ra129.

Shi, Y., Kirwan, P., Smith, J., Robinson, H.P., and Livesey, F.J. (2012c). Human cerebral cortex development from pluripotent stem cells to functional excitatory synapses. Nat Neurosci 15, 477–486, S471.

Song, B., Sun, G., Herszfeld, D., Sylvain, A., Campanale, N.V., Hirst, C.E., Caine, S., Parkington, H.C., Tonta, M.A., Coleman, H.A., et al. (2012). Neural differentiation of patient specific iPS cells as a novel approach to study the pathophysiology of multiple sclerosis. Stem Cell Res 8, 259–273.

Splawski, I., Timothy, K.W., Sharpe, L.M., Decher, N., Kumar, P., Bloise, R., Napolitano, C., Schwartz, P.J., Joseph, R.M., Condouris, K., et al. (2004). Ca(V)1.2 calcium channel dys-function causes a multisystem disorder including arrhythmia and autism. Cell 119, 19–31.

Stefansson, H., Rujescu, D., Cichon, S., Pietilainen, O.P., Ingason, A., Steinberg, S., Fossdal, R., Sigurdsson, E., Sigmundsson, T., Buizer-Voskamp, J.E., et al. (2008). Large recurrent microdeletions associated with schizophrenia. Nature 455, 232–236.

Stone, J.L., O'Donovan, M.C., Gurling, H., Kirov, G.K., Blackwood, D.H., Corvin, A., Craddock, N.J., Gill, M., Hultman, C.M., and Lichtenstein, P. (2008). Rare chromosomal deletions and duplications increase risk of schizophrenia. Nature 455, 237–241.

Sullivan, P.F., Kendler, K.S., and Neale, M.C. (2003). Schizophrenia as a complex trait: evidence from a meta-analysis of twin studies. Arch Gen Psychiatry 60, 1187–1192.

Sun, Y., Pollard, S., Conti, L., Toselli, M., Biella, G., Parkin, G., Willatt, L., Falk, A., Cattaneo, E., and Smith, A. (2008). Long-term tripotent differentiation capacity of human neural stem (NS) cells in adherent culture. Mol Cell Neurosci 38, 245–258.

Takahashi, K., Tanabe, K., Ohnuki, M., Narita, M., Ichisaka, T., Tomoda, K., and Yamanaka, S. (2007). Induction of pluripotent stem cells from adult human fibroblasts by defined factors. Cell 131, 861–872.

Takahashi, K., and Yamanaka, S. (2006). Induction of pluripotent stem cells from mouse embryonic and adult fibroblast cultures by defined factors. Cell 126, 663–676.

Takashima, S., Becker, L.E., Armstrong, D.L., and Chan, F.W. (1981). Abnormal Neuronal Development in the Visual-Cortex of the Human-Fetus and Infant with Downs-Syndrome - a Quantitative and Qualitative Golgi-Study. Brain Res 225, 1–21.

Thomas, K.R., and Capecchi, M.R. (1987). Site-directed mutagenesis by gene targeting in mouse embryo-derived stem cells. Cell 51, 503–512.

Thomson, J.A., Itskovitz-Eldor, J., Shapiro, S.S., Waknitz, M.A., Swiergiel, J.J., Marshall, V.S., and Jones, J.M. (1998). Embryonic stem cell lines derived from human blastocysts. Science 282, 1145–1147.

Urbach, A., Bar-Nur, O., Daley, G.Q., and Benvenisty, N. (2010). Differential modeling of fragile X syndrome by human embryonic stem cells and

induced pluripotent stem cells. Cell Stem Cell 6, 407–411.

Vacano, G.N., Duval, N., and Patterson, D. (2012). The use of mouse models for understanding the biology of down syndrome and aging. Curr Gerontol Geriatr Res 2012, 717315.

van der Worp, H.B., Howells, D.W., Sena, E.S., Porritt, M.J., Rewell, S., O'Collins, V., and Macleod, M.R. (2010). Can animal models of disease reliably inform human studies? PLoS Med 7, e1000245.

Verlinsky, Y., Strelchenko, N., Kukharenko, V., Rechitsky, S., Verlinsky, O., Galat, V., and Kuliev, A. (2005). Human embryonic stem cell lines with genetic disorders. Reprod Biomed Online 10, 105–110.

Vierbuchen, T., Ostermeier, A., Pang, Z.P., Kokubu, Y., Sudhof, T.C., and Wernig, M. (2010). Direct conversion of fibroblasts to functional neurons by defined factors. Nature 463, 1035–1041.

Walsh, T., McClellan, J.M., McCarthy, S.E., Addington, A.M., Pierce, S.B., Cooper, G.M., Nord, A.S., Kusenda, M., Malhotra, D., Bhandari, A., et al. (2008). Rare structural variants disrupt multiple genes in neurodevelopmental pathways in schizophrenia. Science 320, 539–543.

Wang, H., and Doering, L.C. (2012). Induced pluripotent stem cells to model and treat neurogenetic disorders. Neural Plast 2012, 346053.

Weick, J.P., Held, D.L., Bonadurer, G.F., 3rd, Doers, M.E., Liu, Y., Maguire, C., Clark, A., Knackert, J.A., Molinarolo, K., Musser, M., et al. (2013). Deficits in human trisomy 21 iPSCs and neurons. Proc Natl Acad Sci U S A 110, 9962–9967.

Wichterle, H., Lieberam, I., Porter, J.A., and Jessell, T.M. (2002). Directed differentiation of embryonic stem cells into motor neurons. Cell 110, 385–397.

Williams, C.A., Driscoll, D.J., and Dagli, A.I. (2010). Clinical and genetic aspects of Angelman syndrome. Genet Med 12, 385–395.

Williams, L.A., Davis-Dusenbery, B.N., and Eggan, K.C. (2012). SnapShot: directed differentiation of pluripotent stem cells. Cell 149, 1174–1174 e1171.

Wilson, S.W., and Rubenstein, J.L. (2000). Induction and dorsoventral patterning of the telencephalon. Neuron 28, 641–651.

Wiseman, F.K., Alford, K.A., Tybulewicz, V.L., and Fisher, E.M. (2009). Down syndrome--recent progress and future prospects. Hum Mol Genet 18, R75–R83.

Woods, C.G., Bond, J., and Enard, W. (2005). Autosomal recessive primary microcephaly (MCPH): a review of clinical, molecular, and evolutionary findings. Am J Hum Genet 76, 717–728.

Yang, J., Cai, J., Zhang, Y., Wang, X., Li, W., Xu, J., Li, F., Guo, X., Deng, K., Zhong, M., et al. (2010). Induced pluripotent stem cells can be used to model the genomic imprinting disorder Prader-Willi syndrome. J Biol Chem 285, 40303–40311.

Ye, Z., Zhan, H., Mali, P., Dowey, S., Williams, D.M., Jang, Y.Y., Dang, C.V., Spivak, J.L., Moliterno, A.R., and Cheng, L. (2009). Human-induced pluripotent stem cells from blood cells of healthy donors and patients with acquired blood disorders. Blood 114, 5473–5480.

Yingling, J., Youn, Y.H., Darling, D., Toyo-Oka, K., Pramparo, T., Hirotsune, S., and Wynshaw-Boris, A. (2008). Neuroepithelial stem cell proliferation requires LIS1 for precise spindle orientation and symmetric division. Cell 132, 474–486.

Yoo, A.S., Sun, A.X., Li, L., Shcheglovitov, A., Portmann, T., Li, Y., Lee-Messer, C., Dolmetsch, R.E., Tsien, R.W., and Crabtree, G.R. (2011). MicroRNA-mediated conversion of human fibroblasts to neurons. Nature 476, 228–231.

Zhang, S.C., Wernig, M., Duncan, I.D., Brustle, O., and Thomson, J.A. (2001). In vitro differentiation of transplantable neural precursors from human embryonic stem cells. Nat Biotechnol 19, 1129–1133.

11

ANIMAL MODELS FOR NEURODEVELOPMENTAL DISORDERS

HALA HARONY-NICOLAS AND JOSEPH D. BUXBAUM

Seaver Autism Center for Research and Treatment, Departments of Psychiatry, Neuroscience, and Genetics and Genomic Sciences, The Friedman Brain Institute and the Mindich Child Health and Development Institute, Icahn School of Medicine at Mount Sinai, New York, NY, USA

11.1 ANIMAL MODELS – WHAT ARE THEY GOOD FOR?

Using animal models, we have the power to investigate a hypothesis around the pathological effect of specific disease-associated genes, while overcoming confounds common in human studies. These include, but are not limited to, the restricted number of participating subjects and the inability to perfectly control environmental or other factors that could interfere with the interpretation of the findings. Animal models provide us with unlimited supply of high number of subjects to attain significant results and with the ability to conduct controlled experiments, manipulating one variable at a time. In regard of neurodevelopmental disorders, where the brain is often the focus of the research studies, the use of animal models is essential and complementary to studies in humans for multiple reasons. Animal models can be used for more invasive approaches (e.g., electrophysiological recordings necessary for the study of brain activity) and for the acquisition of brain tissues for molecular, morphological, and brain structural studies. Although human postmortem tissues from subjects with neurodevelopmental disorders are available, their usage is limited to a few approaches and is further constrained by the availability and quality of the tissues. In addition, these tissues are not useful for developmental studies, which can be carried in animal models, especially with their relatively short gestation period, lifespan, and reproductive cycle. Animal models are also widely applied for drug discovery research. This includes the basic steps in target identifications, which evolves from basic research in these models, and drug screening, which is followed by preclinical studies of drug safety and efficacy. One of the

The Genetics of Neurodevelopmental Disorders, First Edition. Edited by Kevin J. Mitchell.
© 2015 John Wiley & Sons, Inc. Published 2015 by John Wiley & Sons, Inc.

most intriguing findings in recent years is the observation that cetrain phenotypes, caused by mutations in some neurodevelopmental genes, can be reversed by reactivating the gene, even in adulthood (Silva and Ehninger, 2009). Such studies cannot be approached in humans. In addition, mutagenesis to identify modifier loci will always be restricted to animal models, but yet has the potential to identify important pathways for intervention (see subsequent sections). Altogether, animal models represent a key tool in understanding the pathobiology of neurodevelopmental disorders and in developing optimal pharmacological treatments for these disorders.

11.2   DEFINING VALIDITY

Traditionally, there have been three ways for relating to the validity of a model system: face, construct, and predictive validity (note, however, that these terms are used differently in other branches of science). In the context of neurodevelopmental disorders, face validity refers to the ability of a model to successfully capture aspects of the observed phenotype. This is, of course, a subjective assessment and hence subject to strong bias and ever-changing norms. For example, much is made about social deficits in mice as showing face validity to autism; however, this is an artificial construct. That, for example, when a mouse spends less time with familiar, as compared to a novel, conspecific, this is somehow related to the social deficits in autism, is certainly open to debate. Yet, such tests have become almost required for rodent models of autism. Moreover, as discussed subsequently, there is little evidence that specific gene mutations in human are exclusively present with this or that phenotype. Thus, there is no strong *priori* reason to assume that pathological changes in brain development will necessarily produce only one specific behavioral phenotype.

Construct validity refers to the use of a proven biological cause in a model system. For example, the introduction of a mutation in a gene known to cause a specific neurodevelopmental disorder, or the exposure of an animal to an agent known to cause such a disorder would be examples of approaches with construct validity. Construct validity can also reflect current biases. As discussed further below, the field of neurodevelopmental disorders research went through a long period of candidate gene approaches, but most of those early findings were likely in error. Models with mutations in such genes were thought to have construct validity, which would be challenged now. Clearly, the more solid the data on a given biological cause, the more one would ascribe construct validity to a model incorporating that biological cause.

Predictive validity is a measure of the degree to which a treatment in a model system predicts effective treatment in humans. The universe of model systems is littered with extensive and compelling treatment studies in models with both construct and face validity, with little or no subsequent evidence for predictive validity. The example of early cancer research is an instructive one. After the transplantation of *bona fide* human cancer cells (construct validity) into mice, leading to cancerous lesions that for all intents and purposes look like the human counterparts (face validity), treatments that were effective in those mice often were overwhelmingly ineffective in patients (lack of predictive validity). The failure rate for cancer drugs overall has been estimated as higher than that for all therapies, in spite of what is very compelling face and/or construct validity. Focusing on the psychiatry field, one of the reasons leading to such a high failure rate relies in the approach adopted for evaluating predictive validity of new models, where the criteria for responsiveness to a newly tested drugs are based on the output measures obtained from a routinely applied drug. This approach would reveal, if at all, new drugs with a mechanism of action similar to those already in use.

11.3   IF YOU HAD TO CHOOSE JUST ONE …

A current trend in research of neurodevelopmental disorders is the use of models with construct validity. There are several reasons for this trend. First, discoveries as to etiology are currently incredibly successful and a functional follow up of such findings is a logical next step. Second, historical efforts in models with face validity did not produce very many insights into neurodevelopmental disorders (for example, studies of forward genetics in mouse social behavior). Third, and, in our perspective, most importantly, defining face validity is fraught with biases, while, the etiologically-based approaches allow for unbiased findings of associated phenotypes (particularly intermediate phenotypes, which we would prefer to call intervening phenotypes). It goes without saying that if there were models with proven predictive validity, they would be ideal but, until that time, it would appear that construct validity is a direction most likely to lead to improved therapeutics (see examples below). It is of course the hope that models with construct validity will also show aspects of both face and predictive validity.

11.4 UNDERSTANDING PENETRANCE AND VARIABLE EXPRESSIVITY

For any etiological cause of neurodevelopmental disorders, one must consider the two related parameters of penetrance and variable expressivity. Penetrance is defined in genetics as the proportion of individuals carrying a specific genetic variant that also express a particular phenotype. Variable expressivity is a term meant to capture the diversity of phenotypes associated with a specific genetic variant. To take concrete examples, there are no examples of mutations in genes that are 100% penetrant for an autism phenotype. None of the monogenic disorders that are associated with high risk for autism (e.g., Fragile X, Rett, and Phelan-McDermid syndromes) are 100% penetrant for autism. In contrast, many such mutations are highly penetrant (and, in some examples, even completely penetrant) for a profound neurodevelopmental disorder. For example, the same X-linked *NLGN4* mutations can lead to intellectual disability (ID) with or without autism or less

severe developmental disorders (Laumonnier et al., 2004). Hence, if one considers a broader range of phenotypes (i.e., incorporating variable expressivity), penetrance can be much higher for a given genetic variant (for example see (Kirov et al., 2014; Stefansson et al., 2014)). The causes of reduced penetrance and variable expressivity are not completely understood but can include other modifier genetic loci (including genetic "background"), somatic or mitochondrial changes, and environmental or stochastic effects, some of which may be mediated by epigenetic effects.

When one considers the incomplete penetrance and variable expressivity associated with human mutations, it is surprising the degree to which the field of neurodevelopmental disorders research still emphasizes particular phenotypic manifestations in model systems. It should be clear that since a proportion of patients with, for example, *FMR1*, *MECP2*, *SHANK3*, or (as noted earlier) *NLGN4* mutations do not have autism, expecting that a corresponding animal model must have social abnormalities, communication deficits, and repetitive behaviors is a departure from evidence-driven face validity. Going even further, some loci with high risk for ID and autism also confer high risk for schizophrenia [e.g., copy number variation (CNV) at 16p11.2 or 22q11] – clearly it is not realistic to assume that a mouse model recapitulating such CNV must *necessarily* have an autism and/or a schizophrenia phenotype.

11.5 WHAT SHOULD WE EXPECT TO OBSERVE?

We recently took an unbiased look at both human and mouse phenotypes (MPs) associated with genes that, when mutated, are highly penetrant for neurodevelopmental disorders, and found that neurological phenotypes were the more common behavioral findings (Buxbaum et al., 2012). The list of genes we analyzed had all been associated with autism (syndromic or not). We classified four types of neurobiological phenotypes associated with disruption of a large proportion of the autism genes, including, (1) changes in brain and neuronal morphology, (2) electrophysiological changes, (3) neurological changes, and (4) higher-order behavioral changes. We think that it was significant that in both mouse and human databases, many of the behavioral alterations were neurological changes (for example, sensory alterations, motor abnormalities, and seizures), as opposed to higher-order behavioral changes (for example, learning and memory or social behavior changes). Similarly, a recent study using autism associated *de novo* CNV, and looking for MPs associated with the disrupted genes, observed seven classes of changes: abnormal ear physiology & abnormal hearing physiology, abnormal synaptic transmission, presence of seizures, abnormal motor capabilities/coordination/movement, abnormal emotion/affect behavior, abnormal learning/memory/conditioning, and abnormal social/conspecific interaction (Noh et al., 2013). In considering recent findings, that neurological changes (specifically, motor) are predictors of autism risk in high-risk infants [e.g., (Bhat et al., 2012)], the convergent findings of predominant neurological signs in both mice and patients with mutations in autism genes appear particularly relevant.

Since we are considering neurodevelopmental disorders broadly in this chapter, one can also look at similar approaches with genes implicated in ID but not yet autism, or genes implicated in epilepsy. To look at ID, we made use of a gene list compiled by Dr. Catalina Betancur and used in a prior publication [see (Neale et al., 2012) and the supplement there for a list of these genes]. Carrying out analyses identical to those we used before (Buxbaum et al., 2012), we observed strikingly similar patterns of phenotypes in the mouse and human phenotype databases. ID genes, such as autism genes, when mutated, produce neuronal and brain morphology changes, sensory changes, and motor abnormalities [see Table 11.1 for the top 25 enriched MP terms]. Structural changes and neurological features were also prominent

among enriched terms when examining the human phenotype databases (data not shown).

For epilepsy, we took all genes from a curated website (http://epilepsy.hardwicklab.org/list.php) and ran the enrichment analyses. Seizures and abnormalities in electrophysiology were prominent as expected, but sensory and motor abnormalities were common, and there was evidence for morphological changes (see Table 11.2 for the top 30 enriched terms).

11.6 A PROPOSED FOUR-TIERED ANALYSIS OF ANIMAL MODELS FOR NEURODEVELOPMENTAL DISORDERS

Altogether, we think the overlapping findings between autism, ID, and epilepsy provide a useful roadmap for analysis of animal models for neurodevelopmental disorders. The models can be (1) scored for morphological changes in neural cells and in brain regions, (2) examined for alterations in brain activity and connectivity, and can also be examined for changes in a broad array of behaviors, including those we classified as (3) neurological behaviors and those we classified as (4) higher order behaviors. This four-tiered approach provides opportunities to identify expected and unexpected phenotypes, including intermediate/intervening phenotypes that can be very useful for understanding pathophysiology, and for considering neurobiologically driven novel therapeutics. This approach also simplifies the integration of analyses across model systems. Cellular models (including induced pluripotent stem cells) could be analyzed for morphological and electrophysiological changes. Simple animal models (such as *C.elegans* and *Drosophila*) could be analyzed at these levels and at a higher level for sensory and neurological changes, while more complex animal models could be analyzed at all four levels. Specific examples of analyses at these four tiers can be found in our prior publication (Buxbaum et al., 2012), which could be expanded upon to better capture epilepsy and ID-related phenotypes and which should also include modern systems level analyses (see next section).

TABLE 11.1 **Enrichment of MP terms associated with mice with disruptions in ID genes** (*See insert for color representation of this table*)

ID	Name	*P*-value	Term in query	Term in genome
MP:0003632	Abnormal nervous system morphology	1.76E-16	108	1987
MP:0002152	Abnormal brain morphology	5.46E-10	72	1217
MP:0002882	Abnormal neuron morphology	1.65E-09	69	1157
MP:0002092	Abnormal eye morphology	5.70E-09	58	884
MP:0000788	Abnormal cerebral cortex morphology	1.12E-08	29	249
MP:0003861	Abnormal nervous system development	2.98E-08	58	919
MP:0008540	Abnormal cerebrum morphology	4.41E-08	37	420
MP:0005391	Vision/eye phenotype	1.36E-07	58	953
MP:0006069	Abnormal retinal neuronal layer morphology	3.63E-07	27	249
MP:0003728	Abnormal retinal photoreceptor layer morphology	9.80E-07	20	141
MP:0000428	Abnormal craniofacial morphology	1.90E-06	51	825
MP:0005382	Craniofacial phenotype	1.90E-06	51	825
MP:0000787	Abnormal telencephalon morphology	2.07E-06	41	573
MP:0003727	Abnormal retinal layer morphology	2.84E-06	28	292
MP:0003633	Abnormal nervous system physiology	1.17E-05	72	1490
MP:0001004	Abnormal retinal photoreceptor morphology	2.19E-05	18	135
MP:0003956	Abnormal body size	5.12E-05	82	1870
MP:0000783	Abnormal forebrain morphology	8.82E-05	44	729
MP:0003731	Abnormal retinal outer nuclear layer morphology	1.63E-04	15	105
MP:0010832	Lethality during fetal growth through weaning	1.77E-04	78	1782
MP:0006207	Embryonic lethality during organogenesis	2.61E-04	44	756
MP:0000952	Abnormal CNS glial cell morphology	2.70E-04	21	213
MP:0001265	Decreased body size	4.04E-04	73	1647
MP:0002066	Abnormal motor capabilities/coordination/ movement	4.46E-04	65	1392
MP:0000913	Abnormal brain development	5.08E-04	36	562

11.7 AN ADDED DIMENSION

While the proposed four-tiered analysis was based on publications to date, modern methods have been developed to examine rodents at the systems level. There are too few examples of systems level analyses in the older literature for this to be examined in an unbiased manner, but clearly one major advantage of animal models over both cellular models and studies in patients is the ability to look at such a level, including genome-wide expression analyses in multiple brain regions followed by co-expression analyses, as well as systems electrophysiological analyses, including in awake and behaving animals. As an example, synchrony deficits have been observed in

studies of *Fmr1* knockout mice using systems electrophysiological analyses. A first study showed that inhibitory postsynaptic currents were less synchronous in the somatosensory cortex (barrel cortex) of *Fmr1* knockout, consistent with altered fast-spiking inhibitory circuitry in these animals (Gibson et al., 2008). More recently, recordings from pyramidal neurons in the somatosensory cortex revealed reductions in synchronized synaptic inhibition and coordinated spike synchrony in response to the group I metabotropic glutamate receptor (mGluR) agonist 3,5-dihydroxyphenylglycine (DHPG) (Paluszkiewicz et al., 2011). *In vitro* studies with wild-type and mutant neuroligin-3 (*Nlgn3*) have demonstrated a role for Nlgn3 expression on synchrony. Expression of mutant

TABLE 11.2 Enrichment of MP terms associated with mice with disruptions in epilepsy genes (*See insert for color representation of this table*)

ID	Name	*P*-value	Term in query	Term in genome
MP:0002064	Seizures	2.87E-32	36	279
MP:0003633	Abnormal nervous system physiology	2.18E-22	51	1490
MP:0002272	Abnormal nervous system electrophysiology	3.57E-22	28	242
MP:0009357	Abnormal seizure response to inducing agent	7.62E-20	22	135
MP:0003216	Absence seizures	1.44E-16	13	31
MP:0000947	Convulsive seizures	1.01E-15	19	130
MP:0000948	Nonconvulsive seizures	1.56E-15	13	36
MP:0004994	Abnormal brain wave pattern	2.94E-15	14	49
MP:0003635	Abnormal synaptic transmission	5.18E-15	29	483
MP:0009745	Abnormal behavioral response to xenobiotic	7.02E-14	21	218
MP:0002206	Abnormal CNS synaptic transmission	1.90E-12	25	410
MP:0000950	Abnormal seizure response to pharmacological agent	2.10E-12	15	94
MP:0001516	Abnormal motor coordination/ balance	3.37E-12	29	613
MP:0002066	Abnormal motor capabilities/coordination/movement	1.49E-11	40	1392
MP:0001392	Abnormal locomotor behavior	3.09E-11	34	973
MP:0003492	Abnormal involuntary movement	4.10E-11	27	566
MP:0003491	Abnormal voluntary movement	2.38E-10	34	1041
MP:0002067	Abnormal sensory capabilities/reflexes/nociception	3.47E-10	26	564
MP:0008840	Abnormal spike wave discharge	1.43E-09	8	18
MP:0002906	Increased susceptibility to pharmacologically induced seizures	1.60E-09	12	74
MP:0003997	Tonic-clonic seizures	2.52E-09	11	58
MP:0003313	Abnormal locomotor activation	6.31E-09	27	696
MP:0001961	Abnormal reflex	1.06E-08	22	442
MP:0002063	Abnormal learning/memory/conditioning	2.07E-08	22	457
MP:0000743	Muscle spasm	2.44E-08	10	52
MP:0000745	Tremors	3.26E-08	16	212
MP:0009046	Muscle twitch	3.63E-08	10	54
MP:0001405	Impaired coordination	7.99E-08	18	303
MP:0000243	Myoclonus	9.50E-08	8	28
MP:0002152	Abnormal brain morphology	1.46E-07	33	1217

Nlgn3 does not promote synchrony to the degree of wild-type Nlgn3, and this could be traced to less complex network cytoarchitecture *in vitro* (Gutierrez et al., 2009). The application of multiunit recordings to awake and behaving models of autism will provide a means for revealing the deficits in neural microcircuits and neural synchrony within and between brain structures, thus enhancing our understanding of the relationship between cellular and behavioral manifestations (Del Pino et al., 2013; Sigurdsson et al., 2010).

11.8 CONVERGENT FINDINGS?

One argument for using similar assays across diverse animal models for disease is to determine whether there are findings that are shared across models. The more common a given disorder-related or intermediate/intervening phenotype is, the more useful it would be to target for pharmacotherapies as it might be that the treatment would be effective across a broader range of etiologies. However, we do need to manage expectations in this domain. Our prior analyses (Buxbaum et al., 2012) make it clear that different genetically modified mice show differing phenotypes, even when robust and reproducible assays are used. One clear example is that of electrophysiological changes: common measures such as hippocampal long-term potentiation (LTP) or long-term depression (LTD) differed across mice with mutations in various autism genes. Specific comparisons of two models by a single laboratory showed divergent electrophysiological findings as well, with *Fmr1* knockout mice displaying enhanced LTD and *Tsc2* heterozygous mice displaying reduced LTD (Auerbach et al., 2011). In these studies, a positive allosteric modulator (PAM) of metabotropic glutamate receptors was effective at reversing deficits in the *Tsc2* heterozygotes, while a negative allosteric modulator (NAM) was effective in *Fmr1* knockouts. This reminds us that the widely cited excitation/inhibition imbalance hypotheses for both epilepsy and autism spectrum disorder (ASD) would, as we put it before, "either have to be so nonspecific as to be not falsifiable, or, if specific, would not be supported by the data" (Buxbaum et al., 2012). A recent imaging study of 26 different genetically modified mice with relevance to autism, found divergent structural imaging findings (Ellegood et al., 2015). The authors proposed that the mouse models could be loosely organized into three main groups, which included a group where many brain regions tend to be larger than in controls, a group in which they tend to be smaller, and a third that was more variable. We give an example subsequently where a single agent shows efficacy in two different mouse models for neurodevelopmental disorders, which is an important area of convergence. In summary, convergent phenotypes would be tremendously important and will no doubt be identified, but are not likely to hold true for *all* possible etiologies of a given class of neurodevelopmental disorder.

11.9 GENERATING A GENETICALLY MODIFIED ANIMAL MODEL – TARGETING A GENE OR LOCUS

The steps toward generating a genetically modified animal model can be divided into choosing the gene or locus and choosing the most relevant targeting strategy. Note that while we will focus on genetically modified models, there is some overlap in strategy when considering other etiological models. Choosing a gene or locus sounds like an almost trivial step as there are any number of both interesting and relevant genes and loci that have been implicated in neurodevelopmental disorders. However, for every *bona fide* gene in the literature, there are currently as many that have not stood the test of time. Hence extreme caution is warranted.

One source of constant confusion is around genetic findings. In psychiatric disorders, like other complex disorders (Hirschhorn et al., 2002), candidate gene findings have not replicated in the vast number of cases. For autism, there is now good evidence that all common variant/common gene findings published to date have either greatly overestimated relative risk findings or are in fact false positives. To take an example of a gene that we have some affinity toward, *SLC25A12* has been associated with autism in three studies (but not in others) and, most importantly, the same single nucleotide polymorphism (SNP) was associated in all three studies with the same direction (Segurado et al., 2005; Turunen et al., 2008). We suggest that this represents some of the strongest evidence for a candidate gene in autism and yet, this gene was not found in three genome wide association studies (Anney et al., 2010; Wang et al., 2009; Weiss et al., 2009) (note also that the top findings from these three studies did not overlap). Most importantly, the genotype relative risk (GRR) that we estimated for the disorder-associated variant (> 2.0 for homozygotes) is simply not compatible with any findings of GRR in autism

(Devlin et al., 2011). In fact, this latter study shows that SNPs with effect sizes > 1.5 are not likely to be identified in autism (and more recent studies by the Psychiatric Genetic Consortium extend this even further such that SNPs with effect sizes > 1.2 are not likely to be identified in autism). It then becomes a simple exercise to look at published SNP association studies and ask whether the effect size is compatible with these findings. If not, then the original findings have greatly overestimated the effect size or are false positives. Note that, at least in autism, no published SNP studies to date are sufficiently powered (for example, 80% powered) to detect a variant with relative risk of 1.2 [see (Devlin et al., 2011)] so skepticism is warranted around published SNP association in autism. Even if the published findings are true, the effect size is likely to be overestimated, hence the construct validity of the model would be challenged, although such a model would still be useful for understanding gene function.

For rare genetic variations, there are two main sources of information. The first comes from careful analysis of recurrent variations by clinical geneticists [see (Betancur, 2011) for a curated list in autism]. The other comes from gene discovery carried out either on a candidate gene or genome-wide level, using chromosome microarray (for CNV) or sequencing (for mutations). However, only recently have rigorous genome-wide statistical approaches been applied in neurodevelopmental disorders. In earlier studies, before we appreciated just how much rare variation occurs in the human population, the mere fact that a deleterious variation occurred in a gene was almost sufficient evidence to identify it as genetically implicated in a neurodevelopmental disorder. Now, however, we have very good estimates of the rate of mutation of specific bases in the genome (Neale et al., 2012) and we can rigorously identify neurodevelopmental disorders genes. New and statistically convincing findings are being made at an accelerated rate and large consortia have been organized to enhance this process (e.g., (Epi4K, 2012; Buxbaum et al., 2012; De Rubeis et al., 2014; Iossifov et al., 2014).

11.10   TARGETING STRATEGIES

In model systems in common use, there are methods for overexpressing or disrupting genes of interest. There are also methods for deleting or duplicating larger regions, as a means of modeling a clinically relevant CNV. These latter methods depend on extensive synteny between species; yet, interesting animal models have been developed for many CNV associated with neurodevelopmental disorders.

One question that needs to be considered carefully when targeting a gene or a locus in an animal model surrounds the spectrum of human mutations. In many cases, these mutations lead to a clear change in gene dosage leading to the manifestation of the phenotype. For example, for many genes, loss of a functional copy of the gene is a clear cause of the disorder and hence simple gene disruption strategies are appropriate. By contrast, there are rarer examples, where gain-of-function of the gene is the leading cause for the disease and, for these, a knockin approach would be called for.

Mice have been the primary mammalian model because methods for gene targeting were developed and perfected in mice. However, new methods, making use of new approaches, including zinc finger nucleases (ZFNs), transcription activator like effector nucleases (TALENs), or clustered regulatory interspaced short palindromic repeat (CRISPR)/Cas based RNA-guided DNA endonucleases (Le Provost et al., 2010; Li et al., 2013; Shen et al., 2013) now permit gene disruption in multiple diverse organisms including rats, rabbits, and others. Notably, there has been a recent explosion in interest in genetically modified rat models for neurodevelopmental disorders because rats are more tractable for complex neurobiological analyses and are in wider use for pharmacokinetic and pharmocodynamic studies.

11.11   PAYING ATTENTION TO GENOTYPE

One area where there remains a surprising divergence is the degree to which the genotype of the human disorder is considered. Many human disorders are haploinsufficiency syndromes and, hence, the most relevant animal models would lack just one copy of the gene; however, in many instances studies are published that primarily or exclusively focus on knockouts (lacking two copies of the gene). Such studies would undoubtedly shed light on the function of a gene, but it can certainly be the case where phenotypes are different with loss of one or both copies of a gene and where therapies that successfully rescue a heterozygous model have little or no impact on a complete knockout. There are of course both recessive and X-linked disorders (the latter in males) where there are no functional copies of the relevant gene. In these cases, complete knockouts are the ideal model.

11.12 STRAIN EFFECTS AND MODIFIER LOCI

Laboratory mice are inbred, meaning that they are homozygous at every locus in the genome. This extraordinary and unnatural state certainly complicates the construct, face, and predictive validity of the models. Behaviors, even in wild-type animals, differ considerably across strains. There are robust strain effects on phenotypes observed in genetically modified mice, which contribute to this confounding, as noted below. However, this fact can, in certain situations, be used to facilitate the identification of modifier loci through the use of quantitative trait locus (QTL) analyses.

One recent example of strain effects is that around *Fmr1* knockouts. Mice with a targeted disruption of *Fmr1* are among the most widely studied models for a neurodevelopmental disorder. A recent study, looking at knockout *Fmr1* mice on multiple mixed genetic backgrounds, showed that there are some interesting phenotypes that are only present on specific backgrounds (Spencer et al., 2011). For example, contextual fear conditioning was decreased in only one F1 strain, while social behaviors could be enhanced or reduced in different F1 strains. Such differences could be

mediated by modifier loci in the genome of one of the strains.

In epilepsy, there are numerous examples for modifier loci/QTL findings, although many have not been reduced to the underlying genes. A recent example in Dravet syndrome began with the observation that the severity of the phenotype associated with *Scn1a* haploinsufficiency is profoundly influenced by strain (a prerequisite for QTL analyses), going from no overt phenotype on the 129S6/SvEvTac background to spontaneous seizures and early lethality on the (C57BL/6J × 129S6/SvEvTac) F1 background (Miller et al., 2013). Modifier loci on murine chromosomes 5, 7, 8 and 11 were identified and some genes, including gamma-aminobutyric acid (GABA) receptor subunit genes and calcium, chloride, and potassium channel genes, that underlay the peaks, showed alterations in expression or regulation and hence might contribute to the severity of the phenotype.

Another approach for identifying modifier loci in multiple organisms makes use of mutagenesis. One recent example for Rett syndrome is illustrative (Buchovecky et al., 2013). The authors characterized one (out of five identified) dominant suppressor strain, created by *N*-ethyl-*N*-nitrosourea (ENU) mutagenesis, in which the symptoms of Mecp2 loss were ameliorated. They identified, in this strain, a nonsense mutation in the *Sqle* gene, which encodes for squalene epoxidase, a rate-limiting enzyme in cholesterol biosynthesis. The authors then showed that lipid metabolism was perturbed in *Mecp2* knockout mice and that statins ameliorate motor symptoms and increase lifespan in these mice. It is noteworthy to mention that similarly to the observation that some genetic variants express their effect under specific genetic background, the effect of other variants may only be observed under specific environmental conditions. Therefore some phenotypes may reveal themselves only in the presence of specific environmental triggers and stressors. This highlights the importance of developing more studies that focus on the role that gene−environment interaction plays in psychiatric disorders in particular and other disorders and disease in general.

11.13   RODENTS AREN'T EVERYTHING

Genetic models currently in use to study neurodevelopmental disorders include vertebrates as well as invertebrates. In the latter group, *C. elegans* and *D. melanogaster*, have been both used as useful models in mechanistic studies of neurodevelopmental disorders. Their rapid generation time, low maintenance cost, and the simplified genetic manipulation in these organisms are all advantageous when considering a disease model (Bessa et al., 2013; Furukubo-Tokunaga, 2009). Moreover, with its relatively simple brain structures, *Drosophila* has become an efficient tool for studying a variety of monogenic forms of neurodevelopmental disorders, including Angelman syndrome, Rett syndrome, neurofibromatosis type 1, and fragile X syndrome. Findings from these studies have enhanced our knowledge about the affected molecular pathways and the neural circuits that can serve as candidates for therapeutic intervention strategies (Gatto et al., 2014; Braat and Kooy, 2015). Furthermore, the advances in behavioral tasks, applied in these models, to test cognition, including context generalization (Liu et al., 1999), associative learning (Davis, 1996; Wolf et al., 1998) and attention [reviewed in (van Swinderen, 2011)], have also contributed to our understanding of the consequences of mutations/deletions in a single gene on a subset of behaviors relevant to neurodevelopmental disorders. The *Drosophila* Angelman syndrome model, for example, shows deficient locomotor climbing activity, disruption in the circadian rhythmicity, and long-term associative olfactory memory (Wu et al., 2008) all of which are of relevance for symptoms seen in patients with Angelman syndrome, including gait ataxia/limb tremulousness, cognitive impairments, and disrupted sleep (Williams et al., 2010). Studies from the *Drosophila* neurofibromatosis type 1 disease model, shed a light on the role of the causative gene, NF1, in the regulation of

escape flight response as well as in circadian rhythmicity and long-term memory (Guo et al., 2000; The et al., 1997; Williams et al., 2001). Recently, social interaction measures, which are of relevance to autism, have also been introduced in this model organism. For example, social interaction analysis in the *Drosophila* model for Fragile X showed that *dfmr1* mutant flies interact less among each other compared to their interaction with wild-type flies, indicating a decreased sociability (Bolduc et al., 2010).

11.14   NEUROBIOLOGICALLY-DRIVEN THERAPEUTICS IN NEURODEVELOPMENTAL DISORDERS

The ultimate promise of animal models is the development of novel treatments. The degree to which a given model sheds light on pathophysiological mechanisms and then leads to novel therapeutic approaches, which ideally are verified in the same model system, is the ultimate test of the utility of the model. Recently, there has been enormous excitement in the field as pathophysiological mechanisms have been identified in model systems leading to new clinical trials. The evolving studies in Fragile X syndrome are well known (Krueger and Bear, 2011), but it is important to note that there are several additional examples. Our own work on *Shank3*-deficient mice highlighted more immature synapses, as defined biochemically, and identified synaptic plasticity deficits and motor deficits (Bozdagi et al., 2010). We then showed that insulin-like growth factor-1 (IGF-1) ameliorated both LTP deficits and motor deficits in the *Shank3* heterozygotes (Bozdagi et al., 2013) and this formed the basis for a first pilot clinical trial with IGF-1 in PMS, which has shown benefits with IGF-1 on core symptoms of ASD, suggesting a potentially disease-modifying effect, and forming the basis for larger studies to inform the efficacy of IGF-1 in kids with Shank3-deficiency (Kolevzon et al., 2014). Notably, independent clinical studies on IGF-1 in Rett syndrome has provided clinical evidence for the efficacy of IGF-1 (Khwaja et al

2014 et al., 2011), thus increasing the interest in this compound and suggesting a broader application in other monogenic forms of ASD.

While it is relatively easy to conceptualize treating a monogenic disorder, it is more difficult to consider specific interventions for contiguous gene syndromes. There are dozens of recurrent chromosomal abnormalities and CNVs associated with neurodevelopmental disorders (Betancur, 2011; Cooper et al., 2011) where many of these likely represent contiguous gene syndromes, some of which were modeled in rodents. Ts65DN mice, for example, were generated to contain a translocation of a large portion of chromosome 16, which encompasses large regions syntenic to human chromosome 21, thus creating a mice model that is trisomic for about two thirds of the human chromosome 21 genes. These mice show excess inhibition in the dentate gyrus, and systemic dosing with a $GABA_A$ antagonist has demonstrated beneficial effects on synaptic plasticity (reversing deficits in the induction of LTP) and cognition (reversing deficits in working memory and in object recognition memory) (Fernandez et al., 2007). A phase I clinical trial with an inverse agonist of the $GABA_A$ receptor 5, a subtype of $GABA_A$ receptor relatively abundant in the hippocampus (Rudolph and Knoflach, 2011) is currently being carried out in young adults with Down syndrome by Hoffmann-La Roche (NCT01436955).

11.15 CONCLUSIONS

Model systems represent key tools in understanding the pathobiology of neurodevelopmental disorders, and methods to develop and analyze such models continue to evolve at a rapid pace. The identification of highly penetrant genetic variants that underlie neurodevelopmental disorders provides an easy path to models with construct validity. There are several examples of neurobiologically driven clinical trials that arose from such models, and there is good reason to be optimistic that over the next years, novel treatments for these disorders will emerge.

REFERENCES

Anney, R., Klei, L., Pinto, D., Regan, R., Conroy, J., Magalhaes, T.R., Correia, C., Abrahams, B.S., Sykes, N., Pagnamenta, A.T., *et al.* (2010). A genome-wide scan for common alleles affecting risk for autism. Hum Mol Genet 19, 4072–4082.

Auerbach, B.D., Osterweil, E.K., and Bear, M.F. (2011). Mutations causing syndromic autism define an axis of synaptic pathophysiology. Nature 480, 63–68.

Bessa, C., Maciel, P., and Rodrigues, A.J. (2013). Using C. elegans to decipher the cellular and molecular mechanisms underlying neurodevelopmental disorders. Mol Neurobiol 48, 465–489.

Betancur, C. (2011). Etiological heterogeneity in autism spectrum disorders: more than 100 genetic and genomic disorders and still counting. Brain Res 1380, 42–77.

Bhat, A.N., Galloway, J.C., and Landa, R.J. (2012). Relation between early motor delay and later communication delay in infants at risk for autism. Infant Behav Dev 35, 838–846.

Bolduc, F.V., Valente, D., Nguyen, A.T., Mitra, P.P., and Tully, T. (2010). An assay for social interaction in Drosophila Fragile X mutants. Fly 4, 216–225.

Bozdagi, O., Sakurai, T., Papapetrou, D., Wang, X., Dickstein, D.L., Takahashi, N., Kajiwara, Y., Yang, M., Katz, A.M., Scattoni, M.L., *et al.* (2010). Haploinsufficiency of the autism-associated Shank3 gene leads to deficits in synaptic function, social interaction, and social communication. Mol Autism 1, 15.

Bozdagi, O., Tavassoli, T., and Buxbaum, J.D. (2013). Insulin-like growth factor-1 rescues synaptic and motor deficits in a mouse model of autism and developmental delay. Mol Autism 4, 9.

Braat, S., and Kooy, R.F. (2015). Insights into GABAAergic system deficits in fragile X syndrome lead to clinical trials. Neuropharmacology 88, 48–54.

Buchovecky, C.M., Turley, S.D., Brown, H.M., Kyle, S.M., McDonald, J.G., Liu, B., Pieper, A.A., Huang, W., Katz, D.M., Russell, D.W., *et al.* (2013). A suppressor screen in Mecp2 mutant mice implicates cholesterol metabolism in Rett syndrome. Nat Genet 45, 1013–1020.

Buxbaum, J.D., Betancur, C., Bozdagi, O., Dorr, N.P., Elder, G.A., and Hof, P.R. (2012). Optimizing the phenotyping of rodent ASD models:

enrichment analysis of mouse and human neurobiological phenotypes associated with high-risk autism genes identifies morphological, electrophysiological, neurological, and behavioral features. Mol. Autism 3, 1.

Buxbaum, J.D., Daly, M.J., Devlin, B., Lehner, T., Roeder, K., State, M.W.; Autism Sequencing Consortium. (2012). The autism sequencing consortium: large-scale, high-throughput sequencing in autism spectrum disorders. Neuron.

Cooper, G.M., Coe, B.P., Girirajan, S., Rosenfeld, J.A., Vu, T.H., Baker, C., Williams, C., Stalker, H., Hamid, R., Hannig, V., *et al.* (2011). A copy number variation morbidity map of developmental delay. Nat Genet 43, 838–846.

Davis, R.L. (1996). Physiology and biochemistry of Drosophila learning mutants. Physiol Rev 76, 299–317.

De Rubeis, S., He, X., Goldberg, A.P., Poultney, C.S., Samocha, K., Cicek, A.E., Kou, Y., Liu, L., Fromer, M., Walker, S., et al., (2014). Synaptic, transcriptional and chromatin genes disrupted in autism. Nature.

Del Pino, I., Garcia-Frigola, C., Dehorter, N., Brotons-Mas, J.R., Alvarez-Salvado, E., Martinez de Lagran, M., Ciceri, G., Gabaldon, M.V., Moratal, D., Dierssen, M., *et al.* (2013). Erbb4 deletion from fast-spiking interneurons causes schizophrenia-like phenotypes. Neuron 79, 1152–1168.

Devlin, B., Melhem, N., and Roeder, K. (2011). Do common variants play a role in risk for autism? Evidence and theoretical musings. Brain Res 1380, 78–84.

Ellegood, J., Anagnostou, E., Babineau, B.A., Crawley, J.N., Lin, L., Genestine, M., DiCicco-Bloom, E., Lai, J.K., Foster, J.A., Penagarikano, O., et al. (2015). Clustering autism: using neuroanatomical differences in 26 mouse models to gain insight into the heterogeneity. Molecular psychiatry 120, 118–125.

Epi4K (2012). Epi4K: gene discovery in 4,000 genomes. Epilepsia 53, 1457–1467.

Fernandez, F., Morishita, W., Zuniga, E., Nguyen, J., Blank, M., Malenka, R.C., and Garner, C.C. (2007). Pharmacotherapy for cognitive impairment in a mouse model of Down syndrome. Nat Neurosci 10, 411–413.

Furukubo-Tokunaga, K. (2009). Modeling schizophrenia in flies. Prog Brain Res 179, 107–115.

Gatto, C.L., Pereira, D., and Broadie, K. (2014). GABAergic circuit dysfunction in the Drosophila Fragile X syndrome model. Neurobiology of disease 65, 142–159.

Gibson, J.R., Bartley, A.F., Hays, S.A., and Huber, K.M. (2008). Imbalance of neocortical excitation and inhibition and altered UP states reflect network hyperexcitability in the mouse model of fragile X syndrome. J Neurophysiol 100, 2615–2626.

Guo, H.F., Tong, J., Hannan, F., Luo, L., and Zhong, Y. (2000). A neurofibromatosis-1-regulated pathway is required for learning in Drosophila. Nature 403, 895–898.

Gutierrez, R.C., Hung, J., Zhang, Y., Kertesz, A.C., Espina, F.J., and Colicos, M.A. (2009). Altered synchrony and connectivity in neuronal networks expressing an autism-related mutation of neuroligin 3. Neuroscience 162, 208–221.

Hirschhorn, J.N., Lohmueller, K., Byrne, E., and Hirschhorn, K. (2002). A comprehensive review of genetic association studies. Genet Med 4, 45–61.

Iossifov, I., O'Roak, B.J., Sanders, S.J., Ronemus, M., Krumm, N., Levy, D., Stessman, H.A., Witherspoon, K.T., Vives, L., Patterson, K.E., et al., (2014) The contribution of de novo coding mutations to autism spectrum disorder. Nature.

Khwaja, O.S., Ho, E., Barnes, K.V., O'Leary, H.M., Pereira, L.M., Finkelstein, Y., Nelson, C.A. 3rd, Vogel-Farley, V., DeGregorio, G., et al., (2014). Safety, pharmacokinetics, and preliminary assessment of efficacy of mecasermin (recombinant human IGF-1) for the treatment of Rett syndrome. Proc Natl Acad Sci.

Kirov, G., Rees, E., Walters, J.T., Escott-Price, V., Georgieva, L., Richards, A.L., Chambert, K.D., Davies, G., Legge, S.E., Moran, J.L., *et al.* (2014). The penetrance of copy number variations for schizophrenia and developmental delay. Biol Psychiatry 75, 378–385.

Kolevzon, A., Bush, L., Wang, A.T., Halpern, D., FranK, Y., Grodberg, D., Rapaport, R., Tavassoli, T., Chaplin, W., Soorya, L., et al. (2014). A pilot controlled trial of insulin-like growth factor-1 in children with Phelan-McDermid syndrome. Molecular autism.

Krueger, D.D., and Bear, M.F. (2011). Toward fulfilling the promise of molecular medicine in fragile X syndrome. Annu Rev Med 62, 411–429.

Laumonnier, F., Bonnet-Brilhault, F., Gomot, M., Blanc, R., David, A., Moizard, M.P., Raynaud,

M., Ronce, N., Lemonnier, E., Calvas, P., *et al.* (2004). X-linked mental retardation and autism are associated with a mutation in the NLGN4 gene, a member of the neuroligin family. Am J Hum Genet 74, 552–557.

Le Provost, F., Lillico, S., Passet, B., Young, R., Whitelaw, B., and Vilotte, J.L. (2010). Zinc finger nuclease technology heralds a new era in mammalian transgenesis. Trends Biotechnol 28, 134–141.

Li, D., Qiu, Z., Shao, Y., Chen, Y., Guan, Y., Liu, M., Li, Y., Gao, N., Wang, L., Lu, X., *et al.* (2013). Heritable gene targeting in the mouse and rat using a CRISPR-Cas system. Nat Biotechnol 31, 681–683.

Liu, L., Wolf, R., Ernst, R., and Heisenberg, M. (1999). Context generalization in Drosophila visual learning requires the mushroom bodies. Nature 400, 753–756.

Miller, A.R., Hawkins, N.A., McCollom, C.E., and Kearney, J.A. (2013). Mapping genetic modifiers of survival in a mouse model of Dravet syndrome. Genes, Brain Behav

Neale, B.M., Kou, Y., Liu, L., Ma'ayan, A., Samocha, K.E., Sabo, A., Lin, C.F., Stevens, C., Wang, L.S., Makarov, V., *et al.* (2012). Patterns and rates of exonic de novo mutations in autism spectrum disorders. Nature 485, 242–245.

Noh, H.J., Ponting, C.P., Boulding, H.C., Meader, S., Betancur, C., Buxbaum, J.D., Pinto, D., Marshall, C.R., Lionel, A.C., Scherer, S.W., *et al.* (2013). Network topologies and convergent aetiologies arising from deletions and duplications observed in individuals with autism. PLoS Genet 9, e1003523.

Paluszkiewicz, S.M., Olmos-Serrano, J.L., Corbin, J.G., and Huntsman, M.M. (2011). Impaired inhibitory control of cortical synchronization in fragile X syndrome. J Neurophysiol 106, 2264–2272.

Rudolph, U., and Knoflach, F. (2011). Beyond classical benzodiazepines: novel therapeutic potential of GABAA receptor subtypes. Nat Rev Drug Discov 10, 685–697.

Segurado, R., Conroy, J., Meally, E., Fitzgerald, M., Gill, M., and Gallagher, L. (2005). Confirmation of association between autism and the mitochondrial aspartate/glutamate carrier SLC25A12 gene on chromosome 2q31. Am J Psychiatry 162, 2182–2184.

Shen, Y., Xiao, A., Huang, P., Wang, W.Y., Zhu, Z.Y., and Zhang, B. (2013). [TALE nuclease engineering and targeted genome modification]. Yi chuan 35, 395–409.

Silva, A.J., Ehninger, D. (2009). Adult reversal of cognitive phenotypes in neurodevelopmental disorders. J Neurodev Disord 2, 150–157.

Sigurdsson, T., Stark, K.L., Karayiorgou, M., Gogos, J.A., and Gordon, J.A. (2010). Impaired hippocampal-prefrontal synchrony in a genetic mouse model of schizophrenia. Nature 464, 763–767.

Spencer, C.M., Alekseyenko, O., Hamilton, S.M., Thomas, A.M., Serysheva, E., Yuva-Paylor, L.A., and Paylor, R. (2011). Modifying behavioral phenotypes in Fmr1KO mice: genetic background differences reveal autistic-like responses. Autism Res 4, 40–56.

Stefansson, H., Meyer-Lindenberg, A., Steinberg, S., Magnusdottir, B., Morgen, K., Arnarsdottir, S., Bjornsdottir, G., Walters, G.B., Jonsdottir, G.A., Doyle, O.M., *et al.* (2014). CNVs conferring risk of autism or schizophrenia affect cognition in controls. Nature 505, 361–366.

The, I., Hannigan, G.E., Cowley, G.S., Reginald, S., Zhong, Y., Gusella, J.F., Hariharan, I.K., and Bernards, A. (1997). Rescue of a Drosophila NF1 mutant phenotype by protein kinase A. Science 276, 791–794.

Turunen, J.A., Rehnstrom, K., Kilpinen, H., Kuokkanen, M., Kempas, E., and Ylisaukko-Oja, T. (2008). Mitochondrial aspartate/glutamate carrier SLC25A12 gene is associated with autism. Autism Res 1, 189–192.

van Swinderen, B. (2011). Attention in Drosophila. Int Rev Neurobiol 99, 51–85.

Wang, K., Zhang, H., Ma, D., Bucan, M., Glessner, J.T., Abrahams, B.S., Salyakina, D., Imielinski, M., Bradfield, J.P., Sleiman, P.M., *et al.* (2009). Common genetic variants on 5p14.1 associate with autism spectrum disorders. Nature 459, 528–533.

Weiss, L.A., Arking, D.E., Daly, M.J., and Chakravarti, A. (2009). A genome-wide linkage and association scan reveals novel loci for autism. Nature 461, 802–808.

Williams, C.A., Driscoll, D.J., and Dagli, A.I. (2010). Clinical and genetic aspects of Angelman syndrome. Genet Med 12, 385–395.

Williams, J.A., Su, H.S., Bernards, A., Field, J., and Sehgal, A. (2001). A circadian output in Drosophila mediated by neurofibromatosis-1 and Ras/MAPK. Science 293, 2251–2256.

Wolf, R., Wittig, T., Liu, L., Wustmann, G., Eyding, D., and Heisenberg, M. (1998). Drosophila mushroom bodies are dispensable for visual, tactile, and motor learning. Learn Mem 5, 166–178.

Wu, Y., Bolduc, F.V., Bell, K., Tully, T., Fang, Y., Sehgal, A., and Fischer, J.A. (2008). A Drosophila model for Angelman syndrome. Proc Natl Acad Sci U S A 105, 12399–12404.

12

CASCADING GENETIC AND ENVIRONMENTAL EFFECTS ON DEVELOPMENT: IMPLICATIONS FOR INTERVENTION

ESHA MASSAND AND ANNETTE KARMILOFF-SMITH

Centre for Brain and Cognitive Development, Department of Psychological Sciences, School of Sciences, Birkbeck, University of London, 32 Torrington Square, London, WC1E 7HX UK

12.1 INTRODUCTION

It is a truism that development involves contributions from both genes and the environment, but the respective roles of each, their complex interactions, and their influence on typical or atypical developmental trajectories, are still not fully understood. In this chapter, we will summarize what is known about the genetics of a selection of neurodevelopmental disorders. We will then consider the influence that children themselves have on their environment, and the role of the environment on the developing child. The *emergent* phenotypes of individuals with neurodevelopmental disorders are then discussed, with a particular focus on the neuroconstructivist perspective and how basic-level deficits early in development cascade over

developmental time to result in the phenotypic outcome. We conclude with a discussion of some forms of intervention for children with neurodevelopmental disorders, and the learning theories that underpin them.

12.2 NEURODEVELOPMENTAL DISORDERS OF KNOWN VERSUS UNKNOWN GENETIC ORIGIN

The genetic basis of several neurodevelopmental disorders is relatively well understood. For example, it is known that the origin of Williams syndrome (WS) is caused by the hemizygous microdeletion of some 28 genes on the long arm of chromosome 7q11.23, impacting synaptic regulation. Phenotypically the

The Genetics of Neurodevelopmental Disorders, First Edition. Edited by Kevin J. Mitchell.
© 2015 John Wiley & Sons, Inc. Published 2015 by John Wiley & Sons, Inc.

disorder is characterized by an uneven profile with seriously impaired spatial and numerical cognition, but relatively proficient language and face processing (Karmiloff-Smith et al., 2004; Martens et al., 2008). They also present with an overly friendly, disinhibited social profile, with abnormal activation in amygdala/orbitofrontal cortical regions (Meyer-Lindenberg et al., 2005). Twenty-two of the 28 deleted genes in the WS critical region are expressed in the brain (Osborne, 2012), with brain size only reaching 80% of typical brains. So, it is likely that the WS brain develops structurally, functionally, and biochemically differently from typical brains (Karmiloff-Smith, 2010; Karmiloff-Smith et al., 2012). The mapping of individual genes in the WS critical region to specific aspects of the socio-cognitive outcome continues to be the focus of several studies, although such correlations turn out to be extremely complex (Gray et al., 2006; Karmiloff-Smith et al., 2003, 2012; Karmiloff-Smith et al., 2012; Smith et al., 2009; Tassabehji et al., 1999).

The majority of individuals with Trisomy 21 or Down syndrome (DS) have a third copy of the entire chromosome 21, with a small percentage presenting with partial trisomy (Korbel et al., 2009). Like WS, DS impacts many aspects of brain development from the outset, including defects in neurogenesis, neurite sprouting, mitochondrial function, as well as amyloid-β pepide production, which begins in utero and is linked to the Amyloid Precursor Protein gene, triplicated on chromosome 21 (Bahn et al., 2002; Busciglio and Yankner, 1995; Lott et al., 2006). Wide individual differences exist in the cognitive phenotypes of individuals with DS but, in general, DS gives rise to global intellectual impairment, deficits in learning, memory, attention, and language. Where individuals with WS have stronger verbal than spatial skills, those with DS tend to present with the opposite pattern. However, although at birth the brains of individuals with DS are similar to typically developing babies (Lott and Dierssen, 2010), from 6 months of age differences in volume and in the myelination of specific brain areas become apparent, with overall brain size

reaching approximately 80% of typical brains (Nadel, 2003).

Fragile X syndrome (FXS) is caused by a mutation in the FMR1 gene on the X chromosome, in which the DNA segment – the CGG triplet repeat – is expanded to over 200 repeats. This results in allelic inactivation and a complete loss of a protein that is important for synaptic plasticity. The gene involved is called the fragile X mental retardation gene (FMR1) and the missing protein the "fragile X mental retardation protein" (FMRP). The mutation results in seizures and a disruption to the functioning of the nervous system. Individuals with FXS usually have delayed speech and language, intellectual disability, anxiety, and hyperactive behaviors, with a substantial proportion of them developing autistic-like traits. Recent research has shown that mothers who are carriers of a pre-mutation of the FMR1 gene with less repeats (between 55 and 200 repeats) and who have seemingly normal intelligence, turn out to have subtle impairments (Cornish et al., 2008), stressing the importance of in-depth measures of cognitive function beyond standardized tests.

Interestingly, genetically identical conditions can lead to radically different phenotypes, depending on the parent of origin. Angelman syndrome and Prader–Will syndrome both derive from a loss of gene activity in the *same* critical region of chromosome 15 (15q11–q13) (Pembrey et al., 1989). In typically developing individuals, this region contains two copies of the UBE3A gene, but in the brain of individuals with Angelman syndrome only one (the maternal copy) is active. If the paternal copy of the same 15q11–q13 critical region is partly or entirely deleted, the individual develops a different neurodevelopmental disorder, Prader–Willi syndrome. Angelman syndrome is characterized by developmental delay, problems with movement or balance, lack of speech or a minimal use of words, and an outwardly happy demeanour with frequent laughing or smiling. By contrast, Prader–Willi syndrome, while also characterized by developmental delay, gives rise to extreme and insatiable appetite leading to obesity, hypotonia (low muscle tone), short stature and hypogonadism (resulting in delayed or no puberty). The fact that both Angelman syndrome and Prader–Willi syndrome arise from mutations in the exact same region of chromosome 15 (Clayton-Smith, 2006) provides striking evidence of the complexities of gene expression when parent of origin has to be taken into account.

Aforementioned are a few examples of neurodevelopmental disorders of known genetic origin, which in principle can be diagnosed in the initial stages of development. This opens the possibility of very early treatment that might re-channel developmental trajectories over time. By contrast, infants who are later diagnosed with a disorder of unknown genetic origin, as is currently the case for Autism Spectrum Disorder (ASD), Specific Language Impairment (SLI), or dyslexia, are rarely if ever identified in early infancy. This means that it is considerably later in their development only once the child starts to display characteristic phenotypes of the disorder, that they can be targeted for intervention.

Autism Spectrum Disorders are characterized by deficits in social and reciprocal interaction, imaginative play, with individuals often displaying restricted and repetitive behaviors (Frith, 1991). While the actual genes involved in ASD remain unknown, research is uncovering many candidate genes (Geschwind, 2011), and studies of monozygotic and dizygotic twins have allowed researchers to quantify the genetic/environmental contributions to the disorder (Hallmayer et al., 2011; Rosenberg et al., 2009). Indeed, there is a twofold higher concordance rate for ASD in identical twins than in fraternal twins. Studies of recurrence rates of autism have also indicated a twofold increase in the probability of ASD diagnosis for infant siblings who have one or more older siblings with ASD (Ozonoff et al., 2011). Indeed, a major effort is currently underway to identify autism-specific biological, neural, or cognitive markers in these infant siblings (Elsabbagh and Johnson, 2010). Moreover, recent studies have suggested that each of the phenotypic characteristics of ASD – communication, social interaction, and repetitive behaviors – is likely to be underpinned by different sets of genes (Happé and Ronald, 2008; Robinson et al., 2012).

While these studies point to a strong genetic contribution to the neurodevelopmental disorder, the origins of ASD are likely to lie in multiple genes of small effect across the population. For example, copy number gene variations (CNVs) have been implicated, some of which have been found to be exclusive to subgroups of individuals with ASD (Gai et al., 2011). Many of these mutations affect biological processes such as synapse function, neurotransmission and brain development. The current state of genetics in ASD suggests that there may be numerous different pathways, each genetically different, but with a common phenotypic outcome.

Similarly, the genetic origins of SLI and dyslexia remain to be elucidated. Some researchers have sought to link such disorders to single genes, such as the case of the FOXP2 gene. A British family (KE) had yielded several generations of children with serious speech and language impairments. When affected family members were identified as having a mutation on the FOXP2 gene on chromosome 7 (Lai et al., 2001), some hailed this as the discovery of the gene explaining the evolution of human language (Gopnik and Crago, 1991; Pinker, 2001). But in-depth molecular analyses of FOXP2 in humans (Groszer et al., 2008), and *foxp2* in chimpanzees (Enard et al., 2002), in birds (Bolhuis et al., 2000; Haesler et al., 2004) and in mice (Lai et al., 2003) revealed that this gene is widely expressed in many regions of the brain and that its function seems to lie in contributing to the rapid coordination of sequential processing and its timing. It turns out that *foxp2* is expressed more during bird song *learning* than during subsequent adult song production (Haesler et al., 2004), and that its expression in the mouse brain, while in many regions initially, becomes increasingly confined to motor regions such as the cerebellum (Lai et al., 2003). In the human case, the reason why the mutation affects speech/language more obviously than other cognitive domains is because speech/language is the human domain in which the rapid coordination of sequential processing and its timing is the most critical (Karmiloff-Smith, 2013; Karmiloff-Smith et al., 2012). But FOXP2 is not specific to the language domain. It also affects other domains, albeit more subtly. Indeed, it was shown that affected KE family members also had problems with imitating nonlinguistic articulatory movement sequences, as well as with fine motor control and the perception/production of rhythm (Alcock et al., 2000), suggesting a domain-relevant effect of differing impact. Moreover, if one takes a domain-relevant rather than domain-specific view, the question asked of animal models is not: "What animal behavior is most like human language?", but: "Which domain-relevant processes in this species' repertoire require the coordination and timing of rapid movement sequences?" – a very different type of question. It also encourages the researcher of human *FOXP2* mutations to hypothesize impairments, beyond the obvious deficits in oral language, involving other capacities that call on the coordination and timing of rapid movement sequences, for example, manual sign language, the playing of the piano/violin, and so forth. This fosters a broader examination of the contribution of mutated genes to the overall human phenotype rather than a mere focus on a single domain such as language (Karmiloff-Smith, 2013).

12.3   ENVIRONMENTAL INFLUENCES

The frequently debated question of which aspects of human cognition are likely due to nurture (environment) as opposed to nature (genes) arises when Behaviorists or Nativists attempt simply to dichotomize the influences of these sources of variation. However, neuro-constructivists (Karmiloff-Smith, 1998, 2009; Dekker and Karmiloff-Smith, 2011; Elman et al., 1996; Mareschal et al., 2007) emphasize the multidirectional interactions of these sources of gene, environment, brain, cognition, and behavior variation, as well as the process of ontogeny itself (Karmiloff-Smith, 1998) in shaping developmental outcomes.

Both environmental and genetic influences impact brain development, often with similar phenotypic expression, suggesting that the environment also plays a crucial role in the development of the child. For example, there is evidence to suggest that low socioeconomic status (SES) can have detrimental effects on the functioning of frontal cortex in infants as young as 6 months of age (Tomalski et al., 2013). Furthermore, in typically developing children, differences in mother/child interaction styles have been shown either to foster or hinder cognitive development (Karmiloff-Smith et al., 2010). Evidence such as this indicates that the early environment impacts brain and cognitive development in profound and measurable ways.

The environment in which a child with a genetic mutation develops is likely to undergo subtle changes, compared to the environment that surrounds a typically developing child (Karmiloff-Smith, 2009; Karmiloff-Smith et al., 2012). This is because the atypically developing infant needs special attention, and because parental expectations of their child's abilities change once they are informed that their child has a syndrome. Yet, characterizing the subtle differences in such environments is far from straight forward, with few studies yielding quantifiable data. The environment is modified in several other subtle ways. For example, John and Mervis (2010) studied vocabulary learning in toddlers with DS compared to healthy controls and found striking group differences in the amount that the toddlers were allowed to overgeneralize terms. In contrast to parents of typically developing toddlers, parents of those with DS corrected their toddlers' overgeneralizations immediately. A temporary period of language overgeneralization in the typical case encourages the creation of categories, such that when allowed to call all four-legged animals "dog", children implicitly create the category "animal". By contrast, by immediately correcting labels, parents of toddlers with DS curtail such overgeneralizations, due probably to their natural fear that their child's lower intelligence might mean that they will fail to learn the correct terms. Assumptions such as these may cause parents to produce a less varied environment for the child to explore and to use a less varied linguistic repertoire. Such subtle environmental changes in the context of language acquisition may contribute to the explanation of why category formation is usually weaker in individuals with neurodevelopmental disorders (Karmiloff-Smith et al., 2012).

Other subtle differences probably exist in the environments of individuals with neurodevelopmental disorders, and these differences are likely to be reciprocal. In other words, the child will have an influence on their environment, which in turn influences their development, which then further alters the environment, and so on. Such differences are likely to accumulate over time, with cascading effects that result in an environment that ultimately differs substantially from that of a typically developing child. We are then faced with the challenge of elucidating how a genetic mutation, which changes expression over time, paired with an altered environment, which changes over time, work together to shape the phenotypic outcome.

The fact that the environment impacts on the child's developmental trajectory is clear. However, the fine details of this impact remain to be elucidated. For example, how do different neurodevelopmental disorders impact the child's environment specifically, and to what extent? How can researchers uncover the precise influence of atypically developing children on their social, linguistic, cognitive, or physical environments? What is the impact of these altered environmental components on the development of the (already atypical) child?

In other words, environments are not static, whether a child is growing up typically or atypically. Thus, a *dynamic* notion of the changing environment is critical to fully understand neurodevelopmental disorders (Karmiloff-Smith et al., 2012).

12.4 PHENOTYPES ARE EMERGENT

Just like the environment, the human brain is also dynamic. Phenotypes *emerge* over time,

not from a mere process of maturation, but from complex multilevel interactions during development. From the outset, the brain of an atypically developing infant is likely to develop somewhat differently from the brain of a typically developing child, with cascading effects over developmental time. Thus, researchers can no longer use the static adult neuropsychological model of "preserved/intact/impaired" modules. Indeed, studies of neurodevelopmental disorders have often been based on an interpretation of the mature adult brain, without concern for the dynamic nature of neural and cognitive development (Karmiloff-Smith, 1998, 2013). Tracing these unique developmental pathways is critical to the understanding of neurodevelopmental disorders, particularly where the developmental outcome is highly variable as, for example, in Autism Spectrum Disorder. In these studies, the behavioral research has often attempted to characterize the social and communication impairment of only older children. However, these later deficits are likely to be rooted in more basic-level processes early in infancy and to result in a developmental trajectory that is atypical in numerous ways, rather than being described as "intact" or "impaired" relative to typical controls. Most neurodevelopmental disorders impact brain development from the very outset. If we take a neuroconstructivist stance (Karmiloff-Smith, 1998; Karmiloff-Smith et al., 2012; Mareschal et al., 2007; Farran and Karmiloff-Smith, 2012), the atypicalities observed in developmental disorders must be traced back to their underpinnings in early development and emphasis placed not only on deficits within one part of the system, but on cross-domain interactions and differences over time.

The tendency for researchers to interpret better scores in task A than in task B as absolute, that is, intact versus impaired, rather than relative differences, ignores the fact that the performance on both A and B may be below chronological age, that is, "performance on task A is significantly better than on task B, during this developmental period" slips to a conclusion such as, "domain A is intact, domain

B is impaired, in this syndrome." This tendency within the developmental disorders literature is particularly worrying given that it implies that the brain of an atypically developing individual is directly comparable to that of a typically developed adult human brain. This is unlikely to obtain, given everything that we already know about both the typically and atypically developing brain as well as the evidence of atypical environments for individuals with genetic disorders described in the preceding section. What is required is a clear distinction between the develop*ed* brain and the develop*ing* brain.

A further risk is that when overt behavioral responses in an atypically developing group are the same as in a typically developing group, this leads to the assumption that the same cognitive and/or neural process underlies that behavior in the two populations. One such example is the investigation of face processing in WS. It had been shown that face processing scores in WS are in the normal range, that is, not behaviorally different from those of chronologically aged-matched typically developing controls. Using standardized tests such as the Benton Test of Face Recognition (Bellugi et al., 1994) and the Rivermead Test of Face Memory (Udwin and Yule, 1991), the proficiency of face processing in individuals with WS has been widely replicated (Annaz et al., 2008; Rossen et al., 1996). However, this is at the behavioral level. Are the cognitive and brain processes underlying this proficient behavior the same as, or different from, their age-matched counterparts? Electrophysiological measures showed that individuals with WS fail to display the neural specialization of face processing observed in healthy controls (Grice et al., 2003; Cohen-Kadosh and Johnson, 2007), suggesting that behavioral scores within the normal range do not necessarily signal comparable underlying brain processes.

A further example comes from studies of recognition memory in individuals with ASD, in which comparable behavioral performance between healthy controls and the atypical groups have been shown to be underpinned by different neural processes. Although memory difficulties are not a defining feature of ASD, research on memory in this population has revealed a characteristic pattern of performance across tasks. High-functioning individuals with ASD show proficient immediate memory, cued recall and recognition, with behavioral scores such as typical controls in all these aspects of memory. This suggests at first glance that memory processes in ASD are intact (Bowler et al., 2000). However, using event-related potentials in a recognition memory study, Massand et al., (2013) showed that the underlying neural processes were different. Individuals with ASD were presented with a list of words to study and subsequently asked to rate at test whether a word was "Old" (i.e., they had seen it before during the study phase), or "New" (presented for the first time). Amplitude deflections in the ERP were measured as participants made their recognition judgment. For typically developing individuals, positive deflections in ERPs for old words relative to new words are consistently observed (Rugg and Curran, 2007). However, despite comparable behavioral performance, the ERP for individuals with ASD was both more negative and shorter lasting compared to age and IQ-matched controls. Thus, once again we observe that for individuals with genetic disorders, behavioral performance within the normal range can camouflage an atypical developmental trajectory.

The electrophysiology findings from the two aforementioned studies suggest that the responses given by individuals with WS in face processing tasks, or by individuals with ASD in recognition memory tasks, are qualitatively different in neural terms from those made by typically developing controls. How did the individual with the genetic disorder arrive at this point in their developmental trajectory? Did they display atypical responses during an earlier phase of their development, which cascade to result in the present neural differences alongside behavioral similarities? Was this response compensated for in early or late development by the atypical process, or not differentiated from other systems (as has been suggested for the memory function of individuals with ASD; Massand et al., 2013). In other words, have such processes been shaped differently across time in individuals with genetic disorders and those developing typically?

To reiterate, in order to understand the phenotypic outcome of a genetic disorder, we need to trace its full developmental trajectory from infancy onward. It is crucial to consider how all the different parts of a multi-level, complex system interact at different time points. This is particularly important when predicting or tracing the emergent outcomes for individuals with neurodevelopmental disorders, which are likely the result of subtle or more obvious changes that cascade and accumulate over developmental time.

Clearly, the microcircuitry of the brain is not hard-wired or static, but instead plastic, self-structuring, and dynamic, changing over developmental time, interacting at multiple levels, including the genetic, cognitive, behavioral, and environmental levels (Casey, 2002; Johnson, 2001). Further evidence in support of this comes from research on zebra finches. Studies of the neural and epigenetic consequences of song listening and song production in these birds have shown how gene expression is greatest during learning (Bolhuis et al., 2000). In this study, the amount of gene expression was a function of how many elements of the song were imitated from the chick's tutor, and thus not fixed or predetermined by the bird's genes. Likewise, the location of gene expression can change over time. A study of the mouse brain (Lai et al., 2003) showed that expression of the *foxp2* gene was initially widespread and then became increasingly restricted to motor circuits, particularly the cerebellum. Similarly, there is evidence that maternal behavior toward rodent pups influences patterns of gene expression. A study by Kaffman and Meaney (2007) revealed that the amount of grooming and stroking by the mother rat changed the chemistry of genes involved in the pup's response to stress and that this was a permanent change, impacting on the pup's brain development and behavior. These kinds of environment/gene interactions suggest that epigenesis is not genetically determined, but rather under only very broad genetic control (Gottlieb, 2007).

Studies of brain processing in typically developing infants have yielded a similar picture: *gradual* specialization of brain areas for processing different kinds of stimuli. Take the example of face processing. Initially brain activity is widespread for processing all types of input, with different regions competing (Johnson, 2001; Neville, 2006), but progressively there is a specialization of face processing areas to the fusiform gyrus in right hemisphere (de Haan et al., 2002; Johnson, 2001). In typically developing individuals, this happens slowly over the first year of life and continues even into adolescence. These emergent cortical networks are the product of dynamic interactions between changing processes. The neonate brain may be regionally differentiated in terms of neuron type, neuron density, and so forth, but this is not to say that it is genetically determined. Rather, these early differences between brain regions are more relevant to particular types of processing and progressively become specialized, emerging over the course of development (see Karmiloff-Smith et al., 2012 for a full discussion).

The process of synaptic pruning usually leads to an increase in specialization and localization of brain circuits in typically developing individuals (Huttenlocher and Dabholkar, 1997; Johnson, 2001; Neville and Mills, 1997). If it were the case that in certain disorders the brain failed to specialize, we could hypothesize that brain activity would continue to show more widespread activity throughout development compared to typically developing controls. And, indeed, electrophysiological activity turns out to be more widespread in some tasks in adults with ASD compared to controls (Massand et al., 2013). Similar outcomes hold for individuals with FXS, whose synaptic densities remain well above the normal range (Comery et al., 1997), suggesting that they have undergone less pruning compared to typically developing individuals. It is possible that early pruning atypicalities (too little or too much too early) may turn out to be a feature of many neurodevelopmental disorders (Oliver et al., 2000; Thomas et al., 2011).

These considerations move our thoughts far from the notion of genetically determined brain regions and pre-specialization. Low-level subtle differences in early functioning, (e.g., visual or auditory processing) and in the environment (e.g., poverty, stress or subtle differences in parent's communication and interaction with the infant) cascade over time on the developing system and contribute significantly to a difference across the child's ontogeny and developmental trajectory. Without a clear appreciation of these subtle differences, we are unlikely to fully understand the phenotypic outcomes of individuals with genetic or environmentally-induced neurodevelopmental disorders.

12.5 IMPLICATIONS FOR INTERVENTION

The main goal of intervention is to promote the improvement of skills that are either delayed or deviant, that is, developing atypically. Pharmacological and genetic interventions are frequently researched, mainly in the form of tests on animal models, but the translation to the human case is not always obvious. In this section, we focus on nonmedical interventions, albeit stressing that all forms of intervention require very in-depth post-intervention testing to ascertain whether subtle impairments do not remain. For example, it was claimed that phenylketonuria (PKU), an autosomal recessive metabolic disorder which, when untreated, gives rise to mental retardation and seizures, could be totally cured if treated by a strict diet early in infancy. However, more recent research has revealed subtle cognitive deficits that remain across the lifespan even in treated PKU (Diamond, 2007). Likewise, as we saw in an earlier section, premutation carriers of the FXS gene were thought to be normal, yet in-depth research has uncovered a number of subtle impairments (Cornish et al., 2008).

Given our discussion in the preceding sections, we argue that intervention is likely to offer its best outcome when administered as early as possible after an individual is first diagnosed, so that the effects of the intervention on basic-level deficits cascade over time on the developing higher-level cognitive phenotype.

This might include intervention for attention, memory, motor skills, communication skills, impulsivity, and so on. Such intervention is clearly easier to target in neurodevelopmental disorders of known genetic origin. By contrast, in cases where there is no known genetic mutation, early diagnosis and intervention is more difficult. Often it is the atypical behaviors that the child demonstrates during their later development that signal cause for concern, but for this to be the case, the developmental trajectory must be atypical enough for it to be observed in the child's emerging phenotype. For example, autism spectrum disorders are rarely diagnosed firmly and given targeted intervention before the age of 3, and yet basic-level impairments are likely to be present much earlier in development. This has indeed recently been shown to be the case in studies of at-risk infants in families where an older child has already been diagnosed with ASD (Elsabbagh and Johnson, 2010). To avoid subtle forms of impairment cascading over time and compounding difficulties for children, alongside their other neurodevelopmental problems, we argue that it is crucial that intervention take place as early as possible in the developmental trajectory.

12.5.1 Some Basic Forms of Intervention

Effective intervention requires a solid scientific understanding of the neural and cognitive processes underlying each specific syndrome, although there is likely to be some overlap between the interventions used for different disorders (for example, where the disorders share some characteristic traits). It is also critical to distinguish behavioral proficiency from underlying neural and/or cognitive processes. Indeed, a child may display normal-like behavior after an intervention despite the fact that the processes underpinning the behavior may remain different from those of healthy controls. For instance, in Williams syndrome, individuals can be taught to count to 100 successfully, without, however, understanding cardinality nor what counting is for (Ansari et al., 2003).

Semel and Rosner (2003) suggest five basic forms of intervention, including:

(1) task-specific interventions in clinical settings; (2) naturalistic training situations during normal activities in the child's home or school; (3) compensatory strategies, which use a child's existing strengths in one domain, say language, to bootstrap a weak domain, say spatial navigation; (4) environmental manipulations where complex tasks are broken down artificially into their component parts; and (5) what they call "control mechanisms," an example of which is to use direct verbal instruction to guide the behavior of the individual.

Applied Behavior Analysis (ABA) is often linked to intervention in ASD, but it has also been used to treat a wide range of other behavioral and developmental disorders. ABA focuses on the basic principles of learning such as *positive reinforcement* (when behavior is followed by a reward, the behavior is more likely to be repeated). The method utilizes techniques to bring about meaningful changes in the individual's behavior and to reduce those behaviors that can harm or interfere with learning. A recent systematic review of research in children with ASD suggests that many do best with 25 hours or more per week of comprehensive intervention to address social communication, language, play skills, and maladaptive behaviors (Maglione et al., 2012). Like those described earlier, the techniques can be used in a range of situations, such as structured contexts like the classroom, or less structured ones such as meal times at home. Some ABA therapy sessions involve one-on-one interaction between the therapist and individual, while others include group therapy sessions. The efficacy of intensive ABA programs has been far less studied in adolescents and adults compared to young children. Examples of types of ABA therapy include (1) *Discrete Trial Learning,* which focuses on breaking a skill into smaller parts and teaching one sub-skill at a time (Smith, 2001) and (2) *Pivotal Response Teaching,* which aims to increase production of appropriate communicative and play behaviors using naturalistic and motivational procedures.

12.6 LEARNING THEORIES DRIVING BEHAVIORAL INTERVENTIONS

Learning theories describe how information is absorbed, processed, and retained (i.e., learnt). Some principles of ABA therapy are based upon the Behaviorist learning theory and view learning as a process of change in an individual's behavior. Behaviorism (Watson, 1913; 1878–1959) roots learning in the acquisition of new behaviors through conditioning, that is, a system of rewards and punishment. There are two types of conditioning, *Classical Conditioning*, where the behavior is akin to a reflex response to a stimulus, and *Operant Conditioning*, where there is some reinforcement of the behavior by reward or punishment.

Cognitive theorists argue, by contrast, that mere changes in behavior do not constitute learning. They view learning as an internal process where focus is placed on building the representations underlying intelligent thought. Cognitive theory assumes that memory is an organized system of processing, and that an individual's stored knowledge plays a key role in their learning. The theory interprets learning in terms of patterns of behavior rather than isolated behaviors.

Constructivism emphasizes the role of active learners, rather than passive observers, in constructing knowledge (e.g., Piaget, 1971). *Constructivists* believe that the ability of an individual is largely built upon what they already understand, and argue that acquiring new knowledge is a process of individually tailored *construction,* that is, "active learners" construct knowledge for themselves, assimilating new information into their current and past experience(s), and accommodating their knowledge to aspects of the new information. For intervention to be effective, Constructivists maintain that first a deep understanding is required of what children already have in their knowledge repertoire and therefore of what to build upon. Intervention based upon constructivist theory makes room for dynamic online development of the intervention protocol, taking constant account of the changing development of the child. It is not strictly planned in advance. It also emphasizes the need for free exploration, that is, active learning, discovery, and knowledge building, within a given framework.

Finally, *Neuroconstructivism* focuses on how very early basic-level processes might cascade over developmental time on the resulting neurocognitive phenotype. It thus advocates training very early in development on these more domain-general processes. For example, Baron-Cohen (1998) argues for a theory-of-mind module that might emerge from lower-level systems for detecting eye gaze, intentionality, and shared attention. So training would focus on these lower-level systems rather than the more sophisticated theory-of-mind computations. Likewise in language acquisition, van der Lely (2005) maintains that both syntax and phonology rely on a common computational property operating over linguistic representations, which is claimed to be atypical in individuals with Specific Language Impairment. However, the intervention implications here remain very domain-specific (complex computations operating solely on linguistic representations) and do not consider possible interactions with nonlinguistic parts of the developing system over time. Indeed, the theorizing is based on the claim that the grammatical neurocircuitry underlying language is a developmentally unique higher cognitive system in the functional architecture of the brain, which can be selectively impaired (Fonteneau and van der Lely, 2007). This is contrary to the neuroconstructivist vision that considers multiple cross-circuit interactions early on in development, which progressively become specialized as higher-level cognition emerges over time.

Nonetheless, the notion of impaired versus intact brain systems in uneven cognitive profiles might be considered useful for intervention, even if theoretically it underplays the role of development. If an individual has scores in the normal range in a particular domain, surely there is no need to consider intervention in that domain? The Nativist would probably agree, but the Neuroconstructivist, believing in cross-domain interactions, would not rule out

intervention also in a proficient domain. For instance, take an individual who presents with a serious deficit in, say, number processing, yet scores in the normal range in face processing tasks – two seemingly very distinct higher-level cognitive domains. It would be tempting in such a case to tailor remediation solely to the domain of number. But that misses the very point of the Neuroconstructivist framework. Once one explores multiple, low-level interacting processes that underpin face processing and number early on in development, this leads to a more dynamic view of intervention. Take the case of Williams syndrome. In adulthood, the proficient behavior of individuals with WS on face processing tasks turns out to be due to a focus on features. Now, if an infant cannot plan saccades and therefore has sticky fixation (as is the case for infants with WS, Brown et al., 2003), then they are more likely to fixate on features than to rapidly process the configuration of a face. And, despite scores in the normal range on standardized face-processing tasks, the neural and cognitive processes underlying proficient face processing in WS are atypical compared to controls (Grice et al., 2001, 2003; Mills et al., 2000). Thus, intervention may well be necessary in face processing in WS, that is, in a domain even where the outcome gives rise to scores in the normal range. Only a study of very early development can reveal this. Moreover, early on in development, domains are not isolated from one another in their developmental trajectories; specialization is the outcome of development over time. Number, too, is influenced by deficits in visual scanning and planning of saccades. Infants with WS fail to scan numerical displays as fully as required in order to discriminate changes in number (van Herwegen et al., 2008). So intervention for number and for face processing might *both* start out by stimulating saccadic eye movements, and not with number or face processing training at all.

Attention training is another area of potential neuroconstructivist intervention in that it serves a special cross-domain role in early infancy (Cornish et al., 2007; Wass et al., 2011). Depending on the syndrome, early attention training could be in the auditory and/or visual domains, and such interventions might cascade subsequently on several higher-level cognitive domains.

None the less, the comparison of intervention on basic-level deficits very early in life versus the same intervention carried out in later development remains to elucidate whether developmental trajectories are still open to change and cascading effects even in later development.

12.7 CONCLUDING THOUGHTS

For decades, the notion of plasticity tended to be reserved for the human system's response to damage. By contrast, it has become abundantly clear that development—whether typical or atypical, whether human or nonhuman—is fundamentally characterized by plasticity for learning, with the infant brain dynamically structuring and re-structuring itself over the course of ontogeny. While some macrostructures such as the overall six-layer structure of cortex may be under general genetic constraints, much of the microcircuitry of cortex turns out to be the result of complex multilevel interactions between genes and environment over developmental time. We thus advocate a Neuroconstructivist approach to the theoretical and practical understanding of genetic disorders and to the planning of very early intervention strategies.

REFERENCES

Alcock, K.J., Passingham, R.E., Watkins, K., and Vargha-Khademm, F. (2000). Pitch and timing abilities in inherited speech and language impairment. Brain Lang 75, 34–46.

Annaz, D., Karmiloff-Smith, A., and Thomas, M.C. (2008). The importance of tracing developmental trajectories for clinical child neuropsychology. In: J. Reed, and J. Warner Rogers, eds. Child Neuropsychology: Concepts, Theory and Practice (pp. 7–18), Hoboken, US: Wiley Blackwell.

Ansari, D., Donlan, C., Thomas, M., Ewing, S., Peen, T., and Karmiloff-Smith, A. (2003). What makes counting count? Verbal and visuo-spatial contributions to typical and atypical number development. J Exp Child Psychol 85, 50–62.

Bahn, S., Mimmack, M., Ryan, M., Caldwell, M.A., Jauniaux, E., Starkey, M., Svendsen, C.N., Emson, P. (2002). Neuronal target genes of the neuron-restrictive silencer factor in neurospheres derived from fetuses with Down's syndrome: a gene expression study. Lancet 359, 310–315.

Baron-Cohen, S. (1998). Does the study of autism justify minimalist innate modularity? Learn Individ Differ 10, 179–191

Bellugi, U., Wang, P.P., and Jernigan, T.L. (1994). Williams syndrome: an unusual neuropsychological profile. In: S.H. Broman, and J. Grafman, eds. Atypical cognitive deficits in developmental disorders: implications for brain function (pp. 23–56). Hillsdale, NJ: Lawrence Erlbaum Associates.

Bolhuis, J.J., Zijlstra, G.G.O., den Boer-Visser, A.M., and van der Zee, E.A. (2000). Localized neuronal activation in the zebra finch brain is related to the strength of song learning. Proc Natl Acad Sci U S A. 97(5), 2282–2285.

Brown, J., Johnson, M.H., Paterson, S., Gilmore, R., Gsödl, M., Longhi, E., and Karmiloff-Smith, A. (2003). Spatial representation and attention in toddlers with Williams syndrome and Down syndrome. Neuropsychologia 41, 1037–1046.

Bowler, D.M., Gardiner, J.M., and Grice, S.J. (2000). Episodic Memory and Remembering in Adults with Asperger Syndrome. J Autism Dev Disord 30 (4), 295–304.

Busciglio, B.A., and Yankner, J. (1995). Apoptosis and increased generation of reactive oxygen species in Down's syndrome neurons in vitro. Nature 378, 776–779.

Casey, B.J., (2002). Neuroscience - Windows into the human brain. Science 296, 1408–1409.

Clayton-Smith, J., (2006). 15q11-13 phenotypes: Angelman and Prader-Willi syndromes. J Med Genet 43 (1), S41.

Cohen-Kadosh, K., and Johnson, M.H. (2007). Developing a cortex specialized for face perception. Trends Cogn Sci 11, 367–369.

Comery, T. A., Harris, J. B., Willems, P. J., Oostra, B. A., Irwin, S. A., Weiler, I. J. & Greenough, W. T. (1997). Abnormal dendritic spines in fragile X knockout mice: maturation and pruning deficits. Proceedings of the National Academy of Sciences, 94, 5401–5404.

Cornish, K.M., Li, L., Kogan, C.S., Jacquemont, S., Turk, J., Dalton, A., Hagerman, R.J., and Hagerman, P.J. (2008). Age-dependent cognitive changes in carriers of the fragile X syndrome. Cortex 44 (6), 628–636.

Cornish, K., Scerif, G., and Karmiloff-Smith, A. (2007). Tracing syndrome-specific trajectories of attention across the lifespan. Cortex 43, 672–685.

De Haan, M., Pascalis, O., and Johnson, M.H. (2002). Specialization of neural mechanisms underlying face recognition in human infants. J. Cognitive Neurosci. 14(2), 199–209.

Dekker, T.M., and Karmiloff-Smith, A. (2011). The dynamics of ontogeny: a neuroconstructivist perspective on genes, brains, cognition and behavior. Prog Brain Res 189, 22–33. DOI: 10.1016/B978-0-444-53884-0.00016-6.

Diamond, A. (2007). Consequences of variations in genes that affect dopamine in prefrontal cortex. Cereb Cortex 17, 161–170.

Elman, J.L., Bates, E., Johnson, M.H., Karmiloff-Smith, A., Parisi, D., and Plunkett, K. (1996). Rethinking innateness: A connectionist perspective on development. Cambridge, MA: MIT Press.

Elsabbagh, M., and Johnson, M.H. (2010). Getting answers from babies about autism. Trends Cogn Sci 14, 81–87

Enard, W., Przeworski, M., Fisher, S.E., Lai, S.L., Wiebe, V., Kitano, T., et al. (2002). Molecular evolution of FOXP2, a gene involved in speech and language. Nature 418, 869–872

Farran, E.K., and Karmiloff-Smith, A., eds (2012). Neurodevelopmental Disorders Across the Lifespan: A Neuroconstructivist Approach. Oxford: Oxford University Press.

Fonteneau, C., and van der Lely, H.J.K. (2007). Electrical brain responses in language-impaired children reveal grammar-specific deficits. PLoS One, 3(3), e1832. DOI: 10.1371/journal.pone.0001832

Frith, U. (1991). Autism and Asperger Syndrome. London: Cambridge University Press.

Gai, X., Xie, H.M., Perin, J.C., Takahashi, N., Murphy, K., Wenocur, A.S., D'arcy, M., O'Hara, R.J., Goldmuntz, E., Grice, D.E., Shaikh, T.H., Hakonarson, H., Buxbaum, J.D., Elia, J., and White, P.S. (2011).Rare structural variation of synapse and neurotransmission genes in autism. Mol Psychiatry 17, 402–411.

Geschwind, D.H. (2011). Genetics of autism spectrum disorders. Trends Cogn Sci 15(9), 409–416.

Gopnik, M., and Crago, M.B. (1991). Familial aggregation of a developmental language disorder. Cognition 39 (1), 1–50.

Gottlieb, G. (2007). Probabilistic epigenesis. Dev Sci 10, 1–11.

Gray, V., Karmiloff-Smith, A., Funnell, E., and Tassabehji, M. (2006). In-depth analysis of spatial cognition in Williams Syndrome: a critical assessment of the role of the LIMK1 gene. Neuropsychologia 44(5), 679–685.

Grice, S.J., de Haan, M., Halit, H., Johnson, M.H., Csibra, G., Grant, J., and Karmiloff-Smith, A. (2003). ERP abnormalities of visual perception in Williams syndrome. Neuroreport 14, 1773–1777

Grice, S., Spratling, M.W., Karmiloff-Smith, A., Halit, H., Csibra, G., de Haan, M., et al. (2001). Disordered visual processing and oscillatory brain activity in autism and Williams syndrome. Neuroreport 12, 2697–2700.

Groszer, M., Keays, D.A., Deacon, R.M.J., de Bono, J.P., Prasad-Mulcare, S., Gaub, S., et al. (2008). Impaired synaptic plasticity and motor learning in mice with a point mutation implicated in human speech deficits. Curr Biol 18, 354–362.

Hallmayer, J., Cleveland, S., Torres, A., Phillips, J., Cohen, B., Torigoe, T., Miller, J., Fedele, A., Collins, J., Smith, K., Lotspeich, L., Croen, L.A., Ozonoff, S., Lajonchere, C., Grether, J.K., Risch, N. (2011). Arch Gen Psychiatry 68 (11), 1095–1102. PMID: 21727249

Haesler, S., Wada, K., Nshdejan, A., Morrisey, E.E., Lints, T., Jarvis, E.D., and Scharff, C. (2004). FoxP2 expression in avian vocal learners and non-learners. J Neurosci 24(13), 3164–3175. DOI: 10.1523/JNEUROSCI.4369-03.2004

Happé, F., and Ronald, A. (2008). 'Fractionable Autism Triad': A Review of Evidence from Behavioural, Genetic, Cognitive and Neural Research. Neuropsychol Rev 18, 287–304.

Huttenlocher, P.R., and Dabholkar, A.S. (1997). Regional differences in synaptogenesis in human cerebral cortex. J Comp Neurol 387, 167–178.

Johnson, M.H. (2001). Functional brain development in humans. Nat Rev Neurosci 2, 475–483.

John, A.E., and Mervis, C.B. (2010). Comprehension of the communicative intent behind pointing and gazing gestures by young children with Williams syndrome or Down syndrome. J Speech Lang Hear Res 53, 950–960.

Kaffman, A., and Meaney, M.J. (2007). Neurodevelopmental sequelae of postnatal maternal care in rodents: Clinical and research implications of molecular insights. J Child Psychol Psychiatry 48(3–4), 224–244.

Karmiloff-Smith, A. (1998). Development itself is the key to understanding developmental disorders. Trends Cogn Sci 2(10), 389–398.

Karmiloff-Smith, A. (2009). Nativism vs neuroconstructivism: Rethinking developmental disorders. Dev Psychol 45, 56–63.

Karmiloff-Smith, A. (2010). Neuroimaging of the developing brain: taking "developing" seriously. Hum Brain Mapp 31 (6), 934–941.

Karmiloff-Smith, A., (2013). Challenging the use of adult neuropsychological models for explaining neurodevelopmental disorders: Developed versus developing brains. Q J Exp Psychol 66 (1), 1–14.

Karmiloff-Smith, A., Aschersleben, G., de Schonen, T., Elsabbagh, M., Hohenberger, A., and Serres, J. (2010). Constraints on the timing of infant cognitive change: Domain-specific or domain-general? Eur J Dev Sci 4(1), 31–45.

Karmiloff-Smith, A., Broadbent, H. Farran, E.K., Longhi, E., D'Souza, D., Metcalfe, K., Tassabehji, M., Wu, R., Senju, A., Happé, F., Turnpenny, P. and Sansbury, F. (2012). Social cognition in Williams syndrome: genotype/phenotype insights from partial deletion patients. Front Psychol 3, 168. DOI: 10.3389/fpsyg.2012.00168

Karmiloff-Smith, A., Grant, J., Ewing, S., Carette, M.J., Metcalfe, K., Donnai, D., Read, A.P., Tassabehji, M. (2003). Using case study comparisons to explore genotype-phenotype correlations in Williams-Beuren syndrome. J Med Genet 40(2), 136–140.

Karmiloff-Smith, A., Thomas, M.S.C., Annaz, D., Humphreys, K., Ewing, S., Brace, N., van Duuren, M., Pike, G., Grice, S., and Campbell, R. (2004). Exploring the Williams Syndrome Face Processing Debate: The importance of building developmental trajectories. J Child Psychol Psyc 45 (7), 1258–1274.

Korbel, J.O., Tirosh-Wagner, T., Urban, A.E., Chen, X.N., Kasowsk, M., Dai, L., Grubert, F., Erdman, C., Gao, M.C., Lange, K., Sobel, E.M., Barlow, G.M., Aylsworth, A.S., Carpenter, N.J., Clark, R.D., Cohen, M.Y., Doran, E., Falik-Zaccai, T., Lewin, S.O., Lott, I.T., McGillivray, B.C., Moeschler, J.B., Pettenati, M.J., Pueschel, S.M., Rao, K.W., Shaffer, L.G., Shohat, M., Van Riper,

A.J., Warburton, D., Weissman, S., Gerstein, M.B., Snyder, M., and Korenberg, J.R. (2009). The Genetic Architecture of Down Syndrome Phenotypes Revealed by High Resolution Analysis of Human Segmental Trisomies. Proc Natl Acad Sci U S A, 106(29), 12031–12036.

Lai, C.S., Fisher, S.E., Hurst, J.A., Vargha-Khadem, F., Monaco, A.P. (2001). A forkhead-domain gene is mutated in a severe speech and language disorder. Nature 413, 519–523.

Lott, I.T., and Dierssen, M. (2010). Cognitive deficits and associated neurological complications in individuals with Down's syndrome. Lancet Neurol 9, 623–633.

Lai, C.S., Gerrelli, D., Monaco, A.P., Fisher, S.E., and Copp, A.J. (2003). FOXP2 expression during brain development coincides with adult sites of pathology in a severe speech and language disorder. Brain 126, 2455–2462.

Lott, I.T., Head, E., Doran, E., Busciglio, J. (2006). Beta-amyloid, oxidative stress and down syndrome. Curr Alzheimer Res 3, 521–528.

Maglione, M.A., Gans, D., Das, L., Timbie, J., Kasari, C., (2012). Nonmedical interventions for children with ASD: recommended guidelines and further research needs. Pediatrics 130(Suppl 2) S169–S178. [PMID: 23118248]

Mareschal, D., Johnson, M.H., Sirois, S., Spratling, M., Thomas, M., and Westermann, G. (2007). Neuroconstructivism, Vol. I: How the brain constructs cognition. Oxford, UK: Oxford University Press.

Martens, M.A., Wilson, S.J., and Reutens, D.C. (2008). Research review: Williams syndrome: a critical review of the cognitive, behavioral, and neuroanatomical phenotype. J Child Psychol Psyc 49, 576–608.

Massand, E., Jemel, B., Mottron, L., and Bowler, D.M. (2013). ERP correlates of recognition memory in autism spectrum disorder. J Autism Dev Disord. Online First.

Meyer-Lindenberg, A., Hariri, A.R., Munoz, K.E., et al. (2005). Neural correlates of genetically abnormal social cognition in Williams syndrome. Nat Neurosci 8, 991–993.

Mills, D.L., Alvarez, T.D., St. George, M., Appelbaum, L.G., Bellugi, U., and Neville, H. (2000). Electrophysiological studies of face processing in Williams syndrome. J Cogn Neurosci 12, 47–64.

Nadel, L. (2003). Down's syndrome: a genetic disorder in biobehavioral perspective. Genes Brain Behav 2,156–166.

Neville, H.J. (2006). Different profiles of plasticity within human cognition. In: Y. Munakata, and M. Johnson eds. Processes of change in brain and cognitive development: Attention and Performance XXI (pp. 287–314) London: Oxford University Press.

Neville, H.J., and Mills, D.L., (1997). Epigenesis of Language. Ment Retard Dev Disabil Res Rev 3, 282–292.

Oliver, A., Johnson, M.H., Karmiloff-Smith, A., and Pennington, B. (2000). Deviations in the emergence of representations: A neuroconstructivist framework for analyzing developmental disorders. Dev Sci 3, 1–23.

Osborne L.R. (2012). Genes: the gene expression approach. In: E.K. Farran, and A. Karmiloff-Smith eds. Neurodevelopmental Disorders Across the Lifespan: A Neuroconstructivist Approach (pp. 59–81). Oxford: Oxford University Press.

Ozonoff, S., Young, G., Carter, A., Messinger, D., Yirmiya, N., Zwaigenbaum, L., Bryson, S., Carver, L.J., Constantino, J.N., Dobkins, K., Hutman, T., Iverson, J.M., Landa, R., Rogers, S.J., Sigman, M., and Stone, W.L. (2011). Recurrence risk for autism spectrum disorders: a Baby Siblings Research Consortium study. Pediatrics 128, 488–495.

Pembrey, M., Fennell, S.J., Van Den Berghe, J., Fitchett, M., Summers, D., Btler, L. Clarke, C., Griffiths, M., Thompsn, E., Super, M., and Baraitser, M. (1989). The association of Angelman's syndrome with deletions within 15q11-13. J Med Genet 26, 73–77.

Piaget, J. (1971). Genetic epistemology. New York: W.W. Norton.

Pinker, S. (2001). Words and rules: The ingredients of language. New York, NY: Basic Books.

Robinson E.B., Koenen, K.C., McCormick, M.C., Munir, K., Hallett, V., Happe, F., Plomin, R., and Ronald, A. (2012). A multivariate twin study of autistic traits in 12-year-olds: Testing the fractionable autism triad hypothesis. Behav Genet 42 (2), 245–255

Rossen, M.L., Jones, W., Wang, P.P., and Klima, E.S. (1996). Face processing: remarkable sparing in Williams syndrome. Special Issue, Genet Counsel 6 (1), 138–140.

Rosenberg, R., Law, J., Yenokyan, G., McGready, J., Kaufmann, W., and Law, P. (2009). Characteristics and Concordance of Autism Spectrum Disorders Among 277 Twin Pairs. Arch Pediat Adolesc

Med 163 (10), 907–914. DOI: 10.1001/archpediatrics.2009.98

Rugg, M.D., and Curran, T. (2007). Event-related potentials and recognition memory. Trends Cogn Sci 11, 251–257.

Semel, E., and Rosner, S. (2003). Understanding Williams Syndrome. Mahwah NJ: Lawrence Erlbaum Associates.

Smith, T. (2001) Discrete Trial Training in the Treatment of Autism. Focus on Autism and Other Developmental Disabilities, 16 (2), 86–92.

Smith, A.D., Gilchrist, I.D., Hood, B. Tassabehji, M., and Karmiloff-Smith, A. (2009). Inefficient search of large-scale space in Williams Syndrome: Further insights on the role of LIMK1 deletion in deficits of spatial cognition. Perception 38 (5), 694–701.

Tassabehji, M., Metcalfe, K., Karmiloff-Smith, A., Carette, M.J., Grant, J., Dennis, N., Reardon, W., Splitt, M., Read, A.P., and Donnai D. (1999). Williams syndrome: Use of chromosomal microdeletions as a tool to dissect cognitive and physical phenotypes. Am J Hum Genet 64, 118–125.

Thomas, M.S., Knowland, V.C., and Karmiloff-Smith, A. (2011). Mechanisms of developmental regression in autism and the broader phenotype: A neural network modeling approach. Psychol Rev 118(4), 637–654.

Tomalski, P., Moore, D.G., Ribeiro, H., Axelsson, E.L., Murphy, E., Karmiloff-Smith, A., et al. (2013). Socio-economic status and functional brain development: Associations in early infancy. Dev Sci 16(5), 676–687.

Udwin, O., and Yule, W. (1991). A cognitive and behavioural phenotype in Williams syndrome. J Clin Exp Neuropsyc 13 (2), 232–244.

van der Lely, H.K.J. (2005). Domain-specific cognitive systems: Insight from grammatical specific language impairment. Trends Cogn Sci 9, 53–59.

Van Herwegen, J., Ansari, D., Xu, F., and Karmiloff-Smith, A. (2008). Small and large number processing in infants and toddlers with Williams syndrome. Dev Sci 11, 637–643.

Watson, J.B. (1913). Psychology as the Behaviorist Views it. Psychol Rev 20, 158–177.

Wass, S., Porayska-Pomsta, K., and Johnson, M.H. (2011). Training Attentional Control in Infancy. Curr Biol 21 (18), 1543–1547.

13

HUMAN GENETICS AND CLINICAL ASPECTS OF NEURODEVELOPMENTAL DISORDERS

GHOLSON J. LYON[1,2,3] AND JASON O'RAWE[1,4]

[1]*Stanley Institute for Cognitive Genomics, Cold Spring Harbor Laboratory, Cold Spring Harbor, NY, 11724 USA*
[2]*Institute for Genomic Medicine, Utah Foundation for Biomedical Research, E 3300 S, Salt Lake City, UT, 84106 USA*
[3]*Department of Psychiatry, Stony Brook University, 100 Nicolls Road, Stony Brook, NY, 11794 USA*
[4]*Graduate Program in Genetics, Stony Brook University, Stony Brook, NY, 11794 USA*

13.1 INTRODUCTION

"Our incomplete studies do not permit actual classification; but it is better to leave things by themselves rather than to force them into classes which have their foundation only on paper"

– Edouard Seguin
(Seguin, 1866)

"The fundamental mistake which vitiates all work based upon Mendel's method is the neglect of ancestry, and the attempt to regard the whole effect upon offspring, produced by a particular parent, as due to the existence in the parent of particular structural characters;

while the contradictory results obtained by those who have observed the offspring of parents apparently identical in certain characters show clearly enough that not only the parents themselves, but their race, that is their ancestry, must be taken into account before the result of pairing them can be predicted"

– Walter Frank Raphael Weldon
(Weldon, 1902).

There are ~12 billion nucleotides in every cell of the human body, and there are ~25–100 trillion cells in each human body. Given somatic mosaicism, epigenetic changes, and environmental differences, no two human beings are the same, particularly as there are only ~7 billion

The Genetics of Neurodevelopmental Disorders, First Edition. Edited by Kevin J. Mitchell.
© 2015 John Wiley & Sons, Inc. Published 2015 by John Wiley & Sons, Inc.

people on the planet. One of the next great challenges for studying human genetics will be to acknowledge and embrace complexity (Allchin, 2005; Bearn, 1993; Comfort, 2012; Grillo et al., 2013; Misteli, 2013; Radick, 2011; Sabin et al., 2013; Scriver, 2007; Tennessen et al., 2012; Terwilliger and Weiss, 2003; Weiss and Terwilliger, 2000). Every human *is* unique, and the study of human disease phenotypes (and phenotypes in general) will be greatly enriched by moving from a deterministic to a more stochastic/probabilistic model (Freund et al., 2013; Gigerenzer, 2002; Gigerenzer and Galesic, 2012; Gigerenzer et al., 2010; Kurz-Milcke et al., 2008; Sokal, 2012). The dichotomous distinction between "simple" and "complex" diseases is completely artificial, and we argue instead for a model that considers a spectrum of diseases that are variably manifesting in each person. The rapid adoption of whole genome sequencing (WGS) and the Internet-mediated networking of people promise to yield more insight into this century-old debate (Bateson and Mendel, 1902; Lyon and Segal, 2013; Lyon and Wang, 2012; Nielsen, 2012; Olby, 1989; Provine, 2001; Weldon, 1902). Comprehensive ancestry tracking and detailed family history data, when combined with WGS or at least cascade-carrier screening (McClaren et al., 2010), might eventually facilitate a degree of genetic prediction for some diseases in the context of their familial and ancestral etiologies. However, it is important to remain humble, as our current state of knowledge is not yet sufficient, and in principle, any number of nucleotides in the genome, if mutated or modified in a certain way and at a certain time and place, might influence some phenotype during embryogenesis or postnatal life (Batista and Chang, 2013; Cartault et al., 2012; Dickel et al., 2013; Hansen et al., 2013; Kapusta et al., 2013; Keller, 2010; Khoddami and Cairns, 2013; Ledford, 2013; Maxmen, 2013; Memczak et al., 2013; Mercer and Mattick, 2013; Miura et al., 2013; Moreau et al., 2013; Ning et al., 2013; Pennacchio et al., 2013; Perrat et al., 2013; Sabin et al., 2013; Salzman et al., 2012; Wilusz and Sharp, 2013).

In this chapter, we will traverse contemporary understandings of the genetic architecture of human disease, and explore the clinical implications of the current state of our knowledge. Many molecular models have been postulated as being important in genetic disease, and, despite our incomplete knowledge of the genetic workings of many diseases, significant progress has been made over the past 50 years. Many different classes of genetic mutations have been implicated as being involved in predisposition to certain diseases, and we are continually uncovering other means by which genetics plays an important role in human disease, such as with somatic genetic mosaicism. An explosion in the development of new biomedical techniques, molecular technologies, and analytical tools has enriched our knowledge of the many molecular bases of disease, underscored by the fact that we now exist in a world where each person can be characterized on the level of their "genome," "transcriptome," and "proteome." We discuss these exciting new developments and the current applications of these technologies, their limitations, their implications for prenatal diagnosis, and implantation genetics, as well as future prospects.

13.2 CLINICAL CLASSIFICATIONS AND THE GENETIC ARCHITECTURE OF DISEASE

"Those who have given any attention to congenital mental lesions, must have been frequently puzzled how to arrange, in any satisfactory way, the different classes of this defect which may have come under their observation. Nor will the difficulty be lessened by an appeal to what has been written on the subject. The systems of classification are generally so vague and artificial, that, not only do they assist but feebly, in any mental arrangement of the phenomena represented, but they completely fail in exerting any practical influence on the subject."

– John Langdon Down
(Down, 1995)

As most clinicians know from experience, it is quite difficult to characterize the range of human experience in the two-dimensional world of the printed page, as we are attempting to do here. In addition, classifications can sometimes lead people to try to force round pegs into square holes, and so we are reluctant to further promulgate these classifications. Such classifications include terms such as: "Mendelian," "complex disease," "penetrance," "expressivity," "oligogenic," and "polygenic." For example, some have used the word "Mendelian" to refer to a disease that appears to be "caused" by mutations in a single gene. As such, cystic fibrosis, Huntington's disease, and Fragile X are all diseases that some people refer to as being "caused" by mutations occurring in single genes. However, the expression of the phenotype within these diseases is extremely variable, depending in part on the exact mutations in each gene, and it is not at all clear that any mutation really and truly "causes" any phenotype, at least not according to thoughtful definitions of causation that we are aware of (Fins, 2009; Hume and Selby-Bigge, 1896). For example, some children with certain mutations in *CFTR* may only have pancreatitis as a manifestation of cystic fibrosis, without any lung involvement (Corleto et al., 2010; Derikx and Drenth, 2010), and there is evidence that mutations in other genes in the genomes can have a modifying effect on the phenotype (Emond et al., 2012; Rosendahl et al., 2013). In the case of Huntington's, there is extreme variability in the expression of the phenotype, both in time, period, and scope of illness, and all of this is certainly modified substantially by the number of trinucleotide repeats (Orr and Zoghbi, 2007), genetic background (Tome et al., 2013) and environmental influences (Ciancarelli et al., 2013). Even in the case of whole chromosome disorders, such as Down Syndrome, there is ample evidence of substantial phenotypic expression differences, modified again by genetic background (Ackerman et al., 2012; Li et al., 2012), somatic mosaicism (Papavassiliou et al., 2009), and environmental influences (Dodd and Shields, 2005; Solomon, 2012), including synaptic and brain plasticity

(Freund et al., 2013; Maffei, 2012; Maffei et al., 2012; Maffei and Turrigiano, 2008; Wang et al., 2013). The same is true for genomic deletion and duplication syndromes, such as velocardiofacial syndrome and other deletions (Guris et al., 2006; Iascone et al., 2002; Liao et al., 2004; McDonald-McGinn et al., 2013; Moreno-De-Luca et al., 2013a; Stalmans et al., 2003). And, of course, there is constant interaction of the environment with a person, both prenatally and postnatally. As just one example, cretinism is related to a lack of iodine in the mother's diet, and there is incredibly variable expression of this illness based in part on the amount of iodine deficiency and how this interacts with fetal development (Zimmermann, 2012).

The words "penetrance" and "expressivity" can be defined as:

- *Penetrance*: The number of individuals in a population carrying a disease predisposing allele that are also categorically defined as being affected by the associated disease.

- *Expressivity*: The extremeness, or number of symptoms, in the presentation of a disease in the context of individuals who have the associated disease predisposing allele."

Unfortunately, these two separate terms have led to a great deal of confusion in the field, and this sort of categorical thinking tends to miss complexity. Some use the word "penetrance" when they really mean "expressivity" of disease in any one person. As such, perhaps we should get rid of the two terms altogether and just discuss the expression of each trait in the context of a phenotypic spectrum, which is of course what led Walter Frank Raphael Weldon to establish the field of biometry (Jamieson and Radick, 2013; McIntyre, 2008; Sokal and Rohlf, 2012). Another way to express this point is to say that we have yet to characterize the full breadth of expression for virtually any mutation in humans, as we have not systematically sequenced or karyotyped any genetic alteration in thousands to millions of randomly selected people from a whole range of ethnic classes, that is, clans (Bittles and Black, 2010; Lupski et al., 2011).

There is an ongoing clash of world-views, with some wanting to believe that single mutations predominately drive outcome while others are explicitly acknowledging the importance of substantial phenotypic modification via genetic background and/or environmental influence(s) (Beaudet, 2013; Bernal and Jirtle, 2010; Burga et al., 2011; Casanueva et al., 2012; Comfort, 2001, 2012; Dolinoy et al., 2006; Keller, 2010; Weinhouse et al., 2011). Some recent population-based sequencing efforts have shown the complexity of demonstrating how much any one genetic variant contributes to disease in any one particular individual, and we disagree with overly simplistic and artificial categorizations of mutations as "causative," "pathogenic" or "nonpathogenic" (Andreasen et al., 2013a; Andreasen et al., 2013b; Refsgaard et al., 2012; Risgaard et al., 2013).

It is very likely that there will be a continuum of disease, given that the "effect size" of any particular mutation will obviously vary according to genetic background and environment, as demonstrated repeatedly in model organisms (Bernal and Jirtle, 2010; Blount et al., 2012; Casanueva et al., 2012; Dolinoy et al., 2006; Greenspan, 2008, 2009, 2012; Holmes and Summers, 2006; Kendler and Greenspan, 2006; Meyer et al., 2012a; van Swinderen and Greenspan, 2005; Weinhouse et al., 2011). Thus, while a mutation associated with hemochromatosis or breast cancer might have high expression in one particular pedigree or clan, that same mutation may have very low expression in another pedigree, clan or group of unrelated people (Kohane et al., 2012). The reasons for variable expression can be myriad and are currently unknown in many instances; however, problems start to appear when scientists attempt to invoke a third allele as necessary and perhaps sufficient for the expression of any symptoms from within a typical disease. This disease model has been most clearly advocated for Bardet–Biedl syndrome, in which the authors contend that some subjects have zero disease symptoms while possessing two autosomal recessive mutations in a known "disease gene"; the authors also show that some affected people have a mutation in another gene,

that is, a third allele, which they speculate is necessary and perhaps sufficient for expression of any symptoms of the disease (Eichers et al., 2004; Katsanis et al., 2001; Katsanis et al., 2002). However, this model has been challenged by others (Abu-Safieh et al., 2012; Laurier et al., 2006; Mykytyn et al., 2003; Nakane and Biesecker, 2005; Smaoui et al., 2006), and at least one group maintains that all people that they have studied with two autosomal recessive mutations have some manifestations of disease but with variable expression, that is, one person might only have retinitis pigmentosa whereas another person might have the full-blown symptoms of Bardet–Biedl syndrome (Abu-Safieh et al., 2012). One wonders whether the debate about triallelism might really just be a semantic one due to problems with the phenotyping of "unaffected" people, particularly if these people were not evaluated longitudinally. Detailed online longitudinal characterizations of all such reportedly "unaffected" people could aid in documenting, with some degree of certainty, that these people did indeed have zero symptoms of Bardet–Biedl syndrome, as that would be further proof that mutations are not deterministic. Said another way, this would be a demonstration of the enormous variability in expression for mutations that do contribute more to a phenotype in some people with their own genetic backgrounds and environmental differences, and this observation ought to have dramatic implications for any ideas concerning prenatal diagnosis and "prediction" of any genotype/phenotype relationship (discussed more subsequently).

Surprisingly, a precise definition of the term "oligogenic" is not apparent or consistent in the world literature. Some people have invoked the term "oligogenic" to mean an interaction between mutations in two genes to collectively "cause" a disease, such as with this aforementioned case of triallelism in Bardet–Biedl syndrome (Beales et al., 2003). These authors define oligogenic inheritance as occurring "when specific alleles at more than one locus affect a genetic trait by causing and/or modifying the severity and range of a phenotype" (Beales et al., 2003). Another case in point involves the 22q11.2 locus, also known as velocardiofacial syndrome. This deletion does not involve only a single gene, but rather ~30–40 number of genes, depending on the exact size of the deletion interval. The phenotypic manifestations can be incredibly heterogeneous, illustrated by the fact that some ~30% develop psychotic symptoms and get labeled as "schizophrenic" (Philip and Bassett, 2011). Of course, heuristic diagnoses for schizophrenia are usually made based on certain semantic criteria, so it is likely that subthreshold symptoms are not counted (or perhaps not even detected). But, at least one has the advantage of knowing which people possess the deletion, allowing one to perform detailed phenotyping to determine whether subthreshold symptoms were missed within a family, and this has indeed been done in the case of a well-known translocation involving *DISC1* (Blackwood et al., 2001; Hamshere et al., 2005). Unfortunately, genome-wide studies are not yet performed routinely for people with "idiopathic schizophrenia", so it has been difficult to identify and group many people by genotype(s). As we discuss subsequently, we believe that the routine clinical use of exome and eventually WGS might finally enable this to occur, assuming that aggregation of genotype and phenotype data is allowed on a massive scale.

The definition of "polygenic" literally means "many genes," including the combined effects of dozens (or perhaps even hundreds) of different mutations in different genes on a particular phenotype, although it is sometimes not very clear whether these multiple genes are meant to be spread across individuals or within individuals. We tend to favor the definition involving multiple mutations within the same individual somehow contributing toward phenotypic development. Height has historically been characterized as being a polygenic phenotype, with GWAS studies implicating the possible involvement of hundreds of loci (Berndt et al., 2013; Visscher et al., 2010). Height is an easily measured phenotype and is generally described as being distributed continuously within human populations, modified of course by gender and ancestral backgrounds. If one looks at height in males or females of a certain ethnic background and from the same geographic locale, one can typically draw a semi-Gaussian (normal) function, but with tails that deviate from what is expected, encompassing rare cases of dwarfism and gigantism. We tend to also think that a single vertical measurement does not capture the true phenotypic variability involving height, as this measurement does not adequately capture the variability that exists in the many determinants of height (i.e., bone dimensions, age, environment, etc.). So, for a trait that seems conceptually simple to measure, there exists difficulty in uncovering its genetic component(s) due, in part, to uncharacterized uncertainty (variability) introduced at the phenotypic measurement level. If we now consider psychometrically defined traits, a large amount of further uncertainty is introduced at the phenotypic measurement level, as we are still unable to accurately characterize even a single measurement for most psychiatric disorders. These difficulties are underscored by the fact that psychiatric definitions are ephemeral and can change in a dramatic fashion over the course of even a few years. It seems premature to argue that schizophrenia, for example, is Gaussian in nature (Visscher et al., 2011). We would argue that we simply do not know enough about the phenotypic expression of the many different diseases that this amorphous concept of "schizophrenia" encompasses to be able to make any conclusions regarding its genetic inheritance on a population or individual level (Mitchell, 2012). Until there is substantial evidence to support another viewpoint, it is therefore important to treat each family as a special case. One must study people within families to determine whether some people in families have illness due to mutations with variable expression, modified by genetic background and environmental influences.

There have been numerous reviews concerning the ongoing debate for common and rare variants, with arguments made for various "camps" of thought, including the common disease-common variant (CDCV) model, the infinitesimal model, the rare allele model and the broad sense heritability model (Gibson, 2011). Frankly, these models are simply semantic and reductionistic arguments that do not reflect the complexity of the human condition, and we are not sure that arguing for and against various models is useful, given that these models are basically straw men artificially constructed to be knocked down. This is very similar to the psychiatric literature in which several people decided, about 100 years ago, to introduce various names (or models) for certain diseases, such as the words "schizophrenia" (Bleuler, 1958) and "manic-depressive illness or bipolar" (Kraepelin, 1921). It is quite apparent to most clinicians that the phenotypic heterogeneity of these illnesses is so tremendous as to render these names basically moot and not particularly useful. This is akin to 50 years ago when people simply stated that someone had "cancer." Now, it is not useful to say only that someone has cancer, as there are literally hundreds of molecular etiologies for cancer, divided up not only by organ expression but also by specific pathways in the cell (Sporn, 2011). We anticipate that in 50 years, these terms "schizophrenia" and "bipolar" will be replaced by much more precise molecularly defined terms, as is occurring now in the cancer field (Mukherjee, 2010; Vogelstein et al., 2013). Locus heterogeneity will likely play an important role in most diseases, but particularly in psychiatric disease, given the extensive phenotypic heterogeneity. Some of this complexity has been documented in reports of individual people (Eichenbaum, 2013; Luria, 1972, 1976; Lyon, 2008; Lyon et al., 2008; Lyon and Coffey, 2009; Penrose, 1963; Ratiu et al., 2004; Sacks, 1995, 1998; Van Horn et al., 2012; Ward, 1998; Worthey et al., 2011), and a review by one of us of the literature related to schizophrenia (Lyon et al., 2011) rendered the distinct impression that we really hardly know anything about the mechanistic basis of these many illnesses that we currently lump together as "schizophrenia." This is primarily due to overly broad descriptions and categorizations of these illnesses into these artificially named syndromes, despite the obvious heterogeneous and inconsistent nature of these categorizations. Remarkably, bipolar and schizophrenia have been artificially "split" into different syndromes (Craddock and Owen, 2010; Williams et al., 2011), in spite of the existence of a well documented literature demonstrating overlap in at least some families with symptoms from both "syndromes" (Lichtenstein et al., 2009).

Oddly enough, some diseases such as Fragile X, Rett Syndrome, and other now molecularly defined disorders are sometimes removed from the "nonsyndromic idiopathic autism" camp, leaving the remaining disorders still eligible for a semantic debate about which "genetic model" they fit into (Reiss, 2009). One wonders if the same thing has occurred for velocardiofacial syndrome, with its relevance to schizophrenia, given the overwhelming evidence that the single 22q11.2 deletion event predisposes its carriers to some version of "schizophrenia" with some exhibiting anywhere between 20 and 30% of the symptoms currently being defined as consistent with "schizophrenia"(Philip and Bassett, 2011). All of these disorders were at one point labeled as "idiopathic" until molecular lesions associated with them were identified. It has been known by at least some researchers and clinicians for quite some time that there are likely many minor physical anomalies in people labeled as "nonsyndromic" (Aldridge et al., 2011; Miles, 2011), all of which is further proof of the substantial phenotypic expression differences of all disorders. Therefore, the dichotomous use of the words "syndromic" and "nonsyndromic" is completely artificial and does not reflect the reality or complexity of the situation in any one person.

A recent paper using exome sequencing to study hypertension pedigrees made the following statements: "These findings demonstrate the utility of exome sequencing in disease gene identification despite the combined complexities of locus heterogeneity, mixed models of transmission and frequent de novo mutation. Gene identification was complicated by the combined effects of locus heterogeneity, two modes of transmission at one locus, and few informative meioses. Many so far unsolved Mendelian traits may have similar complexities. Use of control exomes as comparators for analysis of mutation burden may be broadly applicable to discovery of such loci" (Boyden et al., 2012). This paper illustrates exactly what we are discussing earlier, in terms of the possible heterogeneity of many illnesses on many levels, making it impossible to predict (or even need) any particular model that may or may not fit the disease. It is far better to allow the data to speak for themselves.

13.3 DE NOVO MUTATIONS, GERMLINE MOSAICISM, AND OTHER COMPLEXITIES

Although the concept of somatic mosaicism has been in the literature for many years (Bakker et al., 1989; Hall, 1988; Hollander, 1975; Sastry et al., 1965; Vig, 1978), it is really only recently that more people are beginning to realize that it might be much more extensive in humans than previously thought (Baugher et al., 2013; Biesecker and Spinner, 2013; Choate et al., 2010; Coufal et al., 2011; Huisman et al., 2013; Jongmans et al., 2012; Kurek et al., 2012; Lindhurst et al., 2012; Lindhurst et al., 2011; Lyon and Wang, 2012; Macosko and McCarroll, 2012; Margari et al., 2013; Shirley et al., 2013; Steinbusch et al., 2013; Tanaka et al., 2012; Weiss, 2005; Yamada et al., 2012). In fact, hardly anything is truly known regarding the extent of somatic mosaicism in humans and its effect on phenotype in even well studied diseases. For example, little is known regarding pathogenesis of the phenotype in people with trisomy 21 mosaicism and Down syndrome, although there is likely variation in phenotype associated with the percentage of trisomic cells and their tissue-specificity (Hulten et al., 2010; Iourov et al., 2008; Kovaleva, 2010). A more recent study looked at this issue of somatic mosaicism in Timothy syndrome type 1 (TS-1), which is a rare disorder that affects multiple organ systems and has a high incidence of sudden death due to profound QT prolongation and resultant ventricular arrhythmias.

All previously described cases of TS-1 are associated with a missense mutation in exon 8A (p.G406R) of the L-type calcium channel gene (Ca(v)1.2, *CACNA1C*). Most cases reported in the literature represent highly affected people who present early in life with severe cardiac and neurological manifestations, but these authors found somatic mosaicism in people with TS-1 with less severe manifestations than the typical person with TS-1 (Etheridge et al., 2011). There are therefore likely large ascertainment biases, given that people with subtler phenotypes are likely not coming to anyone's attention. The implications of these findings with somatic mosaicism are that one cannot currently predict phenotype from genotype, particularly in the absence of any comprehensive characterization of which tissues are mutated in any one person. Also, putative "de novo" mutations can instead represent cases of parental mosaicism (including in the germline), which could be revealed by careful genotyping of parental tissues other than peripheral blood lymphocytes. In fact, we are increasingly becoming aware of many instances of germline mosaicism, in which a mutation is not present or is present only at a very low level in the blood sample from a parent, but clearly must be in their germline, as they have two or more children with the same mutation that must therefore have originated through the parent's germline (Aldred et al., 2000; Barbosa et al., 2008; Chaturvedi et al., 2000; Evans et al., 2006; Frank and Happle, 2007; Hosoki et al., 2005; Jongmans et al., 2008; Mari et al., 2005; Meyer et al., 2012b; Parodi et al., 2008; Pauli et al., 2009; Rand et al., 2012; Sato et al., 2006; Sbidian et al., 2010; Shanske et al., 2012; Slavin et al., 2012; Sol-Church et al., 2009; Tajir et al., 2013; Trevisson et al., 2014; Venancio et al., 2007; Wuyts et al., 2005). Clearly, we are truly ignorant concerning the extent of diversity brought about by somatic mosaicism, and it is therefore far too simplistic to assume that a single blood draw truly represents the entire genome of a human being, with anywhere from 25 to 100 trillion cells in their body divided up among multiple organs and other tissue systems. Of course, even the words "whole genome sequencing" are misleading, as there might very well be millions to trillions of similar (but not the exact same) genomes in each person's body.

13.4   RARE AND COMPENSATORY MUTATIONS

There is an increasingly rich literature regarding rare mutations with seemingly large phenotypic effects (Boyden et al., 2002; Jonsson et al., 2012; Styrkarsdottir et al., 2013; Williams, 2004). An example of this is Liam Hoekstra, known as the world's strongest toddler when he was age 3, and who has an extremely rare mutation in the gene encoding myostation, leading to myostatin-related muscle hypertrophy with increased muscle mass and reduced body fat. However, the effects of these mutations have mainly been reported in the context of particular genetic backgrounds, and so our knowledge of the expression of these mutations in the context of any number of genetic backgrounds is lacking. It is likely that there can be, and are, many genomic elements that act in concert to influence these traits in a phenotypic spectrum. Of course, compensatory mutations can be explored in the context of other organisms (Esvelt et al., 2011; Fu et al., 2013a; Leconte et al., 2013), but human migration and breeding is certainly not something that can be experimentally manipulated!

There are many disabling psychiatric syndromes, which have been lumped under certain artificial categories, such as schizophrenia, Tourette Syndrome (TS), obsessive compulsive disorder (OCD), and attention deficit hyperactivity disorder (ADHD). A very good way forward is to study these syndromes in large families living in the same geographic region, so as to control for ancestry differences, minimize environmental influences, and focus on specific genotypes in these families. It is possible that a low number of genetic mutations will be shared in a relatively small combination (on the order of 1–3 such variants) among affected relatives within some pedigrees, and that these variants will not be present in the same combination in

unaffected relatives or in other families with very little to no neuropsychiatric disorders (Crepel et al., 2010; Fullston et al., 2011; Girirajan et al., 2012; Lyon and Wang, 2012; Mitchell, 2012; Mitchell and Porteous, 2011; Shi et al., 2013). An alternative is that some affected people in these families have these illnesses due to additive and/or epistatic interactions among dozens to hundreds of loci within each person (Klei et al., 2012; Zuk et al., 2012). The currently classified syndromes of schizophrenia, obsessive compulsive disorder (OCD), attention deficit hyperactivity disorder (ADHD), autism and other mental illnesses are quite heterogeneous within and between families, and these symptoms have also been observed in known single locus disorders such as Fragile X and 22q11.2 velocardiofacial syndrome (Girirajan et al., 2012; Mitchell, 2012).

Some of these syndromes are referred to as "complex" diseases simply because the presentation is so incredibly heterogeneous that is it very likely that there will be multiple different genetic and environmental explanations. One possible genetic explanation is that some symptoms of severe mental illness may emerge in a particular family due to a genetic constellation including dozens to hundreds of loci acting in each person either additively or via epistasis (and possibly modified by environment; G x E), which some refer to as the "polygenic" model (Anney et al., 2012; Klei et al., 2012; Visscher et al., 2011; Zuk et al., 2012), as previously discussed. If true, for predictive efforts in any particular family, the solution will ultimately require WGS to tease out the numerous mutations involved. On the other hand, some discuss this concept of "many rare variants of large effect," which they refer to as the "oligogenic" model of inheritance (Gagnon et al., 2011; Schaaf et al., 2011), as previously discussed. Some families have deleterious copy number variants (Elia et al., 2010; Gai et al., 2012; Girirajan et al., 2012; Malhotra and Sebat, 2012; Shaikh et al., 2011), and de novo single nucleotide mutations have recently been implicated as important for spontaneous "singleton" cases in at least some families (Iossifov et al.,

2012; Neale et al., 2012; Novarino et al., 2012; O'Roak et al., 2012b; Sanders et al., 2012; Xu et al., 2012). There could also be a set of families with single, pair, or triplet interactions among 1–3 gene mutations of high expression that can largely, on their own, contribute to a set of symptoms currently overlapping with named syndromes, such as "autism" and "schizophrenia" (Girirajan et al., 2010). As there is no way of really distinguishing between these two artificially created models in any one particular family, it is reasonable (with current costs) to perform microarray genotyping and WGS as a comprehensive way to ascertain most of the relevant genetic variance in any particular family.

It is becoming generally accepted that at least 5% of the "autisms" appear to be associated with various large copy number variants (Sanders et al., 2011). So, it is likely that some additional portion of the "autisms" will be influenced by other types of mutations, with some evidence pointing to a role for "de novo" mutations in singleton, uninherited cases of autism (Iossifov et al., 2012; Neale et al., 2012; O'Roak et al., 2012a; O'Roak et al., 2012b; Sanders et al., 2012) and other evidence suggesting that there might be multiple genetic and environmental influences in each person (Klei et al., 2012).

13.5 CURRENT ABILITY/APPROACHES

There has been an explosive growth in exome and WGS (Lyon and Wang, 2012), led in part by dramatic cost reductions. The same is true for genotyping microarrays, which are becoming increasingly denser with various markers while maintaining a relatively stable cost (lllumina, 2013). With rapid advancements in sequencing technologies (Schneider and Dekker, 2012) and improved haplotype-phasing (Peters et al., 2012; Williams et al., 2012), high-throughput sequencing (HTS) data on the genomes of a diverse number of species are being generated at an unprecedented rate. The development of bioinformatics tools for handling these data has been somewhat lagged in response, creating a

gap between the massive data being generated, and the ability to fully exploit their biological content. Many short read alignment software tools are now available, along with several single nucleotide variants (SNVs) and copy number variant (CNVs) calling algorithms (Lyon and Wang, 2012). However, there is a paucity of methods that can simultaneously handle a large number of genetic variants and annotate their functional impacts (particularly for a human genome, which typically hosts > 3 million variants), despite the fact that this is an important task in many sequencing applications. Functional interpretation of genetic variants therefore becomes one of the major obstacles to connect sequencing data with biomedical researchers who are willing to embrace the sequencing technology.

In the medical world, WGS has since led to the discovery of the genetic basis of Miller Syndrome (Roach et al., 2010) and in another instance, it was used to investigate the genetic basis of Charcot–Marie–Tooth neuropathy (Lupski et al., 2010), alongside a discussion of the "return of results" (McGuire and Lupski, 2010). In 2011, the diagnosis of a pair of twins with dopa (3, 4-dihydroxyphenylalanine) responsive dystonia (DRD; OMIM #128230) and the discovery that they carried compound heterozygous mutations in the SPR gene encoding sepiapterin reductase led to supplementation of L-dopa therapy with 5-hydroxytryptophan, a serotonin precursor, resulting in clinical improvements in both twins (Bainbridge et al., 2011).

Despite current technological limitations, mutations are continually being identified in research settings (Bamshad et al., 2011; Hedges et al., 2009; Lyon, 2011; Ng et al., 2010a; Ng et al., 2010b; Roach et al., 2010). However, the human genomics community has recognized a number of distinct challenges, including with phenotyping, sample collection, sequencing strategies, bioinformatics analysis, biological validation of variant function, clinical interpretation and validity of variant data, and delivery of genomic information to various constituents (Katsanis and Katsanis, 2013; Lyon and

Wang, 2012). In particular, there is a need for large pedigree sample collection, high-quality sequencing data acquisition, rigorous generation of variant calls, and comprehensive functional annotation of variants (Lyon and Wang, 2012). Empirical estimates seem to suggest that exome sequencing can identify a putative disease associated variant in only about 10–50% of the cases for which it is applied (Lyon and Wang, 2012), and the genetic architecture of most neuropsychiatric illness is still largely undefined and controversial (Klei et al., 2012; Mitchell, 2012; Mitchell and Porteous, 2011; Visscher et al., 2011). The sequencing of entire genomes in large families will create a dataset that can be analyzed and re-analysed for years to come as new biology and new methods emerge. The cost of a whole genome will likely decrease much more rapidly in relation to the cost of exome sequencing, given the relatively fixed labor and reagent costs for capturing the exons in the genome. Also, there is emerging evidence that exon capture and sequencing only achieves high depth of sequencing coverage in about 90% of the exons, whereas WGS does not involve a capture step and thus obtains better coverage on >95% of all exons in the genome. Of course, even the definition of the exome is a moving target, as the research community is constantly annotating and finding new exons not previously discovered (Wu et al., 2013; Zumbo and Mason, 2014), and therefore WGS is a much more comprehensive way to assess coding and noncoding regions of the genome.

It is obvious that in both research and clinical settings, WGS can dramatically impact clinical care, and it is now a matter of economics and feasibility in terms of WGS being adopted widely in a clinical setting (Lyon, 2012; Lyon and Wang, 2012). There are, however, still many challenges in showing how any one mutation can contribute toward a clear phenotype, particularly in the context of genetic background and possible environmental influences (Moreno-De-Luca et al., 2013b). Bioinformatics confounders, such as poor data quality (Nielsen et al., 2011), sequence inaccuracy, and variation introduced by different methodological approaches (O'Rawe et al., 2013) can further complicate biological and genetic inferences. Furthermore, one cannot exclude polygenic and epistatic modes of inheritance (Bloom et al., 2013; Davis et al., 2011; El-Hattab et al., 2010; Kajiwara et al., 1994; Katsanis et al., 2001; Lai et al., 2010; Lemmers et al., 2012). To address these issues, future work will need to focus on evaluating next generation sequencing data coming from multiple sequencing and informatics platforms, and involving multiple other family members. By using a combination of data from many family members and from different sequencing technologies evaluated by a number of bioinformatics pipelines, we can maximize accuracy and thus the biological inference stemming from these data.

13.6 PRENATAL DIAGNOSIS, PREIMPLANTATION GENETIC DIAGNOSIS/SCREENING

"Before a new function can arise, it may be essential for a lineage to evolve a potentiating genetic background that allows the actualizing mutation to occur or the new function to be expressed. Finally, novel functions often emerge in rudimentary forms that must be refined to exploit the ecological opportunities. This three-step process—in which potentiation makes a trait possible, actualization makes the trait manifest, and refinement makes it effective—is likely typical of many new functions."

– Richard Lenski
(Blount et al., 2012)

A great clinical geneticist, John Opitz, observed the following: "More fetuses die prenatally than are born alive. Many die because of genetic conditions, malformations, and syndromes. Most are not autopsied, and in such cases appropriate genetic counseling is not provided or possible. In such "cases" (fetuses, infants) a huge amount of genetic pathology is yet to be discovered (our last frontier!)" (Opitz, 2012).

In this regard, some have suggested a canalization model, which describes phenotypes as being robust to small perturbations, seemingly stuck within "phenotypic canals." Phenotypes may "slosh" against the sides of the canal during development, but with little effect on the final outcome of development (Waddington, 1959, 2012). In such a model, it is only perturbations with a magnitude exceeding a certain threshold that can direct the developmental path out of the canal (see Fig. 13.1 for an illustrative model of canalization). Accordingly, phenotypes are robust up to a limit, with little robustness beyond this limit.

One could argue that the birth of a child in one particular family with a clear phenotype, such as cystic fibrosis, along with previously identified associated mutations, dramatically increases the likelihood that a future child with these same mutations being born in that

same family would have a similar "canalized" phenotype. It is really only in that particular situation in which one could make a somewhat informed prediction of genotype going down one particular phenotypic "canal". And yet, a study in Australia from 2000 to 2004 showed that of the 82 children born with cystic fibrosis (CF) in Victoria, Australia, 5 (6%) were from families with a known history of CF. The authors found that "even when a family history is known, most relatives do not undertake carrier testing. In an audit of cascade carrier testing after a diagnosis of CF through newborn screening, only 11.8% of eligible (nonparent) (82/716) relatives were tested."(McClaren et al., 2011). These same researchers also showed that in a clinical setting, the diagnosis of a baby with CF by newborn screening "does not lead to carrier testing for the majority of the baby's nonparent relatives" (McClaren et al.,

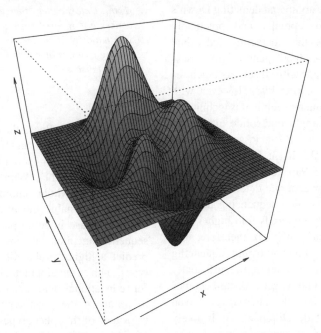

Fig. 13.1 A conceptual model of canalization. The y plane represents a phenotypic spectrum, the x plane represents the canalized progression of development through time, and the z plane represents environmental fluctuations. As any particular phenotype progresses through development, it can encounter environmental fluctuations that either repel (a local maximum) or attract (a local minimum) its developmental path. Either force, if strong enough, can cause a shift in the developmental path, fundamentally altering the end resulting phenotype. *(See insert for color representation of this figure.)*

2010). This is incredibly unfortunate, given that predictions of any reliability ought to include the prior probability of someone being born in that "ancestry group" with the mutations and phenotype of interest.

Despite the aforementioned facts, noninvasive sequencing of fetal genomes is an area of intense interest in genomic medicine, and a cynical person might argue that the rush to implement this technology is driven mainly by financial interests. Current techniques are based on the observation that a small proportion of the cell-free DNA in a pregnant woman's blood is derived from the fetus, so that aneuploidy or genomic sequence of a fetus may be inferred by sequencing of maternal plasma DNA and algorithmic decoupling of maternal and fetal DNA variants. A few companies are already marketing noninvasive prenatal screening (NIPS) tests for noninvasive detection of trisomy 21 associated with Down's syndrome. One can reasonably argue that detecting Down's syndrome is a conceptually and practically much simpler task than detecting individual variants within the fetal genome to assess mutations associated with disorders such as cystic fibrosis and hearing loss. However, with sufficiently high sequence depth, it is technically feasible to detect single nucleotide alterations in a fetal genome, as shown in several recent papers (Cheng et al., 2013; Fan et al., 2012; Kitzman et al., 2012; Papageorgiou and Patsalis, 2013). But, to allow accurate detection of individual variants, very high sequencing depth is required (potentially hundreds-fold higher than sequencing germline genomes); therefore, it is likely that targeted exon capture and sequencing might dominate the market until sufficiently high depth whole-genome sequencing becomes an economically feasible alternative. Given these technological developments, it is likely that some form of fetal genome testing will be available in the next few years. Others have noted that we might be reaching a point in the near-term future where it may be feasible to incorporate genetic, genomic, and transcriptomic data to develop new approaches to fetal

treatment (Bianchi, 2012; Guedj and Bianchi, 2013). One concern is that greed and financial conflicts of interest could lead to indiscriminate marketing and use of NIPS as diagnostic tests, rather than simply as screening, and that this technology will be implemented without any regard for genetic background or environmental differences, alongside a complete misunderstanding of this concept of extreme variability in phenotypic expression.

13.7 IMPLICATIONS FOR ACCEPTANCE, PROGNOSIS AND TREATMENT

"When a complex system starts to dysfunction, it is generally best to fix it early. The alternative often means delaying until the system has degenerated into a disorganized, chaotic mess — at which point it may be beyond repair. Unfortunately, the general approach to cancer has ignored such common sense. The vast majority of cancer research is devoted to finding cures, rather than finding new ways to prevent disease"

– Michael Sporn
(Sporn, 2011).

Prevention of illness through environmental modification has been, and likely always will be, the major driver for global health (Mukherjee, 2010; Sporn, 2011). With this in mind, the sequencing of whole genomes on a large scale promises to enable the discovery and prediction of disease in some people. The ability to sequence an infant at birth and to be able to predict a higher probability of certain phenotypes, such as developmental delay, would allow for educational and behavioral interventions to influence the phenotype, thus altering the trajectory of that phenotype (Bates et al., 2014; McIntyre, 2008; Rickards et al., 2007, 2009; Salem et al., 2012; Velleman and Mervis, 2011). One recent study of chromosomal microarray (CMA) testing found that "among 1792 patients with developmental delay (DD), intellectual disability (ID), multiple congenital anomalies

(MCA), and/or autism spectrum disorders (ASD), 13.1% had clinically relevant results, either abnormal ($n = 131$; 7.3%) or variants of possible significance (VPS; $n = 104$; 5.8%). Abnormal variants generated a higher rate of recommendation for clinical action (54%) compared with VPS (34%; Fisher exact test, $P = 0.01$)" (Coulter et al., 2011). The authors concluded that "CMA results influenced medical management in a majority of patients with abnormal variants and a substantial proportion of those with VPS" thus supporting the use of CMA in this population (Coulter et al., 2011). We agree that the identification of certain CNVs and other mutations can suggest a range of phenotypes that might occur in any one individual with that mutation or mutations.

However, there are some major barriers to the widespread implementation of genomic medicine in the clinic. These include:

1. Lack of public education
2. Lack of physician knowledge about genetics
3. Apathy on the part of the populace in terms of preventive efforts
4. Refusal of insurance companies and governments to pay for genetic testing
5. Focus in our society on treatment, not on early diagnosis and prevention
6. Privacy concerns
7. Limits of our current knowledge

The emphasis should be on diagnosis and prevention, not just on treatment. During the medical training of one of the authors (GJL), two episodes helped to illustrate this. The first involved a 15-year old girl with Type I diabetes, who was hospitalized dozens of times with diabetic ketoacidosis. Literally hundreds of thousands of dollars were spent to repeatedly save her life, but very little time or money was spent on therapy or education to teach her about taking her insulin and ensuring that she did. Unfortunately, in America at least, this is due to a relative lack of reimbursement for such activities, whereas saving someone already in diabetic ketoacidosis is quite lucrative to everyone involved. A second episode involved a 14-year old boy, who had been hospitalized well over 10 times with acute pancreatitis over a ten year period, with very little thought concerning why he had recurring pancreatitis. Finally, someone obtained a genetics consult, and they recommended CF genetic screening, which had never been ordered before due to a prior "negative" sweat test. It turns out that this boy had two rare mutations in *CFTR*, undiagnosed till then, which had been contributing to recurrent pancreatitis. He had never had any lung manifestations, and he had never had a positive sweat test for CF, mainly due to the fact that these mutations appeared to only be exerting effects in his pancreas, not in his skin or lungs. After this diagnosis, this person benefited from pancreatic enzyme supplementation, along with therapy and education. Once again, the reason it took so long to diagnose this person is because the incentive structure in many developed nations is not on early diagnosis and prevention, but rather on treatment of people only once they become severely ill (Brawley and Goldberg, 2012; Makary, 2012). This is illustrated by the fact that there are only about ~1000 medical geneticists in America and ~3000 genetic counselors, for a population of ~315 million, which makes it basically impossible for these limited number of professionals to implement genomic medicine in any meaningful way (Brandt et al., 2013). The numbers of such health-care professionals are even smaller in developing regions of the world, thus making it currently very difficult to provide widespread genetic counseling (Bittles, 2013; Bittles and Black, 2010; Hamamy, 2012). Stepping into this void are direct-to-consumer for-profit genetic testing companies, and this is certainly one disruptive way of trying to help people manage their genetic results online (Chua and Kennedy, 2012; Francke et al., 2013), although financial motives and lack of transparency can create problems (Sterckx et al., 2013).

Privacy concerns have added to the difficulties of implementing genomics-guided medicine. Genetic data have the potential of being informative across a wide variety of human traits and health conditions, and some worry about the potential misuse of these data by insurance agencies as well as by health-care providers (Allain et al., 2012). Genetic testing has historically been focused on targeting and examining a small number of known genetic aberrations (Bakker, 2006); however, since the advent of high-throughput sequencing technologies, the landscape is starting to change. With the emergence of tests that can target and examine all coding regions of the genome, or even the genome in its entirety, testing can now be performed on a more global and exploratory scale. Some people worry about returning the results of such a test, whose findings can have questionable clinical significance, and in response have advocated for selectively restricting the returnable medical content. Others have proposed complicated anonymization techniques that could allow for a safe return of research results to participants whose genome is suspected to contain "clinically actionable" information. One such proposition involves the cryptographic transformation of genomic data in which only by the coalescence of keys held by many different intermediate parties would the identity of the participant be revealed, and only in cases where all parties agree that there is indeed the presence of clinically actionable information (Hunter et al., 2012). These types of recommendations take a more paternalistic approach in returning test results to people, and generally involve a deciding body of people that can range in size from a single medical practitioner to a committee of experts. By contrast, there is a growing movement among the populace to learn more about their own "personalized" health and health care. There has also been a renewed push for the unfiltered sharing and networking of health-related data, which has been facilitated and hastened by the explosion of digitally mediated social networking over the past decade, as well as by efforts from 23andMe (Kranhold et al., 2007) and the Personal Genomes Project (Ball et al., 2012) that aim to popularize and democratize genetic testing. Clearly, between these contrasting

approaches, there is a trade-off between the privacy and personal safety one can expect to retain by either freely acquiring and sharing the full breadth of one's genetic testing data, or by allowing deciding bodies to choose what information you will receive.

Public databases containing human sequence data have grown in magnitude and in number, and relatively comprehensive sequencing data have already been generated and published on thousands of people (Abecasis et al., 2012; Fu et al., 2013b). Similar privacy concerns have since been expressed about the degree of medical and personal privacy that these and other research participants can expect (McGuire and Gibbs, 2006), given that each person is genetically unique. As a demonstration of current vulnerabilities, researchers have shown that the identities of participants can be discovered using these publicly available data (Gymrek et al., 2013). Although these data have been instrumental in furthering our understanding of human genetics, medicine, and biological processes in general, some advocate for caution when sharing and publishing human genetic sequence information (Lowrance and Collins, 2007).

As the cost and difficulty of sequencing continually decreases, a wealth of data are becoming available to researchers, privately funded institutions, and individual consumers. More people are willing to share a larger portion of their personal life in the public arena, and we fully expect that, given the popularization of "personalized" genomic health-related data, more people will want to share these data and offer their own DNA sequence for others to explore. There is a trade-off between the risks inherent in sharing vast quantities of health data, and maintaining personal privacy in the burgeoning age of personalized medicine and genomics. As the technology and science mature, our power to interpret and use these health data for practical and preventative measures will certainly improve. Conventions for privacy and autonomy will likely be driven by popular demand, and could vary from person to person, as all people differ in their desire for privacy and autonomy (see Fig. 13.2 for a conceptual model of this trade-off).

In addition, within the current paradigm of genetic determinism, which stretches back to the time of William Bateson (Radick, 2005, 2013), some people would have us believe that variants can and should be binned into different classes based on clinical utility and validity (Berg et al., 2013; Goddard et al., 2013; Green et al., 2012), without any obvious regard to genetic background or environmental differences. Environment and ancestry matter (Radick, 2005, 2011, 2013; Weldon, 1902), and yet some clinical geneticists trained in the current paradigm of genetic determinism clearly do not wish to acknowledge this. Categorical thinking misses complexity. In fact, one medical academy in America recently released guidelines in which they recommended the "return of secondary findings" for only 57 genes, without any real guidance for the rest of the genome or environmental influences (Green et al., 2013). This is therefore a very conservative set of recommendations, given that there are approximately 20,000 protein-coding genes in the human genome, along with the thousands of other identified, important noncoding elements of the genome (Batista and Chang, 2013; Cartault et al., 2012; Hansen et al., 2013; Kapusta et al., 2013; Khoddami and Cairns, 2013; Ledford, 2013; Maxmen, 2013; Memczak et al., 2013; Mercer and Mattick, 2013; Miura et al., 2013; Moreau et al., 2013; Ning et al., 2013; Perrat et al., 2013; Sabin et al., 2013; Salzman et al., 2012; Wilusz and Sharp, 2013)! As stated earlier, but worth repeating, there are ~12 billion nucleotides of DNA in every cell of the human body, and there are 25–100 trillion cells in each human body. Given genetic modifiers, somatic mosaicism, epigenetic changes, and environmental differences, no two human beings are the same, and therefore the expression of any mutation will be different in each person. At best, phenotypes will follow canalized pathways in direct relatives, such as mother and child, so the analysis of mutations

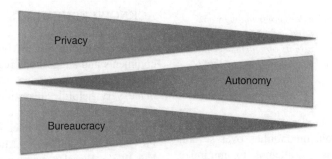

Fig. 13.2 An illustration of the trade-off between privacy and autonomy when receiving results from genetic testing. Models that guarantee an increased level of privacy are generally accompanied by a great deal of bureaucratic and paternalistic decision-making on the part of medical and advisory institutions (left). Models that propose and advocate for increased autonomy when receiving genetic test results come with the risk of reduced privacy (right). A whole genome sequence from a single person could, in principle, inform many aspects of his/her health care as well as allow for the prospect of future health predictions. This leads to speculations on how insurance agencies and health-care providers could/would use this information. One can envision a "sinister scenario" where people are rejected from hospitals and denied insurance based on putative genetic aberrations that may associate with costly, long-term, care. Others worry about the potential implications of results found by genome scale testing, and would rather not know about risks pertaining to untreatable illnesses. Recent movements push for the democratization as well as large-scale adoption of this type of testing for every person, which could help to prove that we are all truly genetically unique and all carry any number of mutations and/or large genetic aberrations that may or may not be associated with disease. In reality, current technologies are far from the realm of genotype to phenotype predictions, and so genetic discrimination could only create illusory economic gains for any institution for the foreseeable future. *(See insert for color representation of this figure.)*

over several generations in the same families is a worthwhile effort. But, how we will ever get to a world of millions of whole genomes shared and analyzed for numerous additive, epistatic interactions and gene by environment interactions, so that we can make any reliable predictions for any one human being, if we are only recommending "return of results" from ~57 genes? We need to sequence and collate online the raw exome and genome data and phenotypic information from thousands and then millions of people, so that we can actually begin to really understand the expression patterns of any mutation in the human genome in particular families. In medicine, people tend to create illusions of certainty, when in fact everything is probabilistic (Gigerenzer, 2002). Some humans like to be told things in a "yes/no" manner, but there always exists a degree of unresolvable uncertainty.

13.8 CONCLUSIONS

"A new scientific truth does not triumph by convincing its opponents and making them see the light, but rather because its opponents eventually die, and a new generation grows up that is familiar with it."

– Max Planck

With the advent of exome and WGS, we need to focus again on families over several generations, so as to attempt to minimize genetic differences, locus heterogeneity and environmental influences. Forging strong ties with families will also enable access to other tissues to continue to study newly discovered loci with many emerging technologies. Some might consider it to be "social activism" to advocate for a more comprehensive collection and collation of human pedigrees, WGS data and phenotypic information. But, in the words of one author: "Scientists, whether we like it or not, are members of society, and we are prone to the ideas and beliefs of the times in which we live (Mole, 2006)." We currently live within a paradigm of genetic determinism, but we should

not be forever condemned to this simplistic mode of thinking. One can imagine or hope that in the not too distant future, each person will be able to keep track of detailed longitudinal phenotyping data on themselves online, and they will be able to link this to records of their relatives, both living and deceased. One can also hope that we are approaching a time where sufficient information is available within many large families for calculating highly accurate probabilistic outcomes (Gigerenzer, 2002; Gigerenzer and Galesic, 2012; Gigerenzer et al., 2010; Kurz-Milcke et al., 2008; Sokal, 2012), at which point we might be able to more effectively alter the trajectory for many diseases. One can see this beginning already to occur in certain geographically isolated clans, such as in Iceland (Jonsson et al., 2012; Styrkarsdottir et al., 2013), so there is some optimism that this can indeed occur on a global level, including in the currently less developed regions of the world (Bittles, 2013).

ACKNOWLEDGEMENTS

We thank the editor, Kevin Mitchell, for detailed comments and suggestions regarding an earlier draft of this manuscript. Others who have made very helpful suggestions include: Anne Buchanan, George Church, Nathaniel Comfort, Jesse Gillis, Nathaniel Pearson, William Provine, Gregory Radick, Michael Stone, and Kai Wang. We also acknowledge members of the Lyon laboratory, particularly Han Fang and Max Doerfel, for their helpful suggestions as well. We would also like to thank Gail Sherman at the CSHL library for her efforts to procure some of the older literature on our behalf.

REFERENCES

Abecasis, G.R., Auton, A., Brooks, L.D., DePristo, M.A., Durbin, R.M., Handsaker, R.E., Kang, H.M., Marth, G.T., and McVean, G.A. (2012). An integrated map of genetic variation from 1,092 human genomes. Nature 491, 56–65.

Abu-Safieh, L., Al-Anazi, S., Al-Abdi, L., Hashem, M., Alkuraya, H., Alamr, M., Sirelkhatim, M.O., Al-Hassnan, Z., Alkuraya, B., Mohamed, J.Y., et al. (2012). In search of triallelism in Bardet-Biedl syndrome. Eur J Hum Genet.

Ackerman, C., Locke, A.E., Feingold, E., Reshey, B., Espana, K., Thusberg, J., Mooney, S., Bean, L.J., Dooley, K.J., Cua, C.L., et al. (2012). An excess of deleterious variants in VEGF-A pathway genes in Down-syndrome-associated atrioventricular septal defects. Am J Hum Genet 91, 646–659.

Aldred, M.A., Bagshaw, R.J., Macdermot, K., Casson, D., Murch, S.H., Walker-Smith, J.A., and Trembath, R.C. (2000). Germline mosaicism for a GNAS1 mutation and Albright hereditary osteodystrophy. J Med Genet 37, E35.

Aldridge, K., George, I.D., Cole, K.K., Austin, J.R., Takahashi, T.N., Duan, Y., and Miles, J.H. (2011). Facial phenotypes in subgroups of prepubertal boys with autism spectrum disorders are correlated with clinical phenotypes. Mol Autism 2, 15.

Allain, D., Friedman, S., and Senter, L. (2012). Consumer awareness and attitudes about insurance discrimination post enactment of the Genetic Information Nondiscrimination Act. Fam Cancer 11, 637–644.

Allchin, D. (2005). The dilemma of dominance. Biol Philos 20, 427–451.

Andreasen, C., Nielsen, J.B., Refsgaard, L., Holst, A.G., Christensen, A.H., Andreasen, L., Sajadieh, A., Haunso, S., Svendsen, J.H., and Olesen, M.S. (2013a). New population-based exome data are questioning the pathogenicity of previously cardiomyopathy-associated genetic variants. Eur J Hum Genet 21, 918–928.

Andreasen, C., Refsgaard, L., Nielsen, J.B., Sajadieh, A., Winkel, B.G., Tfelt-Hansen, J., Haunso, S., Holst, A.G., Svendsen, J.H., and Olesen, M.S. (2013b). Mutations in Genes Encoding Cardiac Ion Channels Previously Associated With Sudden Infant Death Syndrome (SIDS) Are Present With High Frequency in New Exome Data. Can J Cardiol.

Anney, R., Klei, L., Pinto, D., Almeida, J., Bacchelli, E., Baird, G., Bolshakova, N., Bolte, S., Bolton, P.F., Bourgeron, T., et al. (2012). Individual common variants exert weak effects on the risk for autism spectrum disorderspi. Hum Mol Genet 21, 4781–4792.

Bainbridge, M.N., Wiszniewski, W., Murdock, D.R., Friedman, J., Gonzaga-Jauregui, C., Newsham, I.,

Reid, J.G., Fink, J.K., Morgan, M.B., Gingras, M.C., et al. (2011). Whole-genome sequencing for optimized patient management. Sci Transl Med 3, 87re83.

Bakker, E. (2006). Is the DNA Sequence the Gold Standard in Genetic Testing? Quality of Molecular Genetic Tests Assessed. Clin Chem 52, 557–558.

Bakker, E., Veenema, H., Den Dunnen, J.T., van Broeckhoven, C., Grootscholten, P.M., Bonten, E.J., van Ommen, G.J., and Pearson, P.L. (1989). Germinal mosaicism increases the recurrence risk for 'new' Duchenne muscular dystrophy mutations. J Med Genet 26, 553–559.

Ball, M.P., Thakuria, J.V., Zaranek, A.W., Clegg, T., Rosenbaum, A.M., Wu, X., Angrist, M., Bhak, J., Bobe, J., Callow, M.J., et al. (2012). A public resource facilitating clinical use of genomes. Proc Natl Acad Sci U S A 109, 11920–11927.

Bamshad, M.J., Ng, S.B., Bigham, A.W., Tabor, H.K., Emond, M.J., Nickerson, D.A., and Shendure, J. (2011). Exome sequencing as a tool for Mendelian disease gene discovery. Nat Rev Genet 12, 745–755.

Barbosa, R.H., Vargas, F.R., Aguiar, F.C., Ferman, S., Lucena, E., Bonvicino, C.R., and Seuanez, H.N. (2008). Hereditary retinoblastoma transmitted by maternal germline mosaicism. Pediatr Blood Cancer 51, 598–602.

Bates, B.R., Graham, D., Striley, K., Patterson, S., Arora, A., and Hamel-Lambert, J. (2014). Examining antecedents of caregivers' access to early childhood developmental screening: implications for campaigns promoting use of services in Appalachian Ohio. Health Promot Pract 15, 413–421.

Bateson, W., and Mendel, G. (1902). Mendel's principles of heredity a defense Cambridge Eng.: University Press.

Batista, P.J., and Chang, H.Y. (2013). Long noncoding RNAs: cellular address codes in development and disease. Cell 152, 1298–1307.

Baugher, J.D., Baugher, B.D., Shirley, M.D., and Pevsner, J. (2013). Sensitive and specific detection of mosaic chromosomal abnormalities using the Parent-of-Origin-based Detection (POD) method. BMC Genomics 14, 367.

Beales, P.L., Badano, J.L., Ross, A.J., Ansley, S.J., Hoskins, B.E., Kirsten, B., Mein, C.A., Froguel, P., Scambler, P.J., Lewis, R.A., et al. (2003). Genetic interaction of BBS1 mutations with alleles at other BBS loci can result in non-Mendelian

Bardet-Biedl syndrome. Am J Hum Genet 72, 1187–1199.

Bearn, A.G. (1993). Archibald Garrod and the individuality of Man. Oxford, New York: Clarendon Press; Oxford University Press.

Beaudet, A.L. (2013). The utility of chromosomal microarray analysis in developmental and behavioral pediatrics. Child Dev 84, 121–132.

Berg, J.S., Adams, M., Nassar, N., Bizon, C., Lee, K., Schmitt, C.P., Wilhelmsen, K.C., and Evans, J.P. (2013). An informatics approach to analyzing the incidentalome. Genet Med 15, 36–44.

Bernal, A.J., and Jirtle, R.L. (2010). Epigenomic disruption: the effects of early developmental exposures. Birth Defects Res A Clin Mol Teratol 88, 938–944.

Berndt, S.I., Gustafsson, S., Magi, R., Ganna, A., Wheeler, E., Feitosa, M.F., Justice, A.E., Monda, K.L., Croteau-Chonka, D.C., Day, F.R., et al. (2013). Genome-wide meta-analysis identifies 11 new loci for anthropometric traits and provides insights into genetic architecture. Nat Genet 45, 501–512.

Bianchi, D.W. (2012). From prenatal genomic diagnosis to fetal personalized medicine: progress and challenges. Nat Med 18, 1041–1051.

Biesecker, L.G., and Spinner, N.B. (2013). A genomic view of mosaicism and human disease. Nat Rev Genet 14, 307–320.

Bittles, A.H. (2013). Genetics and global healthcare. J R Coll Physicians Edinb 43, 7–10.

Bittles, A.H., and Black, M.L. (2010). Evolution in health and medicine Sackler colloquium: Consanguinity, human evolution, and complex diseases. Proc Natl Acad Sci U S A 107 (Suppl 1), 1779–1786.

Blackwood, D.H., Fordyce, A., Walker, M.T., St Clair, D.M., Porteous, D.J., and Muir, W.J. (2001). Schizophrenia and affective disorders--cosegregation with a translocation at chromosome 1q42 that directly disrupts brain-expressed genes: clinical and P300 findings in a family. Am J Hum Genet 69, 428–433.

Bleuler, E. (1958). Dementia praecox; or, The group of schizophrenias. New York: International Universities Press.

Bloom, J.S., Ehrenreich, I.M., Loo, W.T., Lite, T.L., and Kruglyak, L. (2013). Finding the sources of missing heritability in a yeast cross. Nature 494, 234–237.

Blount, Z.D., Barrick, J.E., Davidson, C.J., and Lenski, R.E. (2012). Genomic analysis of a key innovation in an experimental Escherichia coli population. Nature 489, 513–518.

Boyden, L.M., Choi, M., Choate, K.A., Nelson-Williams, C.J., Farhi, A., Toka, H.R., Tikhonova, I.R., Bjornson, R., Mane, S.M., Colussi, G., et al. (2012). Mutations in kelch-like 3 and cullin 3 cause hypertension and electrolyte abnormalities. Nature 482, 98–102.

Boyden, L.M., Mao, J., Belsky, J., Mitzner, L., Farhi, A., Mitnick, M.A., Wu, D., Insogna, K., and Lifton, R.P. (2002). High bone density due to a mutation in LDL-receptor-related protein 5. N Engl J Med 346, 1513–1521.

Brandt, D.S., Shinkunas, L., Hillis, S.L., Daack-Hirsch, S.E., Driessnack, M., Downing, N.R., Liu, M.F., Shah, L.L., Williams, J.K., and Simon, C.M. (2013). A Closer Look at the Recommended Criteria for Disclosing Genetic Results: Perspectives of Medical Genetic Specialists, Genomic Researchers, and Institutional Review Board Chairs. J Genet Couns.

Brawley, O.W., and Goldberg, P. (2012). How we do harm: a doctor breaks ranks about being sick in America, 1st edn. New York: St. Martin's Press.

Burga, A., Casanueva, M.O., and Lehner, B. (2011). Predicting mutation outcome from early stochastic variation in genetic interaction partners. Nature 480, 250–253.

Cartault, F., Munier, P., Benko, E., Desguerre, I., Hanein, S., Boddaert, N., Bandiera, S., Vellayoudom, J., Krejbich-Trotot, P., Bintner, M., et al. (2012). Mutation in a primate-conserved retrotransposon reveals a noncoding RNA as a mediator of infantile encephalopathy. Proc Natl Acad Sci U S A 109, 4980–4985.

Casanueva, M.O., Burga, A., and Lehner, B. (2012). Fitness trade-offs and environmentally induced mutation buffering in isogenic C. elegans. Science 335, 82–85.

Chaturvedi, L.S., Mittal, R.D., Srivastava, S., Mukherjee, M., and Mittal, B. (2000). Analysis of dinucleotide repeat loci of dystrophin gene for carrier detection, germline mosaicism and de novo mutations in Duchenne muscular dystrophy. Clin Genet 58, 234–236.

Cheng, P., D. Casement, M., Chen, C.F., Hoffmann, R.F., Armitage, R., and Deldin, P.J. (2013). Sleep-disordered breathing in major depressive disorder. J Sleep Res 22, 459–462.

Chua, E.W., and Kennedy, M.A. (2012). Current State and Future Prospects of Direct-to-Consumer Pharmacogenetics. Front Pharmacol 3, 152.

Ciancarelli, I., Tozzi Ciancarelli, M.G., and Carolei, A. (2013). Effectiveness of intensive neurorehabilitation in patients with Huntington's disease. Eur J Phys Rehabil Med 49, 189–195.

Comfort, N.C. (2001). The tangled field: Barbara McClintock's search for the patterns of genetic control. Cambridge, Mass.: Harvard University Press.

Comfort, N.C. (2012). The science of human perfection: how genes became the heart of American medicine. New Haven: Yale University Press.

Corleto, V.D., Gambardella, S., Gullotta, F., D'Apice, M.R., Piciucchi, M., Galli, E., Lucidi, V., Novelli, G., and Delle Fave, G. (2010). New PRSS1 and common CFTR mutations in a child with acute recurrent pancreatitis, could be considered an "Hereditary" form of pancreatitis ? BMC Gastroenterol 10, 119.

Coufal, N.G., Garcia-Perez, J.L., Peng, G.E., Marchetto, M.C., Muotri, A.R., Mu, Y., Carson, C.T., Macia, A., Moran, J.V., and Gage, F.H. (2011). Ataxia telangiectasia mutated (ATM) modulates long interspersed element-1 (L1) retrotransposition in human neural stem cells. Proc Natl Acad Sci U S A 108, 20382–20387.

Coulter, M.E., Miller, D.T., Harris, D.J., Hawley, P., Picker, J., Roberts, A.E., Sobeih, M.M., and Irons, M. (2011). Chromosomal microarray testing influences medical management. Genet Med 13, 770–776.

Craddock, N., and Owen, M.J. (2010). The Kraepelinian dichotomy - going, going … but still not gone. Br J psychiatry 196, 92–95.

Crepel, A., Breckpot, J., Fryns, J.P., De la Marche, W., Steyaert, J., Devriendt, K., and Peeters, H. (2010). DISC1 duplication in two brothers with autism and mild mental retardation. Clin Genet 77, 389–394.

Davis, E.E., Zhang, Q., Liu, Q., Diplas, B.H., Davey, L.M., Hartley, J., Stoetzel, C., Szymanska, K., Ramaswami, G., Logan, C.V., et al. (2011). TTC21B contributes both causal and modifying alleles across the ciliopathy spectrum. Nat Genet.

Derikx, M.H., and Drenth, J.P. (2010). Genetic factors in chronic pancreatitis; implications for diagnosis, management and prognosis. Best Pract Res Clin Gastroenterol 24, 251–270.

Dickel, D.E., Visel, A., and Pennacchio, L.A. (2013). Functional anatomy of distant-acting mammalian enhancers. Philos Trans R Soc Lond B Biol Sci 368, 20120359.

Dodd, K.J., and Shields, N. (2005). A systematic review of the outcomes of cardiovascular exercise programs for people with Down syndrome. Arch Phys Med Rehabil 86, 2051–2058.

Dolinoy, D.C., Weidman, J.R., Waterland, R.A., and Jirtle, R.L. (2006). Maternal genistein alters coat color and protects Avy mouse offspring from obesity by modifying the fetal epigenome. Environ Health Perspect 114, 567–572.

Down, J.L. (1995). Observations on an ethnic classification of idiots. 1866. Ment Retard 33, 54–56.

Eichenbaum, H. (2013). What H.M. taught us. J Cogn Neurosci 25, 14–21.

Eichers, E.R., Lewis, R.A., Katsanis, N., and Lupski, J.R. (2004). Triallelic inheritance: a bridge between Mendelian and multifactorial traits. Ann Med 36, 262–272.

El-Hattab, A.W., Zhang, F., Maxim, R., Christensen, K.M., Ward, J.C., Hines-Dowell, S., Scaglia, F., Lupski, J.R., and Cheung, S.W. (2010). Deletion and duplication of 15q24: Molecular mechanisms and potential modification by additional copy number variants. Genet Med 12, 573–586.

Elia, J., Gai, X., Xie, H.M., Perin, J.C., Geiger, E., Glessner, J.T., D'Arcy, M., deBerardinis, R., Frackelton, E., Kim, C., et al. (2010). Rare structural variants found in attention-deficit hyperactivity disorder are preferentially associated with neurodevelopmental genes. Mol Psychiatry 15, 637–646.

Emond, M.J., Louie, T., Emerson, J., Zhao, W., Mathias, R.A., Knowles, M.R., Wright, F.A., Rieder, M.J., Tabor, H.K., Nickerson, D.A., et al. (2012). Exome sequencing of extreme phenotypes identifies DCTN4 as a modifier of chronic Pseudomonas aeruginosa infection in cystic fibrosis. Nat Genet 44, 886–889.

Esvelt, K.M., Carlson, J.C., and Liu, D.R. (2011). A system for the continuous directed evolution of biomolecules. Nature 472, 499–503.

Etheridge, S.P., Bowles, N.E., Arrington, C.B., Pilcher, T., Rope, A., Wilde, A.A., Alders, M., Saarel, E.V., Tavernier, R., Timothy, K.W., et al. (2011). Somatic mosaicism contributes to phenotypic variation in Timothy syndrome. Am J Med Genet A 155A, 2578–2583.

Evans, J.C., Archer, H.L., Whatley, S.D., and Clarke, A. (2006). Germline mosaicism for a MECP2 mutation in a man with two Rett daughters. Clin Genet 70, 336–338.

Fan, H.C., Gu, W., Wang, J., Blumenfeld, Y.J., El-Sayed, Y.Y., and Quake, S.R. (2012). Non-invasive prenatal measurement of the fetal genome. Nature 487, 320–324.

Fins, J.J. (2009). Deep brain stimulation, deontology and duty: the moral obligation of non-abandonment at the neural interface. J Neural Eng 6, 050201.

Francke, U., Dijamco, C., Kiefer, A.K., Eriksson, N., Moiseff, B., Tung, J.Y., and Mountain, J.L. (2013). Dealing with the unexpected: consumer responses to direct-access BRCA mutation testing. PeerJ 1, e8.

Frank, J., and Happle, R. (2007). Cutaneous mosaicism: right before our eyes. J Clin Invest 117, 1216–1219.

Freund, J., Brandmaier, A.M., Lewejohann, L., Kirste, I., Kritzler, M., Kruger, A., Sachser, N., Lindenberger, U., and Kempermann, G. (2013). Emergence of individuality in genetically identical mice. Science 340, 756–759.

Fu, M., Zhang, X., Lai, X., Wu, X., Feng, F., Peng, J., Zhong, H., Zhang, Y., Wang, Y., Zhou, Q., et al. (2013a). Generation of sequence variants via accelerated molecular evolution methods. Recent Pat DNA Gene Seq 7, 144–156.

Fu, W., O'Connor, T.D., Jun, G., Kang, H.M., Abecasis, G., Leal, S.M., Gabriel, S., Altshuler, D., Shendure, J., Nickerson, D.A., et al. (2013b). Analysis of 6,515 exomes reveals the recent origin of most human protein-coding variants. Nature 493, 216–220.

Fullston, T., Gabb, B., Callen, D., Ullmann, R., Woollatt, E., Bain, S., Ropers, H.H., Cooper, M., Chandler, D., Carter, K., et al. (2011). Inherited balanced translocation t(9;17)(q33.2;q25.3) concomitant with a 16p13.1 duplication in a patient with schizophrenia. Am J Med Genet B Neuropsychiatr Genet 156, 204–214.

Gagnon, F., Roslin, N.M., and Lemire, M. (2011). Successful identification of rare variants using oligogenic segregation analysis as a prioritizing tool for whole-exome sequencing studies. BMC Proc 5(Suppl 9), S11.

Gai, X., Xie, H.M., Perin, J.C., Takahashi, N., Murphy, K., Wenocur, A.S., D'Arcy, M., O'Hara, R.J., Goldmuntz, E., Grice, D.E., et al. (2012). Rare structural variation of synapse and neurotransmission genes in autism. Mol Psychiatry 17, 402–411.

Gibson, G. (2011). Rare and common variants: twenty arguments. Nat Rev Genet 13, 135–145.

Gigerenzer, G. (2002). Calculated risks: how to know when numbers deceive you. New York: Simon & Schuster.

Gigerenzer, G., and Galesic, M. (2012). Why do single event probabilities confuse patients? BMJ 344, e245.

Gigerenzer, G., Wegwarth, O., and Feufel, M. (2010). Misleading communication of risk. BMJ 341, c4830.

Girirajan, S., Rosenfeld, J.A., Coe, B.P., Parikh, S., Friedman, N., Goldstein, A., Filipink, R.A., McConnell, J.S., Angle, B., Meschino, W.S., et al. (2012). Phenotypic heterogeneity of genomic disorders and rare copy-number variants. N Engl J Med 367, 1321–1331.

Girirajan, S., Rosenfeld, J.A., Cooper, G.M., Antonacci, F., Siswara, P., Itsara, A., Vives, L., Walsh, T., McCarthy, S.E., Baker, C., et al. (2010). A recurrent 16p12.1 microdeletion supports a two-hit model for severe developmental delay. Nat Genet 42, 203–209.

Goddard, K.A., Whitlock, E.P., Berg, J.S., Williams, M.S., Webber, E.M., Webster, J.A., Lin, J.S., Schrader, K.A., Campos-Outcalt, D., Offit, K., et al. (2013). Description and pilot results from a novel method for evaluating return of incidental findings from next-generation sequencing technologies. Genet Med 15, 721–728.

Green, R.C., Berg, J.S., Berry, G.T., Biesecker, L.G., Dimmock, D.P., Evans, J.P., Grody, W.W., Hegde, M.R., Kalia, S., Korf, B.R., et al. (2012). Exploring concordance and discordance for return of incidental findings from clinical sequencing. Genet Med 14, 405–410.

Green, R.C., Berg, J.S., Grody, W.W., Kalia, S.S., Korf, B.R., Martin, C.L., McGuire, A.L., Nussbaum, R.L., O'Daniel, J.M., Ormond, K.E., et al. (2013). ACMG recommendations for reporting of incidental findings in clinical exome and genome sequencing. Genet Med 15, 565–574.

Greenspan, R.J. (2008). Seymour Benzer (1921–2007). Curr Biol 18, R106–R110.

Greenspan, R.J. (2009). Selection, gene interaction, and flexible gene networks. Cold Spring Harb Symp Quant Biol 74, 131–138.

Greenspan, R.J. (2012). Biological indeterminacy. Sci Eng Ethics 18, 447–452.

Grillo, E., Lo Rizzo, C., Bianciardi, L., Bizzarri, V., Baldassarri, M., Spiga, O., Furini, S., De Felice, C., Signorini, C., Leoncini, S., et al. (2013). Revealing the complexity of a monogenic disease: rett syndrome exome sequencing. PLoS One 8, e56599.

Guedj, F., and Bianchi, D.W. (2013). Noninvasive prenatal testing creates an opportunity for antenatal treatment of Down syndrome. Prenat Diagn 33, 614–618.

Guris, D.L., Duester, G., Papaioannou, V.E., and Imamoto, A. (2006). Dose-dependent interaction of Tbx1 and Crkl and locally aberrant RA signaling in a model of del22q11 syndrome. Dev Cell 10, 81–92.

Gymrek, M., McGuire, A.L., Golan, D., Halperin, E., and Erlich, Y. (2013). Identifying Personal Genomes by Surname Inference. Science 339, 321–324.

Hall, J.G. (1988). Review and hypotheses: somatic mosaicism: observations related to clinical genetics. Am J Hum Genet 43, 355–363.

Hamamy, H. (2012). Consanguineous marriages: Preconception consultation in primary health care settings. J Community Genet 3, 185–192.

Hamshere, M.L., Bennett, P., Williams, N., Segurado, R., Cardno, A., Norton, N., Lambert, D., Williams, H., Kirov, G., Corvin, A., et al. (2005). Genomewide linkage scan in schizoaffective disorder: significant evidence for linkage at 1q42 close to DISC1, and suggestive evidence at 22q11 and 19p13. Arch Gen Psychiatry 62, 1081–1088.

Hansen, T.B., Jensen, T.I., Clausen, B.H., Bramsen, J.B., Finsen, B., Damgaard, C.K., and Kjems, J. (2013). Natural RNA circles function as efficient microRNA sponges. Nature 495, 384–388.

Hedges, D.J., Burges, D., Powell, E., Almonte, C., Huang, J., Young, S., Boese, B., Schmidt, M., Pericak-Vance, M.A., Martin, E., et al. (2009). Exome sequencing of a multigenerational human pedigree. PLoS One 4, e8232.

Hollander, W.F. (1975). Sectorial mosaics in the domestic pigeon: 25 more years. J Hered 66, 177–202.

Holmes, F.L., and Summers, W.C. (2006). Reconceiving the gene: Seymour Benzer's adventures in phage genetics. New Haven: Yale University Press.

Hosoki, K., Takano, K., Sudo, A., Tanaka, S., and Saitoh, S. (2005). Germline mosaicism of a novel UBE3A mutation in Angelman syndrome. Am J Med Genet A 138A, 187–189.

Huisman, S.A., Redeker, E.J., Maas, S.M., Mannens, M.M., and Hennekam, R.C. (2013). High rate of mosaicism in individuals with Cornelia de Lange syndrome. J Med Genet 50, 339–344.

Hulten, M.A., Jonasson, J., Nordgren, A., and Iwarsson, E. (2010). Germinal and Somatic Trisomy 21 Mosaicism: How Common is it, What are the Implications for Individual Carriers and How Does it Come About? Curr Genomics 11, 409–419.

Hume, D., and Selby-Bigge, L.A. (1896). A treatise of human nature. Oxford,: Clarendon press.

Hunter, L.E., Hopfer, C., Terry, S.F., and Coors, M.E. (2012). Reporting actionable research results: shared secrets can save lives. Sci Transl Med 4, 143cm148.

Iascone, M.R., Vittorini, S., Sacchelli, M., Spadoni, I., Simi, P., and Giusti, S. (2002). Molecular characterization of 22q11 deletion in a three-generation family with maternal transmission. Am J Med Genet 108, 319–321.

Iossifov, I., Ronemus, M., Levy, D., Wang, Z., Hakker, I., Rosenbaum, J., Yamrom, B., Lee, Y.H., Narzisi, G., Leotta, A., et al. (2012). De novo gene disruptions in children on the autistic spectrum. Neuron 74, 285–299.

Iourov, I.Y., Vorsanova, S.G., and Yurov, Y.B. (2008). Chromosomal mosaicism goes global. Mol Cytogenet 1, 26.

Jamieson, A., and Radick, G. (2013). Putting mendel in his place: how curriculum reform in genetics and counterfactual history of science can work together. In: K. Kampourakis, ed. The Philosophy of Biology (pp. 577–595), Netherlands: Springer.

Jongmans, M.C., Hoefsloot, L.H., van der Donk, K.P., Admiraal, R.J., Magee, A., van de Laar, I., Hendriks, Y., Verheij, J.B., Walpole, I., Brunner, H.G., et al. (2008). Familial CHARGE syndrome and the CHD7 gene: a recurrent missense mutation, intrafamilial recurrence and variability. Am J Med Genet A 146A, 43–50.

Jongmans, M.C., Verwiel, E.T., Heijdra, Y., Vulliamy, T., Kamping, E.J., Hehir-Kwa, J.Y., Bongers, E.M., Pfundt, R., van Emst, L., van Leeuwen, F.N., et al. (2012). Revertant somatic mosaicism by mitotic recombination in dyskeratosis congenita. Am J Hum Genet 90, 426–433.

Jonsson, T., Atwal, J.K., Steinberg, S., Snaedal, J., Jonsson, P.V., Bjornsson, S., Stefansson, H.,

Sulem, P., Gudbjartsson, D., Maloney, J., et al. (2012). A mutation in APP protects against Alzheimer's disease and age-related cognitive decline. Nature 488, 96–99.

Kajiwara, K., Berson, E., and Dryja, T. (1994). Digenic retinitis pigmentosa due to mutations at the unlinked peripherin/RDS and ROM1 loci. Science 264, 1604–1608.

Kapusta, A., Kronenberg, Z., Lynch, V.J., Zhuo, X., Ramsay, L., Bourque, G., Yandell, M., and Feschotte, C. (2013). Transposable Elements Are Major Contributors to the Origin, Diversification, and Regulation of Vertebrate Long Noncoding RNAs. PLoS Genet 9, e1003470.

Katsanis, N., Ansley, S.J., Badano, J.L., Eichers, E.R., Lewis, R.A., Hoskins, B.E., Scambler, P.J., Davidson, W.S., Beales, P.L., and Lupski, J.R. (2001). Triallelic inheritance in Bardet-Biedl syndrome, a Mendelian recessive disorder. Science 293, 2256–2259.

Katsanis, N., Eichers, E.R., Ansley, S.J., Lewis, R.A., Kayserili, H., Hoskins, B.E., Scambler, P.J., Beales, P.L., and Lupski, J.R. (2002). BBS4 is a minor contributor to Bardet-Biedl syndrome and may also participate in triallelic inheritance. Am J Hum Genet 71, 22–29.

Katsanis, S.H., and Katsanis, N. (2013). Molecular genetic testing and the future of clinical genomics. Nat Rev Genet 14, 415–426.

Keller, E.F. (2010). The mirage of a space between nature and nurture. Durham N.C.: Duke University Press.

Kendler, K.S., and Greenspan, R.J. (2006). The nature of genetic influences on behavior: lessons from "simpler" organisms. Am J Psychiatry 163, 1683–1694.

Khoddami, V., and Cairns, B.R. (2013). Identification of direct targets and modified bases of RNA cytosine methyltransferases. Nat Biotechnol 31, 458–464.

Kitzman, J.O., Snyder, M.W., Ventura, M., Lewis, A.P., Qiu, R., Simmons, L.E., Gammill, H.S., Rubens, C.E., Santillan, D.A., Murray, J.C., et al. (2012). Noninvasive whole-genome sequencing of a human fetus. Sci Transl Med 4, 137ra176.

Klei, L., Sanders, S.J., Murtha, M.T., Hus, V., Lowe, J.K., Willsey, A.J., Moreno-De-Luca, D., Yu, T.W., Fombonne, E., Geschwind, D., et al. (2012). Common genetic variants, acting additively, are a major source of risk for autism. Mol Autism 3, 9.

Kohane, I.S., Hsing, M., and Kong, S.W. (2012). Taxonomizing, sizing, and overcoming the incidentalome. Genet Med 14, 399–404.

Kovaleva, N.V. (2010). Germ-line transmission of trisomy 21: Data from 80 families suggest an implication of grandmaternal age and a high frequency of female-specific trisomy rescue. Mol Cytogenet 3, 7.

Kraepelin, E. (1921). Manic-depressive insanity and paranoia. Edinburgh: Livingstone.

Kranhold, P., Hanahan, E., Verbinnen, S. (2007). 23andMe Launches Web-Based Service Empowering Individuals to Access and Understand Their Own Genetic Information. (23andMe).

Kurek, K.C., Luks, V.L., Ayturk, U.M., Alomari, A.I., Fishman, S.J., Spencer, S.A., Mulliken, J.B., Bowen, M.E., Yamamoto, G.L., Kozakewich, H.P., et al. (2012). Somatic mosaic activating mutations in PIK3CA cause CLOVES syndrome. Am J Hum Genet 90, 1108–1115.

Kurz-Milcke, E., Gigerenzer, G., and Martignon, L. (2008). Transparency in risk communication: graphical and analog tools. Ann N Y Acad Sci 1128, 18–28.

Lai, J., Li, R., Xu, X., Jin, W., Xu, M., Zhao, H., Xiang, Z., Song, W., Ying, K., Zhang, M., et al. (2010). Genome-wide patterns of genetic variation among elite maize inbred lines. Nat Genet 42, 1027–1030.

Laurier, V., Stoetzel, C., Muller, J., Thibault, C., Corbani, S., Jalkh, N., Salem, N., Chouery, E., Poch, O., Licaire, S., et al. (2006). Pitfalls of homozygosity mapping: an extended consanguineous Bardet-Biedl syndrome family with two mutant genes (BBS2, BBS10), three mutations, but no triallelism. Eur J Hum Genet 14, 1195–1203.

Leconte, A.M., Dickinson, B.C., Yang, D.D., Chen, I.A., Allen, B., and Liu, D.R. (2013). A population-based experimental model for protein evolution: effects of mutation rate and selection stringency on evolutionary outcomes. Biochemistry 52, 1490–1499.

Ledford, H. (2013). Circular RNAs throw genetics for a loop. Nature 494, 415.

Lemmers, R.J.L.F., Tawil, R., Petek, L.M., Balog, J., Block, G.J., Santen, G.W.E., Amell, A.M., van der Vliet, P.J., Almomani, R., Straasheijm, K.R., et al. (2012). Digenic inheritance of an SMCHD1 mutation and an FSHD-permissive D4Z4 allele causes facioscapulohumeral muscular dystrophy type 2. Nat Genet 44, 1370–1374.

Li, H., Cherry, S., Klinedinst, D., DeLeon, V., Redig, J., Reshey, B., Chin, M.T., Sherman, S.L., Maslen, C.L., and Reeves, R.H. (2012). Genetic modifiers predisposing to congenital heart disease in the sensitized Down syndrome population. Circ Cardiovasc Genet 5, 301–308.

Liao, J., Kochilas, L., Nowotschin, S., Arnold, J.S., Aggarwal, V.S., Epstein, J.A., Brown, M.C., Adams, J., and Morrow, B.E. (2004). Full spectrum of malformations in velo-cardio-facial syndrome/DiGeorge syndrome mouse models by altering Tbx1 dosage. Hum Mol Genet 13, 1577–1585.

Lichtenstein, P., Yip, B.H., Bjork, C., Pawitan, Y., Cannon, T.D., Sullivan, P.F., and Hultman, C.M. (2009). Common genetic determinants of schizophrenia and bipolar disorder in Swedish families: a population-based study. Lancet 373, 234–239.

Lindhurst, M.J., Parker, V.E., Payne, F., Sapp, J.C., Rudge, S., Harris, J., Witkowski, A.M., Zhang, Q., Groeneveld, M.P., Scott, C.E., et al. (2012). Mosaic overgrowth with fibroadipose hyperplasia is caused by somatic activating mutations in PIK3CA. Nat Genet 44, 928–933.

Lindhurst, M.J., Sapp, J.C., Teer, J.K., Johnston, J.J., Finn, E.M., Peters, K., Turner, J., Cannons, J.L., Bick, D., Blakemore, L., et al. (2011). A mosaic activating mutation in AKT1 associated with the Proteus syndrome. N Engl J Med 365, 611–619.

lllumina (2013). Genotyping Microarray.

Lowrance, W.W., and Collins, F.S. (2007). Identifiability in Genomic Research. Science 317, 600–602.

Lupski, J.R., Belmont, J.W., Boerwinkle, E., and Gibbs, R.A. (2011). Clan genomics and the complex architecture of human disease. Cell 147, 32–43.

Lupski, J.R., Reid, J.G., Gonzaga-Jauregui, C., Rio Deiros, D., Chen, D.C., Nazareth, L., Bainbridge, M., Dinh, H., Jing, C., Wheeler, D.A., et al. (2010). Whole-genome sequencing in a patient with Charcot-Marie-Tooth neuropathy. N Engl J Med 362, 1181–1191.

Luria, A.R. (1972). The man with a shattered world; the history of a brain wound. New York: Basic Books.

Luria, A.R. (1976). The mind of a mnemonist: a little book about a vast memory. Chicago: H. Regnery.

Lyon, G.J. (2008). Possible varenicline-induced paranoia and irritability in a patient with major depressive disorder, borderline personality disorder, and methamphetamine abuse in remission. J Clin Psychopharmacol 28, 720–721.

Lyon, G.J. (2011). Personal account of the discovery of a new disease using next-generation sequencing. Interview by Natalie Harrison. Pharmacogenomics 12, 1519–1523.

Lyon, G.J. (2012). Guest post: Time to bring human genome sequencing into the clinic.

Lyon, G.J., Abi-Dargham, A., Moore, H., Lieberman, J.A., Javitch, J.A., and Sulzer, D. (2011). Presynaptic regulation of dopamine transmission in schizophrenia. Schizophr Bull 37, 108–117.

Lyon, G.J., Coffey, B., and Silva, R. (2008). Posttraumatic stress disorder and reactive attachment disorder: outcome in an adolescent. J Child Adolesc Psychopharmacol 18, 641–646.

Lyon, G.J., and Coffey, B.J. (2009). Complex tics and complex management in a case of severe Tourette's disorder (TD) in an adolescent. J Child Adolesc Psychopharmacol 19, 469–474.

Lyon, G.J., and Segal, J.P. (2013). Practical, ethical and regulatory considerations for the evolving medical and research genomics landscape. Appl Transl Genomics 2, 34–40.

Lyon, G.J., and Wang, K. (2012). Identifying disease mutations in genomic medicine settings: current challenges and how to accelerate progress. Genome Med 4, 58.

Macosko, E.Z., and McCarroll, S.A. (2012). Exploring the variation within. Nat Genet 44, 614–616.

Maffei, A. (2012). Enriching the environment to disinhibit the brain and improve cognition. Front Cell Neurosci 6, 53.

Maffei, A., Bucher, D., and Fontanini, A. (2012). Homeostatic plasticity in the nervous system. Neural Plast 2012, 913472.

Maffei, A., and Turrigiano, G. (2008). The age of plasticity: developmental regulation of synaptic plasticity in neocortical microcircuits. Prog Brain Res 169, 211–223.

Makary, M. (2012). Unaccountable : what hospitals won't tell you and how transparency can revolutionize health care, 1st U.S. edn. New York: Bloomsbury Press.

Malhotra, D., and Sebat, J. (2012). CNVs: harbingers of a rare variant revolution in psychiatric genetics. Cell 148, 1223–1241.

Margari, L., Lamanna, A.L., Buttiglione, M., Craig, F., Petruzzelli, M.G., and Terenzio, V. (2013). Long-term follow-up of neurological manifestations in a boy with incontinentia pigmenti. Eur J Pediatr.

Mari, F., Caselli, R., Russo, S., Cogliati, F., Ariani, F., Longo, I., Bruttini, M., Meloni, I., Pescucci, C., Schurfeld, K., et al. (2005). Germline mosaicism in Rett syndrome identified by prenatal diagnosis. Clin Genet 67, 258–260.

Maxmen, A. (2013). RNA: The genome's rising stars. Nature 496, 127–129.

McClaren, B.J., Metcalfe, S.A., Aitken, M., Massie, R.J., Ukoumunne, O.C., and Amor, D.J. (2010). Uptake of carrier testing in families after cystic fibrosis diagnosis through newborn screening. Eur J Hum Genet 18, 1084–1089.

McClaren, B.J., Metcalfe, S.A., Amor, D.J., Aitken, M., and Massie, J. (2011). A case for cystic fibrosis carrier testing in the general population. Med J Aust 194, 208–209.

McDonald-McGinn, D.M., Fahiminiya, S., Revil, T., Nowakowska, B.A., Suhl, J., Bailey, A., Mlynarski, E., Lynch, D.R., Yan, A.C., Bilaniuk, L.T., et al. (2013). Hemizygous mutations in SNAP29 unmask autosomal recessive conditions and contribute to atypical findings in patients with 22q11.2DS. J Med Genet 50, 80–90.

McGuire, A.L., and Gibbs, R.A. (2006). No Longer De-Identified. Science 312, 370–371.

McGuire, A.L., and Lupski, J.R. (2010). Personal genome research: what should the participant be told? Trends Genet 26, 199–201.

McIntyre, L.L. (2008). Parent training for young children with developmental disabilities: randomized controlled trial. Am J Ment Retard 113, 356–368.

Memczak, S., Jens, M., Elefsinioti, A., Torti, F., Krueger, J., Rybak, A., Maier, L., Mackowiak, S.D., Gregersen, L.H., Munschauer, M., et al. (2013). Circular RNAs are a large class of animal RNAs with regulatory potency. Nature 495, 333–338.

Mercer, T.R., and Mattick, J.S. (2013). Structure and function of long noncoding RNAs in epigenetic regulation. Nat Struct Mol Biol 20, 300–307.

Meyer, J.R., Dobias, D.T., Weitz, J.S., Barrick, J.E., Quick, R.T., and Lenski, R.E. (2012a). Repeatability and contingency in the evolution of a key innovation in phage lambda. Science 335, 428–432.

Meyer, K.J., Axelsen, M.S., Sheffield, V.C., Patil, S.R., and Wassink, T.H. (2012b). Germline mosaic transmission of a novel duplication of PXDN and MYT1L to two male half-siblings with autism. Psychiatr Genet 22, 137–140.

Miles, J.H. (2011). Autism spectrum disorders--a genetics review. Genet Med 13, 278–294.

Misteli, T. (2013). The cell biology of genomes: bringing the double helix to life. Cell 152, 1209–1212.

Mitchell, K.J. (2012). What is complex about complex disorders? Genome Biol 13, 237.

Mitchell, K.J., and Porteous, D.J. (2011). Rethinking the genetic architecture of schizophrenia. Psychol Med 41, 19–32.

Miura, P., Shenker, S., Andreu-Agullo, C., Westholm, J.O., and Lai, E.C. (2013). Widespread and extensive lengthening of 3' UTRs in the mammalian brain. Genome Res 23, 812–825.

Mole (2006). How we know II: bad dreams. J Cell Sci 119, 197–198.

Moreau, M.P., Bruse, S.E., Jornsten, R., Liu, Y., and Brzustowicz, L.M. (2013). Chronological changes in microRNA expression in the developing human brain. PLoS One 8, e60480.

Moreno-De-Luca, A., Myers, S.M., Challman, T.D., Moreno-De-Luca, D., Evans, D.W., and Ledbetter, D.H. (2013a). Developmental brain dysfunction: revival and expansion of old concepts based on new genetic evidence. Lancet Neurol 12, 406–414.

Moreno-De-Luca, A., Myers, S.M., Challman, T.D., Moreno-De-Luca, D., Evans, D.W., and Ledbetter, D.H. (2013b). Developmental brain dysfunction: revival and expansion of old concepts based on new genetic evidence. Lancet Neurol 12, 406–414.

Mukherjee, S. (2010). The emperor of all maladies: a biography of cancer 1st Scribner hardcover edn. New York: Scribner.

Mykytyn, K., Nishimura, D.Y., Searby, C.C., Beck, G., Bugge, K., Haines, H.L., Cornier, A.S., Cox, G.F., Fulton, A.B., Carmi, R., et al. (2003). Evaluation of complex inheritance involving the most common Bardet-Biedl syndrome locus (BBS1). Am J Hum Genet 72, 429–437.

Nakane, T., and Biesecker, L.G. (2005). No evidence for triallelic inheritance of MKKS/BBS loci in Amish Mckusick-Kaufman syndrome. Am J Med Genet A 138, 32–34.

Neale, B.M., Kou, Y., Liu, L., Ma'ayan, A., Samocha, K.E., Sabo, A., Lin, C.F., Stevens, C., Wang, L.S., Makarov, V., et al. (2012). Patterns and rates of exonic de novo mutations in autism spectrum disorders. Nature 485, 242–245.

Ng, S.B., Bigham, A.W., Buckingham, K.J., Hannibal, M.C., McMillin, M.J., Gildersleeve, H.I., Beck, A.E., Tabor, H.K., Cooper, G.M., Mefford, H.C., et al. (2010a). Exome sequencing identifies MLL2 mutations as a cause of Kabuki syndrome. Nat Genet 42, 790–793.

Ng, S.B., Buckingham, K.J., Lee, C., Bigham, A.W., Tabor, H.K., Dent, K.M., Huff, C.D., Shannon, P.T., Jabs, E.W., Nickerson, D.A., et al. (2010b). Exome sequencing identifies the cause of a mendelian disorder. Nat Genet 42, 30–35.

Nielsen, M.A. (2012). Reinventing discovery: the new era of networked science. Princeton, N.J.: Princeton University Press.

Nielsen, R., Paul, J.S., Albrechtsen, A., and Song, Y.S. (2011). Genotype and SNP calling from next-generation sequencing data. Nat Rev Genet 12, 443–451.

Ning, S., Wang, P., Ye, J., Li, X., Li, R., Zhao, Z., Huo, X., Wang, L., and Li, F. (2013). A global map for dissecting phenotypic variants in human lincRNAs. Eur J Hum Genet.

Novarino, G., El-Fishawy, P., Kayserili, H., Meguid, N.A., Scott, E.M., Schroth, J., Silhavy, J.L., Kara, M., Khalil, R.O., Ben-Omran, T., et al. (2012). Mutations in BCKD-kinase lead to a potentially treatable form of autism with epilepsy. Science.

O'Rawe, J., Guangqing, S., Wang, W., Hu, J., Bodily, P., Tian, L., Hakonarson, H., Johnson, E., Wei, Z., Jiang, T., et al. (2013). Low concordance of multiple variant-calling pipelines: practical implications for exome and genome sequencing. Genome Med 5, 28.

O'Roak, B.J., Vives, L., Fu, W., Egertson, J.D., Stanaway, I.B., Phelps, I.G., Carvill, G., Kumar, A., Lee, C., Ankenman, K., et al. (2012a). Multiplex targeted sequencing identifies recurrently mutated genes in autism spectrum disorders. Science 338, 1619–1622.

O'Roak, B.J., Vives, L., Girirajan, S., Karakoc, E., Krumm, N., Coe, B.P., Levy, R., Ko, A., Lee, C., Smith, J.D., et al. (2012b). Sporadic autism exomes reveal a highly interconnected protein network of de novo mutations. Nature 485, 246–250.

Olby, R. (1989). The dimensions of scientific controversy: the biometric--Mendelian debate. Br J Hist Sci 22, 299–320.

Opitz, J.M. (2012). 2011 William Allan Award: development and evolution. Am J Hum Genet 90, 392–404.

Orr, H.T., and Zoghbi, H.Y. (2007). Trinucleotide repeat disorders. Annu Rev Neurosci 30, 575–621.

Papageorgiou, E.A., and Patsalis, P.C. (2013). Maternal plasma sequencing: a powerful tool towards fetal whole genome recovery. BMC Med 11, 56.

Papavassiliou, P., York, T.P., Gursoy, N., Hill, G., Nicely, L.V., Sundaram, U., McClain, A., Aggen, S.H., Eaves, L., Riley, B., et al. (2009). The phenotype of persons having mosaicism for trisomy 21/Down syndrome reflects the percentage of trisomic cells present in different tissues. Am J Med Genet A 149A, 573–583.

Parodi, S., Bachetti, T., Lantieri, F., Di Duca, M., Santamaria, G., Ottonello, G., Matera, I., Ravazzolo, R., and Ceccherini, I. (2008). Parental origin and somatic mosaicism of PHOX2B mutations in Congenital Central Hypoventilation Syndrome. Hum Mutat 29, 206.

Pauli, S., Pieper, L., Haberle, J., Grzmil, P., Burfeind, P., Steckel, M., Lenz, U., and Michelmann, H.W. (2009). Proven germline mosaicism in a father of two children with CHARGE syndrome. Clin Genet 75, 473–479.

Pennacchio, L.A., Bickmore, W., Dean, A., Nobrega, M.A., and Bejerano, G. (2013). Enhancers: five essential questions. Nat Rev Genet 14, 288–295.

Penrose, L.S. (1963). The biology of mental defect, 3d rev. and reset edn. London: Sidgwick and Jackson.

Perrat, P.N., DasGupta, S., Wang, J., Theurkauf, W., Weng, Z., Rosbash, M., and Waddell, S. (2013). Transposition-driven genomic heterogeneity in the Drosophila brain. Science 340, 91–95.

Peters, B.A., Kermani, B.G., Sparks, A.B., Alferov, O., Hong, P., Alexeev, A., Jiang, Y., Dahl, F., Tang, Y.T., Haas, J., et al. (2012). Accurate whole-genome sequencing and haplotyping from 10 to 20 human cells. Nature 487, 190–195.

Philip, N., and Bassett, A. (2011). Cognitive, behavioural and psychiatric phenotype in 22q11.2 deletion syndrome. Behav Genet 41, 403–412.

Provine, W.B. (2001). The origins of theoretical population genetics, 2nd edn. Chicago: University of Chicago Press.

Radick, G. (2005). Other Histories, Other Biologies. In: Philosophy, Biology and Life (pp. 21–47). Cambridge: Cambridge University Press.

Radick, G. (2011). Physics in the Galtonian sciences of heredity. Stud Hist Philos Biol Biomed Sci 42, 129–138.

Radick, G. (2013). Scientific Inheritance - an Inaugural Lecture from Gregory Radick

Rand, C.M., Yu, M., Jennings, L.J., Panesar, K., Berry-Kravis, E.M., Zhou, L., and Weese-Mayer, D.E. (2012). Germline mosaicism of PHOX2B mutation accounts for familial recurrence of congenital central hypoventilation syndrome (CCHS). Am J Med Genet A 158A, 2297–2301.

Ratiu, P., Talos, I.F., Haker, S., Lieberman, D., and Everett, P. (2004). The tale of Phineas Gage, digitally remastered. J Neurotrauma 21, 637–643.

Refsgaard, L., Holst, A.G., Sadjadieh, G., Haunso, S., Nielsen, J.B., and Olesen, M.S. (2012). High prevalence of genetic variants previously associated with LQT syndrome in new exome data. Eur J Hum Genet 20, 905–908.

Reiss, A.L. (2009). Childhood developmental disorders: an academic and clinical convergence point for psychiatry, neurology, psychology and pediatrics. J Child Psychol Psychiatry 50, 87–98.

Rickards, A.L., Walstab, J.E., Wright-Rossi, R.A., Simpson, J., and Reddihough, D.S. (2007). A randomized, controlled trial of a home-based intervention program for children with autism and developmental delay. J Dev Behav Pediatr 28, 308–316.

Rickards, A.L., Walstab, J.E., Wright-Rossi, R.A., Simpson, J., and Reddihough, D.S. (2009). One-year follow-up of the outcome of a randomized controlled trial of a home-based intervention programme for children with autism and developmental delay and their families. Child Care Health Dev 35, 593–602.

Risgaard, B., Jabbari, R., Refsgaard, L., Holst, A.G., Haunso, S., Sadjadieh, A., Winkel, B.G., Olesen, M.S., and Tfelt-Hansen, J. (2013). High prevalence of genetic variants previously associated with Brugada syndrome in new exome data. Clin Genet 84, 489–495.

Roach, J.C., Glusman, G., Smit, A.F., Huff, C.D., Hubley, R., Shannon, P.T., Rowen, L., Pant, K.P., Goodman, N., Bamshad, M., et al. (2010). Analysis of genetic inheritance in a family quartet by whole-genome sequencing. Science 328, 636–639.

Rosendahl, J., Landt, O., Bernadova, J., Kovacs, P., Teich, N., Bodeker, H., Keim, V., Ruffert, C., Mossner, J., Kage, A., et al. (2013). CFTR, SPINK1, CTRC and PRSS1 variants in chronic pancreatitis: is the role of mutated CFTR overestimated? Gut 62, 582–592.

Sabin, L.R., Delas, M.J., and Hannon, G.J. (2013). Dogma derailed: the many influences of RNA on the genome. Mol Cell 49, 783–794.

Sacks, O.W. (1995). An anthropologist on Mars : seven paradoxical tales, 1st edn. New York: Alfrd A. Knopf.

Sacks, O.W. (1998). The man who mistook his wife for a hat and other clinical tales, 1st Touchstone edn. New York, NY: Simon & Schuster.

Salem, Y., Gropack, S.J., Coffin, D., and Godwin, E.M. (2012). Effectiveness of a low-cost virtual reality system for children with developmental delay: a preliminary randomised single-blind controlled trial. Physiotherapy 98, 189–195.

Salzman, J., Gawad, C., Wang, P.L., Lacayo, N., and Brown, P.O. (2012). Circular RNAs are the predominant transcript isoform from hundreds of human genes in diverse cell types. PLoS One 7, e30733.

Sanders, S.J., Ercan-Sencicek, A.G., Hus, V., Luo, R., Murtha, M.T., Moreno-De-Luca, D., Chu, S.H., Moreau, M.P., Gupta, A.R., Thomson, S.A., et al. (2011). Multiple recurrent de novo CNVs, including duplications of the 7q11.23 Williams syndrome region, are strongly associated with autism. Neuron 70, 863–885.

Sanders, S.J., Murtha, M.T., Gupta, A.R., Murdoch, J.D., Raubeson, M.J., Willsey, A.J., Ercan-Sencicek, A.G., DiLullo, N.M., Parikshak, N.N., Stein, J.L., et al. (2012). De novo mutations revealed by whole-exome sequencing are strongly associated with autism. Nature 485, 237–241.

Sastry, G.R., Cooper, H.B., Jr., and Brink, R.A. (1965). Paramutation and somatic mosaicism in maize. Genetics 52, 407–424.

Sato, N., Ohyama, K., Fukami, M., Okada, M., and Ogata, T. (2006). Kallmann syndrome: somatic and germline mutations of the fibroblast growth factor receptor 1 gene in a mother and the son. J Clin Endocrinol Metab 91, 1415–1418.

Sbidian, E., Feldmann, D., Bengoa, J., Fraitag, S., Abadie, V., de Prost, Y., Bodemer, C., and Hadj-Rabia, S. (2010). Germline mosaicism in keratitis-ichthyosis-deafness syndrome: pre-natal diagnosis in a familial lethal form. Clin Genet 77, 587–592.

Schaaf, C.P., Sabo, A., Sakai, Y., Crosby, J., Muzny, D., Hawes, A., Lewis, L., Akbar, H., Varghese, R., Boerwinkle, E., et al. (2011). Oligogenic heterozygosity in individuals with high-functioning autism spectrum disorders. Hum Mol Genet 20, 3366–3375.

Schneider, G.F., and Dekker, C. (2012). DNA sequencing with nanopores. Nat Biotechnol 30, 326–328.

Scriver, C.R. (2007). The PAH gene, phenylketonuria, and a paradigm shift. Hum Mutat 28, 831–845.

Seguin, E. (1866). Idiocy: and its treatment by the physiological method. New York: William Wood & Co..

Shaikh, T.H., Haldeman-Englert, C., Geiger, E.A., Ponting, C.P., and Webber, C. (2011). Genes and biological processes commonly disrupted in rare and heterogeneous developmental delay syndromes. Hum Mol Genet 20, 880–893.

Shanske, A.L., Goodrich, J.T., Ala-Kokko, L., Baker, S., Frederick, B., and Levy, B. (2012). Germline mosaicism in Shprintzen-Goldberg syndrome. Am J Med Genet A 158A, 1574–1578.

Shi, L., Zhang, X., Golhar, R., Otieno, F.G., He, M., Hou, C., Kim, C., Keating, B., Lyon, G.J., Wang, K., et al. (2013). Whole-genome sequencing in an autism multiplex family. Mol Autism 4, 8.

Shirley, M.D., Tang, H., Gallione, C.J., Baugher, J.D., Frelin, L.P., Cohen, B., North, P.E., Marchuk, D.A., Comi, A.M., and Pevsner, J. (2013). Sturge-Weber syndrome and port-wine stains caused by somatic mutation in GNAQ. N Engl J Med 368, 1971–1979.

Slavin, T.P., Lazebnik, N., Clark, D.M., Vengoechea, J., Cohen, L., Kaur, M., Konczal, L., Crowe, C.A., Corteville, J.E., Nowaczyk, M.J., et al. (2012). Germline mosaicism in Cornelia de Lange syndrome. Am J Med Genet A 158A, 1481–1485.

Smaoui, N., Chaabouni, M., Sergeev, Y.V., Kallel, H., Li, S., Mahfoudh, N., Maazoul, F., Kammoun, H., Gandoura, N., Bouaziz, A., et al. (2006). Screening of the eight BBS genes in Tunisian families: no evidence of triallelism. Invest Ophthalmol Vis Sci 47, 3487–3495.

Sokal, R., and Rohlf, F. (2012). Biometry: the principles and practice of statistics in biological research, 4th edn. New York, NY: H (Freeman & Co).

Sokal, R.R. (2012). Biometry: the principles and practice of statistics in biological research, [Extensively rev.] 4th edn. New York: W.H. Freeman.

Sol-Church, K., Stabley, D.L., Demmer, L.A., Agbulos, A., Lin, A.E., Smoot, L., Nicholson, L., and Gripp, K.W. (2009). Male-to-male transmission of Costello syndrome: G12S HRAS germline mutation inherited from a father with somatic mosaicism. Am J Med Genet A 149A, 315–321.

Solomon, A. (2012). Far from the tree: parents, children and the search for identity, 1st Scribner hardcover edn. New York: Scribner.

Sporn, M.B. (2011). Perspective: The big C - for Chemoprevention. Nature 471, S10–S11.

Stalmans, I., Lambrechts, D., De Smet, F., Jansen, S., Wang, J., Maity, S., Kneer, P., von der Ohe, M., Swillen, A., Maes, C., et al. (2003). VEGF: a modifier of the del22q11 (DiGeorge) syndrome? Nat Med 9, 173–182.

Steinbusch, C.V., van Roozendaal, K.E., Tserpelis, D., Smeets, E.E., Kranenburg-de Koning, T.J., de Waal, K.H., Zweier, C., Rauch, A., Hennekam, R.C., Blok, M.J., et al. (2013). Somatic mosaicism in a mother of two children with Pitt-Hopkins syndrome. Clin Genet 83, 73–77.

Sterckx, S., Cockbain, J., Howard, H., Huys, I., and Borry, P. (2013). "Trust is not something you can reclaim easily": patenting in the field of direct-to-consumer genetic testing. Genet Med 15, 382–387.

Styrkarsdottir, U., Thorleifsson, G., Sulem, P., Gudbjartsson, D.F., Sigurdsson, A., Jonasdottir, A., Jonasdottir, A., Oddsson, A., Helgason, A., Magnusson, O.T., et al. (2013). Nonsense mutation in the LGR4 gene is associated with several human diseases and other traits. Nature 497, 517–520.

Tajir, M., Fergelot, P., Lancelot, G., Elalaoui, S.C., Arveiler, B., Lacombe, D., and Sefiani, A. (2013). Germline mosaicism in Rubinstein-Taybi syndrome. Gene 518, 476–478.

Tanaka, T., Takahashi, K., Yamane, M., Tomida, S., Nakamura, S., Oshima, K., Niwa, A., Nishikomori, R., Kambe, N., Hara, H., et al. (2012). Induced pluripotent stem cells from CINCA syndrome patients as a model for dissecting somatic mosaicism and drug discovery. Blood 120, 1299–1308.

Tennessen, J.A., Bigham, A.W., O'Connor, T.D., Fu, W., Kenny, E.E., Gravel, S., McGee, S., Do, R., Liu, X., Jun, G., et al. (2012). Evolution and functional impact of rare coding variation from deep sequencing of human exomes. Science 337, 64–69.

Terwilliger, J.D., and Weiss, K.M. (2003). Confounding, ascertainment bias, and the blind quest for a genetic 'fountain of youth'. Ann Med 35, 532–544.

Tome, S., Manley, K., Simard, J.P., Clark, G.W., Slean, M.M., Swami, M., Shelbourne, P.F., Tillier, E.R., Monckton, D.G., Messer, A., et al. (2013). MSH3 polymorphisms and protein levels affect CAG repeat instability in Huntington's disease mice. PLoS Genet 9, e1003280.

Trevisson, E., Forzan, M., Salviati, L., and Clementi, M. (2014). Neurofibromatosis type 1 in two siblings due to maternal germline mosaicism. Clin Genet 85, 386–389.

Van Horn, J.D., Irimia, A., Torgerson, C.M., Chambers, M.C., Kikinis, R., and Toga, A.W. (2012). Mapping connectivity damage in the case of Phineas Gage. PLoS One 7, e37454.

van Swinderen, B., and Greenspan, R.J. (2005). Flexibility in a gene network affecting a simple behavior in Drosophila melanogaster. Genetics 169, 2151–2163.

Velleman, S.L., and Mervis, C.B. (2011). Children with 7q11.23 duplication syndrome: speech, language, cognitive, and behavioral characteristics and their implications for intervention. Perspect Lang Learn Educ 18, 108–116.

Venancio, M., Santos, M., Pereira, S.A., Maciel, P., and Saraiva, J.M. (2007). An explanation for another familial case of Rett syndrome: maternal germline mosaicism. Eur J Hum Genet 15, 902–904.

Vig, B.K. (1978). Somatic mosaicism in plants with special reference to somatic crossing over. Environ Health Perspect 27, 27–36.

Visscher, P.M., Goddard, M.E., Derks, E.M., and Wray, N.R. (2011). Evidence-based psychiatric genetics, AKA the false dichotomy between common and rare variant hypotheses. Mol Psychiatry 17, 474–485.

Visscher, P.M., McEvoy, B., and Yang, J. (2010). From Galton to GWAS: quantitative genetics of human height. Genet Res 92, 371–379.

Vogelstein, B., Papadopoulos, N., Velculescu, V.E., Zhou, S., Diaz, L.A., Jr., and Kinzler, K.W. (2013). Cancer genome landscapes. Science 339, 1546–1558.

Waddington, C.H. (1959). Canalization of development and genetic assimilation of acquired characters. Nature 183, 1654–1655.

Waddington, C.H. (2012). The epigenotype. 1942. Int J Epidemiol 41, 10–13.

Wang, L., Kloc, M., Gu, Y., Ge, S., and Maffei, A. (2013). Layer-specific experience-dependent rewiring of thalamocortical circuits. J Neurosci 33, 4181–4191.

Ward, O.C. (1998). John Langdon Down, 1828–1896: a caring pioneer. London; New York, NY: Royal Society of Medicine Press.

Weinhouse, C., Anderson, O.S., Jones, T.R., Kim, J., Liberman, S.A., Nahar, M.S., Rozek, L.S., Jirtle, R.L., and Dolinoy, D.C. (2011). An expression microarray approach for the identification of metastable epialleles in the mouse genome. Epigenetics 6, 1105–1113.

Weiss, K.M. (2005). Cryptic causation of human disease: reading between the (germ) lines. Trends Genet 21, 82–88.

Weiss, K.M., and Terwilliger, J.D. (2000). How many diseases does it take to map a gene with SNPs? Nat Genet 26, 151–157.

Weldon, W.F.R. (1902). Mendel's laws of alternative inheritance in peas. Biometrika 1, 228–254.

Williams, A.L., Patterson, N., Glessner, J., Hakonarson, H., and Reich, D. (2012). Phasing of many thousands of genotyped samples. Am J Hum Genet 91, 238–251.

Williams, H.J., Craddock, N., Russo, G., Hamshere, M.L., Moskvina, V., Dwyer, S., Smith, R.L., Green, E., Grozeva, D., Holmans, P., et al. (2011). Most genome-wide significant susceptibility loci for schizophrenia and bipolar disorder reported to date cross-traditional diagnostic boundaries. Hum Mol Genet 20, 387–391.

Williams, M.S. (2004). Myostatin mutation associated with gross muscle hypertrophy in a child. N Engl J Med 351, 1030–1031; author reply 1030–1031.

Wilusz, J.E., and Sharp, P.A. (2013). Molecular biology: A circuitous route to noncoding RNA. Science 340, 440–441.

Worthey, E.A., Mayer, A.N., Syverson, G.D., Helbling, D., Bonacci, B.B., Decker, B., Serpe, J.M., Dasu, T., Tschannen, M.R., Veith, R.L., et al. (2011). Making a definitive diagnosis: successful clinical application of whole exome sequencing in a child with intractable inflammatory bowel disease. Genet Med 13, 255–262.

Wu, P.Y., Phan, J.H., and Wang, M.D. (2013). Assessing the impact of human genome annotation choice on RNA-seq expression estimates. BMC Bioinf 14(Suppl 11), S8.

Wuyts, W., Biervliet, M., Reyniers, E., D'Apice, M.R., Novelli, G., and Storm, K. (2005). Somatic and gonadal mosaicism in Hutchinson-Gilford progeria. Am J Med Genet A 135, 66–68.

Xu, B., Ionita-Laza, I., Roos, J.L., Boone, B., Woodrick, S., Sun, Y., Levy, S., Gogos, J.A., and Karayiorgou, M. (2012). De novo gene mutations highlight patterns of genetic and neural complexity in schizophrenia. Nat Genet 44, 1365–1369.

Yamada, M., Okura, Y., Suzuki, Y., Fukumura, S., Miyazaki, T., Ikeda, H., Takezaki, S., Kawamura, N., Kobayashi, I., and Ariga, T. (2012). Somatic mosaicism in two unrelated patients with X-linked chronic granulomatous disease characterized by the presence of a small population of normal cells. Gene 497, 110–115.

Zimmermann, M.B. (2012). The effects of iodine deficiency in pregnancy and infancy. Paediatr Perinat Epidemiol 26(Suppl 1), 108–117.

Zuk, O., Hechter, E., Sunyaev, S.R., and Lander, E.S. (2012). The mystery of missing heritability: Genetic interactions create phantom heritability. Proc Natl Acad Sci U S A 109, 1193–1198.

Zumbo, P., and Mason, C.E. (2014). Molecular methods for profiling the RNA world. In Genome Analysis: Current Procedures and Applications. Horizon Press.

14

PROGRESS TOWARD THERAPIES AND INTERVENTIONS FOR NEURODEVELOPMENTAL DISORDERS

Ayokunmi Ajetunmobi[1] and Daniela Tropea[2]

[1]*Nanomedicine and Molecular Imaging Group, Department of Clinical Medicine, School of Medicine, Trinity College Dublin, Dublin, Ireland*
[2]*Department of Psychiatry, Trinity Centre for Health Sciences, St. James Hospital, Dublin 8, Dublin, Ireland*

14.1 INTRODUCTION

Despite growing interdisciplinary efforts in the development of therapies for common neurodevelopmental disorders (NDDs); to date, there are no resolutive treatments for such conditions, and most therapies target specific symptoms rather than the causes of the disorders. In autism, there are drugs that affect irritability, hyperactivity, and attention deficits, but poor results have been obtained in targeting the core features of autism: social and language impairment (Kolevzon, 2012). We see a similar story in schizophrenia where the treatments are merely partially effective, focusing only on the positive symptoms of the disorder, while the negative and cognitive symptoms remain unresolved. The delay in diagnostic and therapeutic interventions reflects the

poor knowledge of the underlying neurobiology of these disorders; therefore, it is fundamental to dissect out the mechanisms behind the onset and progression of the disorders. In some cases, the serendipitous discovery of certain drugs has shed light on the mechanisms involved. Chlorpromazine, a Dopamine (DA) antagonist, which was initially used to reduce the post-operational shock in surgery patients, proved to be very successful in schizophrenia patients pointing at the dopaminergic system as a viable target for therapeutics. Since then, more drugs targeting the dopaminergic system have been developed to reach more specific pathways, but the mechanisms linking dopamine receptor blockade and therapeutic outcome still remain obscure. Certain treatments are used across several disorders (benzodiazepines, fluoexitine) and there is a

The Genetics of Neurodevelopmental Disorders, First Edition. Edited by Kevin J. Mitchell.
© 2015 John Wiley & Sons, Inc. Published 2015 by John Wiley & Sons, Inc.

general consensus that overlapping treatments is a sign of overlapping mechanisms. This can be a misleading principle, considering that NDDs often present similar clinical symptoms, but the biological mechanisms underlying them may be totally different.

In this chapter, we will describe the current therapeutic interventions in clinical or preclinical trials. Starting with genetic discoveries, we will summarize the molecules and signaling pathways that contribute to the pathophysiology of several NDDs, stressing their points of convergence and/or divergence in the molecular targets used for therapeutic intervention. Additionally, we will explore the state-of-the-art tools used for drug discovery and therapeutic intervention, and discuss how each of them can contribute to the research for NDDs.

14.2 GENETICS

In an attempt to uncover the molecular etiology of NDDs, the past decade has witnessed impressive efforts in genetic analysis studies, looking at both variability in repetitions of genomic sequences and single gene analysis. The outcome of these studies revealed that most of the genes implicated in NDDs were not predicted from known biology, and many of them take part in neurodevelopmental processes and synaptic function and plasticity (Mitchell, 2011).

Studies in families have shown that genetic factors play a major role in the development of NDDs; however apart from a few examples of monogenic disorders, in the majority of NDDs, it is not possible to link the clinical outcome to mutations in a single gene, although several risk factors have been identified. To complicate the picture, epidemiological studies show that environmental factors such as maternal infections and malnutrition also contribute to the onset of the disorder, supporting the evidence for gene–environment interaction (Stolp et al., 2012). Strikingly, many of the same genes are emerging across hitherto unrelated neuropsychiatric conditions, such as autism and

schizophrenia, challenging how we conceptualize these disorders (Carroll and Owen, 2009). Without further discussing concepts which are treated in other chapters, we will conclude with the consideration that genetic studies, although remarkably informative, have revealed a picture with additional levels of complexity and demonstrated that it is not possible to build a functional model of disease pathology on the exclusive basis of the genetic data (Fig. 14.1).

Therefore, one of the main quests for the discovery of new treatments is to establish the cellular and molecular mechanisms that underlie each specific condition, identify new biomarkers and their clinical outcome, and establish the right model for understanding the neurobiology of the disorders and testing candidate treatments. In this endeavor, a huge boost in the comprehension of mechanisms for potential therapeutic intervention has come from the study of monogenic

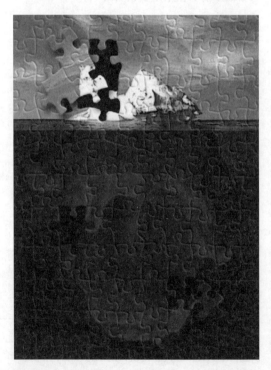

Fig. 14.1 *The hidden knowledge of neurodevelopmental disorders neurobiology.* Genetic studies revealed the molecular underpinnings of the disorders but also showed that there is much more to uncover yet. *(See insert for color representation of this figure.)*

disorders, and this is understandable for several reasons: first, it is easier to identify molecular mechanisms that are altered by the mutation of a single gene, and second, it is possible to create transgenic animal models in the selected gene to study the neurobiology and test candidate treatments. The information derived from single gene disorders can be useful to dissect out the mechanisms of more complex models and to propose new avenues for intervention.

14.3 MOLECULAR PATHWAYS AS TARGETS FOR THERAPEUTIC INTERVENTION

Genetic studies constitute the starting point for research into the molecular mechanisms of NDDs, where many of the genes identified are mostly related to neurodevelopment and synaptic function. However, the challenge for neurobiologists is to uncover the cellular mechanisms that link the gene to synaptic function and to identify the convergent mechanisms across different disorders (Fig. 14.2, Table 14.1).

A clear impairment common to different NDDs is the imbalance of excitatory and inhibitory transmission. The first indication of such impairment comes from clinical observations, which highlight seizures as a common feature across several disorders: seizures are present in Rett syndrome, Down syndrome, Fragile X syndrome, Tuberous sclerosis and 25% of autistic cases (Tuchman and Rapin, 2002), with many current treatments targeting GABAergic pathways. In mice models currently used for studying Down syndrome (Ts65Dn mice), it has been found that some synaptic deficits of the system result from excessive activity of inhibitory neurons (Fernandez and Garner, 2007), and in fact $GABA_A$ and $GABA_B$ receptor antagonists have been shown to improve synaptic deficits in the hippocampus (Kleshevnikov et al., 2008). GABAergic transmission has also been targeted in Fragile X syndrome (Levenga et al., 2010; Olmos-Serrano et al., 2010; Pacey et al., 2009) and neurofibromatosis type 1 (Cui et al., 2008), in addition to tuberous sclerosis where patients

treated with GABA enhancer show relief from epilepsy (Collins et al., 2006; Hancock and Osborne, 1999; Jambaqué et al., 2000).

In most of these examples, the reduction of GABA signaling was used to correct defects of brain plasticity in animal models, however, for the translation of these findings into clinical applications, we need to remember that some patients (Fragile X and Down syndrome) present seizures, and therefore the use of GABA antagonists should be carefully considered.

Along with drugs that target the GABAergic system, there are several treatments based on glutamatergic transmission. In Rett syndrome, dextromethorphan – an NMDA antagonist – is currently in clinical trials and there is compelling evidence that the activation of the glutamatergic system, and in particular NMDA receptors, is reduced. Conversely, activation of NMDA receptors can be used to treat schizophrenia; however the direct activation of NMDA can be dangerous and therefore milder alternatives have been sought. One strategy is to enhance the activation of NMDA with glycine, a coactivator of the NMDA receptor, together with glutamate. Increased concentrations of glycine levels have been obtained with specific blockers of glycine transporters, which indirectly increase glycine concentration (Pinard et al., 2010). Another alternative is to activate metabotropic glutamate receptors (Conn and Jones, 2009), which also ameliorate symptoms of schizophrenia. Similarly, modulators of cholinergic transmission have recently proven to be effective as alternative treatment for schizophrenia (Terry, 2008), possibly due to an indirect modulation of the excitatory transmission.

Proof for the involvement of glutamatergic transmission in NDDs is evident in alterations to the number and morphology of dendritic spines often observed in both postmortem tissue (Bennett, 2011) and animal models (Penzes et al., 2013). Dendritic spines are dendritic protrusions that represent 95% of postsynaptic elements in glutamatergic transmission, and are therefore directly involved in circuit connectivity. Imaging studies have confirmed the

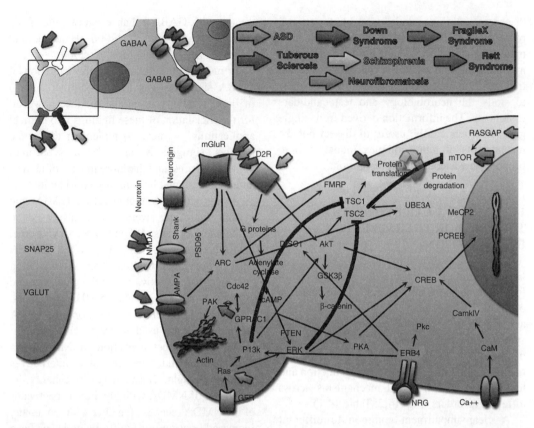

Fig. 14.2 *Molecular mechanisms target of therapeutic interventions in neurodevelopmental disorders (NDDs).* Schematic Representation of circuits (a) and pathways (b) involved in NDDs and currently targeted by approved and in trial drugs. The black arrows connecting two molecules indicate interaction between the molecules without specifying if there is activation or inhibition. The coloured arrows represent current interventions and they point at their molecular target. They are color-coded for specific disorders: pink (ASD), red (Down syndrome), blue (Fragile X), green (Rett syndrome), yellow (schizophrenia), orange (tuberous sclerosis), and purple (neurofibromatosis type 1). Note that the targeted molecules are very limited with respect to the whole machinery. The neuromodulators are dopamine (white), norepinephrine (light grey), serotonin (medium grey), and acetylcholine (black). For detailed information see the text. The same information, together with additional references, is listed in Table 14.1. *(See insert for color representation of this figure.)*

hypothesis of altered connectivity in schizophrenia (Mothersill et al., 2012) and alterations in spines number and morphology have been shown in other disorders (Bennett, 2011; Dölen et al., 2007; Tropea et al., 2009). The shape and number of dendritic spines are strongly dependent on the developmental stage and neuronal activity (Holtmaat and Svoboda, 2009), and the changes are due to reorganization of cytoskeletal actin. Although genetic evidence from several studies point to candidate genes that

are elements of the cytoskeleton (Benitez-King et al., 2004), these molecules are not often targeted for therapeutic intervention. The only exception is represented by members of the PAK (p21-activated kinase) family, which rescue the spine phenotype of Fragile X when inhibited in a mouse model of the disorder (Dolan et al., 2013). Recently Pak inhibitors have been found effective in rescuing cellular phenotypes associated with schizophrenia (Hayashi-Takaji et al., 2014).

TABLE 14.1   Listing of the novel drugs and their molecular target that are currently used in neurodevelopmental disorders

Disease States	Genetic Mutation(s)	Molecular Target(s)	Potential Therapeutic Candidate(s)	References
Rett syndrome	*MECP2*	MeCP2 mGluR	IGF1 Dextromethorphan	Ciucci et al., 2007 clinicaltrials.gov Pini et al., 2012 Tropea et al., 2009
Fragile X syndrome	*FMR1*	FMRP mGluR5 Matrix Metallopro-teinase 9 GABA$_B$R	CTEP MPEP Fenobam AFQ056 (Novartis) RO4917523 (Roche) STX107 GRN-592 Minocycline Ganaxolone Racemic Baclofen	Bear et al., 2004 Berry-Kravis et al., 2009 Bilousova et al., 2009 Heulens et al., 2012 Jacob et al., 2009 Jacquemont et al., 2011 Levenga et al., 2010 Michalon et al., 2012 Pacey et al., 2009 Paribello et al., 2010 Silverman et al., 2012 Su et al., 2011 Thomas et al., 2012
Tuberous sclerosis	*TSC1* *TSC2*	GABA$_A$R mTOR mGluR5	Levetiracetam Rapamycin (everolimus) CDPPB	Auerbach et al., 2011 Collins et al., 2006 Ehninger et al., 2008 Krueger et al., 2010 Meikle et al., 2008 Zeng et al., 2008
Neurofibromatosis Type1	*NF1*	Neurofibromin GABA$_A$R RasGAP	L-655,708 Lovastatin Simvastatin	Acosta et al., 2011 Chabernaud et al., 2012 Cui et al., 2008 Krab et al., 2008 Li et al., 2005 Shilyansky et al., 2010
Schizophrenia	*DISC1* *NRG1*	PDE4B GSK3 GlyT1	Rolipram Haloperidol TDZD-8 RG1678	Clapcote, 2007 Kanes et al., 2007 Lipina et al., 2012 Pinard et al., 2010 Siuciak et al., 2007
Autism Spectrum Disorder	*NLGN* *NRXN* *SHANK*	Neuroligin-Neureglin Complex mGluR5 mTOR MeCP2	CDPPB Rapamycin IGF-1	Auerbach et al., 2011 Blundell et al., 2010 Clifton et al., 2013 Hung et al., 2008 Kim et al., 2008 Tsai et al., 2012 Won et al., 2012

Another system targeted for therapeutic intervention is the metabolism of newly synthesized proteins. This is based on the ability of neurons to respond to stimulation by promoting the synthesis of specific proteins (Kelleher and Bear, 2008). In the case of some disorders, the cell system is overloaded with an excess of protein and the fine modulation of specific newly synthetized proteins is not detectable, leading to a system that is unable to respond to the changes required by external stimulation. This situation has been well described for Fragile X syndrome, where FMRP (fragile x mental retardation protein) controls the synthesis of important proteins involved in cytoskeleton, trafficking, and synaptic function (Ebert and Greenberg, 2013; Wetmore and Garner, 2010) and loss of expression of FMRP in transgenic animal models results in dysregulation of translation of synaptic proteins, associated with developmental deficits in learning and memory.

Additionally, mGluR5 receptors are modulators of protein synthesis and have been suggested to compensate FMRP down-regulation by modulating the activation of mGluR. In fact, partial inhibition of mGluR5 has been proven to ameliorate the symptoms of Fragile X in a mouse model of the disease (Dölen et al., 2007) and mGluR5 modulators are now in clinical trials of Fragile X children.

Another example of the importance of protein metabolism is presented by the enzyme UBE3A, which is involved in ubiquitination and protein degradation and underlies the genetic cause of Angelmann syndrome. UBE3A controls the degradation of important proteins involved in cell function (Mabb et al., 2011) among which there is ARC: a protein involved in trafficking of AMPA receptors. Without the ability to modulate the amount of AMPA receptors at the synaptic level, cells lack an important regulatory system for controlling the response to external stimuli and as a consequence the system is unable to react to changes in activity.

This "rigidity" in the system, can be due to other mechanisms, such as impairment in intracellular signaling and activation of gene transcription. We see this in Neurofibromatosis type 1 and the gene *NF1* which codes for neurofibromin, a Ras GTPase-activating protein, which is a modulator of important cellular pathways such as cAMP (Guo et al., 1997), ERK, and mTOR-mediated protein translation. Mice mutant for *NF1* show impaired learning and memory and long-term potentiation (LTP) deficits (Costa et al., 2002). These deficits can be rescued by lovastatin, which reduces Ras pathway activation.

Several drugs have been tested in animal models for their ability to rescue deficits in synaptic function and plasticity, uncovering shared molecular mechanisms that converge or diverge across different disorders. This is seen in the study by Auerbach et al. (2011), where they show that mGLUR-mediated long-term depression (LTD) is impaired in *Tsc2* mutant mice models for Tuberous Sclerosis, and that this effect is due to a decrease in protein translation required for the activation of LTD. In comparison, the opposite mechanism is observed in Fragile X syndrome, where *Fmr1* mutant mice develop an excess in protein translation causing over-activation of mGLUR-dependent LTD. Interestingly, the defects found in each animal model disappear when the mice are bred to carry both mutations. Since in Fragile X syndrome, inhibition of mGLUR5 rescues LTD, the authors reasoned that the activation of mGluR5 should rescue the opposite phenotype in the Tuberous sclerosis mutants. Indeed CDPPB, a positive allosteric modulator of mGluR5, rescues LTD in *Tsc2* mutant mice. Such approaches could be useful to uncover signaling pathways that are complementary across other disorders. The case of Fragile X and Tuberous Sclerosis is an example of how the genetic etiology of an individual is critical to identifying different, and in this case, opposite-treatments for common clinical symptoms.

Another important pathway for several NDDs is the AKT signaling pathway and the role of mammalian target of rapamycin (mTOR), which is involved in mRNA translation and cellular proliferation (Gipson and Johnston, 2012). mTOR is the molecular target of rapamycin, an immunosuppressor drug that is activated downstream of AKT and is inhibited by the complex formed by TSC1 and TSC2 in tuberous sclerosis. When the complex is inactive, due to the mutation in one of the two genes, the inhibition is released and mTOR becomes active. Therefore, mTOR is a natural target for Tuberous Sclerosis. However, there are other NDDs with an impaired regulation of mTOR. In Neurofibromatosis type 1 (NF1) the redundant activation of Ras produces an activation of PI3K, with a consequent activation of mTOR and the use of rapamycin in animal models of NF1 has shown promising results (Johannessen et al., 2005). Similarly, in *Pten* mutant mice, which are classified as mutants in autism, there is a release of the PI3K inhibition, with a consequent activation of mTOR. Likewise in Fragile X syndrome, the excess in protein synthesis should be reasonably counteracted by mTOR inhibition; however, rapamycin treatment has proven to be of no benefit in *Fmr1* null mice (Osterweil et al., 2010). It is worth mentioning that in Rett syndrome, there is a documented deactivation of the AKT/mTOR pathway (Ricciardi et al., 2011), which explains why activation of IGF1 signaling, with subsequent activation of PI3K pathway, leads to an amelioration of the symptoms of Rett in a mouse model of the disease (Tropea et al., 2009). Interestingly another target of AKT: GSK3β, is also inhibited by disrupted in schizophrenia 1 (DISC1), which is a risk factor for neuropsychiatric conditions, including autism and schizophrenia (Mao et al., 2009). DISC1-mediated inhibition of Gsk3β stabilizes β-catenin. Suppression of DISC1 action causes an interruption of cellular proliferation and a premature exit from the cell cycle, explaining the defects in neuronal proliferation and localization observed in *Disc1* mutant mice.

The AKT signaling pathway is the most striking example of convergence of signaling pathways in different NDDs and this convergence may explain to some extent the overlapping of clinical symptoms. It is likely that specific mutations in different disorders also operate at other molecular levels, which could explain the differences in the phenotypes. One of the challenges for future research is to be able to associate the genetic mutations with specific signaling pathways and to be able to identify the complementary similarities and differences across disorders. Another important factor to take into account is that the impaired pathways may be activated (or inhibited) in specific cellular circuits. For example, a current model that links the glutamatergic hypothesis with GABAergic impairment in schizophrenia focuses on how deficits in NMDA activation may be localized on parvalbumin-positive cells: a specific subset of inhibitory cells that exert their inhibition on the soma of pyramidal neurons. Therefore, impairment of NMDA activation in these cells would result in a decreased inhibition on pyramidal neurons.

Finally, treatments that target neuromodulatory pathways should also be mentioned. Modifiers of such systems are currently used for the treatment of respiratory impairment in Rett syndrome (Roux et al., 2007; Zanella et al., 2008), correction of positive symptoms of schizophrenia (Pratt et al., 2012), and for treating specific symptoms in autism (Wetmore and Garner, 2010). However, neuromodulators may have additional application in NDDs: for example, since acetylcholine and serotonin can affect excitatory and inhibitory transmission, they can be used as an alternative strategy to target the imbalance of excitation/inhibition.

Figure 14.2 and Table 14.1 summarize the current therapeutic treatment with their molecular target and their known correlation to a specific disorder. This is not an exhaustive list and we have not included all the molecules and pathways that are known to be involved in NDDs, but focused on the mechanisms that are targets of therapeutic intervention.

14.4 STRATEGIES FOR INTERVENTION

One of the limiting steps for the identification of a candidate drug is the knowledge of the molecular mechanisms that are dysregulated in the disorder. In order to identify the proper treatment, it is necessary to proceed in ordered steps: the first step is to identify the genetic background of the patient and identify the area of interest of the mutation. In some cases, this can be resolutive; recent evidence shows that mutations in metabolic pathways can lead to intellectual disability (ID), and dietary restrictions and complements can compensate for the genetic deficit. If the deficit is identified early and the treatment is promptly started, there are high chances to prevent the ID, as in the case of phenylketonuria (PKU) (Karnebeek and Stockler, 2012). However, in the majority of cases, the knowledge of the genetic deficit is only partially informative and it is necessary to identify the biological mechanisms disrupted by the mutation. Both animal and cellular models have been useful to link the genetic mutations to the impaired neurobiology and to test candidate treatment (Fig. 14.3).

Once the molecular deficiency has been identified, there are at least two strategies to treating NDDs:

1. To reverse or compensate for the primary molecular/biochemical deficit
2. To correct for the neural systems aberrations that result from neurodevelopmental insults.

The first strategy only works in cases where the requirement for the gene is ongoing; that is, where the clinical defects seen in adults are due to lack of gene function in adults. An example is the blockade of GluR signaling in *FMR1*. Another example is Rett syndrome, where it is possible to rescue the phenotype with overexpression of the mutated gene even in the adult (Guy et al., 2007; Giacometti et al., 2007); however, a constant treatment is required to maintain the benefits (McGraw et al., 2011).

In many cases, it may be too late to correct for altered cell migration, axon guidance, synaptogenesis, or even synaptic plasticity defects that were present during critical periods. We may need, instead, to define the eventual pathophysiological state driving symptoms and

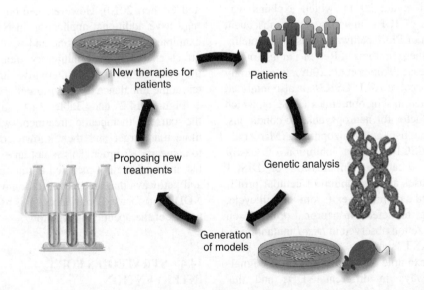

Fig. 14.3 *The cycle of discovery.* The research starts with the patients, who provide the samples for genetic research. Once the genetic factors for neurodevelopmental disorders are identified, researchers generate animal mutants and *in vitro* cellular systems to understand the molecular mechanisms that underlie the genetic dysfunction. Basic research suggests mechanisms and candidate treatments that can be tested in live and *in vitro* models, and, if positive effects are revealed, the treatments can be tested in patients. *(See insert for color representation of this figure.)*

attempt to correct it, indirectly and that is when we have to use the second strategy.

An alternative or complementary strategy is to understand the neurodevelopmental trajectories that lead from neurodevelopmental insults to pathophysiological states and intervene prior to the onset of illness in high-risk individuals. In these cases, genetic screens prenatally or early-postnatally are critical to identify the disorder before the appearance of clinical symptoms.

Considering the heteroegenity of NDDs, there is the possibility that therapies will have to be highly personalized. However, for treating symptoms common to several disorders, there may be some convergence at the level of pathophysiology (or transition to pathophysiological state) that can be targeted, regardless of the primary genetic etiology (e.g., seizures or anxiety). Very likely, a combination of different approaches will be the key, but the validation of the correct strategy will have to be tested in one of the models described in the following sections.

14.5   FINDING THE RIGHT MODEL

Apart from the serendipitous discovery of drugs and mechanisms, much of the information regarding the neuropathology of NDDs and their possible treatments has come from human studies of genetic analysis, *in vivo* imaging, human cell culture lines, and postmortem analysis. All of these approaches have proven highly informative, yet there remain big limitations due to the nature of the disorders. First, the main target area is the brain, which is not easy to access. Second, the onset of the disorder occurs after a period of normal development and it is not possible to reconstruct *a posteriori* if there are precocious signs of the disorders. Third, most of the individuals tested are already under treatment, making it difficult to dissect out the signs of the disease from the effect of the therapies; this is especially true for psychosis and imaging or postmortem studies. It is, therefore, necessary to establish suitable

models for studying the molecular mechanisms of NDDs as well as the onset and the temporal progression of the disease. It is reasonable to think that these models depend on the specific disease, and that more than one model may be considered at the same time.

14.6   ANIMAL MODELS FOR NEURODEVELOPMENTAL DISORDERS

Recent advances in implementing effective therapeutic strategies for NDDs have focused on the creation and characterization of animal models specific for each disease state. These mutants have proven to be useful resources for identifying novel putative candidate genes involved in disease onset, and studying the biological functions of these genes

To effectively make the most of animal studies, it must first be understood that there are some limits in the use of animal models, primarily centered on the anatomical and physiological differences between animals and man, meaning the findings in the mice are not always applicable to man. Furthermore, it is difficult to produce animal models with the same genetic mutations observed in patient variability. However even with these limitations, major benefits have still been found, particularly for monogenic disorders (Zoghbi and Bear, 2012). First, the structure of the nervous system is maintained, and so are the connections between areas and the action of neuromodulators. Second, it is possible to investigate the developmental progression of the disorders, including the onset and the possible prodromal signs of the condition. Finally, which is most relevant to the purpose of this chapter, it is possible to test candidate therapies and to establish their effects on brain circuitry, together with the measurement at the peripheral level (blood tests, cardio-respiratory activity, brain activity, motor behavior). This is particularly important for the use of new proposed therapies.

One of the biggest discoveries from animal studies of NDDs is that, in some cases, a disorder can be rescued even within the adult animal, when the circuitry has already developed. This has shown that, in such cases, the genetic changes do not dramatically alter the basic development of the circuitry and that dysfunctional mechanisms can be corrected. These findings have opened up new avenues for the pharmacological treatment of these disorders and have been used for the pharmacological treatment of pathology and cognitive deficits specific to diseases such as, Rett syndrome (RTT), Fragile X syndrome (FXS), tuberous sclerosis (TS), neurofibromatosis type 1 (NF-1), Schizophrenia (SZ), and autism spectrum disorders (ASD). Here we will limit our description to the therapeutic approach used in animal models, leaving the complete description of the models to other chapters of this book. In all these models, the strategy used has been to correct the phenotype without correcting the genetic defect, and this approach has produced a partial – or total – rescue of some of the symptoms.

14.6.1 Rett Syndrome

Mouse models of RTT have been used to show that reactivation of the native *Mecp2* gene in the adult mutant mice is able to restore phenotypic expression to control conditions, providing evidence that even if the normal development of the brain has been impaired by the expression of a nonfunctional form of MeCP2, there remains the opportunity to re-establish control conditions (Giacometti et al., 2007; Guy et al., 2007). This has been further explored with the systemic treatment of *Mecp2* mutant mice with an active peptide fragment of insulin-like growth factor 1 (IGF1), which modulates the maturation and plasticity of brain circuitry and activates pathways that control synaptic function (Ciucci et al., 2007). Mice studies have revealed that treatments activating IGF1 signaling extends the lifespan of the mice, increases brain weight, ameliorates breathing patterns, reduces irregularity in heart rates and increases locomotor function. In addition, these treatments mitigate against the *Mecp2*-induced deficits in brain maturation, partially restoring spine density and synaptic amplitude as well as

stabilizing cortical plasticity to wild-type levels (Tropea et al., 2008). This translational bridge between genetic association and transgenic mouse model studies has prompted phase 1 clinical trials using IGF1 as a treatment strategy for RTT, with results demonstrating that IGF1 is well tolerated and can be administered to RTT patients with consistent monitoring of the risk parameters (Pini et al., 2012).

14.6.2 Fragile X Syndrome

Since the discovery of the genetic silencing of *FMR1* as the primary cause of FXS, the *Fmr1* knockout mutant mouse model has been the most widely studied mouse model for FXS. Animal models that have been used to determine therapeutic strategies for FXS have primarily targeted the excessive excitation of synapses in group 1 metabotropic glutamate receptor (mGluR5) pathways (Bear et al., 2004), or altered inhibition of synaptic transmission with $GABA_B$ receptor pathways (D'Hulst and Kooy, 2007). *Fmr1* mutant mice with a 50% reduction in mGluR5 expression prevented the appearance of multiple FXS phenotypes, displaying increased spine density, correction to inhibitory avoidance extinction and correction to auditory hypersensitivity (Dölen et al., 2007). Likewise, the prolonged persistent activity in the neocortex to thalamic stimulation in *Fmr1* knockout mice is also corrected by reducing mGluR5 levels by 50%, indicating that aspects of cortical circuit function can be restored to normal levels by reducing mGluR5 signaling (Hays et al., 2011). Furthermore, pharmacological inhibition of mGluR5 with negative allosteric modulators (NAMs) corrects much of the pathophysiology associated with the loss of FMRP in *Fmr1* knockout mice. Inhibition of mGluR5 using the mGluR5 antagonist MPEP corrects the increased prepulse inhibition, auditory hypersensitivity incidence, and locomotor activity in the open field in *Fmr1* knockout mice to wild-type levels (Thomas et al., 2012). MPEP administration also corrects synaptic deficits associated with FXS, reducing average spine length and density in the cortical neurons of

Fmr1 knockout mice at developmental age (Su et al., 2011). The implications of these studies have led to the transfer of therapeutic strategies from bench to bedside with clinical studies assessing the effectiveness of NAM blocking of mGluR5 in FXS with pilot (Jacob et al., 2009) and phase I studies (Berry-Kravis et al., 2009) completed and phase IIb multisite trials in adults and adolescents with FXS are currently underway.

14.6.3 Tuberous Sclerosis

Mice models of *Tsc1* and *Tsc2* mutations have proved effective in developing new therapies for the treatment of TS and the mTOR inhibitor rapamycin has been developed as a promising candidate for TS therapy. Early postnatal inhibition of mTOR with rapamycin significantly improves survival in neuronal *Tsc1* mutant mice displaying substantially improved neurological phenotype in cell size and myelination in addition to improved survival rates (Meikle et al., 2008). Rapamycin treatment also restores late-phase LTP thresholds in Tsc2 hippocampus to levels similar to the control mice (Ehninger et al., 2008). In another study, social dysfunction and behavioral inflexibility of Purkinje cell-specific *Tsc1* mutant mice were also improved by rapamycin (Tsai et al., 2012). Additionally, rapamycin treatment has been effective in rescuing seizure phenotypes in glial specific *Tsc1* mutant mice, preventing seizure onset when treatment is carried out before the manifestation of the symptom and reducing seizure progression when treatment is carried out after seizure onset (Zeng et al., 2008). Together, these animal studies have been a pivotal element in the discovery of a new target for TS therapy in addition to testing for preclinical efficacy of potential drug candidates. Recently, enhancement of mGluR signaling has been proven to be beneficial in rescuing synaptic and behavioral deficits in *TsC2* mutant mice.

14.6.4 Neurofibromatosis Type 1

NF-1 is a common inherited tumor predisposition syndrome in which all affected individuals harbor a germline *NF1* gene mutation. The *NF1* encodes a protein, neurofibromin, which is highly expressed in the brain (Daston et al., 1992). Neurofibromin is a Ras GTPase-activating protein (RasGAP) that suppresses tumor formation and inhibits protein translation via the mTOR pathway. Additionally, Neurofibromin also enhances the adenylyl-cyclase/cyclic AMP pathway that couples neural activity to memory formation (Hyman et al., 2005).

The RasGAP activity of neurofibromin and its role in the increase of GABAergic activity presents a promising therapeutic target for treating NF-1 (Shilyansky et al., 2010). Pharmacological applications that decrease the levels of Ras/ERK signaling have been shown to rescue key electrophysiological and behavioral phenotypes of *Nf1* mutant mice (Li et al., 2005). Prompted by the findings from animal studies, drug therapies designed to reduce aberrant increased Ras/ERK signaling are in clinical development to address cognitive deficits in NF-1 (Acosta et al., 2011; Chabernaud et al., 2012; Krab et al., 2008).

14.6.5 Schizophrenia

Unlike the models described so far, SZ is not a monogenic disorder, and the diagnosis is mostly based on dialogue between the clinician and the patient. For these reasons, it is not possible to propose an animal model of SZ. However, several high penetrant risk factors of the disorder have been identified, and animal models for these genes have been generated. Interestingly, these mice present defects in working memory that can be related to deficits in SZ, and therapies currently used in patients are able to rescue these phenotypes.

Disrupted in schizophrenia 1 (*DISC1*) is a susceptibility gene for major mental disorders. Various strains of *DISC1* mice expressing mutated proteins have been created to explore the role of *DISC1* in psychiatric disorders. These mice have SZ-like behavior, with profound disruption of information processing exhibited by deficits in prepulse inhibition and latent inhibition that were reversed by antipsychotic treatments (haloperidol, rolipram) that are used in patients (Clapcote et al., 2007).

Other risk factors for SZ are genes coding for phosphodiesterases (PDEs) which are a class of key enzymes within the intracellular signal transduction cascade that are produced following activation of many types of membrane-bound receptors. In particular, PDE4B and other PDE4s have been shown to be involved in molecular mechanisms that underlie psychiatric disorders through interaction with DISC1 protein (Millar et al., 2005). Rolipram, a specific PDE4 inhibitor has been shown to display the same behavioral effects in mouse mutants as traditional antipsychotic medications, showing reversals of amphetamine-induced hyperactivity and prepulse inhibition deficits (Kanes et al., 2007; Siuciak et al., 2007). Similarly, glycogen synthase kinase-3 (GSK3), a highly conserved serine/threonine protein kinase has also been implicated in pathology of schizophrenia (Karam et al., 2010). Interestingly, both PDE4B and GSK3 have common binding sites at the N-terminal region of DISC1. Pharmacological and genetic inactivation of GSK-3 reverses prepulse inhibition and latent inhibition deficits as well as normalizing the hyperactivity of *Disc1*-L100P mutant mice. In parallel, interaction between DISC1 and GSK-3α and β is reduced in *Disc1*-L100P mutants (Lipina et al., 2011). Combined treatment of *Disc1*-L100P mice with rolipram and the GSK3 inhibitor TDZD-8 at subthreshold doses can correct prepulse inhibition deficits and spontaneous hyperactivity possibly suggesting synergistic interactions between PDE4, GSK3, and DISC1 in the etiology of schizophrenia (Lipina et al., 2012). Overall, these studies suggest the inhibition of PDE4 and GSK3 is a new approach for therapeutic interventions in schizophrenia.

14.6.6 Autism Spectrum Disorder

Several candidate therapies have focused on targeting disrupted synaptic signaling as determinants of ASD pathology. Positive allosteric modulators of mGluR5 receptors have been suggested for ASD treatment through the enhancement of NMDA receptor function. These modulators increase the function of NMDA receptors only when occupied by the endogenous ligand glutamate, providing high blood-brain barrier penetrance and minimal desensitization. The concept of augmenting NMDA receptor signaling via mGluR potentiation was first proposed for treatments in schizophrenia due to minimized excitotoxicity and the enabling of high-dose administrations (Gregory et al., 2011). In Chinese hamster ovary (CHO) cells expressing human mGluR5, administration of the positive mGluR5 allosteric modulator 3-cyano-*N*-(1,3-diphenyl-1H-pyrazol-5-yl)benzamide (CDPPB), was shown to enhance mGluR5 activity in a concentration-dependent manner. Consequently, behavioral tests on Sprague-Dawley rat models demonstrated alleviation of prepulse inhibition and hyperactivity produced by amphetamine, suggesting the potential use of CDPPB as an antipsychotic agent (Kinney et al., 2005). Additionally, CDPPB has been shown to enhance the performance of wild-type mice in cognitive tasks, indicating a role in synaptic plasticity and learning and memory (Stefani and Moghaddam, 2010; Uslaner et al., 2009). These studies have implicated positive allosteric modulators of mGluR5 as potential therapeutic candidates for autism – as in the study mentioned earlier. Similarly, deficits in social novelty recognition induced by neonatal phencyclidine treatment were reversed with CDPPB treatment and social deficits associated with *Shank2^-/-^* mutant models were rescued by CDPPB treatment (Clifton et al., 2013), implicating hypofunction of mGluRs and NMDA receptors in social impairment (Won et al., 2012). These results suggest that mGluR5 positive allosteric modulators may have the potential to improve social and cognitive impairments associated ASD pathology.

Several new therapies for ASD have also been proposed based on effective treatment from other brain disorders. Dysfunctions in mTOR signaling have significant impacts on normal brain functions, and rapamycin treatment has been shown to alleviate several pathological traits observed in animal models of Alzheimer's disease (Harrison et al., 2009), Parkinson's disease (Tain et al., 2009), and polyglutamine diseases (Berger et al., 2006). Recently, rapamycin has also been suggested as a therapy for ASD given the molecular association between the mTOR pathway and its upstream inhibitory regulators TSC1 and TSC2 (Han and Sahin, 2011). Given the success of rapamycin in ameliorating the cognitive impairments associated with tuberous sclerosis, these studies suggest a role for rapamycin in reversing core symptoms of autism.

Indeed, *Pten* mutant mice, which present symptoms that resemble autism behavior (Zhou and Parada, 2012), when treated with rapamycin show a reduction of the phenotype (Zhou et al., 2009). This is consistent with the molecular mechanisms of *Pten* mutant mice that present a constitutive activation of AKT signaling that can be controlled with rapamycin. This is another example of common treatment for different genetic etiology such as mutations in *Pten* and *Tsc2*.

Similarly, a new approach for alleviating phenotypic traits of ASD in animal models has come from research on Rett syndrome. As previously discussed, IGF-1 has been implicated in Rett syndrome and activation of IGF1 signaling in *Mecp2* mutant models rescues hypoactivity, and respiratory deficits in addition to normalizing impaired spine density, synaptic transmission, and cortical plasticity (Tropea et al., 2008). IGF-1 and IGF binding proteins have been implicated in autism with reduced concentrations of IGF-1 in the cerebrospinal fluid in autistic individuals (Riikonen et al., 2006). As IGF-1 crosses the blood-brain barrier, it may be a viable candidate therapy for ASD. Indeed haploinsufficiency in *SHANK3*, which accounts for 0.5% of ASD cases, leads to deficits in synaptic transmission that can be ameliorated by administration of IGF1 and its active peptide (Bozdagi et al., 2013).

14.7 THE PROMISE OF INDUCED PLURIPOTENT STEM CELLS FOR PERSONALIZED MEDICINE

One of the main concerns for the use of animal models as a sole method for facilitating translational research is that the pathophysiology of these diseases usually arises from heterogeneous combinations of genetic factors producing phenotypic expressions of clinical symptoms. Apart from diseases caused by monogenic mutations, the vast majority of neurodevelopmental disorders have a polygenic etiology, even without considering the influence of extragenetic factors.

Considering the diversity of genetic and environmental origins in individual cases of neurodevelopmental disorders, it is difficult to rely solely on the discoveries and therapeutic strategies developed on animal models of transgenic mutations. There is an increasing appreciation to develop personalized approaches with treatments tailored to the specific pathology and response of individual patients. The development of induced pluripotent stem cells (iPSCs) is rapidly advancing the cause of personalized medicine (Juopperi et al., 2011). Several studies have confirmed at the cellular level that it is possible to replicate some of the results observed in animals. In the case for cells derived from Rett syndrome patients (Marchetto et al., 2010), the authors find decreased expression of markers for synaptic function and altered spontaneous electrical activity as found in animal models (Tropea et al., 2008). Also, the authors find that potential therapies proposed for patients (such as Insulin-like growth factor 1—IGF1) rescue the phenotypes described *in vitro*, therefore, validating the hypothesis that iPSCs can be used to analyse patient phenotype and test candidate treatments. The very same conclusions have been reached for other NDDs such as schizophrenia (Brennand et al., 2011), where alterations in cell morphology have been identified in iPSCs samples derived from patients, and psychotic drugs are able to rescue the phenotype *in vitro*. Additionally, in Fragile X syndrome, the iPSCs technique has been used to generate neuronal cultures derived from patients where a reduction of PSD95 immunostaining and the number of synaptic puncta has been observed (Liu et al., 2012).

Although this new technique has the potential to precisely address patient-specific issues, there are limitations that still need to be resolved in order to pursue the quest for personalized medicine. First, we need to be aware that the neurons derived in culture, even if they have the same DNA sequence, are likely to have different epigenetic modifications. This problem may have limited consequences for X-linked syndromes (i.e., Fragile X- and Rett-syndrome), when the X-chromosome inactivation is opportunely checked and taken into account (Cheung et al., 2012); however, for mutations on autosomal chromosomes, the whole gene expression machinery can be altered and additional controls are required (Robinton and Daley, 2012). Second, the numbers of phenotypes that are visible in a dish are limited due to a still imperfect methodology used to derive more homogeneous classes of neurons (Brennand and Gage, 2011). Apart from the technical limitations, the *in vitro* preparation itself presents some drawbacks with respect to animal models: first, it is not possible to study events related to development; second, the cell types are not homogeneous and not organized in structures; third, it is not possible to evaluate the effects of systemic factors such as the effects of neuromodulators; and fourth it is not possible to study the succession of stages that eventually lead to dysfunction of neural systems. Nonetheless, iPSCs represent a powerful technology for the investigation and testing of the primary molecular biochemical defects leading to some cases of neuropsychiatric conditions. The continued integration of this platform with whole-genome analysis of individual patients suffering from neuropsychiatric illness, will provide an excellent model to explore how risk susceptibility genes functionally interact to result in increased cellular vulnerability leading to disease onset. Such a system could ensure a

high-throughput and reproducible means for the targeted investigation of neuronal function and provide a valuable platform to facilitate the drug discovery process.

Another approach recently explored is the use of olfactory neural precursors (ONPs) for the study of abnormalities in SZ neurons (Benítez-King et al., 2011). ONPs can be derived from the nasal cavity with a noninvasive method, and with their ability to self-renew, they represent a source of neurons from SZ patients and control groups. The advantage of this system is that the neuronal population, even if immature, is homogeneous and therefore allows direct comparison of gene expression and cellular pathways between patients and controls. This system is therefore complementary to the iPSCs in some aspects and it could be explored in NDDs other than schizophrenia.

14.8 NEUROTECHNOLOGIES FOR NEURODEVELOPMENTAL DISORDERS

As previously discussed, understanding the molecular and cellular mechanisms involved in regulating the synaptic processes of regular brain function is critical for gaining new insights into disease etiology and providing the best chance for driving innovation in the introduction of novel treatments. Genetic analysis studies have presented a kaleidoscope of candidate genes implicated in dysfunctional mechanisms of developmental plasticity while animal and human cellular models have expanded on the molecular pathways, which underlie specific processes of synapse development and presented potential targets for therapeutic intervention. The development of novel interfacing neurotechnologies could have significant implications in our understanding of neuronal function, the efficacy of pharmacological intervention and the implementation of intelligent neuroprosthetic devices. This rapidly advancing field presents a unique opportunity to confront the challenges of therapeutic inertia and usher in an era of innovation to the clinical outcomes for NDDs.

14.8.1   Pharmacological Screening

Efficient neurophysiological assessment is an important and necessary step of the drug development process and the ability to predict the effect of new therapies on specific targets allows for accurately judging their potential at a much earlier stage during preclinical analysis. High-throughput platforms for conducting patch-clamp electrophysiology are available, and have been utilized by the pharmaceutical industry for drug development. Recently, the advent of planar multielectrode arrays (MEAs) has emerged as a credible tool for shedding new light on the processes involved in neural circuit formation and function (Liu et al., 2011). An MEA functions by forming a unique electrical interface with neurons that are cultured directly onto the electrode. This technology allows for combining electrophysiological and molecular imaging modalities and the provision of a multiparametric tool for studying the cellular and molecular mechanisms of neural plasticity (He et al., 2009).

By recording the changes in spike activity of individual neurons on an MEA device, the network-level characteristics of substances such as GABA (Suyama et al., 2004), strychnine (Harsch et al., 1997), ethanol (Xia and Gross, 2003), dopamine (Eytan et al., 2004), fluoxetine (Xia et al., 2003), bicuculline (Arnold et al., 2005), and acetylcholine esterase inhibitors (Keefer et al., 2001) have been evaluated. The rapid characterization of neurochemical actions on electrical activity has highlighted MEA potential for biosensor applications in pharmaceutical research, illustrating their use as a high throughput and rapid screening method for pharmacological testing (Gramowski et al., 2004). This could be particularly useful in the screening of drugs targeted at nervous system development through the use of assay screens for important developmental processes such as proliferation, differentiation, neurite outgrowth, and synaptogenesis. Further improvements can be made by combining MEA pharmacological screening with iPSCs opening up vast new territory in the search of effective personalized treatments for neurodevelopmental disorders.

14.8.2   Neurostimulation

Neurostimulation involves the electrical modulation of active neurons through specifically designed neural interfaces that can be either invasive or noninvasive in nature. These technologies serve as a key part of neural prosthetics, potentially providing a unique means of correcting dysfunctional neural circuits. Deep brain stimulation (DBS) is an invasive neurological procedure involving implantable electrode arrays into a specific region of the brain via burr holes through the skull. Each array usually consists of several electrode contacts spanning 10–20 mm. DBS leads are connected via subcutaneous extension wires to one or more implanted pulse generators containing the battery and computer that drives stimulation. Parameters can be set noninvasively and adjusted via a handheld computer interface. DBS has found major applications in movement disorders proving effective in ameliorating the debilitating effect caused by parkinsonian tremors (Castrioto et al., 2011). Based on its effectiveness in these disorders, DBS has also been investigated for psychiatric disorders, enhanced by the development of detailed neuroanatomical models for regulating emotion, cognition, and behavior (Paul and Helen, 2011). The therapeutic principle behind DBS is the electrical modulation of pathological activity within brain networks. As discussed previously, irregular synaptic activity can result in widespread dysfunction throughout an entire neural network leading to pathological changes in function and behavior (Lisman, 2012). As a result, it may be possible to neutralize, disrupt, or drive activity at these pathological sites to re-establish functional integrity and output of the involved circuits leading to a clinical benefit (Lozano et al., 2008).

An alternative modulatory technique is deep transcranial magnetic stimulation (TMS), a noninvasive method of neurostimulation caused by electromagnetic induction of an electric field in the brain (Roth et al., 2007). When of sufficient magnitude and density, this field can depolarize neurons, modulating cortical excitability through repetitive stimulation with defined parameters (Fitzgerald et al., 2006). Standard TMS is mostly applied with an electromagnetic (figure-of-eight) coil, which is able to modulate cortical excitability up to a maximum depth of 1.5–2.5 cm from the scalp; conversely, deep TMS uses the H-coil for clinical applications giving an improved cortical excitability depth of 6 cm from the scalp and can therefore be used to modulate activity of the cerebral cortex and deeper circuits. The first step of treatment administration is the identification of the motor threshold (MT), indicating the lowest stimulation intensity required to evoke a motor potential of at least 50 μV. MT represents a global measure of cortico-spinal excitability of axons, which are activated by the TMS pulse as well as the excitability of cortical and spinal synaptic connections (Paulus et al., 2008). Once the MT is identified, the coil is moved from the motor cortex to the target cortical region. Two quantitative variables are also considered at this point; the frequency, which refers to the effect of the stimulation on cortical excitability, whereby frequencies less than or equal to 1 Hz produce an inhibitory effect and frequencies greater than 1 Hz produce an excitatory effect; and the intensity of electromagnetic stimulation referring to the depth of the stimulation protocol measured in relation to the MT (Fitzgerald et al., 2006).

Several studies have indicated standard TMS to be moderately effective in treating a wide range of neuropsychiatric diseases. For the treatment of the social deficits in autism spectrum disorders, a potential target area is the bilateral medial prefrontal cortex (Enticott et al., 2011); in the treatment of major depressive disorder, bipolar disorder and the negative symptoms of schizophrenia, treatment of the left dorsolateral prefrontal cortex has been identified (Harel et al., 2011; Levkovitz et al., 2009; Levkovitz et al., 2011). Given the capability of greater depth penetration, deep TMS is gaining the attention of the medical community as a possible therapeutic tool in the treatment of numerous NDDs (Bersani et al., 2013).

14.9 BIOLOGICAL MARKERS AND CLINICAL MARKERS

One critical limitation for therapeutic intervention in NDDs is the ability to relate clinical symptoms with the biological findings. The main criteria used in clinical evaluation of autism and psychosis are based on observation and discussion with the patient. Even if some parameters are scored: IQ test, autism disorder observation (ADO), severity of positive and negative symptoms in schizophrenia, there is no evidence that a specific biological marker correlates with one of the clinical parameters used in the evaluation. This is the main dichotomy between the process of drug discovery in models and the clinical applications. Nonetheless, in the last decade, some progress has been made and we can start to see some correlations between biological measures and progression of the disorder.

What are the parameters that we should look to monitor in NDDs in order to check for the progression of the disease and the efficacy of the therapy?

One noninvasive analysis that can be done is at the genetic level. For monogenic disorders such as Rett syndrome or Fragile X syndrome, specific mutations would be very informative for diagnosis; however, genetic analysis is not suitable for monitoring the onset and progression of a disorder, or to evaluate the effect of a drug. The alternative would be to evaluate the expression of RNA transcripts in peripheral tissue; yet in the majority of cases the major changes are more likely to occur in the brain, which is not accessible for analysis in the patient. It is worth mentioning though that recently the expression of miRNA in peripheral blood has shown to be correlated with the expression of other clinical signs (Mellios and Sur, 2012).

At the moment, cellular, anatomical, and genetic studies point to deficits that affect the structure and function of cellular connectivity. Indeed morphological characteristics such as neuronal size and localization, length and morphology of neurites, and shape and size of dendritic spines seem to be affected in NDDs. Of course, these parameters vary according to the specific disorder; postmortem studies show that in schizophrenia there is a decrease in the number of dendritic spines in prefrontal cortex (Bennett, 2011), in Fragile X syndrome the spines present an immature morphology (Dölen et al., 2007), and in Rett syndrome there is a reduction of dendritic spines and proteins related to synapse strength and function (Tropea et al., 2008; for a recent review see Penzes et al., 2011).

The development of *in vivo* imaging has allowed a correlation – to a certain extent – of morphological data with the living patient. Even if it is not possible to measure the number of dendritic spines in the cortex of the living patient (although it is possible in a mutant animal), it is still possible to measure the connectivity with Magnetic Resonance Imaging (MRI); indeed the morphological data of synapse structure in relation to function in the brain of schizophrenic patients have been confirmed with imaging data (Mothersill et al., 2012). Also for Fragile X syndrome, it has been possible to confirm the genetic and molecular studies with structural and functional imaging (Lightbody and Reiss, 2009).

A similar approach can be used to study the contribution of specific molecules in defined brain regions with positron-emission-tomography (PET) analysis (Booij and van Amelsvoort, 2012; Chugani, 2012). Therefore, *in vivo* imaging constitutes a noninvasive method to monitor the progression of the disorder and the efficacy of a candidate treatment through repetitive sessions.

The balance between excitation and inhibition, which is altered in the majority of NDDs, is also reflected in some of the current treatments (Table 14.1, Fig. 14.2). This imbalance produces

alterations in the electrical activity of the brain, as is apparent in syndromes with seizures and detectable with EEG (Angelmann syndrome, Rett syndrome, Fragile X, Down syndrome, tuberous sclerosis, and autism spectrum disorders). In schizophrenia, the rhythmic activity of the brain is disrupted by the decrease in parvalbuminergic signaling (Lisman, 2012), and even areas that are apparently not affected by the disorder, such as the visual cortex, show an alteration in the electric signal as revealed by EEG (Knebel et al., 2011; O'Donoghue et al., 2012).

Another possible parameter for the assessment and treatment of intellectual disability associated with psychiatric disorders is the stimulus-selective response plasticity in the visual cortex (Cooke and Bear, 2012). This phenotype consists of an increase in evoked cortical activity in response to a visual stimulus and it is present in control, but not in SZ patients. Interestingly, the very same phenotype is measurable in animal and in humans, and can, therefore, be used to monitor the disorder in animal mutants. In several studies on NDDs, even if there is not an evident impairment in the visual system, protocols of visual cortical plasticity have been informative for uncovering the neurobiology of the disorder and for testing candidate treatments (Dölen et al., 2007; Tropea, 2008; Yashiro and Philpot, 2008).

Today, one of the issues for neuropsychiatry is to find biological markers that reflect clinical markers, so that they can be used for diagnosis and for monitoring the status of the disorder during development and in response to treatment. Some of the technical tools for solving this issue have been developed and more are in progress and this process can be accelerated if we are open to considering different and complementary approaches.

14.10 CONCLUSIONS

The field of neuropsychiatry is living a unique moment: on one side, the genetic discoveries have enlightened the molecular basis of the disorders, yet they also showed the complexity of genetic etiology. Understanding the neurobiology represents the grand challenge for identifying appropriate treatments (Tropea, 2012). Genetic heterogeneity and overlapping between clinical features are creating a barrier for the discovery of new drugs, and on top of the practical and conceptual difficulties are the costs for the discovery and testing of new treatments.

On the other side, the existence of appropriate models – mostly for monogenic disorders – and advancements in cellular models, imaging modalities, and novel neurotechnologies have proven to be efficient for establishing new therapies for orphan disease and for realizing the potential of personalized diagnosis and intervention. We now have a plethora of tools for advancing the therapeutic intervention in NDDs, and we are eager to use them in the next decade of discoveries. For now, there are three main conclusions that we can derive from the discoveries: first, that basic research is critical for the discovery of novel treatments and the development of new tools. Second, that we need to be open to consider new models for investigation: most of the discoveries comes from investigation in single gene disorders, but valuable models can also be found in mice mutants for high penetrant risk factors. This is particularly useful in the study of psychosis, where it is not easy to define a mouse model of the disorder (Karayiorgou et al., 2012). Finally, that we should be ready to expand our view of molecular mechanisms of NDDs and move from comprehension of genetics to the comprehension of biology, and possibly reconsider the classification of the different disorders according to the molecular mechanisms that are involved rather than the genetic etiology and/or the clinical evaluation.

REFERENCES

Acosta, M., Kardel, P., Walsh, K., Rosenbaum, K., Gioia, G., and Packer, R. (2011). Lovastatin as treatment for neurocognitive deficits in neurofibromatosis type 1: phase I study. Pediatric neurology 45, 241–245.

Arnold, F., Hofmann, F., Bengtson, C., Wittmann, M., Vanhoutte, P., and Bading, H. (2005). Microelectrode array recordings of cultured hippocampal networks reveal a simple model for transcription and protein synthesis-dependent plasticity. The Journal of physiology 564, 3–19.

Auerbach, B., Osterweil, E., and Bear, M. (2011). Mutations causing syndromic autism define an axis of synaptic pathophysiology. Nature 480, 63–68.

Bear, M., Huber, K., and Warren, S. (2004). The mGluR theory of fragile X mental retardation. Trends in neurosciences 27, 370–377.

Benitez-King, G., Ramírez-Rodríguez, G., Ortíz, L., and Meza, I. (2004). The neuronal cytoskeleton as a potential therapeutical target in neurodegenerative diseases and schizophrenia. Current drug targets CNS and neurological disorders 3, 515–533.

Benítez-King, G., Riquelme, A., Ortíz-López, L., Berlanga, C., Rodríguez-Verdugo, M., Romo, F., Calixto, E., Solís-Chagoyán, H., Jímenez, M., Montaño, L., et al. (2011). A non-invasive method to isolate the neuronal linage from the nasal epithelium from schizophrenic and bipolar diseases. Journal of neuroscience methods 201, 35–45.

Bennett, M. (2011). Schizophrenia: susceptibility genes, dendritic-spine pathology and gray matter loss. Progress in neurobiology 95, 275–300.

Berger, Z., Ravikumar, B., Menzies, F., Oroz, L., Underwood, B., Pangalos, M., Schmitt, I., Wullner U., Evert, B., O'Kane, C., et al. (2006). Rapamycin alleviates toxicity of different aggregate-prone proteins. Human molecular genetics 15, 433–442.

Berry-Kravis, E., Hessl, D., Coffey, S., Hervey, C., Schneider, A., Yuhas, J., Hutchison, J., Snape, M., Tranfaglia, M., Nguyen, D., et al. (2009). A pilot open label, single dose trial of fenobam in adults with fragile X syndrome. Journal of medical genetics 46, 266–271.

Bersani, F., Minichino, A., Enticott, P., Mazzarini, L., Khan, N., Antonacci, G., Raccah, R., Salviati, M., Delle Chiaie, R., Bersani, G., et al. (2013). Deep transcranial magnetic stimulation as a treatment for psychiatric disorders: a comprehensive review. Eur Psychiatry: the journal of the Association of European Psychiatrists 28, 30–39.

Bilousova, T., Dansie, L., Ngo, M., Aye, J., Charles, J.R., Ethell, D.W., and Ethell, I.M. (2009). Minocycline promotes dendritic spine maturation and improves behavioural performance in the fragile X mouse model. Journal of Medical Genetics 46, 94–102.

Blundell, J., Blaiss, C., Etherton, M., Espinosa, F., Tabuchi, K., Walz, C., Bolliger, M., Südhof, T., and Powell, C. (2010). Neuroligin-1 deletion results in impaired spatial memory and increased repetitive behavior. The Journal of neuroscience: the official journal of the Society for Neuroscience 30, 2115–2129.

Booij, J., and van Amelsvoort, T. (2012). Imaging as tool to investigate psychoses and antipsychotics. Handb Exp Pharmacol, 299–337.

Bozdagi, O., Tavassoli, T., and Buxbaum, J.D. (2013). Insulin-like growth factor-1 rescues synaptic and motor deficits in a mouse model of autism and developmental delay. Mol Autism 4, 9.

Brennand, K., and Gage, F. (2011). Concise review: the promise of human induced pluripotent stem cell-based studies of schizophrenia. Stem Cells 29, 1915–1922.

Brennand, K., Simone, A., Jou, J., Gelboin-Burkhart, C., Tran, N., Sangar, S., Li, Y., Mu, Y., Chen, G., Yu, D., et al. (2011). Modelling schizophrenia using human induced pluripotent stem cells. Nature 473, 221–225.

Carroll, L., and Owen, M. (2009). Genetic overlap between autism, schizophrenia and bipolar disorder. Genome medicine 1, 102.

Castrioto, A., Lozano, A., Poon, Y.-Y., Lang, A., Fallis, M., and Moro, E. (2011). Ten-year outcome of subthalamic stimulation in Parkinson disease: a blinded evaluation. Archives of neurology 68, 1550–1556.

Chabernaud, C., Mennes, M., Kardel, P., Gaillard, W., Kalbfleisch, M., Vanmeter, J., Packer, R., Milham, M., Castellanos, F., and Acosta, M. (2012). Lovastatin regulates brain spontaneous low-frequency brain activity in neurofibromatosis type 1. Neuroscience letters 515, 28–33.

Cheung, A., Horvath, L., Carrel, L., and Ellis, J. (2012). X-chromosome inactivation in rett syndrome human induced pluripotent stem cells. Frontiers in psychiatry/Frontiers Research Foundation 3, 24.

Chugani, D. (2012). Neuroimaging and neurochemistry of autism. Pediatric clinics of North America 59, 63.

Ciucci, F., Putignano, E., Baroncelli, L., Landi, S., Berardi, N., and Maffei, L. (2007). Insulin-like growth factor 1 (IGF-1) mediates the effects of enriched environment (EE) on visual cortical development. PloS One 2.

Clapcote, S.J., Lipina, T. V., Millar, J. K., Mackie, S., Christie, S., Ogawa, F., Lerch, J. P., Trimble, K., Uchiyama, M., Sakuraba, Y., Kaneda, H., Shiroishi, T., Houslay, M. D., Henkelman, R. M., Sled, J. G., Gondo, Y., Porteous, D. J., Roder, J. C. (2007). Behavioral phenotypes of Disc1 missense mutations in mice. Neuron 54, 387–402.

Clifton, N., Morisot, N., Girardon, S., Millan, M., and Loiseau, F. (2013). Enhancement of social novelty discrimination by positive allosteric modulators at metabotropic glutamate 5 receptors: adolescent administration prevents adult-onset deficits induced by neonatal treatment with phencyclidine. Psychopharmacology 225, 579–594.

Collins, J., Tudor, C., Leonard, J., Chuck, G., and Franz, D. (2006). Levetiracetam as adjunctive antiepileptic therapy for patients with tuberous sclerosis complex: a retrospective open-label trial. Journal of child neurology 21, 53–57.

Conn, P., and Jones, C. (2009). Promise of mGluR2/3 activators in psychiatry. Neuropsychopharmacol: official publication of the American College of Neuropsychopharmacology 34, 248–249.

Cooke, S., and Bear, M. (2012). Stimulus-selective response plasticity in the visual cortex: an assay for the assessment of pathophysiology and treatment of cognitive impairment associated with psychiatric disorders. Biological psychiatry 71, 487–495.

Costa, A., and Grybko, M. (2005). Deficits in hippocampal CA1 LTP induced by TBS but not HFS in the Ts65Dn mouse: a model of Down syndrome. Neuroscience letters 382, 317–322.

Costa, R., Federov, N., Kogan, J., Murphy, G., Stern, J., Ohno, M., Kucherlapati, R., Jacks, T., and Silva, A. (2002). Mechanism for the learning deficits in a mouse model of neurofibromatosis type 1. Nature 415, 526–530.

Cui, Y., Costa, R., Murphy, G., Elgersma, Y., Zhu, Y., Gutmann, D., Parada, L., Mody, I., and Silva, A. (2008). Neurofibromin regulation of ERK signaling modulates GABA release and learning. Cell 135, 549–560.

D'Hulst, C., and Kooy, R. (2007). The GABAA receptor: a novel target for treatment of fragile X? Trends in neurosciences 30, 425–431.

Daston, M., Scrable, H., Nordlund, M., Sturbaum, A., Nissen, L., and Ratner, N. (1992). The protein product of the neurofibromatosis type 1 gene is expressed at highest abundance in neurons,

Schwann cells, and oligodendrocytes. Neuron 8, 415–428.

Dolan, B., Duron, S., Campbell, D., Vollrath, B., Rao, B.S., Ko, H.-Y., Lin, G., Govindarajan, A., Choi, S.-Y., and Tonegawa, S. (2013). Rescue of fragile X syndrome phenotypes in Fmr1 KO mice by the small-molecule PAK inhibitor FRAX486. Proceedings of the National Academy of Sciences of the United States of America 110, 5671–5676.

Dölen, G., Osterweil, E., Rao, B.S., Smith, G., Auerbach, B., Chattarji, S., and Bear, M. (2007). Correction of fragile X syndrome in mice. Neuron 56, 955–962.

Ebert, D., and Greenberg, M. (2013). Activity-dependent neuronal signalling and autism spectrum disorder. Nature 493, 327–337.

Ehninger, D., Han, S., Shilyansky, C., Zhou, Y., Li, W., Kwiatkowski, D., Ramesh, V., and Silva, A. (2008). Reversal of learning deficits in a Tsc2+/- mouse model of tuberous sclerosis. Nature medicine 14, 843–848.

Enticott, P., Kennedy, H., Zangen, A., and Fitzgerald, P. (2011). Deep repetitive transcranial magnetic stimulation associated with improved social functioning in a young woman with an autism spectrum disorder. The journal of ECT 27, 41–43.

Eytan, D., Minerbi, A., Ziv, N., and Marom, S. (2004). Dopamine-induced dispersion of correlations between action potentials in networks of cortical neurons. Journal of neurophysiology 92, 1817–1824.

Fernandez, F., and Garner, C. (2007). Over-inhibition: a model for developmental intellectual disability. Trends in neurosciences 30, 497–503.

Fitzgerald, P., Fountain, S., and Daskalakis, Z. (2006). A comprehensive review of the effects of rTMS on motor cortical excitability and inhibition. Clin Neurophysiol: Off J Int Fed Clin Neurophysiol 117, 2584–2596.

Giacometti, E., Luikenhuis, S., Beard, C., and Jaenisch, R. (2007). Partial rescue of MeCP2 deficiency by postnatal activation of MeCP2. Proceedings of the National Academy of Sciences of the United States of America 104, 1931–1936.

Gipson, T., and Johnston, M. (2012). Plasticity and mTOR: towards restoration of impaired synaptic plasticity in mTOR-related neurogenetic disorders. Neural plasticity 2012, 486402.

Gramowski, A., Jügelt, K., Weiss, D., and Gross, G. (2004). Substance identification by quantitative characterization of oscillatory activity in murine spinal cord networks on microelectrode arrays. The European journal of neuroscience 19, 2815–2825.

Gregory, K., Dong, E., Meiler, J., and Conn, P. (2011). Allosteric modulation of metabotropic glutamate receptors: structural insights and therapeutic potential. Neuropharmacology 60, 66–81.

Guo, H., The, I., Hannan, F., Bernards, A., and Zhong, Y. (1997). Requirement of Drosophila NF1 for activation of adenylyl cyclase by PACAP38-like neuropeptides. Science (New York, NY) 276, 795–798.

Guy, J., Gan, J., Selfridge, J., Cobb, S., and Bird, A. (2007). Reversal of neurological defects in a mouse model of Rett syndrome. Science (New York, NY) 315, 1143–1147.

Han, J., and Sahin, M. (2011). TSC1/TSC2 signaling in the CNS. FEBS letters 585, 973–980.

Hancock, E., and Osborne, J. (1999). Vigabatrin in the treatment of infantile spasms in tuberous sclerosis: literature review. Journal of child neurology 14, 71–74.

Harel, E., Zangen, A., Roth, Y., Reti, I., Braw, Y., and Levkovitz, Y. (2011). H-coil repetitive transcranial magnetic stimulation for the treatment of bipolar depression: an add-on, safety and feasibility study. World J Biol Psychiatry: the official journal of the World Federation of Societies of Biological Psychiatry 12, 119–126.

Harrison, D., Strong, R., Sharp, Z., Nelson, J., Astle, C., Flurkey, K., Nadon, N., Wilkinson, J., Frenkel, K., Carter, C., et al. (2009). Rapamycin fed late in life extends lifespan in genetically heterogeneous mice. Nature 460, 392–395.

Harsch, A., Ziegler, C., and Göpel, W. (1997). Strychnine analysis with neuronal networks in vitro: extracellular array recording of network responses. Biosensors & bioelectronics 12, 827–835.

Hayashi-Takaji, A., Araki, Y., Nakamura, M., Vollrath, B., Duron, S., Yan, Z., Kasai, H., Huganir, R., Campbell, D., and Sawa, A. (2014). PAK inhibitors ameliorate schizophrenia-associated dendritic spine deterioration in vitro and in vivo during late adolescence. Proc Nat Acad Sci USA 111, 6461–6466.

Hays, S., Huber, K., and Gibson, J. (2011). Altered neocortical rhythmic activity states in Fmr1 KO mice are due to enhanced mGluR5 signaling and involve changes in excitatory circuitry. The Journal of neuroscience: the official journal of the Society for Neuroscience 31, 14223–14234.

He, Y., Liu, M.-G., Gong, K.-R., and Chen, J. (2009). Differential effects of long and short train theta burst stimulation on LTP induction in rat anterior cingulate cortex slices: multi-electrode array recordings. Neuroscience bulletin 25, 309–318.

Heulens, I., D'Hulst, C., Van Dam, D., De Deyn, P., and Kooy, R. (2012). Pharmacological treatment of fragile X syndrome with GABAergic drugs in a knockout mouse model. Behavioural brain research 229, 244–249.

Holtmaat, A., and Svoboda, K. (2009). Experience-dependent structural synaptic plasticity in the mammalian brain. Nature reviews Neuroscience 10, 647–658.

Hung, A., Futai, K., Sala, C., Valtschanoff, J., Ryu, J., Woodworth, M., Kidd, F., Sung, C., Miyakawa, T., Bear, M., et al. (2008). Smaller dendritic spines, weaker synaptic transmission, but enhanced spatial learning in mice lacking Shank1. J Neurosci: Off J Soc Neurosci 28, 1697–1708.

Hyman, S., Shores, A., and North, K. (2005). The nature and frequency of cognitive deficits in children with neurofibromatosis type 1. Neurology 65, 1037–1044.

Jacob, W., Gravius, A., Pietraszek, M., Nagel, J., Belozertseva, I., Shekunova, E., Malyshkin, A., Greco, S., Barberi, C., and Danysz, W. (2009). The anxiolytic and analgesic properties of fenobam, a potent mGlu5 receptor antagonist, in relation to the impairment of learning. Neuropharmacology 57, 97–108.

Jacquemont, S., Curie, A., Des Portes, V., Torrioli, M.G., Berry-Kravis, E., Hagerman, R.J., Ramos, F.J., Cornish, K., He, Y., and Paulding, C. (2011). Epigenetic modification of the FMR1 gene in fragile X syndrome is associated with differential response to the mGluR5 antagonist AFQ056. Science Translational Medicine 3, 64ra1.

Jambaqué, I., Chiron, C., Dumas, C., Mumford, J., and Dulac, O. (2000). Mental and behavioural outcome of infantile epilepsy treated by vigabatrin in tuberous sclerosis patients. Epilepsy research 38, 151–160.

Johannessen, C., Reczek, E., James, M., Brems, H., Legius, E., and Cichowski, K. (2005). The NF1 tumor suppressor critically regulates TSC2 and mTOR. Proceedings of the National Academy of Sciences of the United States of America 102, 8573–8578.

Juopperi, T., Song, H., and Ming, G.-L. (2011). Modeling neurological diseases using patient-derived induced pluripotent stem cells. Future neurology 6, 363–373.

Kanes, S., Tokarczyk, J., Siegel, S., Bilker, W., Abel, T., and Kelly, M. (2007). Rolipram: a specific phosphodiesterase 4 inhibitor with potential antipsychotic activity. Neuroscience 144, 239–246.

Karam, C., Ballon, J., Bivens, N., Freyberg, Z., Girgis, R., Lizardi-Ortiz, J., Markx, S., Lieberman, J., and Javitch, J. (2010). Signaling pathways in schizophrenia: emerging targets and therapeutic strategies. Trends in pharmacological sciences 31, 381–390.

Karayiorgou, M., Simon, T.J., and Gogos, J.A. (2010). 22q11. 2 microdeletions: linking DNA structural variation to brain dysfunction and schizophrenia. Nature Reviews Neuroscience 11, 402–416.

Keefer, E., Norton, S., Boyle, N., Talesa, V., and Gross, G. (2001). Acute toxicity screening of novel AChE inhibitors using neuronal networks on microelectrode arrays. Neurotoxicology 22, 3–12.

Kelleher, R., and Bear, M. (2008). The autistic neuron: troubled translation? Cell 135, 401–406.

Kim, J., Jung, S.-Y., Lee, Y., Park, S., Choi, J.-S., Lee, C., Kim, H.-S., Choi, Y.-B., Scheiffele, P., Bailey, C., et al. (2008). Neuroligin-1 is required for normal expression of LTP and associative fear memory in the amygdala of adult animals. Proceedings of the National Academy of Sciences of the United States of America 105, 9087–9092.

Kinney, G., O'Brien, J., Lemaire, W., Burno, M., Bickel, D., Clements, M., Chen, T.-B., Wisnoski, D., Lindsley, C., Tiller, P., et al. (2005). A novel selective positive allosteric modulator of metabotropic glutamate receptor subtype 5 has in vivo activity and antipsychotic-like effects in rat behavioral models. The Journal of pharmacology and experimental therapeutics 313, 199–206.

Knebel, J.-F., Javitt, D., and Murray, M. (2011). Impaired early visual response modulations to spatial information in chronic schizophrenia. Psychiatry research 193, 168–176.

Kolevzon, A. (2012). Current Trends in the Pharmacological treatment of Autism. In The Neuroscience of Autism Spectrum Disorder, Joseph Buxbaum & Patrick Hof, 1st edn (Academic Press: Elsevier), 1.6.

Krab, L., de Goede-Bolder, A., Aarsen, F., Pluijm, S., Bouman, M., van der Geest, J., Lequin, M., Catsman, C., Arts, W., Kushner, S., et al. (2008). Effect of simvastatin on cognitive functioning in children with neurofibromatosis type 1: a randomized controlled trial. JAMA: the journal of the American Medical Association 300, 287–294.

Levenga, J., de Vrij, F., Oostra, B., and Willemsen, R. (2010). Potential therapeutic interventions for fragile X syndrome. Trends in molecular medicine 16, 516–527.

Levkovitz, Y., Harel, E., Roth, Y., Braw, Y., Most, D., Katz, L., Sheer, A., Gersner, R., and Zangen, A. (2009). Deep transcranial magnetic stimulation over the prefrontal cortex: evaluation of antidepressant and cognitive effects in depressive patients. Brain stimulation 2, 188–200.

Levkovitz, Y., Rabany, L., Harel, E., and Zangen, A. (2011). Deep transcranial magnetic stimulation add-on for treatment of negative symptoms and cognitive deficits of schizophrenia: a feasibility study. The international journal of neuropsychopharmacology/official scientific journal of the Collegium Internationale Neuropsychopharmacologicum (CINP) 14, 991–996.

Li, W., Cui, Y., Kushner, S., Brown, R., Jentsch, J., Frankland, P., Cannon, T., and Silva, A. (2005). The HMG-CoA reductase inhibitor lovastatin reverses the learning and attention deficits in a mouse model of neurofibromatosis type 1. Current biology 15, 1961–1967.

Lightbody, A., and Reiss, A. (2009). Gene, brain, and behavior relationships in fragile X syndrome: evidence from neuroimaging studies. Developmental disabilities research reviews 15, 343–352.

Lipina, T., Kaidanovich-Beilin, O., Patel, S., Wang, M., Clapcote, S., Liu, F., Woodgett, J., and Roder, J. (2011). Genetic and pharmacological evidence for schizophrenia-related Disc1 interaction with GSK-3. Synapse (New York, NY) 65, 234–248.

Lipina, T., Wang, M., Liu, F., and Roder, J. (2012). Synergistic interactions between PDE4B and GSK-3: DISC1 mutant mice. Neuropharmacology 62, 1252–1262.

Lisman, J. (2012a). Excitation, inhibition, local oscillations, or large-scale loops: what causes the symptoms of schizophrenia? Curr Opin Neurobiol 22, 537–544.

Lisman, J. (2012b). Excitation, inhibition, local oscillations, or large-scale loops: what causes the symptoms of schizophrenia? Current opinion in neurobiology 22, 537–544.

Liu, J., Koscielska, K., Cao, Z., Hulsizer, S., Grace, N., Mitchell, G., Nacey, C., Githinji, J., McGee, J., Garcia-Arocena, D., et al. (2012). Signaling defects in iPSC-derived fragile X premutation neurons. Human molecular genetics 21, 3795–3805.

Liu, M.-G., Wang, R.-R., Chen, X.-F., Zhang, F.-K., Cui, X.-Y., and Chen, J. (2011). Differential roles of ERK, JNK and p38 MAPK in pain-related spatial and temporal enhancement of synaptic responses in the hippocampal formation of rats: multi-electrode array recordings. Brain research 1382, 57–69.

Lozano, A., Mayberg, H., Giacobbe, P., Hamani, C., Craddock, R., and Kennedy, S. (2008). Subcallosal cingulate gyrus deep brain stimulation for treatment-resistant depression. Biological psychiatry 64, 461–467.

Mabb, A., Judson, M., Zylka, M., and Philpot, B. (2011). Angelman syndrome: insights into genomic imprinting and neurodevelopmental phenotypes. Trends in neurosciences 34, 293–303.

Mao, Y., Ge, X., Frank, C., Madison, J., Koehler, A., Doud, M., Tassa, C., Berry, E., Soda, T., Singh, K., et al. (2009). Disrupted in schizophrenia 1 regulates neuronal progenitor proliferation via modulation of GSK3beta/beta-catenin signaling. Cell 136, 1017–1031.

Marchetto, M.C., Carromeu, C., Acab, A., Yu, D., Yeo, G.W., Mu, Y., Chen, G., Gage, F.H., and Muotri, A.R. (2010). A model for neural development and treatment of Rett syndrome using human induced pluripotent stem cells. Cell 143, 527–539.

McGraw, C.M., Samaco, R.C., and Zoghbi, H.Y. (2011). Adult neural function requires MeCP2. Science 333, 186.

Meikle, L., Pollizzi, K., Egnor, A., Kramvis, I., Lane, H., Sahin, M., and Kwiatkowski, D. (2008). Response of a neuronal model of tuberous sclerosis to mammalian target of rapamycin (mTOR) inhibitors: effects on mTORC1 and Akt signaling lead to improved survival and function. The Journal of neuroscience : the official journal of the Society for Neuroscience 28, 5422–5432.

Mellios, N., and Sur, M. (2012). The emerging role of microRNAs in schizophrenia and autism spectrum disorders. Frontiers in psychiatry / Frontiers Research Foundation 3, 39.

Michalon, A., Sidorov, M., Ballard, T., Ozmen, L., Spooren, W., Wettstein, J., Jaeschke, G., Bear, M., and Lindemann, L. (2012). Chronic pharmacological mGlu5 inhibition corrects fragile X in adult mice. Neuron 74, 49–56.

Millar, J.K., Pickard, B. S., Mackie, S., James, R., Christie, S., Buchanan, S. R., Malloy, M. P, Chubb, J. E., Huston, E., Baillie, G. S., Thomson, P. A., Hill, E. V., Brandon, N. J., Rain, J. C., Camargo, L. M., Whiting, P. J., Houslay, M. D., Blackwood, D. H., Muir, W. J., Porteous, D. J. (2005). DISC1 and PDE4B are interacting genetic factors in schizophrenia that regulate cAMP signaling. Science 310, 1187–1191.

Mitchell, K. (2011). The genetics of neurodevelopmental disease. Current opinion in neurobiology 21, 197–203.

Mothersill, O., Kelly, S., Rose, E., and Donohoe, G. (2012). The effects of psychosis risk variants on brain connectivity: a review. Frontiers in psychiatry / Frontiers Research Foundation 3, 18.

O'Donoghue, T., Morris, D., Fahey, C., Da Costa, A., Foxe, J., Hoerold, D., Tropea, D., Gill, M., Corvin, A., and Donohoe, G. (2012). A NOS1 variant implicated in cognitive performance influences evoked neural responses during a high density EEG study of early visual perception. Human brain mapping 33, 1202–1211.

Olmos-Serrano, J., Paluszkiewicz, S., Martin, B., Kaufmann, W., Corbin, J., and Huntsman, M. (2010). Defective GABAergic neurotransmission and pharmacological rescue of neuronal hyperexcitability in the amygdala in a mouse model of fragile X syndrome. The Journal of neuroscience: the official journal of the Society for Neuroscience 30, 9929–9938.

Osterweil, E., Krueger, D., Reinhold, K., and Bear, M. (2010). Hypersensitivity to mGluR5 and ERK1/2 leads to excessive protein synthesis in the hippocampus of a mouse model of fragile X syndrome. The Journal of neuroscience: the official journal of the Society for Neuroscience 30, 15616–15627.

Pacey, L.K., Heximer, S., and Hampson, D. (2009). Increased GABA(B) receptor-mediated signaling reduces the susceptibility of fragile X knockout mice to audiogenic seizures. Molecular pharmacology 76, 18–24.

Paribello, C., Tao, L., Folino, A., Berry-Kravis, E., Tranfaglia, M., Ethell, I., and Ethell, D. (2010). Open-label add-on treatment trial of minocycline in fragile X syndrome. BMC neurology 10, 91.

Paul, E.H., and Helen, S.M. (2011). Deep brain stimulation for psychiatric disorders. Annual Review of Neuroscience 34, 289–307.

Paulus, W., Classen, J., Cohen, L., Large, C., Di Lazzaro, V., Nitsche, M., Pascual-Leone, A., Rosenow, F., Rothwell, J., and Ziemann, U. (2008). State of the art: pharmacologic effects on cortical excitability measures tested by transcranial magnetic stimulation. Brain stimulation 1, 151–163.

Penzes, P., Buonanno, A., Passafarro, M., Sala, C., and Sweet, R. (2013). Developmental Vulnerability of Synapses and Circuits Associated with Neuropsychiatric Disorders. Journal of neurochemistry 126, 165–182.

Penzes, P., Cahill, M.E., Jones, K.A., VanLeeuwen, J.-E.E., and Woolfrey, K.M. (2011). Dendritic spine pathology in neuropsychiatric disorders. Nature neuroscience 14, 285–293.

Pinard, E., Alanine, A., Alberati, D., Bender, M., Borroni, E., Bourdeaux, P., Brom, V., Burner, S., Fischer, H., Hainzl, D., et al. (2010). Selective GlyT1 inhibitors: discovery of [4-(3-fluoro-5-trifluoro methylpyridin-2-yl)piperazin-1-yl][5-methanesulf onyl-2-((S)-2,2,2-trifluoro-1-methylethoxy)phenyl] methanone (RG1678), a promising novel medicine to treat schizophrenia. Journal of medicinal chemistry 53, 4603–4614.

Pini, G., Scusa, M., Congiu, L., Benincasa, A., Morescalchi, P., Bottiglioni, I., Di Marco, P., Borelli, P., Bonuccelli, U., Della-Chiesa, A., et al. (2012). IGF1 as a potential treatment for Rett syndrome: safety assessment in six Rett patients. Autism research and treatment 2012, 679801.

Pratt, J., Winchester, C., Dawson, N., and Morris, B. (2012). Advancing schizophrenia drug discovery: optimizing rodent models to bridge the translational gap. Nature reviews Drug discovery 11, 560–579.

Ricciardi, S., Boggio, E., Grosso, S., Lonetti, G., Forlani, G., Stefanelli, G., Calcagno, E., Morello, N., Landsberger, N., Biffo, S., et al. (2011). Reduced AKT/mTOR signaling and protein synthesis dysregulation in a Rett syndrome animal model. Human molecular genetics 20, 1182–1196.

Riikonen, R., Makkonen, I., Vanhala, R., Turpeinen, U., Kuikka, J., and Kokki, H. (2006). Cerebrospinal fluid insulin-like growth factors IGF-1 and IGF-2 in infantile autism. Developmental medicine and child neurology 48, 751–755.

Robinton, D., and Daley, G. (2012). The promise of induced pluripotent stem cells in research and therapy. Nature 481, 295–305.

Roth, Y., Amir, A., Levkovitz, Y., and Zangen, A. (2007). Three-dimensional distribution of the electric field induced in the brain by transcranial magnetic stimulation using figure-8 and deep H-coils. Journal of clinical neurophysiology: official publication of the American Electroencephalographic Society 24, 31–38.

Roux, J.-C., Dura, E., Moncla, A., Mancini, J., and Villard, L. (2007). Treatment with desipramine improves breathing and survival in a mouse model for Rett syndrome. The European journal of neuroscience 25, 1915–1922.

Shilyansky, C., Lee, Y.S., and Silva, A.J. (2010). Molecular and cellular mechanisms of learning disabilities: a focus on NF1. Annual review of neuroscience 33, 221.

Silverman, J., Smith, D., Rizzo, S., Karras, M., Turner, S., Tolu, S., Bryce, D., Smith, D., Fonseca, K., Ring, R., et al. (2012). Negative allosteric modulation of the mGluR5 receptor reduces repetitive behaviors and rescues social deficits in mouse models of autism. Science translational medicine 4, 131ra51.

Siuciak, J., Chapin, D., McCarthy, S., and Martin, A. (2007). Antipsychotic profile of rolipram: efficacy in rats and reduced sensitivity in mice deficient in the phosphodiesterase-4B (PDE4B) enzyme. Psychopharmacology 192, 415–424.

Stefani, M., and Moghaddam, B. (2010). Activation of type 5 metabotropic glutamate receptors attenuates deficits in cognitive flexibility induced by NMDA receptor blockade. European journal of pharmacology 639, 26–32.

Stolp, H., Neuhaus, A., Sundramoorthi, R., and Molnár, Z. (2012). The long and the short of it: gene and environment interactions during early cortical development and consequences for long-term neurological disease. Frontiers in psychiatry / Frontiers Research Foundation 3, 50.

Su, T., Fan, H.-X., Jiang, T., Sun, W.-W., Den, W.-Y., Gao, M.-M., Chen, S.-Q., Zhao, Q.-H., and Yi, Y.-H. (2011). Early continuous inhibition of group 1 mGlu signaling partially rescues dendritic spine abnormalities in the Fmr1 knockout mouse model for fragile X syndrome. Psychopharmacology 215, 291–300.

Suyama, K., Daikoku, S., Funabashi, T., and Kimura, F. (2004). Effects of GABA and bicuculline on the electrical activity of rat olfactory placode neurons derived at E13.5 and cultured for 1 week on multi-electrode dishes. Endocrine journal 51, 171–176.

Tain, L., Mortiboys, H., Tao, R., Ziviani, E., Bandmann, O., and Whitworth, A. (2009). Rapamycin activation of 4E-BP prevents parkinsonian dopaminergic neuron loss. Nature neuroscience 12, 1129–1135.

Terry, A. (2008). Role of the central cholinergic system in the therapeutics of schizophrenia. Current neuropharmacology 6, 286–292.

Thomas, A., Bui, N., Perkins, J., Yuva-Paylor, L., and Paylor, R. (2012). Group I metabotropic glutamate receptor antagonists alter select behaviors in a mouse model for fragile X syndrome. Psychopharmacology 219, 47–58.

Tropea, D. (2012). New challenges and frontiers in the research for neuropsychiatric disorders. Frontiers in psychiatry / Frontiers Research Foundation 3, 69.

Tropea, D., Giacometti, E., Wilson, N., Beard, C., McCurry, C., Fu, D., Flannery, R., Jaenisch, R., and Sur, M. (2009). Partial reversal of Rett syndrome-like symptoms in MeCP2 mutant mice. Proceedings of the National Academy of Sciences of the United States of America 106, 2029–2034.

Tropea, D., Van Wart, A., Sur, M. (2008). Molecular mechanisms of experience-dependent plasticity in visual cortex. Phil Trans R Soc B 12, 341–355.

Tsai, P., Hull, C., Chu, Y., Greene-Colozzi, E., Sadowski, A., Leech, J., Steinberg, J., Crawley, J., Regehr, W., and Sahin, M. (2012). Autistic-like behaviour and cerebellar dysfunction in Purkinje cell Tsc1 mutant mice. Nature 488, 647–651.

Tuchman, R., and Rapin, I. (2002). Epilepsy in autism. Lancet neurology 1, 352–358.

Uslaner, J., Parmentier-Batteur, S., Flick, R., Surles, N., Lam, J., McNaughton, C., Jacobson, M., and Hutson, P. (2009). Dose-dependent effect of CDPPB, the mGluR5 positive allosteric modulator, on recognition memory is associated with GluR1 and CREB phosphorylation in the prefrontal cortex and hippocampus. Neuropharmacology 57, 531–538.

van Karnebeek, C.D.M., and Stockler, S. (2012). Treatable inborn errors of metabolism causing intellectual disability: a systematic literature review. Molecular genetics and metabolism 105, 368–381.

Wetmore, D., and Garner, C. (2010). Emerging pharmacotherapies for neurodevelopmental disorders. Journal of developmental and behavioral pediatrics: JDBP 31, 564–581.

Won, H., Lee, H.-R., Gee, H., Mah, W., Kim, J.-I., Lee, J., Ha, S., Chung, C., Jung, E., Cho, Y., et al. (2012). Autistic-like social behaviour in Shank2-mutant mice improved by restoring NMDA receptor function. Nature 486, 261–265.

Xia, Y., Gopal, K., and Gross, G. (2003). Differential acute effects of fluoxetine on frontal and auditory cortex networks in vitro. Brain research 973, 151–160.

Xia, Y., and Gross, G.W. (2003). Histiotypic electrophysiological responses of cultured neuronal networks to ethanol. Alcohol 30, 167–174.

Yashiro, K., and Philpot, B. (2008). Regulation of NMDA receptor subunit expression and its implications for LTD, LTP, and metaplasticity. Neuropharmacology 55, 1081–1094.

Zanella, S., Mebarek, S., Lajard, A.-M., Picard, N., Dutschmann, M., and Hilaire, G. (2008). Oral treatment with desipramine improves breathing and life span in Rett syndrome mouse model. Respiratory physiology & neurobiology 160, 116–121.

Zeng, L.-H., Xu, L., Gutmann, D., and Wong, M. (2008). Rapamycin prevents epilepsy in a mouse model of tuberous sclerosis complex. Annals of neurology 63, 444–453.

Zhou, J., Blundell, J., Ogawa, S., and Kwon, C.H. (2009). Pharmacological inhibition of mTORC1 suppresses anatomical, cellular, and behavioral abnormalities in neural–specific Pten knock-out mice. The Journal of neuroscience: the official journal of the Society for Neuroscience 29, 1773–1783.

Zhou, J., and Parada, L.F. (2012). PTEN signaling in autism spectrum disorders. Current opinion in neurobiology 22, 873–879.

Zoghbi, H., and Bear, M. (2012). Synaptic dysfunction in neurodevelopmental disorders associated with autism and intellectual disabilities. Cold Spring Harbor perspectives in biology 4.

SUBJECT INDEX

Notes: Gene names are listed separately in the Gene Index. Specific chromosomal locations (e.g., 1q21.1, 22q11.2, etc.) are listed under "Chromosomal locations". Where terms occur in a heading or subheading, the page numbers are listed in bold. Figure page numbers are *italicized* and Table page numbers are underlined. Frequently occurring terms such as autism, epilepsy, intellectual disability, schizophrenia, deletion, duplication, etc., are not indexed, as they occur throughout the text.

Abuse, 33
ADHD. *see* Attention-Deficit Hyperactivity Disorder
Age, paternal, 36, **59,** 61, 84, **90,** 113, **115–16,** 210
Agenesis of the corpus callosum, 14, 166, 174, 218
Aggregate score, 76
AKT, **141–2,** 203, 210, *322,* 324–5, 331
Albinism, 163, 164
Allelic heterogeneity. *see* Heterogeneity, allelic
Alpha2-chimaerin, 162
Alzheimer's disease, 240–52
Amish lethal microcephaly, 134
AMPA receptor, 214–16, 324
Amygdala, 168, 218, 276
Aneuploidy, 300
Angelman syndrome, 9, 11, 37, 197, 204, 243, 250, 270, 276–7, 324, 335
Anxiety, 70, 145, 171–2, 214, 276, 327
Apert syndrome, 116
ARC complex, 208, 211
Asperger, H., 31
Asymmetry, fluctuating, 83–4, 86, 88, 89
Ataxia, 13, 29, 35, 250, 270

Ataxia, cerebellar, 13, 35
Attention, 100, 249, 270, 276, 282, 284, 319
Attention-Deficit Hyperactivity Disorder, 8, 10, 13, 30–39, *86,* **99–100,** 145, 170, 207–12, 216, 220, 296
Autophagy, 211
Axon guidance, 40, 137, *142,* 144, **155–76,** 214, 218, 239, 326

Background, genetic, 11, 15, *16,* 31, 56, 70, 74, 98–102, 112, 146, 220, 241–3, 249, 253, 269, 291–303, 326
BAF complex, 219
Baraitser-Winter syndrome, 56, 137
Bardet-Biedl syndrome, 76, 292
Basal ganglia, 135, 171–2
Bateson, W., 69, 71, 290, 303
Bilateral frontal polymicrogyria. *see* Polymicrogyria
Bipolar disorder, 8, 10, 30–40, 93, 145, 198–200, 207, 218, 294, 334
Bleuler, E., 30, 294
Bohring-Opitz syndrome, 55
Brachydactyly mental retardation syndrome, 205, 219

The Genetics of Neurodevelopmental Disorders, First Edition. Edited by Kevin J. Mitchell.
© 2015 John Wiley & Sons, Inc. Published 2015 by John Wiley & Sons, Inc.

Broad autism phenotype, 16, 214
Buffering, 13, 72, 82, 85, 101–102

C. elegans, 70, 158, 264, 270
Canalization, 72, 82, 101, 103, 299
Cancer, 113, 121, 141, 143, 217, 219, 262, 292, 294,
    300
Cannabis, 98, 118–19
Cav1.2, 248–9
CD/CV model, 3, 4, 50, 60
CDPPB, 323, 324, 330
CD/RV model, 50
Cell adhesion, 40, 49, 196, 208–13, 220
Cell cycle, 130, 132, 137, 325
Cell death, 130–33, 173
Cell fate, 132–3, 253
Cell migration. *see* Migration, cell/neuronal
Centrosome, *131, 132–5*
Cerebellum, 139, 144, 168, 212, 277, 281
Cerebral organoids, 251
Cerebral palsy, 29
CFEOM. *see* Congenital fibrosis of the extraocular
    muscles
CGH. *see* Comparative Genome Hybridization
Charcot-Marie-Tooth neuropathy, 297
Chromatin, 17, 133, 197, 204, 209, 218–20
Chromosomal locations
    1p36.11, 204
    2p16.3, 37, 199
    6p21.32, 203
    6p25, *12*
    9p24.3, *205*
    12p13.1, 202
    12p13.33, 201
    16p11.2, *12,* 36, 38, 145, 206, 207, 263
    16p13.1, 36, 38, 51, 207
    16p13.2, 201
    16p13.3, 204
    17p12, 50
    19p13.2, 206
    1q21.1, *12,* 36, 37, 51, 207
    1q42.2, 200
    2q24, 218
    2q24.2, 206
    2q24.3, 202
    2q37.3, 205, 219
    3q29, *12, 37,* 215
    5q14.3, 205, 219
    6q25.3, 204
    7q11.23, 37, 50, 207, 275
    7q36.3, 37, 208
    9q34.3, 205, 208

9q34.11, 203
9q34.13, 204
10q23, *12,* 203
10q23.31, 203
10q24, 199
11q13.3, 200
11q24.2, 61
13q31.1, 170, 199
15q11.2, *12,* 36, 37, 204
15q13.3, *12,* 36, 38, 201, 207
17q11.2, 203
17q12, *12,* 36, 38, 207
17q21.2, 206
17q21.31, 50
18q21.2, 35, 61
22q11.2, *12,* 19, 36, 38, 58, 74, 100, 141, 207,
    293–4, 296
22q11.23, 206
22q13.2, 204
22q13.33, 200, 208, 216
7q35-q36.1, 198
Xp11.4, 200
Xp11.22, 202
Xp11.23, 203
Xp22.3, 53, 199
Xp22.13, 202
Xp21.2-p21.3, 198
Xp22.32-p22.31, 199
Xq13.1, 199–200
Xq22.1, 199
Xq24, 202
Xq25, 201
Xq27.3, 202
Xq28, 198, 203
Xq13-q21, 53, 199
Chromosomal Microarray (CMA), 300–301. *see also*
    Comparative Genome Hybridization
Cilia, **143–4,** 164
Ciliopathy. *see* Cilia
Clinical genetics, 36, 220
Clouston, Thomas, 30
CMA. *see* Chromosomal Microarray (CMA)
CNP. *see* Polymorphism, copy number
CNTNs in Gene Index, 212, 214
CNV, 6, **9–14,** 36, 39, 49–55, 75, 82, 90–102, 116,
    145, 195, **207–16,** 263–4, 268, 271, 277,
    296–7, 301
Cobblestone lissencephaly. *see* Lissencephaly,
    cobblestone
Cockayne syndrome, 132
Coffin-Siris syndrome, 56, 204, 206–207, 219
Cognition, 144, 146, 270–71. 276, 278, 284, 333

Cohen syndrome, 133, 144
Commissure, 157, 165–6, 184
Common Disease/Common Variants model. *see* CD/CV model
Common Disease/Rare Variants model. *see* CD/RV model
Communication, 263, 277, 279, 282–3
Comorbidity, 31–2, 82, 85–8, 170–71
Comparative genome hybridization, 12, 50. *see also* Chromosomal microarray
Congenital cranial dysinnervation disorder, 160–61
Congenital fibrosis of the extraocular muscles, 136, 160–63
Congenital innervation disorder, 160–61
Connectivity, brain/neuronal, 14, 155, 173, 196–7, 214, 240, 247, 249, 264, 321–2, 335
Consanguinity, 39, 53–4, 89, 95. *see also* Inbreeding
Contactin, 196, 212, 214, 218. *see also* CNTNs in Gene Index
Copy number variant. *see* CNV
Corpus callosum, 14, 136, 156, 163, **165–6**, 171, 174, 176, 198, 203–204, 214, 218
Cortex, cerebral, 130–41, 162, 164, 167, 197, 209–210, 215, 240, 244–8, 251–2, 265, 278, 285, 328, 334–5
Cortical dysplasia. *see* Dysplasia, cortical
Cortical malformation. *see* Malformation, cortical
Corticospinal tract, 156, 164
CRASH syndrome, 156, 166
CRISPR/Cas, 268
Cryptic genetic variation, 13, 15, 72, 101, 103
3-cyano-N-(1,3-diphenyl-1H-pyrazol-5-yl)benzamide. *see* CDPPB
Cystic fibrosis, 13, 291, 299–300

De novo mutation. *see* Mutation, de novo
Deep brain stimulation, 333
Deletion. *see* CNV
Delusions, 30, 166, 249
Dementia praecox, 30
Dendritic spines, 211–16, 248, 321–2, 335
Depression, 8, 17, 32, 36, 157, 172, 200
Developmental delay, 11, 33, 36–9, 132, 213, 219–20, 250, 276, 300
Developmental instability (DI), 81–9, 101–103
Developmental variation, 14–15, 81, *86, 87,* 91, 220
Dextromethorphan, 321, 323
Diabetes, 29, 33, 39, 72, 75, 115, 301
Diagnostic and Statistical Manual of Mental Disorders 5 (DSM5), 31
Diffusion tensor imaging, 166–7
DiGeorge syndrome. *see* Velocardiofacial syndrome

Dopamine or dopaminergic, 119, 167, 196, 212, 217, *245,* 246, *322,* 333
Double cortex, 130, 135, *136,* 141
Down syndrome, 50, 83, 95, 133, 145, 157, 174, 240–45, 251, 271, 276, 291, 295, 321, *322,* 335
Dravet syndrome, 13, 202, 213, 216, 269
Drosophila, 70, 84, 114, 161, 168, 264, 270
DTI. *see* Diffusion tensor imaging
Duane syndrome, 156, 160, 162
Duplication. *see* CNV
Dwarfism, 6, 131, 293
Dyslexia, 1, 13, 29–30, 145, 277
Dysmorphology, 36, 37, 55, 131, 133, 137, 141, 198, 207, 214, 219
Dysplasia, cortical, 141, 143, 198, 212
Dyspraxia, 29
Dystroglycan, 137–41, 145, 159
Dystrophin, 11, 137

ECM. *see* Matrix, extracellular
Embryonic stem cell. *see* Stem cell, embryonic
Emergent phenotypes, **17,** 275
Emotional regulation, 29
Encephalopathy, epileptic, 35, 199–205, 216–19
ENCODE Project, 40, 91
Endophenotype, 3, **6–8,** 55, 94, 97–9
Enhancer, 70
Environment, family or shared, 15, 95, 119
Environment, non-shared, 15, 119
Eph-R, 159, 164–7, 175
Ephrin, 159, 164–7, 175
Epigenetic (modifications), 91, 112, 116, 130, 146, 250, 263, 281, 289, 332
Epigenetic landscape, 15, *83*
Epileptic encephalopathy. *see* Encephalopathy, epileptic
Epistasis, 13, 16, **69–74,** 98, 296–8, 304
Epistatic interaction. *see* Epistasis
ES cell. *see* Stem cell, embryonic
Executive function, 3, 17, 97, 98
Exome sequencing. *see* Sequencing, exome
Expressivity, **11,** 19, 74, 208, **263,** 291

Familial amyloid polyneuropathy, 74
Familiality, **5**
Family environment. *see* Environment, family or shared
Fetal alcohol syndrome, 29
FISH, 50
Fisher, R., 71
Fitness, 4, 10, 55–6, 60–61, 75, 82–8, 92, 95
Fluctuating asymmetry. *see* Asymmetry, fluctuating
Fluorescent in situ hybridization. *see* FISH

FMR1 in Gene Index, 202, 240, 250, 263, 276, 326, 328
FMRP. *see* Fragile X, protein
Focal cortical dysplasia, 141, 143
Folate, 29, 34, 112, 114, 115, 120
Folic acid. *see* Folate
Fragile X
   gene (*see* FMR1 in Gene Index)
   protein, 58, 210–19, **250,** 276, 323, 324, **328**
   syndrome, 10–11, 29, 74, 95, 197, 202, 222, 240–43, **250,** 263, 270, 276, 281–2, 291–6, **321–29,** 331–5

GABA, 196, 271, 333
   receptor, 216, 269, 271, 321, 328
GABAergic (system), 168, 244–5, 321, *322,* 323, 329
GCTA, 8, 18
Gene by environment interaction, 14, 304
Gene-by-environment interaction, 14, **117–20,** 304
Genetic background. *see* Background, genetic
Genetic variance. *see* Variance, genetic
Genome-wide association study. *see* GWAS
Genome-wide complex trait analysis. *see* GCTA
Germline, *52,* 57, 59, 143, 249, **295,** 300, 329
Gibson, G., 72
Gigantism, 7, 293
Glia, 129, 142, 244, 265, 329
Glia, midline, 166
Glia, radial, *138,* 244, 255
Globus pallidus, 171
Glutamatergic (system), 167–8, 208–209, 212, 216–19, 244, 321, 325
Glycine, 216, 321
Glycosylation, 139, 169
GnRH neurons, 176
GSK3, 166, 174–5, *322,* 323, 325, 330
GTPase, 56, 162, 203, 208–209, 214, 217–18, 324, 329
Gurdon, J., 242–3
GWAS, **7–9,** 13, 18, **34–5,** 39–40, 60–61, 72–6, 94, 102, 120–21, 167, 212, 293
GxE interaction. *see* Gene by environment interaction

Handedness, 86
Haploinsufficiency, 35, 204–205, 209, 218–20, 269, 331
Haplotype, 7–9, 167–8, 297
Haplotype map. *see* HapMap Project
HapMap Project, 7, 34, 60
Height, 6, 39, 72, 84, 293
Hemimegalencephaly, 141, *142*
Heparan sulfate proteoglycan, 159

Heritability, *3,* 6, 8, 11, 15, 18–19, 32, 35–6, 39, 58, 61, 71, 84–5, 95–6, 118–19, 249, 294
Heterogeneity, allelic, 11, 15
Heterogeneity, clinical or phenotypic, 55, 74, 139, 143, 294
Heterogeneity, genetic/locus, 2–6, 13, **15–18,** 56, 72, 74, 94, 294, 304
Heterotopia, , periventricular nodular, 15, 130, 135–7, 141, 174
Hetrotopia, periventricular nodular, 130, *136,* 137
HGPPS, 156, 162, **165**
High-risk mutation. *see* Mutation, high-risk
Hippocampus, 144, 157, 162, 197, 212, 245, 247, 271, 321, 329
Hirschsprung disease, 6, 13, 16, 20, 55, 74, 76
Homeostasis, circuit or synaptic, 75, 197
Horizontal gaze palsy with progressive scoliosis. *see* HGPPS
hPSC. *see* Stem cell, human pluripotent
HSPG. *see* Heparan sulfate proteoglycan
Huntington's disease, 13, 112, 243, 291
Hyperactivity, 17, 31, 250, 319, 330. *see also* ADHD

IGF1, 221, 270, 323, 325, 328, 331
Immune activation, maternal, 33, 114
Inborn errors of metabolism, 11. *see also* Metabolic disorder/deficiency
Inbreeding, 53, 84, 89–91, 100, 102. *see also* Consanguinity
Infection, 14, 29, **33,** 85, **111–15,** 117, 120–21, 145, 169
Inheritance, autosomal dominant, **55–6,** 162–5, 199, 214–15, 248
Inheritance, digenic, 16, 75
Inheritance, Mendelian, 2, 5, *7,* 13, 29, 34–5, 39, 54, 69, 291, 295
Inheritance, oligogenic, **11,** 16, **74–5,** 291–2, 296
Inheritance, polygenic, **2–7,** 16, 59, 61, 94–5, 101, 120, 211, 291, 293, 296, 298, 331
Inheritance, recessive, 2, 35, 39, 50, **53–5,** 95, 130, 133–9, 144–5, 161, 165, 198–9, 212–13, 216, 251, 269, 282, 292
Intelligence, 53, 88–91, **95–9.** *see also* IQ
Interneuron, 164–5, 171, 197, 212, 245–8
iPS cells. *see* Stem cell, induced pluripotent
IQ, 7, 54, 95–6, 99–100, 119. *see also* Intelligence

Jackson, Hughlings, 30
Joubert syndrome, 143, 156, 164
JSRD. *see* Joubert syndrome

Kabuki syndrome, 55
Kainate receptor, 197

Kanner, L., 31
KBG syndrome, 55
Kleefstra syndrome, 197, 205, 208
Klippel-feil syndrome, 164
Knobloch syndrome, 139
Kraepelin, E., 30–32

Language, 276–9, 283–4
Language impairment, 115, 204–206, 208, 319
Language impairment, specific, 1, 277, 284. *see also*
  Language Impairment
Learning and memory, 114, 168, 197, 219, 251, 264,
  324, 330
Learning disability or disorder, 31, 203, 250
Lesch-Nyhan syndrome, 52, 240, 243
Liability, 3, 8, 18–19, 36, 39, 98
Liability-threshold model, 3
Lig 4 syndrome, 132
Linkage, 2, **5–6,** *12,* 39, 53–4, 56
Lissencephaly, 130, *131,* **134–41**
Lissencephaly, cobblestone, 138–40
Lissencephaly with cerebellar hypoplasia, 138
Locus heterogeneity. *see* Heterogeneity, genetic/locus
Long-term depression. *see* LTD
Long-term potentiation. *see* LTP
LTD, 197, 217, 219, 267, 324
LTP, 168, 197, 217, 267, 270–71, 324, 329

Machine learning, 72–4
Magnetic resonance imaging, 8, 143, 162–3, 166–7,
  335
Magnetic resonance spectroscopy, 90
Malformation, cortical, 11, 129, 135–45
MASA syndrome, 166
Maternal immune activation. *see* Immune activation,
  maternal
Matrix, extracellular, 135–40, 158
Meckel-Gruber syndrome, 143
Megalencephaly, 130, **141–2**
Memory. *see* Learning and memory
Memory impairment, 166, 173
Mendelian. *see* Inheritance, Mendelian
Mental retardation. *see* Retardation, mental
Metabolic disorder/deficiency, 17, 29, 134, 240, 282,
  326
Metabotropic glutamate receptor, 99, 197, 209,
  216–17, 265, 267, 321, 328
mGluR5, 323, 324, 328–30
MIA. *see* Maternal immune activation
Microcephaly, 35, 38, 55, **130–34,** 135, 137, 141,
  144–5, 200 , 205, **251**
Microglia, 173
Microlissencephaly, *131,* 134

Migrant, **33–4,** 113, **116–17,** 119
Migration, cell/neuronal, **135–8,** 158–9, 162–3,
  166–8, 176, 210–14, 218–19, 253, 326
Miller syndrome, 297
Minor physical anomalies, 82–3, 85–6, 95, 294
Mitochondria, 134, 263, 276
Modifier, genetic, 4–5, 9, **11,** 16, 18, 75, 262–3, **269,**
  303
Mosaicism, germline, 57, **295**
Mosaicism, somatic, 141–2, 289–91, **295,** 303
Motor function, 29, 241
Motor neuron, 160–61, 164, 175, 246
Mowat-Wilson syndrome, 55
MPAs. *see* Minor physical anomalies
MRI. *see* Magnetic resonance imaging
MRS. *see* Magnetic resonance spectroscopy
mTOR, 141–3, 203–204, 210, *322,* 324, 324–5,
  329–31
Multielectrode array, 333
Multifactor dimensionality reduction, 73
Multiple sclerosis, 243
Muscular dystrophy, 11, 137–9, 145
Mutation, de novo, 2–5, 10, 36, 50–59, 81, 90, 95–6,
  116, 135, 207–216, 249, 294–7
Mutation, high-risk, 2, 7, 11, 12, 17–18, 20, 73, 75
Mutation load, **81–102**
Mutation, rare, 4, 6, **9–10,** 13–14, 34, 36, 51, 53,
  75–6, 167, 198–206, 208–214, 218, **296,** 301.
  see also Variant, rare
Mutation rate, 36, 39, 51, 55, 58, **59,** 90, 268
Mutation, somatic, 116, **141–3,** 145–6
Mutational target, 4, 56, 196
Mutation-selection balance, 59, 102
Myelin or myelination, 159, 276, 329

NAHR. *see* Non-allelic homologous recombination
Neocortex. *see* Cortex, cerebral
Neural stem cell. *see* Stem cell, neural
Neural tube, 29, 36, 143–4, 160, 244
Neurexin, 36, 196, 198–9, 208, **212,** *322. see also*
  NRXN1 in Gene Index
Neuroconstructivism, 275–9, 284–5
Neurofibromatosis, 203, 209, 217, 270, 321–5, 328,
  329
Neurofibromin, 203, 217, 323, 329. *see also* NF1 in
  Gene Index
Neurogenesis, *131,* 133, *136,* 208, 219, 239–40, 244,
  247, 251, 253, 276
Neuroimaging, 30, 102, 167. *see also* Magnetic
  resonance imaging
Neuroligin, 10, 36, 39, 53, 196, 199, **212,** 216, 265,
  322, *322. see also* NLGN1–4 in Gene Index

Neuronal migration. *see* Migration, cell/neuronal
Neuronal progenitor. *see* Progenitor, neuronal
Neuropilin, **159,** 161, 169
Next-generation sequencing. *see* Sequencing,
　　next-generation
NF1 in Gene Index, 203, 217, 270, 323, 324, 325, 329
Nijmegen Breakage syndrome, 132
NLGN1–4 in Gene Index, 53, 199, 212, 263
NMDA receptor, 175, 197, 201–202, 208, 211, 213,
　　215–18, 321, *322,* 325, 330
Non-allelic homologous recombination, 92
Non-shared environment. *see* Environment,
　　non-shared
Noonan syndrome, 209
NRXN1 in Gene Index, 19, 37, 39, 40, 57, 199, 208,
　　212
NuRD complex, 219
Nutrition, 29, 33, **34, 114,** 121, 320

Obsessive compulsive disorder, 157, 170, 172, 199,
　　213–14, 296
Obstetric complications, 14, **33,** 98, **115**
OCD. *see* Obsessive compulsive disorder
Oculomotor, 136, 156, **160–65**
Olfactory neural precursor, 332
Oligogenic. *see* Inheritance, oligogenic
Oro-facial-digital syndrome, 143

Pachygyria, 134–5, 139
PAK, 322
Parkinson's disease, 175–6, 245–6, 331, 333
Paternal age. *see* Age, paternal
PCDHs in Gene Index, 199, 207, 213, 219
Penetrance, high, 5, *16,* 20, 39–40, 54–5, 75, 94, 263,
　　271, 329, 336
Penetrance, incomplete, 5–6, 10, **11,** 14, *16,* 19, 74,
　　201, 263
Perception, 29, 163
Periventricular nodular heterotopia. *see* Heterotopia,
　　periventricular nodular
Phelan-McDermid syndrome, 200, 208, 216, 263
Phenylketonuria, 282, 326
PKU. *see* Phenylketonuria
Plasticity, synaptic, 39, 58, 168, **196–7,** 202–206,
　　208, 214, 216–18, 221–2, 270–71, 276, 326,
　　330
Plexin, **159,** 161–2, 165–6, **167–9**
Polygene profile or score, 35, 120–21
Polygenic. *see* Inheritance, polygenic
Polymicrogyria, 134–5, **139–41,** 143, 145
Polymorphism, copy number, 94
Polymorphism, single-nucleotide (SNP), 7–9, 13,
　　18–19, 34–6, 50, 60–61, 71–6, 91, 94–6, 99,

102, 119–21, 157, 167–8, 176, 267, 268. *see*
　　also Variant, common
Porencephaly, 139
Postmortem, 146, 162, 168, 173, 239–40, 261, 321,
　　327, 335
Postsynaptic density, 196, 213, 215–17. *see also*
　　Scaffolding proteins
Prader-Willi syndrome, 9, 37, 50, 243, 250, 276–7
Preimplantation genetic diagnosis, 241, **298**
Prenatal diagnosis, 290, 292, **298**
Privacy, 301–303
Progenitor, neuronal, 129–33, 137, 140–42, 146,
　　240, 244–7, 250–52
Proliferation, 116, **129–34,** 137, **141–4,** 158
Proteome or Proteomics, 70, 169–70, 209, 215, 290
Protocadherin, 196, 199, **212–13,** 219. *see also*
　　PCDHs in Gene Index
Pruning, axonal, dendritic or synaptic, 159, 162, 167,
　　173, **176,** 197, 211, 281
Psychosis, 17, 19, 32, 36, 74, 100, 112, 118–19,
　　220–21, 327, 334, 336
Public health, 112, 116, 121

Quantitative trait, 3, 18, 70, 72–3, 121, 269

Rapamycin, 323, 325, 329, 331
Ras pathway, 116, 217, 324. *see also* GTPase
RASopathies, 218
Recurrence risk, 5, 19, 119
Resilience, 81
Retardation, mental, 51, 53, 55–6, 163, 166, 205, 282
Retina, 133, 139, 143, 163–4, 244, 247–8, 265
Retinitis pigmentosa, 2, 143, 292
Rett syndrome, 1, 6, 10, 13, 29, 197, 205, 207, 213,
　　217, 219, 222, 243, 248–9, 269–70, 294,
　　321–3, 325–6, 328, 331–5
Robustness, 15, 299
Runs of heterozygosity, or ROH, 54, 91, 94–6, 99

Scaffolding proteins, 39, 196, 200, 211, 213, **215–16,**
　　218
Schinzel-Giedion syndrome, 55–6
Schizencephaly, 134, 139, 141
Schizoaffective disorder, 32
Schizotypal personality disorder, 32
Season of birth, **33,** 115, **117,** 119–20
Seckel syndrome, 131–2
Segmental duplication, **92–4,** 207–208
Segregation, 2, 5–6, *16,* 18, 36, *52,* 54–5, 94, 119,
　　132, 200
Seizures, 17, 30, 33–6, 39, 75, 130–33, 142–5,
　　201–205, 212, 218, 220–21, 247, 264, 266,
　　269, 276, 282, 321, 327, 329, 335

Selection, evolutionary, 3–5, 9, 51, 59–61, 72, 76, 82, 84, 87, 91–4, 97, 102, 114, 195, 275
Semaphorin, **159,** 161–2, 164–6, **167–9,** 196
Sequencing, exome, *12,* 54–9, 195, 207, 209, 213, 219, 294, 298
Sequencing, next-generation, 10, *12,* 57, 74, 129, 141, 145
Sequencing, whole-genome, 36, 39, 76, 290, 300, *303*
Serotonin, 168, 172, 196, 217, 297, *322,* 325
Shh. *see* Sonic Hedgehog
Sickle-cell anemia, 13
Single nucleotide variant. *see* Variant, single-nucleotide
SLI. *see* Language Impairment, Specific
Smith-Magenis syndrome, 50
SNP. *see* Polymorphism, single-nucleotide
SNV. *see* Variant, single-nucleotide
Social behaviour, deficits or interaction, 3, 29, 31, 112, 168, 249, 262–3, 270, 276–9, 283, 319, 329–30, 334
Socioeconomic status, 84, 278
Somatic mutation. *see* Mutation, somatic
Sonic Hedgehog, 144, 156, 245–7
Sotos syndrome, 208
Specific language impairment. *see* Language Impairment, Specific
Spines, dendritic, 211–16, 248, 321–2, 335
Sporadic cases, 5, 11, *16,* 51, 55, 57–8, 140, 175, 199, 207–208, 213, 215, 219, 249
Stem cell, embryonic, **241–7,** 250
Stem cell, human pluripotent, 241, **243–6, 248,** 252
Stem cell, induced pluripotent, 40, 221, **242–3,** 246, **248–53,** 264, **331–3**
Stem cell, neural, 240, 246–7
Stem cell, pluripotent, 218, 221, **241, 248,** 251
Strabismus, **136, 160, 162–3**
Stress or Stressor, 82, 84–6, 97, 101–102, 114, 117, 119, 269, 281–2
Substance abuse, 95, 103
Substantia nigra, 171
Suppressor, genetic, 70, 269
Synapse formation, 133, **196,** 198–205, 213–18, 220. *see also* Synaptogenesis
Synaptic transmission, 49, 208–209, 211–12, 215, 218, 221, 264, 266, 328, 331
Synaptogenesis, 100, 166–9, 175, **196,** 203, 209, 253, 326, 333. *see also* Synapse formation
Synchrony, neural, 265–6
Synthetic association, 9, 13

TALEN, 268
Tau, 173–4, 240, 252
Temporal lobe epilepsy, 32, 199, 215
Therapy, 18, **221–2,** 248, 262, 267, 269, 283, 297, 301, **319, 326–31,** 333–6
Timothy syndrome, 13, 34, 40, 201, 216, 221, 243, **248–9**
TMS. *see* Transcranial magnetic stimulation
Tourette syndrome, **170,** 199, 207–208, 212–14, 296
Toxoplasmosis, 29, 33, 114
Transcranial magnetic stimulation, 334
Transcription factor, 61, 161, 164, 166, 197, 205–206, 213, **218–20,** 246
Transcriptome, 39, 290, 300
Transdifferentiation, **246**
Translation (mRNA), 17, 49, 75, 197, 202, 210, 216, **217,** 220, *322,* 324, 329
Trauma, 11, 29, 118–19
Trisomy, 50, 83, 133, 240, 251–2, 276, 295, 300
TSC genes in Gene Index, 143, 210
Tuberous sclerosis, 1, 6, 74–5, 143, 197, 204, 217, **321–5, 328–9,** 331, 335. *see also* TSC genes in Gene Index
Tubulin, 135–6, 140, 163
Turner syndrome, 243
Twins or twin studies, 11, 14–15, 18, 20, 32, 74–5, 85, 118–19, 277

Urbanicity, 117–19

Validity (construct, etiological, face or predictive), 18, **262–3,** 268–9, 271
Valproate, 115
Variance, genetic, 8, 15, 18–19, 73, 297
Variant, common, 3–4, **7–9,** 13–14, *16,* **18–19,** 39, 50, **60–61,** 74, **75–6,** 91, 167, 212, 267, 293–4
Variant, copy number. *see* CNV
Variant, rare, 4, 9, *16,* 19, 39, 50, 58, **60–61,** 74, **75,** 91, 94, 99, 195, 293, 296. *see also* Mutation, rare and Variant, rare
Variant, single nucleotide, **10,** 14, **55–61,** 209, 219, 297. *see also* Mutation, rare and Variant, rare
Velocardiofacial syndrome, 1, 32, 36, **38,** 141, 207, 291, 293–4, 296. *see also* 22q11.2
Vitamin D, 115, 117–18, 120

Waddington, C., 15, 72, 82, 299
Williams syndrome, 11, 37, 50, 207, 275, 282, 284
Williams-Beuren syndrome. *see* Williams syndrome
Wilmut, I., 243
Wnt, 144, 156, 161, 196, 219, 245–7

X chromosome, 14, 50, **53,** 101, 135–6, 141, 166, 252, 276, 332
X chromosome inactivation, 135, 332
Xist, 252
X-linked (gene or disorder), **52–3,** 135, 137, 141, 176, 198–203, 207, 213–15, 248, 250, 252, 263, 269, 332

X-linked female-limited epilepsy, 199, 207
X-linked intellectual disability (XLID), 52–3

Y chromosome, 13–14, 76
Yamanaka, S., 243

Zinc finger nuclease, 268

GENE INDEX

Notes: Genes are listed by official gene symbol. Where these occur multiple times per page, the page numbers are in bold. Figure page numbers are *italicized* and Table page numbers are <u>underlined</u>.

A2B, 158
ACTB, 56, 137
ACTG1, 56, 137
ADAM22, 215
ADAM23, 215
AHI1, 144
AKT3, 142
AMT, 54
ANK2, 210
ANK3, 34, 35
ANKRD11, 55
APLP1, 174
APLP2, 174
APP, 174–5
ARCA1, 35
ARFGEF2, 133, 137
ARID1A, <u>204</u>, 219
ARID1B, *12*, <u>204</u>, 219–20
ASPM, 132
ASXL1, 55
ATR, 130–31
ATRIP, 131
AUTS2, 218
AUTSX1, 53
AUTSX2, 53

AUTSX5, 53
AUTSX6, 53

BACE1, <u>157</u>, **173–4**
B3GALNT2, 139
B3GNT1, 139
BRAG1, <u>202</u>, 218

CACNA1A, 216
CACNA1C, 13, 34–5, 40, <u>201</u>, 221, 295
CACNA2D2, 40
CACNA1F, 40
CACNB2, 35
CACNG2, 57
CASK, 196, <u>200</u>, 215, 218
CDKL5, *12*, <u>202</u>, 213, 217
CDK5RAP2, 132
CENPJ, 132
CEP63, 132
CEP135, 132
CEP152, 131
CEP290, 144
CHD2, 219
CHD4, 219
CHD7, 176, 219
CHD8, *12*, 39, 209–10, 219–20

The Genetics of Neurodevelopmental Disorders, First Edition. Edited by Kevin J. Mitchell.
© 2015 John Wiley & Sons, Inc. Published 2015 by John Wiley & Sons, Inc.

CHK1, 130
CHL1, 174, **213–14**
CHMP1A, 133
CHN1, <u>156</u>, 161–2
CHRNA7, *12*, <u>201</u>, 216
CNTN4, 212, 214
CNTN6, 212, 214
CNTNAP2, *12*, 36, <u>198</u>, 207, **212**
CNTNAP3, 212
CNTNAP4, 212
CNTNAP5, 212
COH1, 133, 144
COL3A1, 140
COL4A1, 139
COL18A1, 139
CREBBP, <u>204–206</u>, 219
CRMP1, <u>157</u>, 168
CRMP2, <u>157</u>, 168, **175**
CUL3, 210
CUL4B, <u>202</u>
CXCL12, 161
CXCR4, 161, 167

DAB1, 174
DAG1, 138–9
DCC, <u>156</u>, **158–9**, **163–5**, 174–5
DCX, **135**, <u>136</u>, 137, **141**
DGCR2, 58
DISC1, 10, *12*, 36, 40, <u>156</u>, 166, 174, <u>200</u>, **218**, 221–2, 293, *322*, <u>323</u>, **325**, **329–30**
DLG1, 215
DLG2, 215
DLG3, <u>200</u>, 215
DLGAP1, 215
DLGAP2, 215
DR6, 173
DSCAM, 158
DYNC1H1, 135
DYRK1A, **133**, 145, 209, 210

EHMT1, *12*, 197, <u>205</u>, **208**
ELFN1, 197
EP300, <u>204</u>, 219
EPB41L1, 57
EPHA4, 162, **165**
EPHA7, 165
EPHRINB3, 165

FAT1, 213
FE65, <u>157</u>, 174
FE65L1, <u>157</u>, 174
FGF2, 244, <u>245</u>, 246
FGF8, 161, 176, <u>245</u>, 246

FGFR1, 176
FKRP, 139
FKTN, 139
FLNA, 137
FMR1, *12*, 75, <u>202</u>, 240, **250**, 263, 265, 267, **269**, 276, <u>323</u>, 324–6, **328–9**
FMRP, 210, 211, 213, 217, 219, **250**, 276, *322*, <u>323</u>, 324, 328
FOXP1, 58
FOXP2, **277–8**, 281

GKAP1, 215
GKAP2, 215
GPHN, 39, 216
GPR56, 140
GRIA3, *12*, <u>201</u>, 216
GRIN1, 57
GRIN2A, *12*, <u>201</u>, 216
GRIN2B, 58, <u>202</u>, 210, 218
GRM1, 209
GRM5, 209
GRM7, 209
GRM8, 209

HDAC4, <u>205</u>, 219
HOXA1, 161–2
HPRT, 53, 240–41
HS6ST1, 176

IL1RAPL1, 57, <u>198</u>, 214
IQSEC2, *12*, <u>202</u>, 218
ISPD, 139
ITIH3, 35
ITIH4, 35

KAL1, 176
KATNAL2, 39, 209–10
KIF1A, 57, 135
KIF2A, 135
KIF21A, 136, <u>156</u>, 161–3
KIF5C, 135

LAMA2, 139
LAMB1, 139
LAMC3, 58, 139–40
LAR, 213
LARGE, 139
L1CAM, <u>156</u>, 159, 165–6, <u>198</u>, 213–14
LGI1, <u>199</u>, 214–15
LIS1, **134–5**, 141, 166

MAGI1, 215
MAGI2, 215
MAP1B, <u>156</u>, 163

MBD5, 220
MCPH1, **130**, 132
MECP2, *12*, 53, <u>205</u>, 207, 217, 219–20, 248, 263, 269, *322*, <u>323</u>, **328**, 331
MEF2C, <u>205</u>, 218–19
MET, 161
MHC, 35, **60**
MIR137, 35
MLL2, 55
MTOR, **141–3**, <u>203–206</u>, 210, *322*, <u>323</u>, **324–5**, 329–31
MYO18B, 60

NCAM, 169
NDE1, 134
NETRIN1, 164, 174
NF1, 203, 217, 270, <u>323</u>, 324–5, **329**
NFIA, <u>156</u>
NGL, 213, 217
NHPH1, 144
NIN, 132
NLGN1, 212
NLGN3, *12*, 36, 39, 53, <u>199</u>, 212, 265–6
NLGN4, 39, 53, 263
NRCAM, 159, 164, 213–14
NRG3, 76
NRGN, 61
NRXN1, *12*, 19, 36, <u>37</u>, 39–40, 57, <u>199</u>, 208, 212
NRXN2, 212
NSD1, 208
NTNG1, 213

ODZ4, 35
ORC3, 211

PCDH10, 213, 219
PCDH17, 213
PCDH19, <u>199</u>, 207, **213**
PCDH20, 213
PCNT, 132
PEX7, 54
PHOX2A, 161
PIK3CA, 142
PIK3RC, 142
PLXNA2, <u>157</u>, 167
PLXNB3, <u>157</u>
PNKP, 132
POGZ, 209, 210
POMGNT1, 139, 145
POMGNT2, 139
POMK, 139
POMT1, 139, 145
POMT2, 139

PROK2, 176
PROKR2, 176
PROSAP, 216
PS1, <u>157</u>, 173–5
PS2, 173
PSD95, 213, 215, 218–19, *322*, 332
PTEN, *12*, 197, <u>203</u>, 210, 217, *322*, 325, **331**

RAB39B, 57, <u>203</u>
RAD51, <u>156</u>, 165
RAS, 56, 116, <u>203</u>, 208–10, 217, <u>322</u>, 324–5, 329
RBBP8, 131
RELN, 137, <u>138</u>
RET, 13, 76
ROBO1, <u>157</u>, 158, 168
ROBO2, <u>157</u>, 168
ROBO3, <u>156–7</u>, 161, **165**, 168
RPL10, 53

SALL4, 161
SCN1A, 58, <u>202</u>, 216, 269
SCN2A, *12*, 39, <u>202</u>, 209–11
SDF1, 161
SEMA3A, <u>157</u>, 159, **161**, 162, 165, 168, **175**, 176
SEMA5A, <u>157</u>, 168
SEMA6A, <u>157</u>, 165, 168
SEMA4B, <u>157</u>, 168
SEMA3D, <u>157</u>, 167
SEMA4D, <u>157</u>, 168
SETBP1, 55
SHANK2, <u>200</u>, 216, 330
SHANK3, 36, **57**, <u>200</u>, 208, 216, 221, 263, 270, 331
SHH, 144, <u>156</u>, **245–7**
SLC6A8, 53
SLC25A12, 267
SLC25A19, 134
SLIT, **158–9**, <u>199</u>, 214
SLITRK1, <u>157</u>, **170–72**, <u>199</u>, 214
SLITRK5, <u>157</u>, 171–2, 214
SLITRK6, <u>157</u>, 170, **172**, 214
SMARCA2, <u>205</u>, 219
SMARCA4, <u>206</u>, 219
SMARCB1, <u>206</u>, 219
SMARCE1, <u>206</u>, 219
SRCAP, <u>206</u>, 219
STIL, 132
ST8SIA2, <u>157</u>, 169
STXBP1, *12*, 57, <u>203</u>, 211
SYN1, <u>203</u>
SYNE1, 13, **35**, 40
SYNGAP1, *12*, 56, 57, <u>203</u>, 209, 211, 217, 222

TBR1, *12*, <u>206</u>, 210, **218**, **219**
TCF4, *12*, 13, **35**, 40, 61
TMEM5, 139
TSC1, *12*, 143, <u>204</u>, 217, *322*, <u>323</u>, 325, **329**, 331
TSC2, 75, 143, <u>204</u>, 217, 267, *322*, <u>323</u>, 324–5, **329**, 331
TUBA8, **135**, 163
TUBA1A, 135, 163
TUBB2, 140
TUBB3, **135–6**, <u>156</u>, 161, **163**, 166
TUBB5, **135**, 163
TUBB2B, 135, 163
Tyrosinase, <u>156</u>, 163

UBE3A, *12*, <u>204</u>, 217, 250, 276, *322*, 324
UNC5, 158
UNC5C, 164
UNC5H3, 164

VIPR2, <u>37</u>, 208
VLDLR, 137
VRK2, 35

WDR62, 132, **134**, 140–41
WNT, **144**, <u>156</u>, 161, 219, 245–7

ZEB2, 55
ZNF335, 133
ZNF804A, 34